CORE CONCEPTS IN HEALTH

BRIEF
THIRTEENTH EDITION

Paul M. Insel
Stanford University

Walton T. Roth
Stanford University

Mc Graw Hill Education

5 6 7 8 9 0   DIG DIG   16 15 14

ISBN-13: 978-1-25-911517-2
ISBN-10: 1-25-911517-8

Learning Solutions Consultant: Dave Fleming
Associate Project Manager: Alyssa Gantzert

CONTENTS

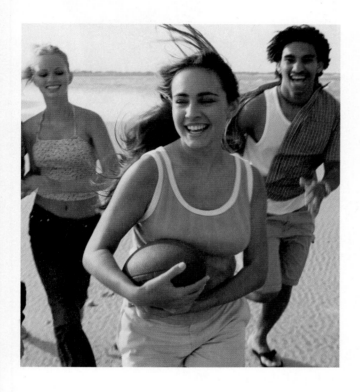

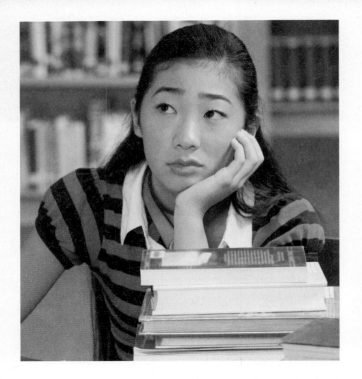

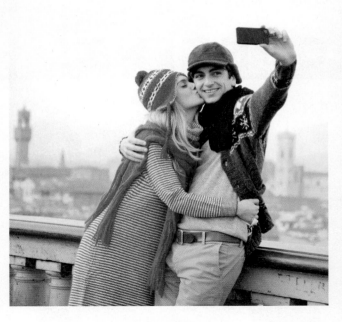

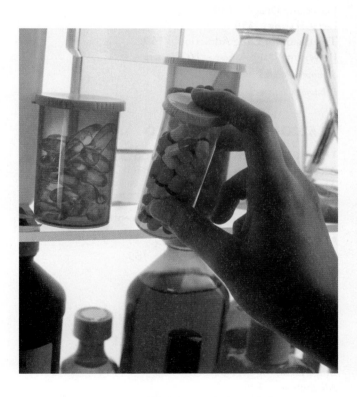

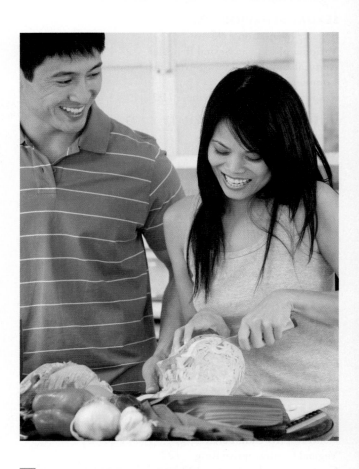

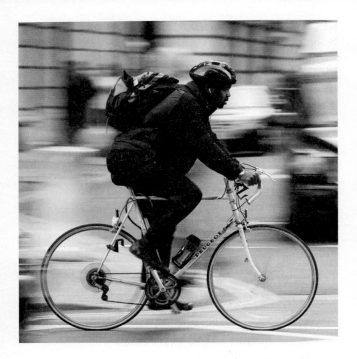

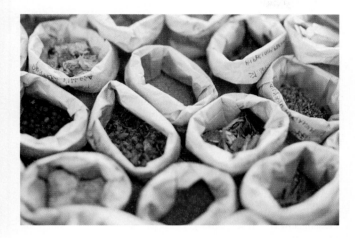

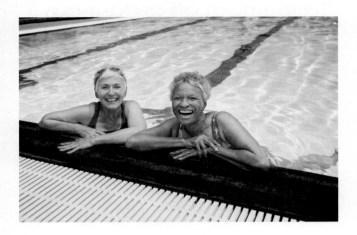

WELLNESS ON CAMPUS

TOPICS OF SPECIAL CONCERN TO WOMEN

TOPICS OF SPECIAL CONCERN TO MEN

*Note: The health issues and conditions listed here include those
that disproportionately influence or affect women or men. For more
information, see the Index under gender, women, men, and any of the
special topics listed here.*

DIVERSITY TOPICS RELATED TO ETHNICITY

*Note: The health issues and conditions listed here include those that
disproportionately influence or affect specific U.S. ethnic groups or for
which patterns may appear along ethnic lines. For more information,
see the Index under ethnicity, culture, names of specific population
groups, and any of the topics listed here.*

THE CORE CONCEPTS IN HEALTH LEARNING SYSTEMS

Connect Core Concepts in Health is an integrated program designed to personalize the science of personal health and to motivate students to build research skills, critical thinking skills, and behavior change skills for lifelong health. The new edition of *Connect Core Concepts in Health* combines the expert content you've come to expect with an increased focus on behavior change and personalization—personal learning styles, personal motivation, and personal responsibility. Highlights of the 13th edition include

- The LearnSmart adaptive testing program, which creates individualized study plans for each student, helping to build a strong foundation of knowledge.

- The latest scientific findings, data, and statistics, with up-to-date coverage of topics ranging from the government's MyPlate food guidance system to the potential positive and negative effects of digital communication technologies to the latest physical activity recommendations.

- A new "Wellness on Campus" feature in every chapter that explores specific health and wellness issues as they pertain to college students.

- A new media bank in Connect, offering easy access to all of the video content available with *Connect Core Concepts in Health*.

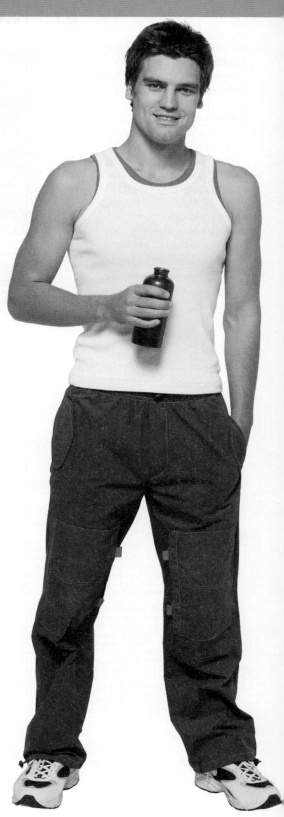

A PERSONAL PLAN FOR LEARNING

McGraw-Hill's LearnSmart is an adaptive learning system designed to help students learn faster, study more efficiently, and retain knowledge for greater success. Through a series of adaptive questions, LearnSmart continually measures and monitors each student's progress. LearnSmart provides each student with a unique, individualized learning path to help him or her increase knowledge and competencies while helping to make class time more interactive and productive.

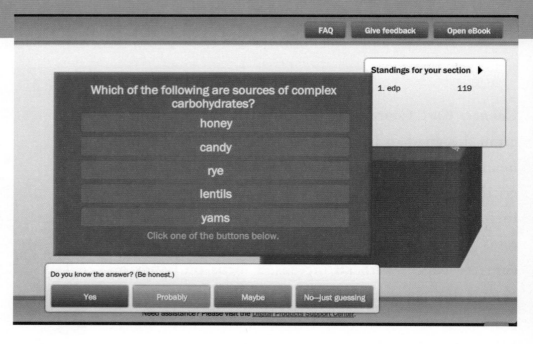

FAQ Give feedback Open eBook

Which of the following are sources of complex carbohydrates?

honey

candy

rye

lentils

yams

Click one of the buttons below.

Standings for your section ▶

1. edp   119

Do you know the answer? (Be honest.)

Yes   Probably   Maybe   No—just guessing

Need assistance? Please visit the Digital Products Support Center.

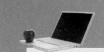

WELLNESS ON CAMPUS
Deliberate Self-Harm

In general, people want to be well and healthy, protect themselves from harm, and try to make use of the guidance that this book gives. But surprisingly, there are individuals—predominantly in their teens and adolescence—who deliberately harm themselves, although in a nonfatal way. One common method is to cut or burn their skin, leaving scars that may serve as visible representation of emotional pain that they shamefully hide beneath their clothes.

Self-cutting and other self-injurious behaviors are not aesthetically motivated. Many report seeking the physical sensations (including pain) produced by a self-inflicted injury, which may temporarily relieve feelings of tension, perhaps through a release of endorphins.

In 2011 a research group led by Alicia Meuret, an associate professor of psychology at Southern Methodist University, conducted surveys on more than 550 college students and found that over 20% had engaged in self-injury at some point, which is consistent with prevalence estimates in other studies on college populations. In examining differences between self-injurers and non-injurers, individuals that had recently engaged in self-harm were significantly more depressed, anxious, and disgusted with themselves. Compared to non-injurers, self-injurers were roughly 4 times more likely to report a history of physical abuse and 11 times more likely to report a history of sexual abuse.

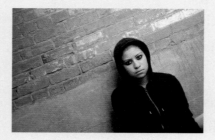

Self-injury is not the same as a suicide attempt, but individuals who repeatedly hurt themselves are more likely to commit suicide than the general population. In any case, self-injury should be taken seriously. If you do it, talk to a counselor. If someone you know does it, try to convince him or her to talk to a counselor.

NEW "Wellness on Campus" features highlight health and wellness issues that are of particular relevance to college students. Topics include alcoholic energy drinks, eating well while on campus, and protecting against STDs.

Connect Core Concepts in Health gives students access to a wealth of interactive online content, including fitness labs and self-assessments, video activities, a fitness and nutrition journal, a behavior change workbook, and practice quizzes with immediate feedback. Additionally, the media-rich eBook available with Connect Plus contains embedded video clips, full-color images, links to discipline-specific sites, key terms and definitions, and behavior change tools.

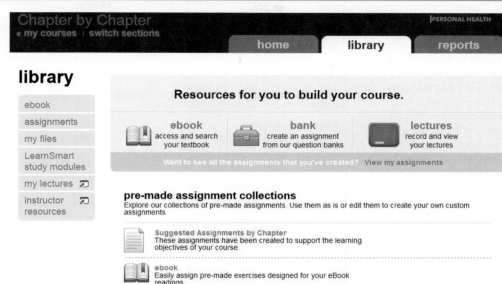

Connect Core Concepts in Health supports student learning with a wealth of print and online features. In addition to the rich set of resources available in Connect, feature boxes in the text highlight issues related to diversity, behavior change, and consumer awareness. The 13th edition features two vibrant transparency sections called "Touring Lifestyle Behaviors" and "Touring the Cardiorespiratory System" designed to engage students and reinforce learning, especially for visual learners.

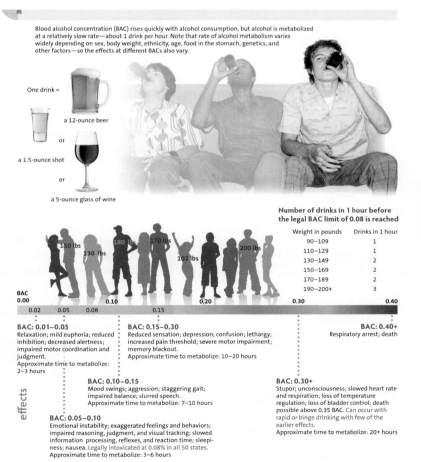

Blood alcohol concentration (BAC) rises quickly with alcohol consumption, but alcohol is metabolized at a relatively slow rate—about 1 drink per hour. Note that rate of alcohol metabolism varies widely depending on sex, body weight, ethnicity, age, food in the stomach, genetics, and other factors—so the effects at different BACs also vary.

One drink =

a 12-ounce beer

or

a 1.5-ounce shot

or

a 5-ounce glass of wine

Number of drinks in 1 hour before the legal BAC limit of 0.08 is reached

Weight in pounds	Drinks in 1 hour
90–109	1
110–129	1
130–149	2
150–169	2
170–189	2
190–200+	3

BAC 0.00   0.02   0.05   0.08   0.10   0.15   0.20   0.30   0.40

effects

BAC: 0.01–0.05
Relaxation; mild euphoria; reduced inhibition; decreased alertness; impaired motor coordination and judgment.
Approximate time to metabolize: 2–3 hours

BAC: 0.05–0.10
Emotional instability; exaggerated feelings and behaviors; impaired reasoning, judgment, and visual tracking; slowed information processing, reflexes, and reaction time; sleepiness; nausea. Legally intoxicated at 0.08% in all 50 states.
Approximate time to metabolize: 3–6 hours

BAC: 0.10–0.15
Mood swings; aggression; staggering gait; impaired balance; slurred speech.
Approximate time to metabolize: 7–10 hours

BAC: 0.15–0.30
Reduced sensation; depression; confusion; lethargy; increased pain threshold; severe motor impairment; memory blackout.
Approximate time to metabolize: 10–20 hours

BAC: 0.30+
Stupor; unconsciousness; slowed heart rate and respiration; loss of temperature regulation; loss of bladder control; death possible above 0.35 BAC. Can occur with rapid or binge drinking with few of the earlier effects.
Approximate time to metabolize: 20+ hours

BAC: 0.40+
Respiratory arrest; death

A PERSONAL APPROACH TO BEHAVIOR CHANGE

An extensive program of Wellness Worksheets help students to evaluate and assess their own health-related behaviors, and to chart their progress in meeting personal health goals. These Wellness Worksheets are available online, where they can be assigned, submitted, and stored electronically.

Wellness Worksheet 93 *Diet and Cancer*

All the information you enter in this exercise will be saved when you exit.

Your diet may include both cancer fighters and cancer promoters. Track your diet for 3 days and select which day you ate any food on one of the following lists.

Potential Cancer Fighters

Orange and yellow vegetables and (some) fruits

Day1	Day2	Day3	
☐	☐	☐	apricots
☐	☐	☐	cantaloupe
☐	☐	☐	carrots
☐	☐	☐	mangoes
☐	☐	☐	papaya
☐	☐	☐	pumpkin
☐	☐	☐	red and yellow peppers
☐	☐	☐	sweet potatoes (yams)
☐	☐	☐	winter squash (acorn, butternut, banana, etc.)
☐	☐	☐	other:

Dark-green leafy vegetables

Day1	Day2	Day3	
☐	☐	☐	beet greens
☐	☐	☐	broccoli rabe
☐	☐	☐	chard
☐	☐	☐	collard greens

Day1	Day2	Day3	
☐	☐	☐	whole grains (whole-grain bread, cereal, and pasta; brown rice; etc.)
☐	☐	☐	legumes (peas, lentils, and beans, including fava, navy, kidney, pinto, black, and lima beans)
☐	☐	☐	apples
☐	☐	☐	asparagus
☐	☐	☐	berries (strawberries, raspberries, blueberries)
☐	☐	☐	chili peppers
☐	☐	☐	grapes
☐	☐	☐	green peppers
☐	☐	☐	honeydew melon
☐	☐	☐	kiwi fruit
☐	☐	☐	onions, garlic, leeks
☐	☐	☐	radishes
☐	☐	☐	soy products (tofu, tempeh, soy milk, miso, soybeans, etc.)
☐	☐	☐	sprouts (alfalfa, broccoli)
☐	☐	☐	tomatoes
☐	☐	☐	watermelon
☐	☐	☐	other:

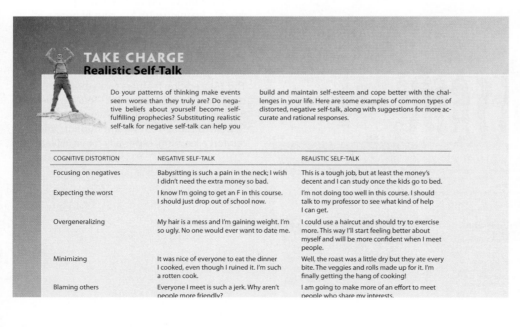

TAKE CHARGE
Realistic Self-Talk

Do your patterns of thinking make events seem worse than they truly are? Do negative beliefs about yourself become self-fulfilling prophecies? Substituting realistic self-talk for negative self-talk can help you build and maintain self-esteem and cope better with the challenges in your life. Here are some examples of common types of distorted, negative self-talk, along with suggestions for more accurate and rational responses.

COGNITIVE DISTORTION	NEGATIVE SELF-TALK	REALISTIC SELF-TALK
Focusing on negatives	Babysitting is such a pain in the neck; I wish I didn't need the extra money so bad.	This is a tough job, but at least the money's decent and I can study once the kids go to bed.
Expecting the worst	I know I'm going to get an F in this course. I should just drop out of school now.	I'm not doing too well in this course. I should talk to my professor to see what kind of help I can get.
Overgeneralizing	My hair is a mess and I'm gaining weight. I'm so ugly. No one would ever want to date me.	I could use a haircut and should try to exercise more. This way I'll start feeling better about myself and will be more confident when I meet people.
Minimizing	It was nice of everyone to eat the dinner I cooked, even though I ruined it. I'm such a rotten cook.	Well, the roast was a little dry but they ate every bite. The veggies and rolls made up for it. I'm finally getting the hang of cooking!
Blaming others	Everyone I meet is such a jerk. Why aren't people more friendly?	I am going to make more of an effort to meet people who share my interests.

"Embracing Wellness," "Ask Yourself," and "Take Charge" sections encourage students to relate material to their own lives, to examine their health-related behaviors, and to take responsibility for those behaviors and change them when necessary. Many of these sections are paired with assignable and assessable activities in Connect.

Effective and lasting behavior change is given even greater emphasis in the 13th edition, with a streamlined pedagogical program focusing on actions student can take now and in the future, a new box program ("Wellness on Campus") focusing on the health and well-being of college students, and a new "Behavior Change Contract" in Chapter 1.

BEHAVIOR CHANGE STRATEGY
Dealing with Social Anxiety

Shyness is often the result of both high anxiety levels and lack of key social skills. To help overcome shyness, you need to learn to manage your fear of social situations and to develop social skills such as appropriate eye contact, initiating topics in conversations, and maintaining the flow of conversations by asking questions and making appropriate responses.

As described in the chapter, repeated *exposure* to the source of one's fear—in this case social situations—is the best method for reducing anxiety. When you practice new behaviors, they gradually become easier and you experience less anxiety.

A counterproductive strategy is avoiding situations that make you anxious. Although this approach works in the short term—you eliminate your anxiety because you escape the situation—it keeps you from meeting new people and having new experiences. Another counterproductive strategy is self-medicating with alcohol or drugs. Being under their influence actually prevents you from learning new social skills and new ways to handle your anxiety.

- Watch your interpretations. Having a stress reaction doesn't mean that you don't belong in the group, that you're unattractive or unworthy, or that the situation is too much for you. Try thinking of yourself as excited or highly alert instead of anxious.

- Avoid cognitive distortions and practice realistic self-talk. Replace your self-critical thoughts with more supportive ones: "No one else is perfect, and I don't have to be either." "It would have been good if I had a funny story to tell, but the conversation was interesting anyway."

- Give yourself a reality check: Ask if you're really in a life-threatening situation (or just at a party), if the outcome you're imagining is really likely (or the worst thing that could possibly happen), or if you're the only one who feels nervous (or if many other people might feel the same way).

- Don't think of conversations as evaluations. Remind yourself that you don't

life—a course you're taking or a hobby you have—to something in the other person's life. Match self-disclosure with self-disclosure.

- Have something to say. Expand your mind and become knowledgeable about current events and local or campus news. If you have specialized knowledge about a topic, practice discussing it in ways that both beginners and experts can understand and appreciate.

- If you get stuck for something to say, try giving a compliment ("Great presentation!" or "I love your earrings.") or performing a social grace (pass the chips or get someone a drink).

- Be an active listener. Reward the other person with your full attention and with regular responses. Make frequent eye contact and maintain a relaxed but alert posture. (See Chapter 4 for more on being an active listener.)

At first, your new behaviors will likely make you anxious. Don't give up—things will

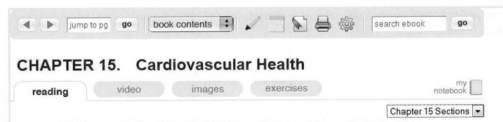

CHAPTER 15. Cardiovascular Health

reading   video   images   exercises

my notebook

Chapter 15 Sections ▼

PROTECTING YOURSELF AGAINST CARDIOVASCULAR DISEASE

There are several important steps you can take now to lower your risk of developing CVD (Figure 15.6). CVD can begin very early in life. For example, fatty streaks (very early atherosclerosis) can be seen on the aorta in children younger than age 10. Also, young adults with relatively low cholesterol levels go on to live substantially longer than those with higher levels. Reducing CVD risk factors when you are young can pay off with many extra years of life and health (see the box "Are You at Risk for CVD?").

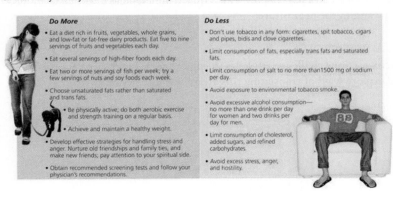

Do More
- Eat a diet rich in fruits, vegetables, whole grains, and low-fat or fat-free dairy products. Eat five to nine servings of fruits and vegetables each day.
- Eat several servings of high-fiber foods each day.
- Eat two or more servings of fish per week; try a few servings of nuts and soy foods each week.
- Choose unsaturated fats rather than saturated and trans fats.
- Be physically active; do both aerobic exercise and strength training on a regular basis.
- Achieve and maintain a healthy weight.
- Develop effective strategies for handling stress and anger. Nurture old friendships and family ties, and make new friends; pay attention to your spiritual side.
- Obtain recommended screening tests and follow your physician's recommendations.

Do Less
- Don't use tobacco in any form: cigarettes, spit tobacco, cigars and pipes, bidis and clove cigarettes.
- Limit consumption of fats, especially trans fats and saturated fats.
- Limit consumption of salt to no more than 1500 mg of sodium per day.
- Avoid exposure to environmental tobacco smoke.
- Avoid excessive alcohol consumption—no more than one drink per day for women and two drinks per day for men.
- Limit consumption of cholesterol, added sugars, and refined carbohydrates.
- Avoid excess stress, anger, and hostility.

With the *Connect Plus* interactive e-Book, students can access *Connect Core Concepts in Health* anywhere, anytime. Among its features are the ability to highlight, take notes, and bookmark key content, providing one place for simple, comprehensive review.

KEY FEATURES AND LEARNING AIDS

The streamlined pedagogical program for the 13th edition maintains important features discussing diversity, behavior change, and personal reflection, while integrating some key material into the body of the chapter. All features that appear with a Connect icon offer a linked Connect activity.

 Diversity Matters features address the ways that our personal backgrounds influence our health strengths, risks, and behaviors.

 Embracing Wellness boxes outline ways that physical health is influenced by *all* of the dimensions of wellness and provide strategies for improvement.

 Critical Consumer sections help students to navigate the numerous and diverse set of health-related products currently available.

 Take Charge boxes challenge students to take meaningful action toward personal improvement.

Behavior Change Strategy sections offer specific behavior management/modification plans related to the chapter topics.

Quick Stat sections focus attention on particularly striking statistics related to the chapter content.

Ask Yourself (Questions for Critical Thinking) sections encourage critical reflection on students' own health-related behaviors.

Tips for Today and the Future end each chapter with a quick, bulleted list of concrete actions readers can take now and in the near future.

Connect to Your Choices sections challenge students to explore their inner motivations for their health choices and to explore ways of translating this awareness into action.

CHAPTER-BY-CHAPTER CHANGES

Chapter 1

+ The discussion of the dimensions of wellness has been thoroughly updated, with the addition of financial wellness, and refined explanations of emotional, interpersonal, and occupation wellness

+ All of the chapter's statistical material has been updated to reflect the latest information on morbidity, mortality, and measures of quality of life

+ The discussion of Healthy People 2020 has been updated with the newest round of objectives and the latest statistics on Americans' progress toward meeting these goals

+ A new Wellness Matters box, "Wellness Matters for College Students," introduces students to the wellness issues most relevant to their age and circumstances

+ A new blank Behavior Change Contract provides a vital tool for tracking and achieving meaningful behavior change

Chapter 2

+ Statistics on stress have been updated throughout, with data from the 2011 American Psychological Association's "Stress in America" survey

+ A new Wellness Matters box, "Coping with News of Traumatic Events," helps students deal with troubling news, whether it be about local, nation, or international events

+ An expanded discussion of the role of spirituality in managing stress includes spiritual engagement beyond the traditional definition of organized religion

Chapter 3

+ A new section on becoming resilient defines psychological resilience and provides tips on building personal resiliency

+ All of the chapter's statistical material has been updated to reflect the latest information on the prevalence of psychological disorders among Americans

+ A new Wellness Matters box, "Deliberate Self-harm," addresses the prevalence of and treatment for deliberate self injury

+ Updated coverage on pharmacological therapy includes the latest drug therapies for depression, psychosis, and ADHD; discussion of the criticisms of drug therapy has been expanded

Chapter 4

+ Self-acceptance added to the discussion of self-concept and self-esteem, including the role adults play in nurturing self-acceptance in children

+ A new section explores the role that emotional intelligence plays in developing and maintaining meaningful relationships; tips included on enhancing one's own emotional intelligence

+ The discussion on ending a relationship has been expanded to include "rebound relationships"

+ A new section addresses the potential positive and negative effects that digital communication has on human relationships

+ The discussion of same-sex marriage has been updated to include the latest state and national legislature

+ Demographic statistics have been updated throughout, with data from the U.S. Census Bureau, the National Center for Health Statistics, and others

Chapter 5

+ A new table on reproductive aging in women outlines the changes that occur in the female reproductive system from puberty to postmenopause

+ A new Wellness Matters box, "Questions to Ask Before Getting Involved in a Sexual Relationship" prompts readers to consider their sexual beliefs, interest, and boundaries before entering a sexual relationship

+ Statistics on Americans' sexual attitudes and behaviors have been thoroughly updated

+ The sections on infertility and infertility treatments have been updated with the latest statistics and medical considerations

+ New information on the causes and survival rates of preterm birth now included in the section on complications of pregnancy

Chapter 6

+ A new Wellness Matters box "Contraception Use and Pregnancy Among College Students" provides the most up-to-date statistics on college-aged populations, including differences among races and ethnicities

+ Sections on the contraceptive ring, contraceptive implants, injectable contraceptives, and IUDS have been updated

- with the latest information on effectiveness and potential side effects
- Statistics on the popularity and effectiveness of available contraceptive methods have been updated throughout
- Information on the current legal status of abortion has been updated to include the latest laws and restrictions
- The most current statistics on abortion rates and methods have been integrated throughout the chapter

Chapter 7

- A new section addresses the rise of synthetic recreational drugs, including "bath salts"
- A new Wellness Matters box, "Drug Use Among College Students," contains the latest statistics and data
- Information on gender differences and drug use has been significantly revised
- The section on the legal consequences of drug use has been updated and expanded

Chapter 8

- A new Wellness Matters box on alcoholic energy drinks details the usage and dangers of these increasingly popular beverages
- The newest data on binge drinking is included, along with discussion of the potentially harmful consequences of the practice
- Material on gender differences and alcohol use has been integrated throughout the chapter
- Statistics on tobacco use updated, with data from the National Survey on Drug Use and Health, the Youth Risk Behavior Strategy, the American Cancer Society, and others
- Updated content on e-cigarettes addresses their composition and the validity of their marketing claims

Chapter 9

- Coverage of U.S. food guidance systems has been updated to reflect new 2010 Dietary Guidelines for Americans
- Coverage of the USDA's new MyPlate added
- The recommended Daily Allowances for calcium and vitamin D have been updated to reflect 2011 revisions to the Dietary Reference Intakes (DRIs) by the Food and Nutrition Board of the Institute of Medicine
- New content on the 2011 Food Safety Modernization Act appears

Chapter 10

- A new, more detailed definition of physical fitness opens the chapter
- All exercise guidelines have been updated to reflect the 2011 statement of the ACSM

- A new section on responders vs. nonresponders to exercise addresses the variety of individual response to any particular exercise program
- A new section describes how to use a heart rate monitor to measure the intensity of exercise

Chapter 11

- Statistics on overweight and obesity in the United States updated, including breakdown by gender and race/ethnicity; all statistics reflect the latest numbers available from the CDC
- Results of the latest research on overweight and obesity addressed throughout the chapter
- Material from the 2010 Dietary Guidelines for Americans on overweight and obesity added, including information on obesogenic environments
- A new Wellness Matters box, "The Freshman 15: Fact or Myth?", addresses the true amount of typical college weight gain and provides tips for maintaining a healthy weight in college

Chapter 12

- Statistics on heart disease updated throughout
- New information appears on optimal cholesterol and LDL levels
- New content addresses the use of statins to reduce the risk of CVD
- A new figure (16.1) provides data on cancer deaths attributable to cigarette smoking
- A new section describes the link between the BRCA gene and breast cancer
- Expanded coverage addresses environmental and industrial pollution as a cause of cancer
- Information on screening and treatment for prostate cancer and ovarian cancer has been updated with the latest medical recommendations
- New information appears on the treatment of melanoma

Chapter 13

- Statistics on top infectious diseases nationwide and worldwide updated with data from the CDC and the WHO
- A new Wellness on Campus box "Meningococcal Meningitis and College Students" provides information on the disease along with vaccination recommendations from the CDC and the American College
- A new section provides coverage of the 2011–2012 controversy over suppression of influenza research
- Statistics on the prevalence of HIV/AIDS and other STDs in the United States and worldwide have been

updated throughout, with breakdown by gender, ethnicity/race, sexual orientation, and sexual behavior; latest numbers available from the CDC, the WHO, and UN-AIDS included

+ Content updates address the latest research on HIV/AIDS and other STDs

+ The new U.S. Preventive Services Task Force and American Cancer Society recommendations for Pap test and HPV test are included

+ New coverage addresses the STD lymphogranuloma venereum

Chapter 14

+ Updated coverage of global warming provides the latest scientific information on the problem and potential solutions

+ Information on renewable energy sources has been significantly updated with the latest usage statistics and technologies

+ A new section addresses the risk and risks of extreme energy sources

+ All statistics have been updated throughout the chapter

Chapter 15

+ A new section on pharmaceuticals and the placebo effect integrates this coverage into the chapter

+ A new Wellness on Campus box guides students through the process of creating a personal health record

Chapter 16

+ Update information on the dangers of distracted driving, including coverage of recent state legislation and the NTSB's recommended ban on the use of portable electronic devises while driving

+ Statistics updated throughout with data from the National Safety Council, Federal Bureau of Investigation, CDC, WHO, and others

Chapter 17

+ A new section on sexual functioning in older adults describes changes that typically occur as we age

+ Expanded information on dementia discusses the latest Alzheimer's research, as well as other common causes of dementia

+ The section on end-of-life care has been considerably revised, including a significantly expanded section on hospice care

+ Material on funeral procedures has been updated to reflect the rising prevalence of cremation in the United States

TEACHING AND LEARNING WITH
CORE CONCEPTS IN HEALTH

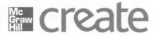

Design your own ideal course materials with McGraw-Hill's 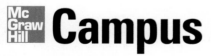 **www.mcgrawhillcreate.com.** Rearrange or omit chapters, combine material from other sources, upload your syllabus or any other content you have written to make the perfect resource for your students. Search thousands of leading McGraw-Hill textbooks to find the best content for your students; then arrange it to fit your teaching style. You can even personalize your book's appearance by selecting the cover and adding your name, school, and course information. When you order a Create book, you receive a complimentary review copy. Get a printed copy in 3 to 5 business days or an electronic copy (e-Comp) via e-mail in about an hour.

> Register today at **www.mcgrawhillcreate.com**, and craft your course resources to match the way you teach.

Campus

McGraw-Hill Campus™ is a new one-stop teaching and learning experience available to users of any learning management system. This institutional service allows faculty and students to enjoy single sign-on (SSO) access to all McGraw-Hill Higher Education materials, including the award-winning McGraw-Hill Connect® platform, from directly within the institution's website. McGraw-Hill Campus provides faculty with instant access to all McGraw-Hill Higher Education teaching materials (e.g., eTextbooks, test banks, PowerPoint slides, animations, and learning objects), allowing them to browse, search, and use any instructor ancillary content in our vast library at no additional cost to instructor or students. Students enjoy SSO access to a variety of free (e.g., quizzes, flash cards, narrated presentations) and subscription-based products (e.g., McGraw-Hill Connect). With this program enabled, faculty and students will never need to create another account to access McGraw-Hill products and services.

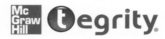

Tegrity Campus is a service that makes class time available around the clock. It automatically captures every lecture in a searchable format for students to review when they study and complete assignments. With a simple one-click start-and-stop process, you capture all computer screens and corresponding audio. Students replay any part of any class with easy-to-use browser-based viewing on a PC or Mac. With Tegrity Campus, students quickly recall key moments by using Tegrity Campus's unique search feature, which lets them efficiently find what they need, when they need it, across an entire semester of class recordings. Help turn all your students' study time into learning moments immediately supported by your lecture. To learn more about Tegrity, watch a 2-minute Flash demo at **http://tegritycampus. mhhe.com.**

INSTRUCTOR SUPPLEMENTS

Find materials you need to get your course up and running on **www.mhhe.com/Inselbrief13e.** There, you will find:

- Course Integrator guide
- Test bank
- PowerPoint slides
- Transparency masters and student handouts
- Health and wellness related weblinks

ACKNOWLEDGEMENTS

Connect Core Concepts in Health has benefited from the thoughtful commentary, expert knowledge, and helpful suggestions of many people. We are deeply grateful for their participation in the project.

Academic Contributors

Philip Insel, M.S. Center for Imaging of Neurodegenerative Disease, VA Medical Center, San Francisco
Stress: The Constant Challenge

Thomas D. Fahey, Ed.D., California State University—Chico
Exercise for Health and Fitness

Philip Takakjian, Ph.D.
Intimate Relationships & Communication

Lisa Medoff, Ph.D., Stanford University
Sexuality, Pregnancy, and Childbirth

Katherine Willoughby, Ph.D., Stanford University
Contraception and Abortion

Sarah Waller, M.D., Stanford University
Sexuality, Pregnancy, and Childbirth

Patrick Zickler, Senior Health and Science Writer, Circle Solutions, Inc.
Drug Use and Addiction

Marcia Seyler, MPH
Alcohol Use and Alcoholism

Omid Fotuhi. Ph.D. University of Waterloo
Tobacco Use

Melissa Bernstein, Ph. D, R.D., L.D., Rosalind Franklin University of Medicine and Science
Nutrition Basics and Weight Management

Tannon Carroll, M.D., M.P.A., Cardiovascular Medicine Fellow, Stanford University Hospital
Cardiovascular Health

Lauren Maeda, M. D., Oncology Fellow, Stanford University
Cancer

Martha Zinuga, Ph.D., University of California, Santa Cruz
Immunity and Infection

Candice McNeil, M.D., Stanford University
Sexually Transmitted Diseases

Dennis Murphy, MBA, Founding Chair, U.S. Green Bldg. Council of California
Environmental Health

Robert Jarski, Ph.D., Professor of Health Sciences, Directory, Complementary Medicine and Wellness Program, Oakland University
Conventional and Complementary Medicine

Michael Hoadley, Ph.D., Assistant Vice-President for Academic Affairs, Center for Academic Technology Support, Eastern Illinois University
Personal Safety

Mary Iten, Ph.D., University of Nebraska at Kearney
Aging

Nancy Kemp, M.D.
Dying and Death

Academic Advisors and Reviewers for the Thirteenth Edition

Kathleen Allison, Lock Haven University of Pennsylvania
Jana Arabas, Truman State University
Paul Bondurant, Macomb Community College
Janis Bowman, Jamestown Community College
Becca Brimhall, Utah Valley University—Orem
Carol Carr-Smith, Community College of Baltimore County—Essex
Allen J. Cone, East Los Angeles College
Brent Damron, Bakersfield College
Nicholas Dicicco, Camden County College
Brian Findley, Palm Beach State College—Lake Worth

Dee Ann Goshgarian, West Hills College—LeMoore

Kyle Hanks, Los Medanos College

Brian Hickey, Florida A&M University

Karen Hunter, Eastern Kentucky University

Matt Hutchins, Indiana State University—Terre Haute

Maureen Johnson, Indiana State University—Terre Haute

Kelly Knee, College of Western Idaho

Rhonna Krouse, College of Western Idaho

Garry Ladd, Southwestern Illinois College

Alison Oberne, University of South Florida—Tampa

Kurt Olson, Modesto Jr. College

Rick Scheidt, Fresno City College

Christine Sholtey, Waubonsee Community College

Rob Turrisi, Penn State University—University Park

Silvia Villasenor, Moreno Valley College

Bonnie Young, Georgia Perimeter College

Personal Health Symposia Participants

Dede Bodnar, San Diego City College

Christine Bouffard, Waubonsee Community College

Curtiss Brown, Solano Community College

Carrie Edwards, Southeastern Louisiana University

Kelly Falcone, Palomar College

Jennifer Fay, Arizona State University

Gabrielle Floyd, Texas Southern University

Jackie Franz, Mercer County Community College

Rachelle Franz, University of Central Oklahoma

Kathy Gilbert, Indiana University

Gilbert Gipson, Virginia State University

Christine Gorman, Kean University

Christine Harrison, Montgomery College—Rockville

Del Helms, Mt. San Jacinto College—Menifee

Kathy Hixon, Northeastern State University

Jerolyn Hughes-Golightly, Alabama A&M University

Don Hume, Kingsborough Community College

Kris Jankovitz, California Polytech State University

Chester Jones, University of Arkansas-Fayetteville

Walt Justice, Southwestern College

Raeann Koerner, Ventura College

Jennifer Langeland (Mills), Western Michigan University

Grace Lartey, Western Kentucky University

Randy Maday, Butte College

Lori Mallory, Johnson County Community College

Michelle McCarthy, San Jose State

Brian McFarlin, University of Houston

Alison Oberne, University of South Florida—Tampa

Caree Oslislo-Wizenberg, Anne Arundel Community College

Kimberly Peabody, Benedict College

Kay Perrin, University of South FL-Tampa Dollie Richards, Salt Lake Community College

Tara Rouse, Pearl River Community College—Poplarville

Linda Rosskopf, Georgia Institute of Technology

Karla Rues, Ozarks Technical Community College

Cindy Shelton, University of Central Arkansas

Jake Silvestri, Hudson Valley Community College

Cynthia Smith, Central Piedmont Community College

John Smith, Springfield College

Jamean Southall, Hampton University

Amanda Tapler, Elon University

Gayle Truitt-Bean, Clarion University of Pennsylvania

Carol Weideman, Western Michigan University—Kalamazoo

Jae Westfall, Ohio State University-Columbus

Virginia White, Riverside City College

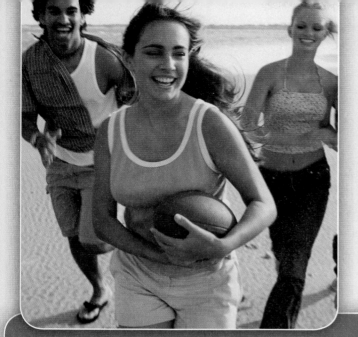

LOOKING AHEAD...

After reading this chapter, you should be able to

- Describe the dimensions of wellness
- Identify major health problems in the United States today
- Describe the influence of gender, ethnicity, income, disability, family history, and environment on health
- Explain the importance of personal decision making and behavior change in achieving wellness
- List some available sources of health information and explain how to think critically about them
- Describe the steps in creating a behavior management plan to change a health-related behavior

1

Taking Charge of Your Health

"How are you?"
"Fine. And you?"
"Fine."
How many times have you had this brief conversation this week—or even today? And how many times have you told someone you were "fine" when in fact you were feeling no better than just all right or even downright miserable? Instead of merely telling people we are "fine," what if we strove to truly feel good—not merely to be free of major illness, but to live life actively, energetically, and fully in a state of optimal personal, interpersonal, and environmental well-being? What if we each took charge of our personal health and wellness? What would it mean to meet a friend in passing and honestly be able to say, "I'm feeling great"?

WELLNESS: NEW HEALTH GOALS

Generations of people have viewed good health simply as the absence of disease, and that view largely prevails today. The word **health** typically refers to the overall condition of a person's body or mind and to the presence or absence of illness or injury. **Wellness**, a relatively new concept, expands our idea of good health to include living rich, meaningful, and energetic life. Beyond the simple presence or absence of disease, wellness can refer to optimal health and vitality—to living life to its fullest.

Wellness involves our making conscious decisions that affect **risk factors** that contribute to disease or injury. Although age and family history are risk factors we cannot control, behaviors such as smoking, exercising, and eating a healthful diet are well within our control.

The Dimensions of Wellness

Experts have defined seven dimensions of wellness, which are listed in Table 1.1, along with some of the qualities and behaviors associated with each dimension.

These dimensions are interrelated. Each one has an effect on the others. Further, the process of achieving wellness is continuing and dynamic (Figure 1.1), involving change and growth. Wellness is not static. Ignoring any dimension of wellness can be harmful. But the encouraging aspect of wellness is that you can actively pursue it.

Physical Wellness   Your physical wellness includes not just your body's overall condition and the absence of disease, but your fitness level and your ability to care for yourself. The higher your fitness level is, the higher your level of physical wellness will be. Similarly, as you develop the ability to take care of your own physical needs, you ensure greater physical wellness. To achieve optimum physical wellness, you need to make choices that will help you avoid illnesses and injuries.

Table 1.1 — Examples of Qualities and Behaviors Associated with the Dimensions of Wellness

PHYSICAL	EMOTIONAL	INTELLECTUAL	INTERPERSONAL	SPIRITUAL	ENVIRONMENTAL	FINANCIAL
■ Eating well	■ Optimism	■ Openness to new ideas	■ Communication skills	■ Capacity for love	■ Having abundant, clean natural resources	■ Basic understanding of how money works
■ Exercising	■ Trust	■ Capacity to question	■ Capacity for intimacy	■ Compassion	■ Maintaining sustainable development	■ Living within one's means
■ Avoiding harmful habits	■ Self-esteem	■ Ability to think critically	■ Ability to establish and maintain satisfying relationships	■ Forgiveness	■ Recycling whenever possible	■ Avoiding debt, especially for unnecessary items
■ Practicing safe sex	■ Self-acceptance	■ Motivation to master new skills	■ Ability to cultivate support system of friends and family	■ Altruism	■ Reducing pollution and waste	■ Save for the future and for potential emergencies
■ Recognizing symptoms of disease	■ Self-confidence	■ Sense of humor		■ Joy		
■ Getting regular checkups	■ Ability to understand and accept one's feelings	■ Creativity		■ Fulfillment		
■ Avoiding injuries	■ Ability to share feelings with others	■ Curiosity		■ Caring for others		
		■ Lifelong learning		■ Sense of meaning and purpose		
				■ Sense of belonging to something greater than oneself		

Emotional Wellness   Trust, self-confidence, optimism, satisfying relationships, and self-esteem are some of the qualities of emotional wellness. Emotional wellness is dynamic, and involves the ups and downs of living. No one can achieve an emotional "high" all the time. Emotional wellness fluctuates with your intellectual, physical, spiritual, social, and interpersonal health. Maintaining emotional wellness requires exploring thoughts and feelings. One of the best ways to achieve emotional wellness is to share your emotional problems with others. If it's a risk, it's a risk worth taking. Achieving emotional wellness means finding solutions to emotional problems, with professional help if necessary.

Intellectual Wellness   Those who enjoy intellectual wellness constantly challenge their minds. An active mind is essential to wellness because it detects problems, finds solutions, and directs behavior. Throughout their lifetimes people who enjoy intellectual wellness never stop learning. They not only seek and relish new experiences and challenges but often discover new things about themselves.

Interpersonal Wellness   Satisfying and supportive relationships are important to physical and emotional wellness. Learning good communication skills, developing the capacity for intimacy, and cultivating a supportive network are all important to interpersonal (or social) wellness. Social wellness requires participating in and contributing to your community and to society.

> **TERMS**
>
> **health**   The overall condition of body or mind and the presence or absence of illness or injury.
>
> **wellness**   Optimal health and vitality, encompassing all the dimensions of well-being.
>
> **risk factor**   A condition that increases one's chances of disease or injury.

FIGURE 1.1 The wellness continuum.
The concept of wellness includes vitality in seven interrelated dimensions, all of which contribute to overall wellness.

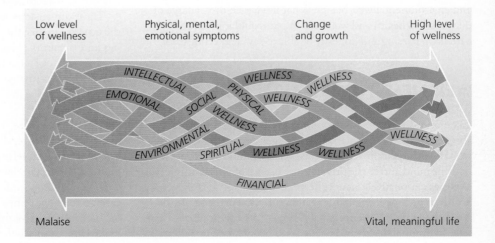

Low level of wellness   Physical, mental, emotional symptoms   Change and growth   High level of wellness

INTELLECTUAL   EMOTIONAL   SOCIAL   PHYSICAL   WELLNESS   WELLNESS   WELLNESS   WELLNESS   ENVIRONMENTAL   WELLNESS   SPIRITUAL   WELLNESS   WELLNESS   WELLNESS   FINANCIAL

Malaise   Vital, meaningful life

Spiritual Wellness   To enjoy spiritual wellness is to possess a set of guiding beliefs, principles, or values that give meaning and purpose to your life, especially in difficult times. The spiritually well person focuses on the positive aspects of life and finds spirituality to be an antidote for negative feelings such as cynicism, anger, and pessimism. Organized religions help many people develop spiritual health. Religion, however, is not the only source or form of spiritual wellness. Many people find meaning and purpose in their lives on their own—through nature, art, meditation, or good works—or with their loved ones.

Environmental Wellness   Your environmental wellness is defined by the livability of your surroundings. Personal health depends on the health of the planet—from the safety of the food supply to the degree of violence in society. Your physical environment can support your wellness or diminish it. To improve your environmental wellness, you can learn about and protect yourself against hazards in your surroundings and work to make your world a cleaner and safer place.

Financial Wellness   Financial wellness refers to your ability to live within your means and manage your money in a way that gives you peace of mind. It includes balancing your income and expenses, staying out of debt, saving for the future, and understanding your emotions about money. For more on this topic, see the "Financial Wellness" box.

Other Aspects of Wellness   Many experts consider occupational wellness to be an additional important dimension of wellness. *Occupational wellness* refers to the level of happiness and fulfillment you gain through your work. An occupationally well person enjoys his or her work, feels a connection with others in the workplace, and takes advantage of the opportunities to learn and be challenged. To achieve occupational wellness, set career goals that reflect your personal values.

New Opportunities for Taking Charge

Wellness is a fairly new concept. A century ago, Americans considered themselves lucky just to survive to adulthood. A child born in 1900, for example, could expect to live only about 47 years. **Morbidity** and **mortality rates** (rates of illness and death, respectively) from common **infectious diseases** (such as pneumonia, tuberculosis, and diarrhea) were much higher than Americans experience today.

Since 1900, **life expectancy** has nearly doubled, due largely to the development of vaccines and antibiotics to fight infections, and to public health measures such as water purification and sewage treatment to improve living conditions. But even though life expectancy has increased, poor

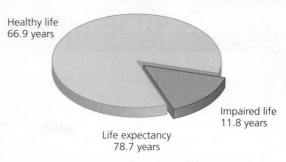

FIGURE 1.2   Quantity of life versus quality of life. Years of healthy life as a proportion of life expectancy in the U.S. population.
SOURCE: National Center for Health Statistics. 2012. Deaths: Preliminary data for 2010 (data release). *National Vital Statistics Report* 60(4).

health will limit most Americans' activities during the last 15% of their lives, resulting in some sort of **impaired life** (Figure 1.2). Today a different set of diseases has emerged as our major health threat, and heart disease, cancer, and stroke are now the three leading causes of death for Americans (Table 1.2). Treating such **chronic diseases** is costly and difficult.

The good news is that people have some control over whether they develop chronic diseases. People make choices every day that increase or decrease their risks for such diseases. Each of us can take personal responsibility for **lifestyle choices** that include behaviors such as smoking, diet, exercise, and alcohol use. As Table 1.3 makes clear, lifestyle factors contribute to many deaths in the United States, and people can influence their own health risks.

The need to make good choices is especially true for teens and young adults. For Americans aged 15–24, for example, the top three causes of death are unintentional injuries (accidents), homicide, and suicide (Table 1.4).

QUICK STATS

72% of American men are overweight.
—NIH, 2011

TERMS

morbidity rate   The relative incidence of disease among a population.

mortality rate   The number of deaths in a population in a given period of time; usually expressed as a ratio, such as 75 deaths per 1000 members of the population.

infectious disease   A disease that can spread from person to person, caused by microorganisms such as bacteria and viruses.

life expectancy   The period of time a member of a given population is expected to live.

impaired life   The period of a person's life when he or she may not be able to function fully due to disease or disability.

chronic disease   A disease that develops and continues over a long period of time, such as heart disease or cancer.

lifestyle choice   A conscious behavior that can increase or decrease a person's risk of disease or injury; such behaviors include smoking, exercising, eating a healthful diet, and others.

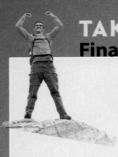

TAKE CHARGE
Financial Wellness

With the news full of stories of home fore-closures, credit card debt, and personal bankruptcies, it has become painfully clear that many Americans do not know how to manage their finances. You can avoid such stress—and gain financial peace of mind—by developing skills that contribute to financial wellness.

Financial wellness means having a healthy relationship with money. It involves knowing how to manage your money, using self-discipline to live within your means, using credit cards wisely, staying out of debt, meeting your financial obligations, having a long-range financial plan, and saving.

Learn to Budget

Although the word *budget* may conjure up thoughts of deprivation, a budget is really just a way of tracking where your money goes and making sure you're spending it on the things that are most important to you. To start one, list your monthly income and your expenditures. If you aren't sure where you spend your money, track your expenses for a few weeks or a month. Then organize them into categories, such as housing, food, transportation, entertainment, services, personal care, clothes, books and school supplies, health care, credit card and loan payments, and miscellaneous. Use categories that reflect the way you actually spend your money. Knowing where your money goes is the first step in gaining control of it.

Now total your income and expenditures. Are you taking in more than you spend, or vice versa? Are you surprised by your spending patterns? Use this information to set guidelines and goals for yourself. If your expenses exceed your income, identify ways to make some cuts. If you have both a cell phone and a land line, for example, consider whether you can give one up. If you spend money on movies and restaurants, consider less expensive options like having a weekly game night with friends or organizing an occasional potluck.

Be Wary of Credit Cards

College students are prime targets for credit card companies, and most undergraduates have at least one card. In fact, many college students use credit cards to live beyond their means, not just for convenience. According a recent report, half of all students have four or more cards, and the average outstanding balance on undergraduate credit cards is over $3000.

The best way to avoid credit card debt is to have just one card, to use it only when necessary, and to pay off the entire balance every month. Make sure you understand terms like *APR* (annual percentage rate—the interest you're charged on your balance),

credit limit (the maximum amount you can borrow), *minimum monthly payment* (the smallest payment your creditor will accept each month), *grace period* (the number of days you have to pay your bill before interest or penalties are charged), and *over-the-limit* and *late fees* (the amount you'll be charged if your payment is late or if you go over your credit limit).

Get Out of Debt

If you have credit card debt, stop using your cards and start paying them off. If you can't pay the whole balance, at least try to pay more than the minimum payment each month. It can take a very long time to pay off a loan by making only the minimum payments. For example, paying off a credit card balance of $2000 at 10% interest with monthly payments of $20 would take 203 months—17 years. To see for yourself, check out an online credit card calculator like http://cgi.money.cnn.com/tools/debtplanner/debtplanner.jsp. And remember: By carrying a balance and incurring finance charges, you are also paying back much more than your initial loan.

Start Saving

The same miracle of compound interest that locks you into years of credit card debt can work to your benefit if you start saving early (for an online compound interest calculator, visit http://www.interestcalc.org). Experts recommend "paying your-self first" every month—that is, putting some money into savings before you start paying your bills, depending on what your budget allows. You may want to save for a large purchase, or you may even be looking ahead to retirement. If you work for a company with a 401(k) retirement plan, contribute as much as you can every pay period.

Become Financially Literate

Although modern life requires financial literacy, most Americans have not received any kind of basic financial training. For this reason, the U.S. government has established the Financial Literacy and Education Commission (www.MyMoney.gov) to help Americans develop financial literacy and learn how to save, invest, and manage their money better. The consensus is that developing lifelong financial skills should begin in early adulthood, during the college years, if not earlier.

SOURCES: Federal Deposit Insurance Corporation. 2010. *Money Smart: A Financial Education Program* (http://www.fdic.gov/consumers/consumer/moneysmart/young.html); Plymouth State University. 2012. *Student Monetary Awareness and Responsibility Today!* (http://www.plymouth.edu/office/financial-aid/smart/); U.S. Financial Literacy and Education Commission. 2012. *MyMoney.gov* (http://www.mymoney.gov).

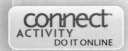

connect
ACTIVITY
DO IT ONLINE

Table 1.2   Leading Causes of Death in the United States, 2010

RANK	CAUSE OF DEATH	NUMBER OF DEATHS	PERCENTAGE OF TOTAL DEATHS*	DEATH RATE†	LIFESTYLE FACTORS
	All causes	2,465,932	100.0	798.7	
1	Heart disease	599,444	24.3	192.9	D I S A
2	Cancer	573,855	23.3	185.9	D I S A
3	Chronic lower respiratory diseases	137,789	5.6	44.6	■ ■ S ■
4	Stroke	129,180	5.2	41.8	D I S A
5	Unintentional injuries (accidents)	118,043	4.9	38.2	■ I S A
6	Alzheimer's disease	83,308	3.8	27.0	■ ■ ■ ■
7	Diabetes mellitus	68,905	2.8	22.3	D I S ■
8	Kidney disease	50,472	2.1	16.3	D I S A
9	Influenza and pneumonia	50,003	2.0	16.2	■ ■ S ■
10	Intentional self-harm (suicide)	37,793	1.5	12.2.9	■ ■ ■ A
11	Septicemia (systemic blood infection)	34,843	1.4	11.3	■ ■ ■ A
12	Chronic liver disease and cirrhosis	31,802	1.3	10.34	■ ■ ■ A
13	Hypertension (high blood pressure)	26,577	1.1	8.6	D I S A
14	Parkinson's disease	21,963	0.8	7.1	■ ■ ■ ■
15	Pneumonitis due to solids and liquids	17,001	0.7	5.5	■ ■ ■ A
	All other causes	488,954	19.0	158.5	■ ■ ■ ■

Key
D Diet plays a part.
I Inactive lifestyle plays a part.
S Smoking plays a part.
A Excessive alcohol use plays a part.

NOTE: Although not among the overall top 15 causes of death, HIV/AIDS (8,352 deaths in 2010) is a major killer. In 2010 HIV/AIDS was the 11th leading cause of death for Americans aged 15–24 years and the 7th leading cause of death for those aged 25–44 years.

*Percentages may not sum to 100% due to rounding.
† Age-adjusted death rate per 100,000 persons.

SOURCE: National Center for Health Statistics. 2012. Deaths: Preliminary data for 2010 (data release). *National Vital Statistics Report* 60(4).

Promoting Health and Preventing Disease

People are a nation's most important resource. The creativity, vitality, and prosperity of a country depend on the health of its people. Governments as well as communities find it in their long-term interests to promote health and prevent disease. The World Health Organization (WHO) defines **health promotion** as "the process of enabling people to increase control over their health and its determinants, and thereby improve their health." The primary means of promoting health are public health policies and agencies that identify and discourage unhealthy and high-risk behaviors and that encourage and provide incentives for judicious health behaviors. Many college campuses have health promotion programs or activities.

In the United States, the National Insitutes of Health (NIH) and the Centers for Disease Control and Prevention (CDC) are federal agencies charged with promoting the public's health. NIH is the primary federal agency for conducting and supporting medical research. NIH scientists investigate ways to prevent disease as well as the causes, treatments, and cures for common and rare diseases. Composed of 27 institutes and centers, the NIH provides leadership and financial support to researchers in every state as well as around the world. The NIH translates research results into interventions and communicates research findings to patients, health care providers, and the public.

Disease prevention is a major focus of public health promotion. Working at disease prevention, the CDC collaborates

> **TERMS**
>
> **health promotion**   The process of enabling people to increase control over their health and its determinants, and thereby improve their health.
>
> **disease prevention**   The process of providing tools that people and communities need to protect their health by reducing risks; promoting health; preventing disease, injury, and disability; and preparing for new health threats.

Table 1.3 — Key Contributors to Death among Americans

	NUMBER OF DEATHS PER YEAR	PERCENTAGE OF TOTAL DEATHS PER YEAR
Tobacco	443,000	18.0
Obesity*	111,909	4.5
Alcohol consumption	25,440	1.0
Microbial agents	50,003	2.0
Toxic agents	55,000	2.3
Motor vehicles	35,080	1.4
Firearms	11,015	0.5
Sexually transmitted diseases	20,000	0.8
Illicit drug use	37,792	1.5

NOTE: The factors listed here are defined as lifestyle and environmental factors that contribute to the leading killers of Americans. Microbial agents include bacterial and viral infections like influenza and pneumonia; toxic agents include environmental pollutants and chemical agents such as asbestos.

*The number of deaths due to obesity is an area of ongoing controversy and research. Recent estimates have ranged from 112,000 to 365,000.

SOURCES: Centers for Disease Control and Prevention. 2008. Smoking-attributable mortality, years of potential life lost, and productivity losses—United States, 2000–2004. *Morbidity and Mortality Weekly Report* 57(45): 1226–1228; Flegal, K. M. 2010. *Supplemental Analyses for Estimates of Excess Deaths Associated with Underweight, Overweight, and Obesity in the U.S. Population* (http://www.cdc.gov/nchs/data/hestat/excess_deaths/excess_deaths.htm); National Center for Health Statistics. 2012. Deaths: final data for 2009 (data release). *National Vital Statistics Report* 60(3).; National Center for Health Statistics. 2012. Deaths: Preliminary data for 2010 (data release). *National Vital Statistics Report* 60(4).

with partners throughout the nation and the world to provide tools that people and communities need to protect their health through health promotion; prevention of disease, injury, and disability; and preparedness for new health threats. Prevention research focuses on identifying risk factors and protective factors for diseases, disorders, and injuries; identifying high-risk behaviors; and developing, managing, and evaluating preventive interventions.

The Healthy People Initiative

The national Healthy People initiative aims to prevent disease and improve Americans' quality of life. *Healthy People* reports, published each decade since 1980, set national health goals based on 10-year agendas. The initiative's most recent iteration, *Healthy People 2020*, was developed in 2008–2009 and released to the public in 2010. *Healthy People 2020* envisions "a society in which all people live long, healthy lives" and proposes the eventual achievement of the following broad national health objectives:

- *Eliminate preventable disease, disability, injury, and premature death.* This objective involves activities such as taking more concrete steps to prevent diseases and injuries among individuals and groups, promoting healthy lifestyle choices, improving the nation's preparedness for emergencies, and strengthening the public health infrastructure.
- *Achieve health equity, eliminate disparities, and improve the health of all groups.* This objective involves identifying, measuring, and addressing health differences between individuals or groups that result from a social or economic disadvantage.
- *Create social and physical environments that promote good health for all.* This objective involves the use of health interventions at many different levels (such as anti-smoking campaigns by schools, workplaces, and local agencies), improving the situation of undereducated and poor Americans by providing a broader array of educational and job opportunities, and actively developing healthier living and natural environments for everyone.
- *Promote healthy development and healthy behaviors across every stage of life.* This objective involves taking a cradle-to-grave approach to health promotion by encouraging disease prevention and healthy behaviors in Americans of all ages.

In a shift from the past, *Healthy People 2020* emphasizes the importance of health determinants—factors that affect the health of individuals, demographic groups, or entire

Table 1.4 — Leading Causes of Death among Americans Aged 15–24

RANK	CAUSE OF DEATH	NUMBER OF DEATHS	PERCENTAGE OF TOTAL DEATHS
1	Accidents:	12,015	40.7
	Transport	7,209	24.4
	Nontransport	4,806	16.3
2	Homicide	4,651	15.8
3	Suicide	4,559	15.5
4	Cancer	1,594	5.4
5	Heart disease	984	3.3
	All causes	29,504	

SOURCE: National Center for Health Statistics. 2012. Deaths: Preliminary data for 2010. *National Vital Statistics Report* 60(4).

| Table 1.5 | Selected *Healthy People 2020* Objectives |

OBJECTIVE	ESTIMATE OF CURRENT STATUS (%)	GOAL (%)
Reduce the proportion of adults who are sedentary and engage in no leisure-time physical activity.	36.2	32.6
Increase the proportion of adults who are at a healthy weight.	30.8	33.9
Increase the proportion of adults with mental health disorders who receive treatment.	58.7	64.6
Reduce the proportion of adults who use cigarettes.	20.6	12.0
Increase the proportion of adults who get sufficient sleep.	69.6	70.9
Reduce the proportion of adults with hypertension.	29.9	26.9
Reduce the proportion of adults who drank excessively in the previous 30 days.	28.1	25.3
Increase the proportion of persons who use the Internet to communicate with their health care providers.	13	15
Increase the proportion of persons with health insurance.	83	100

SOURCE: Institute of Medicine. 2011. *Leading Health Indicators for Healthy People 2020.* Washington, DC: The National Academies Press.

populations. Health determinants are social (including factors such as ethnicity, education level, or economic status) and environmental (including natural and human-made environments). Thus one goal is to improve living conditions in ways that reduce the impact of negative health determinants.

Examples of individual health promotion goals from *Healthy People 2020*, along with estimates of how well Americans are tracking toward achieving those goals, appear in Table 1.5.

Health Issues for Diverse Populations

Americans are a diverse people. Our ancestry is European, African, Asian, Pacific Islander, Latin American, and Native American. We live in cities, suburbs, and rural areas and work in every imaginable occupation.

When it comes to health, most differences among people are insignificant; most health issues concern us all equally. We all need to eat well, exercise, manage stress, and cultivate satisfying personal relationships. We need to know how to protect ourselves from heart disease, cancer, sexually transmitted diseases, and injuries. We need to know how to use the health care system.

But some of our differences, as individuals and as members of groups, have important implications for health. Some of us, for example, have a genetic predisposition for developing certain health problems, such as high cholesterol. Some of us have grown up eating foods that raise our risk of heart disease or obesity. Some of us live in an environment that increases the chance that we will smoke cigarettes or abuse alcohol. These health-related differences among individuals and groups can be biological—that is, determined genetically—or cultural—acquired as patterns of behavior through daily interactions with our families, communities, and society. Many health conditions are a function of biology and culture combined. A person can have a genetic predisposition for a disease, for example, but won't actually develop the disease itself unless certain lifestyle factors are present, such as tobacco use or a poor diet.

> When it comes to wellness, **personal responsibility can make the difference.**

Health-related differences among groups can be identified and described in the context of several different dimensions. Those highlighted by the Healthy People initiative are gender, ethnicity, income and education, disability, geographic location, and sexual orientation.

Sex and Gender   Sex and gender profoundly influence wellness. The WHO defines **sex** as the biological and physiological characteristics that define men and women. These characteristics are related to chromosomes and their effects on reproductive organs and the functioning of the body. Menstruation in women and the presence of testicles in men are examples of sex-related characteristics.

Gender is defined as roles, behaviors, activities, and attributes that a given society considers appropriate for men and women. A person's gender is rooted in biology and physiology, but it is shaped by experience and environment—how society responds to individuals based on their sex. Examples of gender-related characteristics that affect wellness include higher rates of smoking and drinking among men and lower earnings among women (compared with men doing similar work).

Both sex and gender have important effects on wellness, but they can be difficult to separate (see Table 1.6). For example, in the early 20th century, more women began smoking with changes in culturally defined ideas about women's behavior (a gender issue). Because women are more vulnerable to the toxins in tobacco smoke (a sex issue), their cancer rates also increased. Although men are more biologically likely than women to suffer from certain diseases (a sex issue), men are less likely to visit their physicians for regular exams (a gender issue). As a

TERMS

sex   The biological and physiological characteristics that define men and women.

gender   The roles, behaviors, activities, and attributes that a given society considers appropriate for men and women.

Table 1.6 Women's Health, Men's Health

HEALTH ISSUES	WOMEN	MEN
Life expectancy	On average, live about five years longer but have higher rates of disabling health problems such as arthritis, osteoporosis, and Alzheimer's disease.	Have a shorter life expectancy but lower rates of disabling health problems.
Height and weight	Shorter on average, with a lower proportion of muscle; tend to have a "pear" shape with excess body fat stored in the hips; obesity is more common in women than men.	Taller on average, with a higher proportion of muscle; tend to have an "apple" shape with excess body fat stored in the abdomen.
Skills and fluencies	Score better on tests of verbal fluency, speech production, fine motor skills, and visual and working memory.	Score better on tests of visual-spatial ability (such as the ability to imagine the relationships between shapes and objects when rotated in space).
Heart attacks	Experience heart attacks about 10 years later than men, on average, with a poorer 1-year survival rate; more likely to experience atypical heart attack symptoms (such as fatigue and difficulty breathing) or "silent" heart attacks that occur without chest pain.	Experience heart attacks about 10 years earlier than women, on average, with a better 1-year survival rate; more likely to have "classic" heart attack symptoms (such as chest pain).
Stroke	More likely to have a stroke or die from one, but also more likely to recover language ability after a stroke that affects the left side of the brain.	Less likely to die from a stroke, but also more likely to suffer permanent loss of language ability after a stroke that affects the left side of the brain.
Immune response	Stronger immune systems; less susceptible to infection by certain bacteria and viruses, but more likely to develop autoimmune diseases such as lupus.	Weaker immune systems; more susceptible to infection by certain bacteria and viruses, but less likely to develop autoimmune diseases.
Smoking	Lower rates of smoking than men, but higher risk of lung cancer at a given level of exposure to smoke.	Higher rates of smoking and spit tobacco use.
Alcohol	Become more intoxicated at a given level of alcohol intake.	Become less intoxicated at a given level of alcohol intake, but are more likely to use or abuse alcohol or to develop alcoholism.
Stress	More likely to react to stress with a "tend-and-befriend" response that involves social support; may have a longevity advantage because of a reduced risk of stress-related disorders.	More likely to react to stress with aggression or hostility; this pattern may increase the rate of stress-related disorders.
Depression	More likely to suffer from depression and to attempt suicide.	Lower rates of depression than women and less likely to attempt suicide, but four times more likely to succeed at suicide.
Headaches	More commonly suffer migraines and chronic tension headaches.	More likely to suffer from cluster headaches.
Sexually transmitted diseases (STDs)	More likely to be infected with an STD during a heterosexual encounter; more likely to suffer severe, long-term effects from STDs, such as chronic infection and infertility.	Less likely to be infected with an STD during a heterosexual encounter.

result, 55% of American men have not seen their doctors for checkups in the past year, and 29% of men say they wait as long as possible before seeing a doctor—even when they are sick. About one in three American men don't have a regular health care provider, compared to about one in five American women.

Ethnicity Compared with the U.S. population as a whole, American ethnic minorities have higher rates of death and disability from many causes. These disparities result from a complex mix of genetic variations, environmental factors, and health behaviors.

Some diseases are concentrated in certain gene pools, the result of each ethnic group's relatively distinct history. Sickle-cell disease is most common among people of African ancestry. Tay-Sachs disease afflicts people of Eastern European Jewish

One in three American men and **one in five** American women have no regular health care provider.

heritage and French Canadian heritage. Cystic fibrosis is more common among Northern Europeans. In addition to biological differences, many cultural differences occur along ethnic lines. Ethnic groups may vary in their traditional diets; their family and interpersonal relationships; their attitudes toward tobacco, alcohol, and other drugs; and their health beliefs and practices. All of these factors have implications for wellness (see the "Health Disparities among Ethnic Americans" box for more information).

The federal government collects population and health information on five broad ethnic minority groups in American society. Each group has some specific health concerns:

- *Latinos* are a diverse group, with roots in Mexico, Puerto Rico, Cuba, and South and Central America. Many

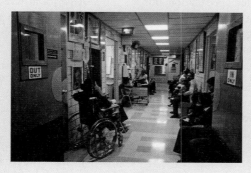

Among America's ethnic groups, striking disparities exist in health status, access to and quality of health care, and life expectancy.

For example, the estimated life expectancy of black Americans (75.1) is about four years shorter than that of whites (79.0). Blacks also have the highest age-adjusted death rate (898 deaths per 100,000 population) of any ethnic group. Whites have the second-highest death rate (741), followed by Native Americans/Alaska Natives (626), Hispanics (558), and Asian Americans/Pacific Islanders (424).

In studying and attempting to understand the underlying causes of health disparities, it is often helpful to separate the many potential contributing factors.

Income and Education

As noted in the chapter, poverty and low educational attainment are the most important factors underlying health disparities. However, when groups with similar incomes and levels of education are compared, ethnic disparities persist. Consider the following examples:

- *Overall health.* People living in poverty report worse health than people with higher incomes. Within the latter group, however, African Americans and Latinos rate their health as "bad" more frequently than do whites.

- *Infant mortality.* Rates of infant deaths go down as the education level of mothers goes up. Among mothers who are college graduates, however, African Americans have significantly higher rates of infant mortality than whites, Latinos, and Asian Americans. Overall, the rate of infant mortality among blacks is more than double that of whites, Asian Americans, or Hispanics.

Access to Appropriate Health Care

The health care reform bill passed by Congress in 2010 mandated insurance coverage for 32 million Americans without insurance. Major coverage expansion begins in 2014. The legislation should reduce the number of people without access to health care and without information about services and preventive care.

Although people with low incomes have tended to receive poorer-quality health care, disparities among ethnic minorities persist even at higher income levels. For example, among nonpoor Americans, many more Latinos than whites or African Americans report no usual source of health care and no health care visits within the past year. Ongoing studies continually find that racial minorities have less access to better health care (such as complex surgery at high-volume hospitals) and receive lower-quality care than whites.

Factors affecting such disparities may include the following:

- *Local differences in the availability of high-tech health care and specialists.* Minorities, regardless of income, may be more likely to live in medically underserved areas.

- *Problems with communication and trust.* People whose primary language is not English are more likely to be uninsured and to have trouble communicating with health care providers. They may also have problems interpreting health information from public health education campaigns. Language and cultural barriers may be compounded by an underrepresentation of minorities in the health professions.

- *Cultural preferences relating to health care.* Groups may vary in their assessment of when it is appropriate to seek medical care and what types of treatments are acceptable.

Culture and Lifestyle

As described in the chapter, ethnic groups may vary in health-related behaviors such as diet, tobacco and alcohol use, coping strategies, and health practices—and these behaviors can have important implications for wellness, both positive and negative. For example, African Americans are more likely to report consuming five or more servings of fruits and vegetables per day than people from other ethnic groups. American Indians report high rates of smoking and smoking-related health problems.

Cultural background can be an important protective factor. For example, poverty is strongly associated with increased rates of depression, but some groups, including Americans born in Mexico or Puerto Rico, have lower rates of mental disorders at a given level of income and appear to have coping strategies that provide special resilience.

Discrimination

Racism and discrimination are stressful events that can cause psychological distress and increase the risk of physical and psychological problems. Discrimination can contribute to lower socioeconomic status and its associated risks. Bias in medical care can directly affect treatment and health outcomes.

Conversely, research shows that better health care results when doctors ask patients detailed questions about their ethnicity. (Most medical questionnaires ask patients to put themselves in a vague racial or ethnic category, such as Asian or Caucasian.) Armed with more information about patients' backgrounds, medical professionals may find it easier to detect some genetic diseases or to overcome language or cultural barriers.

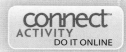

Latinos are of mixed Spanish and American Indian descent or of mixed Spanish, Indian, and African American descent. Latinos on average have lower rates of heart disease, cancer, and suicide than the general population, but higher rates of infant mortality and a higher overall birth rate; other areas of concern include gallbladder disease and obesity. At current rates, about one in two Latinas will develop diabetes in her lifetime.

- *African Americans* have the same leading causes of death as the general population, but they have a higher infant mortality rate and lower rates of suicide and osteoporosis. Health issues of special concern for African Americans include high blood pressure, stroke, diabetes, asthma, and obesity. African American men are at significantly higher risk of prostate cancer than men in other groups, and early screening is recommended for them.

- *Asian Americans* include people who trace their ancestry to countries in the Far East, Southeast Asia, or the Indian subcontinent, including Japan, China, Vietnam, Laos, Cambodia, Korea, the Philippines, India, and Pakistan. Asian Americans have a lower death rate and a longer life expectancy than the general population. They have lower rates of coronary heart disease and obesity. However, health differences exist among these groups. For example, Southeast Asian men have higher rates of smoking and lung cancer, and Vietnamese American women have higher rates of cervical cancer.

- *American Indians and Alaska Natives* typically embrace a tribal identity, such as Sioux, Navaho, or Hopi. American Indians and Alaska Natives have lower death rates from heart disease, stroke, and cancer than the general population, but they have higher rates of early death from causes linked to smoking and alcohol use, including injuries and cirrhosis. Diabetes is a special concern for many groups; for example, the Pimas of Arizona have the highest known prevalence of diabetes of any population in the world.

> **QUICK STATS**
>
> For **75%** of measured criteria, poor Americans typically receive lower-quality health care than more affluent Americans.
>
> —*National Healthcare Disparities Report*, 2010

- *Native Hawaiian and other Pacific Islander Americans* trace their ancestry to the original peoples of Hawaii, Guam, Samoa, and other Pacific Islands. Pacific Islander Americans have a higher overall death rate than the general population and higher rates of diabetes and asthma. Smoking and obesity are special concerns for this group.

Income and Education Inequalities in income and education underlie many of the health disparities among Americans. In fact, poverty and low educational attainment are far more important predictors of poor health than any ethnic factor. Income and education are closely related, and groups with the highest poverty rates and least education have the worst health status. These Americans have higher rates of infant mortality, traumatic injury, violent death, and many diseases, including heart disease, diabetes, tuberculosis, HIV infection, and some cancers. They are more likely to eat poorly, be overweight, smoke, drink, and use drugs. They are exposed to more day-to-day stressors and have less access to health care services.

Disability People with disabilities have activity limitations, need assistance, or perceive themselves as having a disability. About one in five people in the United States has some level of disability, and the rate is rising, especially among younger segments of the population. People with disabilities are more likely to be inactive and overweight. They report more days of depression than people without disabilities. Many also lack access to health care services.

Geographic Location About one in four Americans currently lives in a rural area—a place with fewer than 10,000 residents. People living in rural areas are less likely to be physically active, to use safety belts, or to obtain screening tests for preventive health care. They have less access to timely emergency services and much higher rates of some diseases and injury-related death than people living in urban areas. They are also more likely to lack health insurance. Children living in dangerous neighborhoods—rural or urban—are four times more likely to be overweight than children living in safer areas.

Sexual Orientation The 1–5% of Americans who identify themselves as homosexual or bisexual make up a diverse community with varied health concerns. Their emotional wellness and personal safety are affected by factors relating to personal, family, and social acceptance of their sexual orientation. Gay, lesbian, bisexual, and transgender teens are more likely to engage in risky behaviors such as unsafe sex and drug use; they are also more likely to be depressed and to attempt suicide. HIV/AIDS is a major concern for gay men, and gay men and lesbians may have higher rates of substance abuse, depression, and suicide.

Ask Yourself

QUESTIONS FOR CRITICAL THINKING AND REFLECTION

How often do you feel exuberant? Vital? Joyful? What makes you feel that way? Conversely, how often do you feel downhearted, de-energized, or depressed? What makes you feel that way? Have you ever thought about how you might increase experiences of vitality and decrease experiences of discouragement?

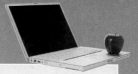

If you are like most college students, you probably feel pretty good about your health right now. Most college students are in their late teens or early twenties, lead active lives, have plenty of friends, and look forward to a future filled with opportunity. With all these things going for you, why shouldn't you feel good?

A Closer Look

Although most college-age people look healthy, appearances can be deceiving. Each year, thousands of students lose productive academic time to physical and emotional health problems—some of which can continue to plague them for life.

The following table shows the top 10 health issues affecting students' academic performance, according to the Spring 2011 American College Health Association–National College Health Assessment II.

HEALTH ISSUE	STUDENTS AFFECTED (%)
Stress	27.5
Sleep difficulties	19.4
Anxiety	19.1
Cold/flu/sore throat	16.4
Work	13.3
Internet use/computer games	12.4
Depression	11.9
Concern for a friend/family member	11.0
Relationship difficulties	10.5
Extracurricular activities	9.5

Each of these issues is related to one or more of the seven dimensions of wellness, and most can be influenced by choices students make daily. Although some troubles—such as the death of a friend—cannot be controlled, other physical and emotional concerns can be minimized by choosing healthy behaviors. For example, there are many ways to manage stress, the top health issue affecting students. By reducing unhealthy choices (such as using alcohol to relax) and by increasing healthy choices (such as using time management techniques), even busy students can reduce the impact of stress on their lives.

The survey also estimated that, based on students' reporting of their height and weight, nearly 33% of college students are either overweight or obese. Although heredity plays a role in determining one's weight, lifestyle is also a factor in weight and weight management.

In many studies over the past few decades, a large percentage of students have reported behaviors such as these:

- Overeating
- Snacking on junk food
- Frequently eating high-fat foods
- Using alcohol and binge drinking

Clearly, eating behaviors are often a matter of choice. Although students may not see (or feel) the effects of their dietary habits today, the long-term health risks are significant. Overweight and obese persons run a higher-than-normal risk of developing diabetes, heart disease, and cancer later in life. We now know with certainty that improving one's eating habits, even a little, can lead to weight loss and improved overall health.

Other Choices, Other Problems

Students commonly make other unhealthy choices. Here are some examples from the 2011 National College Health Assessment II:

- About 48% of students reported that they did not use a condom the last time they had vaginal intercourse.
- About 15% of students had seven or more drinks the last time they partied.
- About 15% of students had smoked cigarettes at least once during the past month.

What choices do you make in these situations? Remember: It's never too late to change. The sooner you trade an unhealthy behavior for a healthy one, the longer you'll be around to enjoy the benefits.

SOURCE: American College Health Association. 2011. *American College Health Association–National College Health Assessment II: Reference Group Executive Summary Spring 2011.* Hanover, MD: American College Health Association. Reprinted by permission of the American College Health Association.

CHOOSING WELLNESS

Wellness is something everyone can have. Achieving it requires knowledge, self-awareness, motivation, and effort, but the benefits last a lifetime. Optimal health comes mostly from a healthy lifestyle—patterns of behavior that promote and support your health now and as you get older. In the pages that follow, you'll find current information and suggestions you can use to build a healthier lifestyle; also, see the "Wellness Matters for College Students" box.

Factors That Influence Wellness

Our behavior, family health history, environment, and access to health care are all important influences on wellness. These factors, which vary for both individuals and groups, can interact in ways that produce either health or disease.

Health Habits   Research continually reveals new connections between our habits and health. For example, heart disease is associated with smoking, stress, a hostile attitude, a poor diet, and being sedentary. Poor health habits take hold before many Americans reach adulthood.

The effect of human activity on the environment has gradually become clear over several generations, and awareness has grown about environmental issues like air and water pollution, resource depletion, waste disposal, and overpopulation.

Only in the last few years, however, has climate change attracted intensive attention worldwide. Most scientists agree that human activity—specifically, the burning of fossil fuels for energy and the release of greenhouse gases into the atmosphere—has caused changes that are raising Earth's temperature and threatening the health of the planet and its living systems. The evidence includes melting ice caps, shifting weather patterns, species extinctions, and a gradual increase in worldwide temperatures. Scientists are trying to determine how high Earth's temperature can climb before a tipping point is reached when damage becomes irreversible.

As governments and industry only begin to address (and some continue to deny) the issue of climate change, you may wonder if it is possible for individuals to make a difference in improving our climate. The answer is yes. In fact, some believe we have moved past the time when we can depend on experts to solve environmental problems. In-

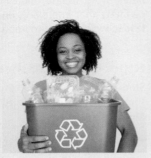

stead a broader understanding of environmental issues by the general public is needed, along with the willingness to make different choices in everyday life. Of course government at every level must lead the way, but there are hundreds of actions each of us can take to reduce our impact on the environment. Here are just a few:

- **Drive less.** Walk, bike, and take public transportation more.

- **Use less energy.** Use less heat, hot water, and air conditioning, and turn off lights and electronic devices, including power strips and chargers, when not in use.

- **Buy energy-efficient products**—from cars to appliances to compact fluorescent lightbulbs.

- **Eat responsibly.** Buy locally grown foods to reduce the amount of fuel needed to transport food, as well as air pollution and greenhouse gas emissions. Eating organically keeps petroleum-based pesticides and chemicals out of the food chain and water supply.

- **Measure your personal carbon footprint** with an online calculator, and learn what you can do to reduce it.

Chapter 14 explores various aspects of environmental health and literacy and discusses environmental issues in detail. Achieving a balance between global development and environmental protection is the great challenge facing the 21st century and all world citizens.

Other habits, however, are beneficial. Regular exercise can help prevent heart disease, high blood pressure, diabetes, osteoporosis, and depression. Exercise can also reduce the risk of colon cancer, stroke, and back injury. A balanced and varied diet helps prevent many chronic diseases. As we learn more about how our actions affect our bodies and minds, we can make informed choices for a healthier life.

Heredity/Family History Your **genome** consists of the complete set of genetic material in your cells—about 25,000 genes, half from each of your parents. **Genes** control the production of proteins that serve both as the structural material for your body and as the regulators of all your body's chemical reactions and metabolic processes. The human genome varies only slightly from

QUICK STATS

8% of Americans have diabetes, but about one-fourth of them don't know it.

—American Diabetes Association, 2012

person to person, and many of these differences do not affect health. However, some differences have important implications for health, and knowing your family's health history can help you determine which conditions may be of special concern for you.

Errors in our genes are responsible for about 3500 clearly hereditary conditions, including sickle-cell disease and cystic fibrosis. Altered genes also play a part in heart disease, cancer, stroke, diabetes, and many other common conditions. However, in these more common and complex disorders, genetic alterations serve only to increase an individual's risk, and the disease itself results from the interaction of many genes with other factors. An example of the power of behavior and environment can be seen in the more than 60% increase in the incidence of diabetes that has occurred among Americans since 1990. This huge increase is not due to any sudden change in our genes; it is the result of increasing rates of obesity caused by poor dietary choices and lack of physical activity.

Environment Your environment includes substances and conditions in your home, workplace, and community. Are you

TERMS

genome The complete set of genetic material in an individual's cells.

gene The basic unit of heredity; a section of genetic material containing chemical instructions for making a particular protein.

frequently exposed to environmental tobacco smoke or the radiation in sunlight? Do you live in an area with high rates of crime and violence? Do you have access to nature? Today environmental influences on wellness also include conditions in other countries and around the globe, particularly weather and climate changes occurring as a result of global warming (see the box titled "The Environmental Challenge").

Access to Health Care　Adequate health care helps improve both quality and quantity of life through preventive care and the treatment of disease. For example, vaccinations prevent many dangerous infections, and screening tests help identify key risk factors and diseases in their early treatable stages. As described earlier in the chapter, inadequate access to health care is tied to factors such as low income and lack of health insurance. Cost is one of many issues surrounding the development of advanced health-related technologies.

Taking Personal Responsibility for Your Wellness

In many cases, behavior can tip the balance toward good health, even when heredity or environment is a negative factor. For example, breast cancer can run in families, but it also may be associated with being overweight and inactive. A woman with a family history of breast cancer is less likely to develop the disease if she controls her weight, exercises regularly, and has regular mammograms to help detect the disease in its early, most treatable stage.

Similarly, a young man with a family history of obesity can maintain a normal weight by being careful to balance calorie intake against activities that burn calories. If your life is highly stressful, you can lessen the chances of heart disease and stroke by learning ways to manage and cope with stress. If you live in an area with severe air pollution, you can reduce the risk of lung disease by not smoking. You can also take an active role in improving your environment. Behaviors like these enable you to make a difference in how great an impact heredity and environment will have on your health.

REACHING WELLNESS THROUGH LIFESTYLE MANAGEMENT

As you consider the behaviors that contribute to wellness—being physically active, choosing a healthful diet, and so on—you may be doing a mental comparison with your own behaviors. If you are like most young adults, you probably have some healthy habits and some habits that place your health at risk. For example, you may be physically active and have a healthful diet but indulge in binge drinking on weekends. You may be careful to wear your safety belt in your car but smoke cigarettes or use chewing tobacco. Moving in the direction of wellness means cultivating healthy behaviors and working to overcome unhealthy ones. This approach to lifestyle management is called **behavior change.**

As you may already know from experience, changing an unhealthy habit (such as giving up cigarettes) can be harder than it sounds. When you embark on a behavior change plan, it may seem like too much work at first. But as you make progress, you will gain confidence in your ability to take charge of your life. You will also experience the benefits of wellness—more energy, greater vitality, deeper feelings of appreciation and curiosity, and a higher quality of life.

The rest of this chapter outlines a general process for changing unhealthy behaviors that is backed by research and that has worked for many people. The following sections offer many specific strategies and tips for change.

Getting Serious about Your Health

Before you can start changing a wellness-related behavior, you have to know that the behavior is problematic and that you *can* change it. To make good decisions, you need information about relevant topics and issues, including what resources are available to help you change.

Examine Your Current Health Habits　Have you considered how your current lifestyle is affecting your health today and how it will affect your health in the future? Do you know which of your current habits enhance your health and which detract from it? Begin your journey toward wellness with self-assessment: Think about your own behavior, and talk with friends and family members about what they have noticed about your lifestyle and your health. Challenge any unrealistically optimistic attitudes or ideas you may hold—for example, "To protect my health, I don't need to worry about quitting smoking until I'm 40 years old" or "Being overweight won't put *me* at risk for diabetes." Health risks are very real and can become significant while you're young; health habits are important throughout life.

Many people start to consider changing a behavior when friends or family members express concern, when a landmark event occurs (such as turning 30), or when new information raises their awareness of risk. If you find yourself reevaluating some of your behaviors as you read this text, take advantage of the opportunity to make a change in a structured way.

> Moving in the direction of wellness means **cultivating healthy behaviors and overcoming unhealthy ones**.

behavior change　A lifestyle management process that involves cultivating healthy behaviors and working to overcome unhealthy ones.

TERMS

Choose a Target Behavior Changing any behavior can be demanding. This is why it's a good idea to start small by choosing one behavior you want to change—called a **target behavior**—and working on it until you succeed. Your chances of success will be greater if your first goal is simple, such as resisting the urge to snack between classes. As you change one behavior, make your next goal a little more significant, and build on your success.

Learn about Your Target Behavior Once you've chosen a target behavior, you need to learn its risks and benefits for you—both now and in the future. Ask these questions:

- How is your target behavior affecting your level of wellness today?
- What diseases or conditions does this behavior place you at risk for?
- What effect would changing your behavior have on your health?

As a starting point, use this text and the resources listed in the "For More Information" section at the end of each chapter. See the "Evaluating Sources of Health Information" box for additional guidelines.

Find Help Have you identified a particularly challenging target behavior or mood—something like alcohol addiction, binge eating, or depression—that interferes with your ability to function or places you at a serious health risk? If so, you may need help to change a behavior or condition that is too deeply rooted or too serious for self-management. Don't let the problem's seriousness stop you; many resources are available to help you solve it. On campus, the student health center or campus counseling center can provide assistance. To locate community resources, ask your physician or look on the Internet.

Building Motivation to Change

Knowledge is necessary for behavior change, but it isn't usually enough to make people act. Millions of people have sedentary lifestyles, for example, even though they know it's bad for their health. This is particularly true of young adults, who may not be motivated to change because they feel healthy despite their unhealthy behaviors. To succeed at behavior change, you need strong motivation. Here are some ways to boost your motivation.

Examine the Pros and Cons of Change Health behaviors have short-term and long-term benefits and costs. Consider the benefits and costs of an inactive lifestyle:

- Short-term, such a lifestyle allows you more time to watch TV, use social media, do your homework, and hang out with friends, but it leaves you less physically fit and less able to participate in recreational activities.

- Long-term, it increases the risk of heart disease, cancer, stroke, and premature death.

To successfully change your behavior, you must believe that the benefits of change outweigh the costs.

Carefully examine the pros and cons of continuing your current behavior and of changing to a healthier one. Focus on the effects that are most meaningful to you, including those that are tied to your personal identity and values. For example, if you see yourself as an active person who is a good role model for others, then adopting behaviors such as engaging in regular physical activity and getting adequate sleep will support your personal identity. If you value independence and control over your life, then quitting smoking will be consistent with your values and goals. To complete your analysis, ask friends and family members about the effects of your behavior on them. For example, a younger sister may say that your smoking habit influenced her decision to start smoking.

The short-term benefits of behavior change can be an important motivating force. Although some people are motivated by long-term goals, such as avoiding a disease that may hit them in 30 years, most are more likely to be moved to action by shorter-term, more personal goals. Feeling better, doing better in school, improving at a sport, reducing stress, and increasing self-esteem are common short-term benefits of health behavior change.

Boost Self-Efficacy When you start thinking about changing a health behavior, a big factor in your eventual success is whether you have confidence in yourself and in your ability to change. **Self-efficacy** refers to your belief in your ability to successfully take action and perform a specific task. Strategies for boosting self-efficacy include developing an internal locus of control, using visualization and self-talk, and getting encouragement from supportive people.

LOCUS OF CONTROL Who do you believe is controlling your life? Is it your parents, friends, or school? Is it "fate?" Or is it you? **Locus of control** refers to the figurative "place" a person designates as the source of responsibility for the events in his or her life. People who believe they are in control of their own lives are said to have an *internal locus of control*. Those who believe that factors beyond their control determine the course of their lives are said to have an *external locus of control*.

> To change a behavior, you need to recognize that **you can take control of your actions**.

TERMS

target behavior An isolated behavior selected as the object for a behavior change program.

self-efficacy The belief in one's ability to take action and perform a specific task.

locus of control The figurative "place" a person designates as the source of responsibility for the events in his or her life.

CRITICAL CONSUMER
Evaluating Sources of Health Information

Believability of Health Information Sources

Surveys indicate that college students are smart about evaluating health information. They trust the health information they receive from health professionals and educators and are skeptical about popular information sources, such as magazine articles and websites.

How good are you at evaluating health information? Here are some tips.

General Strategies

Whenever you encounter health-related information, take the following steps to make sure it is credible:

- **Go to the original source.** Media reports often simplify the results of medical research. Find out for yourself what a study really reported, and determine whether it was based on good science. What type of study was it? Was it published in a recognized medical journal? Was it an animal study or did it involve people? Did the study include a large number of people? What did the authors of the study actually report?

- **Watch for misleading language.** Reports that tout "break-throughs" or "dramatic proof" are probably hype. A study may state that a behavior "contributes to" or is "associated with" an outcome; this does not prove a cause-and-effect relationship.

- **Distinguish between research reports and public health advice.** Do not change your behavior based on the results of a single report or study. If an agency such as the National Cancer Institute urges a behavior change, however, you should follow its advice. Large, publicly funded organizations issue such advice based on many studies, not a single report.

- **Remember that anecdotes are not facts.** A friend may tell you he lost weight on some new diet, but individual success stories do not mean the plan is truly safe or effective. Check with your doctor before making any serious lifestyle changes.

- **Be skeptical.** If a report seems too good to be true, it probably is. Be wary of information contained in advertisements. An ad's goal is to sell a product, even if there is no need for it.

- **Make choices that are right for you.** Friends and family members can be a great source of ideas and inspiration, but you need to make health-related choices that work best for you.

Internet Resources

Online sources pose special challenges; when reviewing a health-related website, ask these questions:

- **What is the source of the information?** Websites maintained by government agencies, professional associations, or established academic or medical institutions are likely to present trustworthy information. Many other groups and individuals post accurate information, but it is important to look at the qualifications of the people who are behind the site. (Check the home page or click the "About Us" link.)

- **How often is the site updated?** Look for sites that are updated frequently. Check the "last modified" date of any web page.

- **Is the site promotional?** Be wary of information from sites that sell specific products, use testimonials as evidence, appear to have a social or political agenda, or ask for money.

- **What do other sources say about a topic?** Be cautious of claims or information that appear at only one site or come from a chat room, bulletin board, newsgroup, or blog.

- **Does the site conform to any set of guidelines or criteria for quality and accuracy?** Look for sites that identify themselves as conforming to some code or set of principles, such as those established by the Health on the Net Foundation or the American Medical Association. These codes include criteria such as use of information from respected sources and disclosure of the site's sponsors.

For lifestyle management, an internal locus of control is an advantage because it reinforces motivation and commitment. An external locus of control can sabotage efforts to change behavior. For example, if you believe that you are destined to die of breast cancer because your mother died from the disease, you may view monthly breast self-exams and regular checkups as a waste of time. In contrast, if you believe that you can take action to reduce your risk of breast cancer despite hereditary factors, you will be motivated to follow guidelines for early detection of the disease.

If you find yourself attributing too much influence to outside forces, gather more information about your wellness-related behaviors. List all the ways that making lifestyle changes will improve your health. If you believe you'll succeed, and if you recognize that you are in charge of your life, you're on your way to wellness.

VISUALIZATION AND SELF-TALK One of the best ways to boost your confidence and self-efficacy is to visualize yourself successfully engaging in a new, healthier behavior. Imagine yourself going for an afternoon run three days a week or no longer smoking cigarettes. Also visualize yourself enjoying all the short-term and long-term benefits

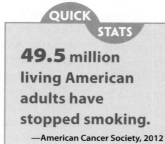

QUICK STATS

49.5 million living American adults have stopped smoking.
—American Cancer Society, 2012

that your lifestyle change will bring. Create a new self-image: What will you and your life be like when you become a regular exerciser or a nonsmoker?

You can also use *self-talk*, the internal dialogue you carry on with yourself, to increase your confidence in your ability to change. Counter any self-defeating patterns of thought with more positive or realistic thoughts: "I am a strong, capable person, and I can maintain my commitment to change." (See Chapter 3 for more about self-talk.)

ROLE MODELS AND SUPPORTIVE PEOPLE   Social support can make a big difference in your level of motivation and your chances of success. Perhaps you know people who have reached the goal you are striving for. They could be role models or mentors for you, providing information and support for your efforts. Gain strength from their experiences, and tell yourself, "If they can do it, so can I." Find a buddy who wants to make the same changes you do and who can take an active role in your behavior change program. For example, an exercise buddy can provide companionship and encouragement when you might be tempted to skip your workout.

IDENTIFY AND OVERCOME BARRIERS TO CHANGE   Don't let past failures at behavior change discourage you. They can be a great source of information you can use to boost your chances of future success. Make a list of the problems and challenges you faced in any previous behavior change attempts. To this, add the short-term costs of behavior change that you identified in your analysis of the pros and cons of change. Once you've listed these key barriers to change, develop a practical plan for overcoming each one. For example, if you always smoke when you're with certain friends, decide in advance how you will turn down the next cigarette you are offered.

Enhancing Your Readiness to Change

The transtheoretical, or "stages of change," model has been shown to be an effective approach to lifestyle self-management. According to this model, you move through distinct stages as you work to change your target behavior. It is important to determine what stage you are in now so that you can choose appropriate strategies for progressing through the cycle of change. This approach can help you enhance your readiness and intention to change. Read the following sections to determine what stage you are in for your target behavior.

Precontemplation   People at this stage do not think they have a problem and do not intend to change their behavior. They may be unaware of the risks associated with their behavior or may deny them. They may have tried unsuccessfully to change in the past and may now think the situation is hopeless. They may also blame other people or external factors for their problems. People in the precontemplation stage believe that there are more reasons or more important reasons not to change than there are reasons to change.

Contemplation   People at this stage know they have a problem and intend to take action within six months. They

acknowledge the benefits of behavior change but are also aware of the costs of changing. To be successful, people must believe that the benefits of change outweigh the costs. People in the contemplation stage wonder about possible courses of action but don't know how to proceed. There may also be specific barriers to change that appear too difficult to overcome.

Preparation   People at this stage plan to take action within a month or may already have begun to make small changes in their behavior. They may be engaging in their new, healthier behavior but not yet regularly or consistently. They may have created a plan for change but may be worried about failing.

Action   During the action stage, people outwardly modify their behavior and their environment. The action stage requires the greatest commitment of time and energy, and people in this stage are at risk for relapsing into old, unhealthy patterns of behavior.

Maintenance   People at this stage have maintained their new, healthier lifestyle for at least six months. Lapses may have occurred, but people in maintenance have been successful in quickly reestablishing the desired behavior. The maintenance stage can last months or years.

Termination   For some behaviors, a person may reach the sixth and final stage of termination. People at this stage have exited the cycle of change and are no longer tempted to lapse back into their old behavior. They have a new self-image and total self-efficacy with regard to their target behavior.

Dealing with Relapse

People seldom progress through the stages of change in a straightforward, linear way. Rather, they tend to move to a certain stage and then slip back to a previous stage before resuming their forward progress. Research suggests that most people make several attempts before they successfully change a behavior, and four out of five people experience some degree of backsliding. For this reason, the stages of change are best conceptualized as a spiral in which people cycle back through previous stages but are farther along in the process each time they renew their commitment.

If you experience a lapse (a single slip) or a relapse (a return to old habits), don't give up. Relapse can be demoralizing, but it is not the same as failure; failure means stopping before you reach your goal and never changing your target behavior. During the early stages of the change process, it's a good idea to plan for relapse so you can avoid guilt and self-blame and get back on track quickly.

If relapses keep occurring or you can't seem to control them, you may need to return to a previous stage of the behavior change process. If this is necessary, reevaluate your goals and strategy. A different or less stressful approach may help you avoid setbacks when you try again.

Date	November 5			Day	M	TU	W	TH	F	SA	SU

Time of day	M/S	Food eaten	Cals.	H	Where did you eat?	What else were you doing?	How did someone else influence you?	What made you want to eat what you did?	Emotions and feelings?	Thoughts and concerns?
7:30	M	1 C Crispix cereal 1/2 C skim milk coffee, black 1 C orange juice	110 40 — 120	3	home	reading newspaper	alone	I always eat cereal in the morning	a little keyed up & worried	thinking about quiz in class today
10:30	S	1 apple	90	1	hall outside classroom	studying	alone	felt tired & wanted to wake up	tired	worried about next class
12:30	M	1 C chili 1 roll 1 pat butter 1 orange 2 oatmeal cookies 1 soda	290 120 35 60 120 150	2	campus food court	talking	eating w/ friends; we decided to eat at the food court	wanted to be part of group	excited and happy	interested in hearing everyone's plans for the weekend
	M/S = Meal or snack			H = Hunger rating (0–3)						

FIGURE 1.3 Sample health journal entries.

Developing Skills for Change: Creating a Personalized Plan

Once you are committed to making a change, it's time to put together a plan of action. Your key to success is a well-thought-out plan that sets goals, anticipates problems, and includes rewards.

1. Monitor Your Behavior and Gather Data
Keep a record of your target behavior and the circumstances surrounding it. Record this information for at least a week or two. Keep your notes in a health journal or notebook or on your computer (see the sample journal entries in Figure 1.3). Record each occurrence of your behavior, noting the following:

- What the activity was
- When and where it happened
- What you were doing
- How you felt at that time

If your goal is to start an exercise program, track your activities to determine how to make time for workouts.

2. Analyze the Data and Identify Patterns
After you have collected data on the behavior, analyze the data to identify patterns. When are you most likely to overeat? What events trigger your appetite? Perhaps you are especially hungry at midmorning or when you put off eating dinner until 9:00. Perhaps you overindulge in food and drink when you go to a particular restaurant or when you're with certain friends. Note the connections between your feelings and such external cues as time of day, location, situation, and the actions of others around you.

3. Be "SMART" about Setting Goals
If your goals are too challenging, you will have trouble making steady progress and will be more likely to give up altogether. If, for example, you are in poor physical condition, it will not make sense to set a goal of being ready to run a marathon within two months. If you set goals you can live with, it will be easier to stick with your behavior change plan and be successful.

Experts suggest that your goals meet the "SMART" criteria; that is, your behavior change goals should be

- *Specific.* Avoid vague goals like "eat more fruits and vegetables." Instead state your objectives in specific terms, such as "eat two cups of fruit and three cups of vegetables every day."
- *Measurable.* Recognize that your progress will be easier to track if your goals are quantifiable, so give your goal a number. You might measure your goal in terms of time (such as "walk briskly for 20 minutes a day"), distance ("run two miles, three days per week"), or some other amount ("drink eight glasses of water every day").
- *Attainable.* Set goals that are within your physical limits. For example, if you are a poor swimmer, it might not be possible for you to meet a short-term fitness goal by swimming laps. Walking or biking might be better options.
- *Realistic.* Manage your expectations when you set goals. For example, it may not be possible for a long-time smoker to quit cold turkey. A more realistic approach might be to use nicotine replacement patches or gum for several weeks while getting help from a support group.
- *Time frame–specific.* Give yourself a reasonable amount of time to reach your goal, state the time frame in your behavior change plan, and set your agenda to meet the goal within the given time frame.

Using these criteria, a sedentary person who wants to improve his health and build fitness might set a goal of being able to run three miles in 30 minutes, to be achieved within a time frame of six months. To work toward that goal, he might set a number of smaller, intermediate goals that are easier to achieve. For example, his list of goals might look like this:

WEEK	FREQUENCY (DAYS/WEEK)	ACTIVITY	DURATION (MINUTES)
1	3	Walk < 1 mile	10–15
2	3	Walk 1 mile	15–20
3	4	Walk 1–2 miles	20–25
4	4	Walk 2–3 miles	25–30
5–7	3–4	Walk/run 1 mile	15–20
⋮			
21–24	4–5	Run 2–3 miles	25–30

4. Devise a Plan of Action Develop a strategy that will support your efforts to change. Your plan of action should include the following steps:

• *Get what you need.* Identify resources that can help you. For example, you can join a community walking club or sign up for a smoking cessation program. You may also need to buy some new running shoes or nicotine replacement patches. Get the items you need right away; waiting can delay your progress.

• *Modify your environment.* If there are cues in your environment that trigger your target behavior, try to control them. For example, if you normally have alcohol at home, getting rid of it can help prevent you from indulging. If you usually study with a group of friends in an environment that allows smoking, try moving to a nonsmoking area. If you always buy a snack at a certain vending machine, change your route so you don't pass by it.

• *Control related habits.* You may have habits that contribute to your target behavior. Modifying these habits can help change the behavior. For example, if you usually plop down on the sofa while watching TV, try putting an exercise bike in front of the set so you can burn calories while watching your favorite programs.

• *Reward yourself.* Giving yourself instant, real rewards for good behavior will reinforce your efforts. Plan your rewards; decide in advance what each one will be and how you will earn it. Tie rewards to achieving specific goals or subgoals. For example, you might treat yourself to a movie after a week of avoiding snacks. Make a list of items or events to use as rewards. They should be special to you and preferably unrelated to food or alcohol.

• *Involve the people around you.* Tell family and friends about your plan, and ask them to help. To help them respond appropriately to your needs, create a specific list of dos and don'ts. For example, ask them to support you when you set aside time to exercise or avoid second helpings at dinner.

• *Plan for challenges.* Think about situations and people that might derail your program, and develop ways to cope

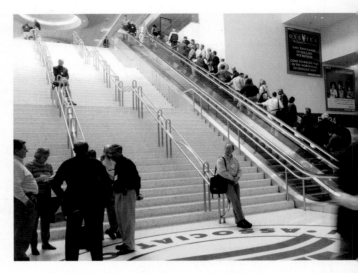

Your environment contains powerful cues for both positive and negative lifestyle choices. Identifying and using the healthier options available to you throughout the day is a key part of a successful behavior change program.

with them. For example, if you think it will be hard to stick to your usual exercise program during exams, schedule short bouts of physical activity (such as a brisk walk) as stress-reducing study breaks.

5. Make a Personal Contract A serious personal contract— one that commits you to your word—can result in a better chance of follow-through than a casual, offhand promise. Your contract can help prevent procrastination by specifying important dates and can also serve as a reminder of your personal commitment to change.

Your contract should include a statement of your goal and your commitment to reaching it. The contract should also include details, such as the following:

• The date you will start
• The steps you will take to measure your progress
• The strategies you plan to use to promote change
• The date you expect to reach your final goal

Have someone—preferably someone who will be actively helping you with your program—sign your contract as a witness.

Figure 1.4 shows a sample behavior change contract for someone who is committing to eating more fruit every day.

You can apply the general behavior change planning framework presented in this chapter to any target behavior. Additional examples of behavior change plans appear in the Behavior Change Strategy sections at the end of many chapters in this text. In these sections, you will find specific plans for quitting smoking, starting an exercise program, and making other positive lifestyle changes.

Putting Your Plan into Action

When you're ready to put your plan into action, you need commitment—the resolve to stick with the plan no matter

Behavior Change Contract

1. I, __Tammy Lau__, agree to __increase my consumption of fruit from__ __1 cup per week to 2 cups per day.__

2. I will begin on _____10/5_____ and plan to reach my goal of __2 cups__ __of fruit per day__ by __12/7__

3. To reach my final goal, I have devised the following schedule of mini-goals. For each step in my program, I will give myself the reward listed.

I will begin to have ½ cup of fruit with breakfast	10/5	see movie
I will begin to have ½ cup of fruit with lunch	10/26	new cd
I will begin to substitute fruit juice for soda 1 time per day	11/16	concert

   My overall reward for reaching my goal will be __trip to beach__

4. I have gathered and analyzed data on my target behavior and have identified the following strategies for changing my behavior: __Keep the__ __fridge stocked with easy-to-carry fruit. Pack fruit in my backpack__ __every day. Buy lunch at place that serves fruit.__

5. I will use the following tools to monitor my progress toward my final goal: __Chart on fridge door__ __Health journal__

   I sign this contract as an indication of my personal commitment to reach my goal: _____Tammy Lau_____ _____9/28_____

   I have recruited a helper who will witness my contract and __also increase__ __his consumption of fruit; eat lunch with me twice a week.__
   _____Eric March_____ _____9/28_____

FIGURE 1.4   A sample behavior change contract.

what temptations you encounter. Remember all the reasons you have to make the change—and remember that *you* are the boss. Use all your strategies to make your plan work. Make sure your environment is change-friendly, and get as much support and encouragement from others as possible. Keep track of your progress in your health journal, and give yourself regular rewards. And don't forget to give yourself a pat on the back—congratulate yourself, notice how much better you look or feel, and feel good about how far you've come and how you've gained control of your behavior.

BEING HEALTHY FOR LIFE

Your first few behavior change projects may never go beyond the planning stage. Those that do may not all succeed. But as you begin to see progress and changes, you'll start to experience new and surprising positive feelings about yourself. You'll probably find that you're less likely to buckle under stress. You may accomplish things you never thought possible— winning a race, climbing a mountain, quitting smoking. Being healthy takes extra effort, but the paybacks in energy and vitality are priceless.

Once you've started, don't stop. Remember that maintaining good health is an ongoing process. Tackle one area at a time, but make a careful inventory of your health strengths and weaknesses and lay out a long-range plan. Take on the easier problems first, and then use what you have learned to attack more difficult areas. Keep informed about the latest health news and trends; research is constantly providing new information that directly affects daily choices and habits.

You can't completely control every aspect of your health. At least three other factors—heredity, health care, and environment—play important roles in your well-being. After you quit smoking, for example, you may still be inhaling smoke from other people's cigarettes. Your resolve to eat better foods may suffer a setback when you have trouble finding healthy choices on campus.

But you can make a difference—you can help create an environment around you that supports wellness for everyone. You can support nonsmoking areas in public places. You can speak up in favor of more nutritious foods and better physical fitness facilities. You can provide nonalcoholic drinks at your parties.

You can also work on larger environmental challenges: air and water pollution, traffic congestion, overcrowding and overpopulation, global warming and climate change, toxic and nuclear waste, and many others. These difficult issues need the attention and energy of people who are informed and who care about good health. On every level, from personal to planetary, we can all take an active role in shaping our environment.

Ask Yourself

QUESTIONS FOR CRITICAL THINKING AND REFLECTION

Have you tried to change a behavior in the past, such as exercising more or quitting smoking? How successful were you? Do you feel the need to try again? If so, what would you do differently to improve your chances of success?

connect™

Connect to Your Choices

Have you ever thought about why you make the lifestyle choices you do? Many factors can influence our lifestyle choices, some not as obvious as others. Do you have a lot of the same lifestyle behaviors you had in high school, when you were living at home, such as watching TV or playing video games? Are you strongly influenced by your peers or roommates when it comes to eating and exercise patterns? Do you drink or smoke just because you have the freedom to do so?

What are the external factors that influence your choices about your lifestyle behaviors? What are your inner motivations and core values, and how do they affect your choices? Based on what you learned in this chapter, will you make some different choices in the future? If so, what will they be?

Go online to Connect to complete this activity: www.mcgraw-hillconnect.com

SUMMARY

- Wellness is the ability to live life fully, with vitality and meaning. Wellness is dynamic and multidimensional. It incorporates physical, emotional, intellectual, spiritual, interpersonal, environmental, and financial dimensions.

- As chronic diseases have become the leading cause of death in the United States, people have recognized that they have greater control over, and greater responsibility for, their health than ever before.

- The Healthy People initiative seeks to achieve a better quality of life for all Americans. The program's broad goals are to eliminate preventable disease, disabilities, injury, and premature death; achieve health equity for all groups; create social and physical environments that promote good health for all; and promote healthy development and healthy behaviors across every stage of life.

- Health-related differences among people that have implications for wellness can be described in the context of gender, ethnicity, income and education, disability, geographic location, and sexual orientation.

- Although heredity, environment, and health care all play roles in wellness and disease, behavior can mitigate their effects.

- To make lifestyle changes, you need information about yourself, your health habits, and resources available to help you change.

- You can increase your motivation for behavior change by examining the benefits and costs of change, boosting self-efficacy, and identifying and overcoming key barriers to change.

- The "stages of change" model describes six stages that people move through as they try to change their behavior: precontemplation, contemplation, preparation, action, maintenance, and termination.

- You can develop a specific plan for change by (1) monitoring behavior by keeping a journal; (2) analyzing those data; (3) setting specific goals; (4) devising strategies for modifying the environment, rewarding yourself, and involving others; and (5) making a personal contract.

- To start and maintain a behavior change program, you need commitment, a well-developed plan, social support, and a system of rewards.

- Although we cannot control every aspect of our health, we can make a difference in helping create an environment that supports wellness for everyone.

FOR MORE INFORMATION

BOOKS

Duhigg, C. 2012. *The Power of Habit: Why We Do What We Do in Life and Business.* New York: Random House. *An entertaining and intelligent exploration of how habits control our lives and how we can take charge of our habits to change our lives; includes both current research and a wealth of real-life stories.*

Komaroff, A. L., ed. 2005. *Harvard Medical School Family Health Guide.* New York: Free Press. *Provides consumer-oriented advice for the prevention and treatment of common health concerns.*

Litin, S.C. (ed.). 2009. *Mayo Clinic Family Health Book,* 4th ed. New York: HarperCollins Publishers. *A complete health reference for every stage of life, covering thousands of conditions, symptoms, and treatments.*

Murat, B., and G. Stewart. 2009. *Do I Need to See the Doctor? The Home-Treatment Encyclopedia—Written by Medical Doctors—That Lets You Decide,* 2nd ed. New York: John Wiley & Sons. *Fully illustrated, easy-to-read guide to hundreds of common symptoms and ailments, designed to help consumers determine whether they can treat themselves or should seek professional medical attention.*

Prochaska, J. O., J. C. Norcross, and C. C. DiClemente. 1995. *Changing for Good: The Revolutionary Program That Explains the Six Stages of Change and Teaches You How to Free Yourself from Bad Habits.* New York: Morrow. *Outlines the authors' model of behavior change and offers suggestions and advice for each stage of change.*

NEWSLETTERS

Consumer Reports on Health (800-274-7596;
    http://www.consumerreports.org/health/home.htm)
Harvard Health Publications (877-649-9457;
    http://www.health.harvard.edu)
Mayo Clinic Health Letter (800-333-9037;
    http://healthletter.mayoclinic.com)
University of California, Berkeley, Wellness Letter (800-829-9170;
http://www.wellnessletter.com)

ORGANIZATIONS, HOTLINES, AND WEBSITES

The Internet addresses listed here were accurate at the time of publication.

Centers for Disease Control and Prevention. Through phone, fax, and the Internet, the CDC provides a wide variety of health information. http://www.cdc.gov

Federal Trade Commission: Consumer Protection—Health. Includes on-line brochures about a variety of consumer health topics, including fitness equipment, generic drugs, and fraudulent health claims.

http://www.ftc.gov/bcp/menus/consumer/health.shtm

Healthfinder. A gateway to online publications, websites, support and self-help groups, and agencies and organizations that produce reliable health information.

http://www.healthfinder.gov

Healthy People 2020. Provides information on Healthy People objectives and priority areas.

http://www.healthypeople.gov

MedlinePlus. Provides links to news and reliable information about health from government agencies and professional associations; also includes a health encyclopedia and information about prescription and over-the-counter drugs.

http://www.nlm.nih.gov/medlineplus/

National Health Information Center (NHIC). Puts consumers in touch with the organizations that are best able to provide answers to health-related questions.

http://www.health.gov/nhic

National Institutes of Health. Provides information about all NIH activities as well as consumer publications, hotline information, and an A-to-Z listing of health issues with links to the appropriate NIH institute.

http://www.nih.gov

National Wellness Institute. Serves professionals and organizations that promote health and wellness.

http://www.nationalwellness.org

National Women's Health Information Center. Provides information and answers to frequently asked questions.

http://www.womenshealth.gov

Office of Minority Health. Promotes improved health among racial and ethnic minority populations.

http://minorityhealth.hhs.gov

Surgeon General. Includes information on activities of the Surgeon General and the text of many key reports on such topics as tobacco use, physical activity, and mental health.

http://www.surgeongeneral.gov

World Health Organization (WHO). Provides information about health topics and issues affecting people around the world.

http://www.who.int/en

SELECTED BIBLIOGRAPHY

American Cancer Society. 2012. *Cancer Facts and Figures—2012.* Atlanta: American Cancer Society.

American College Health Association. 2011. *American College Health Association—National College Health Assessment II: Reference Group Executive Summary Spring 2011.* Hanover, MD: American College Health Association.

American Heart Association. 2012. *Heart Disease and Stroke Statistics—2012 Update.* Dallas: American Heart Association.

Barr, D. A. 2008. *Health Disparities in the United States: Social Class, Race, Ethnicity, and Health.* Baltimore: The Johns Hopkins University Press.

Bennett, I. M., et al. 2009. The contribution of health literacy to disparities in self-rated health status and preventive health behaviors in older adults. *Annals of Family Medicine* 7(3): 204–211.

Centers for Disease Control and Prevention. 2008. Racial/ethnic disparities in self-rated health status among adults with and without disabilities—United States, 2004–2006. *Morbidity and Mortality Weekly Report* 57(39): 1069–1073.

Centers for Disease Control and Prevention. 2010. *Racial and Ethnic Approaches to Community Health (REACH U.S.): Finding Solutions to Health Disparities, 2010* (http://www.cdc.gov/chronicdisease/resources/publications/AAG/reach.htm).

Fisher, E. G., et al. 2011 Behavior matters. *American Journal of Preventive Medicine* 40(5): e15–30.

Flegal, K. M., et al. 2007. Cause-specific excess deaths associated with underweight, overweight, and obesity. *Journal of the American Medical Association* 298(17): 2028–2037.

Flegal, K. M., et al. 2010. Prevalence and trends in obesity among U.S. adults, 1999–2008. *Journal of the American Medical Association* 303(3): 235–241.

Herd, P., et al. 2007. Socioeconomic position and health: The differential effects of education versus income on the onset versus progression of health problems. *Journal of Health and Social Behavior* 48(3): 223–238.

Horneffer-Ginter, K. 2008. Stages of change and possible selves: Two tools for promoting college health. *Journal of American College Health* 56(4): 351–358.

Kohl, H. K., et al. 201. Healthy people: A 2020 vision for the social determinants approach. *Health Education & Behavior* 38(6): 551–557.

National Center for Health Statistics. 2010. Health behaviors of adults: United States, 2005–07. *Vital and Health Statistics* 10(245).

National Center for Health Statistics. 2011. *Health, United States, 2010.* Hyattsville, MD: National Center for Health Statistics.

National Center for Health Statistics. 2012. Deaths: preliminary data for 2010. *National Vital Statistics Report* 60(4).

O'Loughlin, J., et al. 2007. Lifestyle risk factors for chronic disease across family origin among adults in multiethnic, low-income, urban neighborhoods. *Ethnicity and Disease* 17(4): 657–663.

Pinkhasov, R. M., et al. 2010. Are men shortchanged on health? Perspective on health care utilization and health risk behavior in men and women in the United States. *International Journal of Clinical Practice* 64(4): 475–487.

Printz, C. 2012. Disparities in cancer care: Are we making progress? A look at how researchers and organizations are working to reduce cancer health disparities. *Cancer* 118(4): 867–868.

Rotimi, C. N. 2012. Health disparities in the genomic era: The case for diversifying ethnic representation. *Genomic Medicine* 4(8): 65.

UC Berkeley. 2011 Update. *Evaluating Web Pages: Techniques to Apply and Questions to Ask* (http://www.lib.berkeley.edu/TeachingLib/Guides/Internet/Evaluate.html).

Vaccaro, J. A., and F. G. Huffman. 2012. Reducing health disparities: Medical advice received for minorities with diabetes. *Journal of Health and Human Services Administration* 34(4): 389–417.

Walker, B., and C. P. Mouton. 2008. Environmental influences on cardiovascular health. *Journal of the National Medical Association* 100(1): 98–102.

Williams, D. R. 2012. Miles to go before we sleep: Racial inequities in health. *Journal of Health and Social Behavior* 53(3): 279–295.

BEHAVIOR CHANGE STRATEGY
Blank Behavior Change Strategy Contract

1. I, _____, agree to _____
_____

2. I will begin on _____ and plan to reach my goal of _____
_____ by _____

3. To reach my final goal, I have devised the following schedule of mini-goals. For each step in my program, I will give myself the reward listed.

_____   _____   _____
_____   _____   _____
_____   _____   _____
_____   _____   _____
_____   _____   _____
_____

My overall reward for reaching my goal will be _____

4. I have gathered and analyzed data on my target behavior and have identified the following strategies for changing my behavior:
_____
_____

5. I will use the following tools to monitor my progress toward my final goal:
_____
_____

I sign this contract as an indication of my personal commitment to reach my goal: _____
_____

I have recruited a helper who will witness my contract and _____
_____
_____

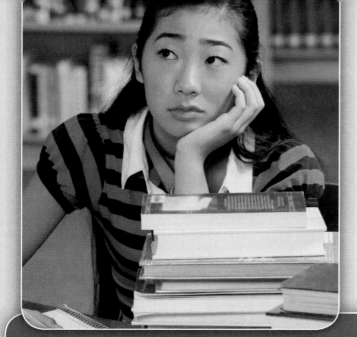

LOOKING AHEAD...

After reading this chapter, you should be able to

- Explain what stress is and how people react to it—physically, emotionally, and behaviorally

- Describe the relationship between stress and disease

- List common sources of stress

- Describe techniques for preventing and managing stress

- Put together a plan for successfully managing the stress in your life

Stress: The Constant Challenge

2

Like the term *wellness*, *stress* is a word many people use without understanding its precise meaning. Stress is popularly viewed as an uncomfortable response to a negative event, which probably describes *nervous tension* more than the cluster of physical and psychological responses that actually constitute stress. In fact, stress is not limited to negative situations; it is also a response to pleasurable physical challenges and the achievement of personal goals. Whether stress is experienced as pleasant or unpleasant depends largely on the situation and the individual. Because learning effective responses to stress can enhance psychological health and help prevent a number of serious diseases, stress management can be an important part of daily life.

As a college student, you may be in one of the most stressful times of your life. This chapter explains the physiological and psychological reactions that make up the stress response and describes how these reactions can put your health at risk. The chapter also presents methods of managing stress.

WHAT IS STRESS?

In common usage, the term *stress* refers to two different things: situations that trigger physical and emotional reactions, *and* the reactions themselves. This text uses the more precise term **stressor** for a physical or psychological event that triggers physical and emotional reactions and the term **stress response** for the reactions themselves. A first date and a final exam are examples of stressors; sweaty palms and a pounding heart are symptoms of the stress response. We'll use the term **stress** to describe the general physical and emotional state that accompanies the stress response. So a person taking a final exam experiences stress.

Each individual's experience of stress depends on many factors, including the nature of the stressor and how it is perceived. Stressors take many different forms. Some occur suddenly and don't last long or repeat, like a fire in the building you live in. Others, like air pollution or quarreling parents, can continue for a long time. The memory of a stressful occurrence can itself be a stressor years after the event, such as the memory of the loss of a loved one. Responses to stressors can include a wide variety of physical, emotional, and behavioral changes. A short-term response might be an upset stomach or insomnia, whereas a long-term response might be a change in your personality or social relations.

Physical Responses to Stressors

Imagine a close call: As you step off the curb, a car careens toward you. With just a fraction of a second to spare, you leap safely out of harm's way. In that split second of danger and in the moments following it, you experience a predictable series of physical reactions. Your body goes from a relaxed state to one prepared for physical action to cope with a threat to your life.

Two systems in your body are responsible for your physical response to stressors: the nervous system and the endocrine system. Through rapid chemical reactions affecting almost every part of your body, you are primed to act quickly and appropriately in time of danger.

Actions of the Nervous System

The **nervous system** consists of the brain, spinal cord, and nerves. Part of the nervous system is under voluntary control, as when you tell your arm to reach for a chocolate. The part that is not under conscious supervision—for example, the part that controls the digestion of the chocolate—is the **autonomic nervous system.** In addition to digestion, it controls your heart rate, breathing, blood pressure, and hundreds of other involuntary functions.

The autonomic nervous system consists of two divisions:

- The **parasympathetic division** is in control when you are relaxed. It aids in digesting food, storing energy, and promoting growth.
- The **sympathetic division** is activated during times of arousal, including exercise, and when there is an emergency, such as severe pain, anger, or fear.

Sympathetic nerves use the neurotransmitter **norepinephrine** to exert their actions on nearly every organ, sweat gland, blood vessel, and muscle to enable your body to handle an emergency. The sympathetic division commands your body to stop storing energy and to use it in response to a crisis.

Actions of the Endocrine System

During stress, the sympathetic nervous system triggers the **endocrine system.** This system of glands, tissues, and cells helps control body functions by releasing **hormones** and other chemical messengers into the bloodstream to influence metabolism and other body processes. These chemicals act on a variety of targets throughout the body. Along with the nervous system, the endocrine system prepares the body to respond to a stressor.

The Two Systems Together

How do both systems work together in an emergency? Let's go back to your near collision with a car. Both reflexes and higher cognitive areas in your brain quickly make the decision that you are facing a threat, and your body prepares to meet the danger. Chemical messages and the actions of sympathetic nerves cause the release of key hormones, including **cortisol** and **epinephrine.** These hormones trigger the physiological changes shown in Figure 2.1, including these:

- Heart and respiration rates accelerate to speed oxygen through the body.
- Hearing and vision become more acute.
- The liver releases extra sugar into the bloodstream to boost energy.
- Perspiration increases to cool the skin.
- The brain releases **endorphins**—chemicals that can inhibit or block sensations of pain—in case you are injured.

Taken together, these nearly instantaneous physical changes are called the **fight-or-flight reaction.** They give you the heightened reflexes and strength you need to dodge the car or deal with other stressors. Although these physical changes may vary in intensity, the same basic set of physical reactions occurs in response to any type of stressor—positive or negative, physical or psychological.

The Return to Homeostasis

Once a stressful situation ends, the parasympathetic division of your autonomic nervous system takes command and halts the stress response. It restores **homeostasis,** a state in which blood pressure, heart rate, hormone levels, and other vital functions are maintained within a narrow range of normal. Your parasympathetic nervous system calms your body down, slowing a rapid heartbeat, drying sweaty palms, and returning breathing to normal.

TERMS

stressor Any physical or psychological event or condition that produces physical and emotional reactions.

stress response The physical and emotional reactions to a stressor.

stress The general physical and emotional state that accompanies the stress response.

nervous system The brain, spinal cord, and nerves.

autonomic nervous system The branch of the nervous system that controls basic body processes; consists of the sympathetic and parasympathetic divisions.

parasympathetic division A division of the autonomic nervous system that moderates the excitatory effect of the sympathetic division, slowing metabolism and restoring energy supplies.

sympathetic division A division of the autonomic nervous system that reacts to danger or other challenges by accelerating body processes.

norepinephrine A neurotransmitter released by the sympathetic nervous system into specific tissues to increase their function in the face of increased activity; when released by the brain, causes arousal (increased attention, awareness, and alertness); also called *noradrenaline.*

endocrine system The system of glands, tissues, and cells that secrete hormones into the bloodstream to influence metabolism and other body processes.

hormone A chemical messenger produced in the body and transported in the bloodstream to target cells or organs for specific regulation of their activities.

cortisol A steroid hormone secreted by the cortex (outer layer) of the adrenal gland; also called *hydrocortisone.*

epinephrine A hormone secreted by the medulla (inner core) of the adrenal gland that affects the functioning of organs involved in responding to a stressor; also called *adrenaline.*

endorphins Brain secretions that have pain-inhibiting effects.

fight-or-flight reaction A defense reaction that prepares a person for conflict or escape by triggering hormonal, cardiovascular, metabolic, and other changes.

homeostasis A state of stability and consistency in an individual's physiological functioning.

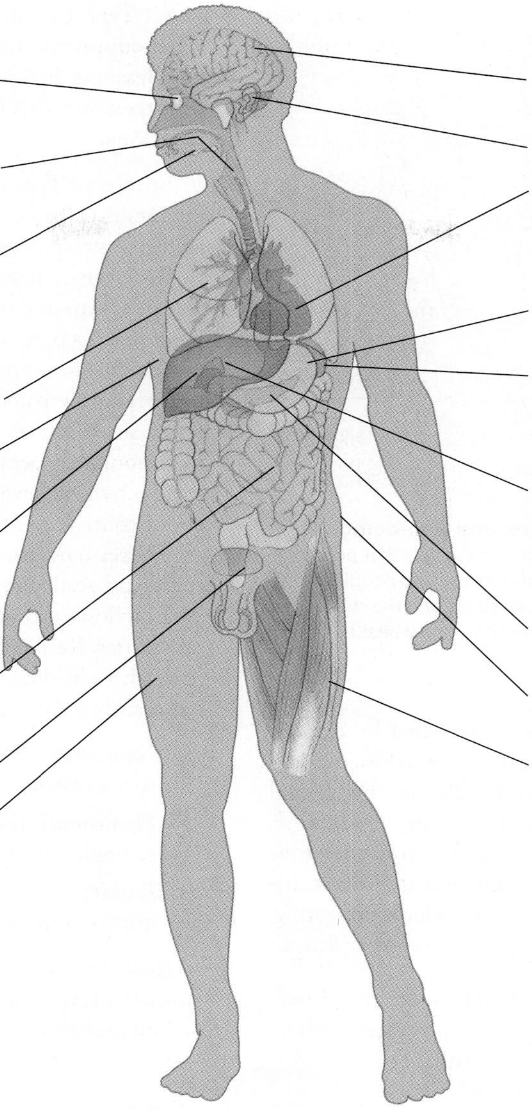

Pupils dilate to admit extra light for more sensitive vision.

Mucous membranes of nose and throat shrink, while muscles force a wider opening of air passages to allow easier airflow.

Secretion of saliva and mucus decreases; digestive activities have a low priority in an emergency.

Air passages dilate to allow more air into lungs.

Perspiration increases, especially in armpits, groin, hands, and feet, to flush out waste and cool the overheating body by evaporation.

Liver releases sugar into bloodstream to provide energy for muscles and brain.

Muscles of intestines stop contracting because digestion has halted.

Bladder relaxes. Emptying of bladder contents releases excess weight, making it easier to flee.

Blood vessels in skin and internal organs contract; those in skeletal muscles dilate. This increases blood pressure and delivery of blood to where it is most needed.

Endorphins are released to block any distracting pain.

Hearing becomes more acute.

Heart accelerates rate of beating, increases strength of contraction to allow more blood flow where it is needed.

Digestion, an unnecessary activity during an emergency, halts.

Spleen releases more red blood cells to meet an increased demand for oxygen and to replace any blood lost from injuries.

Adrenal glands stimulate secretion of epinephrine, increasing blood sugar, blood pressure, and heart rate; also spur increase in amount of fat in blood. These changes provide an energy boost.

Pancreas decreases secretions because digestion has halted.

Fat is removed from storage and broken down to supply extra energy.

Voluntary (skeletal) muscles contract throughout the body, readying them for action.

FIGURE 2.1 The fight-or-flight reaction. In response to a stressor, the autonomic nervous system and the endocrine system prepare the body to deal with an emergency.

Gradually your body resumes its normal "housekeeping" functions, such as digestion and temperature regulation. Damage that may have been sustained during the fight-or-flight reaction is repaired. The day after you narrowly dodge the car, you wake up feeling fine. In this way, your body can grow, repair itself, and acquire new reserves of energy. When the next crisis comes, you'll be ready to respond again instantly.

The Fight-or-Flight Reaction in Modern Life The fight-or-flight reaction is a part of our biological heritage, and it's a survival mechanism that has served humans well. In modern life, however, it is often absurdly inappropriate. Many of the stressors we face in everyday life do not require a physical response—for example, an exam, a mess left by a roommate, or a stoplight. The fight-or-flight reaction prepares the body for physical action regardless of whether such action is a necessary or appropriate response to a particular stressor.

Emotional and Behavioral Responses to Stressors

We all experience a similar set of physical responses to stressors, which make up the fight-or-flight reaction. These responses, however, vary from person to person and from one situation to another. People's perceptions of potential stressors—and of their reactions to such stressors—also vary greatly. A certain amount of stress, if coped with appropriately, can help promote optimal performance (Figure 2.2).

Effective and Ineffective Responses Common emotional responses to stressors include anxiety, depression, and fear. Although emotional responses are determined in part by inborn personality or temperament, we often can moderate or learn to control them. Coping techniques are discussed later in the chapter.

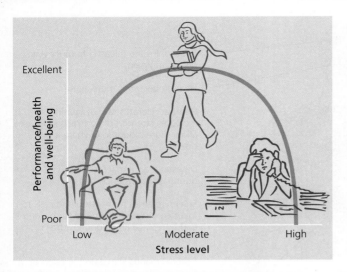

FIGURE 2.2 Stress level, performance, and well-being.
A moderate level of stress challenges individuals in a way that promotes optimal performance and well-being. Too little stress, and people are not challenged enough to improve; too much stress, and the challenges become stressors that can impair physical and emotional health.

Behavioral responses to stressors—controlled by the **somatic nervous system,** which manages our conscious actions—are entirely under our control. Effective behavioral responses such as talking, laughing, exercising, meditating, learning time management skills, and becoming more assertive can promote wellness and enable us to function at our best. Ineffective behavioral responses to stressors include overeating, expressing hostility, and using tobacco, alcohol, or other drugs.

Personality and Stress   Some people seem to be nervous, irritable, and easily upset by minor annoyances. Others are calm and composed even in difficult situations. Scientists remain unsure just why this is or how the brain's complex emotional mechanisms work. But **personality**—the sum of cognitive, behavioral, and emotional tendencies—clearly affects how people perceive and react to stressors. To investigate the links among personality, stress, and wellness, researchers examine different clusters of characteristics, or "personality types":

- *Type A.* People with Type A personality are described as ultracompetitive, controlling, impatient, aggressive, and even hostile. Type A people have a higher perceived stress level and more problems coping with stress. They react explosively to stressors and are upset by events that others would consider only annoyances. Studies indicate that certain characteristics of the Type A pattern—anger, cynicism, and hostility—increase the risk of heart disease.

- *Type B.* The Type B personality is relaxed and contemplative. Type B people are less frustrated by daily events and more tolerant of the behavior of others.

- *Type C.* The Type C personality is characterized by anger suppression, difficulty expressing emotions, feelings of hopelessness and despair, and an exaggerated response to minor stressors. This heightened response may impair immune functions.

Studies of Type A and C personalities suggest that expressing emotions is beneficial, but habitually expressing exaggerated stress responses or hostility is unhealthy.

Researchers have also looked for personality traits that enable people to deal more successfully with stress. One such trait is *hardiness*, a particular form of optimism. People with a hardy personality view potential stressors as challenges and opportunities for growth and learning, rather than as burdens. They see fewer situations as stressful and react less intensely to stress than nonhardy people might. Hardy people are committed to their activities, have a sense of inner purpose and an inner locus of control, and feel at least partly in control of their lives.

The term *resilience* refers to personality traits associated with social and academic success in at-risk populations, such as people from low-income families and those with mental or physical disabilities. Resilient people tend to set goals and face adversity through individual effort. There are three basic types of resilience, and each one determines how a person responds to stress:

- *Nonreactive resilience*, in which a person does not react to a stressor.

- *Homeostatic resilience*, in which a person may react strongly but returns to baseline functioning quickly.

- *Positive growth resilience*, in which a person learns and grows from the stress experience.

Resilience is associated with emotional intelligence and violence prevention.

You probably can't change your basic personality, but you can change your typical behaviors and patterns of thinking. You can also use positive stress management techniques like those described later in the chapter.

Cultural Background   Young adults from around the world come to America for a higher education; most students finish college with a greater appreciation for other cultures and worldviews. The clash of cultures, however, can be a big source of stress for many students—especially when it leads to disrespectful treatment, harassment, or violence. It is important to remember that everyone's reaction to stress is influenced by his or her family and

somatic nervous system   The branch of the peripheral nervous system that governs motor functions and sensory information, largely under conscious control.

personality   The sum of behavioral, cognitive, and emotional tendencies.

TERMS

cultural background. Learning to accept and appreciate the cultural backgrounds of other people is both a mind-opening experience and a way to avoid stress over cultural differences.

Gender   Our **gender role**—the activities, abilities, and behaviors our culture expects of us based on our sex—can affect our experience of stress. Some behavioral responses to stressors, such as crying or openly expressing anger, may be deemed more appropriate for one gender than the other.

Strict adherence to gender roles, however, can limit one's response to stress and can itself become a source of stress. Gender roles can also affect one's perception of a stressor. If a man derives most of his self-worth from his work, for example, retirement may be more stressful for him than for a woman whose self-image is based on several different roles.

In early 2012 the American Psychological Association released the results of its "Stress in America 2011" survey. The survey shows the different views American men and women have of their personal stress. In the latest survey, about 45% of both men and women said they were dissatisfied with their lives, but when asked to rate their stress levels on a scale of 1–10, women generally reported a significantly higher level of stress than men. The survey also shows that women are more likely than men to cope with stress through behaviors such as reading, spending time with friends, or meditating. Men are more likely to manage stress by playing sports.

Levels of testosterone (the primary male hormone, responsible for many masculine traits) increase in men from puberty onward, so men tend to have higher blood pressure than women of the same age. This factor contributes to greater wear on the male circulatory system, sometimes increasing a man's risk for cardiovascular disease. A part of the brain that regulates emotions, the amygdala, is sensitive to testosterone. This may be one reason why men are more likely than women to find certain situations (such as social interactions) to be stressful.

Conversely, women have higher levels of oxytocin (a hormone involved in social interaction and mood regulation) and are more likely to respond to stressors by seeking social support. This coping response may give women a longevity advantage over men by decreasing the risk of some stress-related disorders. It does not, however, free women from stress-related ailments, and women are more likely than men to suffer stress-related hypertension, depression, and obesity.

Experience   Past experiences can profoundly influence the evaluation of a potential stressor. Consider someone who has had a bad experience giving a speech in the past. He or she is much more likely to perceive an upcoming speech as stressful than someone who has had positive public speaking experiences.

STRESS AND HEALTH

According to the American Psychological Association, 76% of the general population report suffering physical symptoms related to stress (such as tense muscles or headaches), and 71% report nonphysical symptoms. The role of stress in health is

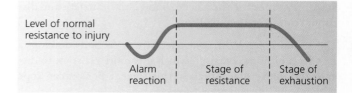

FIGURE 2.3 The general adaptation syndrome. During the alarm phase, a lower resistance to injury is evident. With continued stress, resistance to injury is actually enhanced. With prolonged exposure to repeated stressors, exhaustion sets in, with a return of low resistance levels seen during acute stress.

complex, but evidence suggests that stress can increase vulnerability to many ailments. Several theories have been proposed to explain the relationship between stress and disease.

The General Adaptation Syndrome

Biologist Hans Selye was one of the first scientists to develop a comprehensive theory of stress and disease. Based on his work in the 1930s and 1940s, Selye coined the term **general adaptation syndrome (GAS)** to describe what he believed to be a universal and predictable response pattern to all stressors. As mentioned earlier, some stressors (such as attending a party) are pleasant, and others (such as getting a bad grade) are unpleasant. In the GAS theory, the stress triggered by a pleasant stressor is called **eustress;** stress brought on by an unpleasant stressor is called **distress.** The sequence of physical responses associated with GAS is the same for eustress and distress and occurs in three stages (Figure 2.3):

• *Alarm.* The alarm stage includes the complex sequence of events brought on by the fight-or-flight reaction. At this stage, the body is more susceptible to disease or injury because it is geared up to deal with a crisis. Someone in this

Ask Yourself

QUESTIONS FOR CRITICAL THINKING AND REFLECTION

Think of the last time you faced a significant stressor. How did you respond? List the physical, emotional, and behavioral reactions you experienced. Did these responses help you deal with the stress, or did they interfere with your efforts to handle it?

TERMS

gender role   A culturally expected pattern of behavior and attitudes determined by a person's sex.

general adaptation syndrome (GAS)   A pattern of stress responses consisting of three stages: alarm, resistance, and exhaustion.

eustress   Stress resulting from a pleasant stressor.

distress   Stress resulting from an unpleasant stressor.

stage may experience headaches, indigestion, anxiety, and disrupted eating or sleep patterns.

• *Resistance.* With continued stress, the body develops a new level of homeostasis in which it is more resistant to disease and injury than usual. In this stage, a person can cope with normal life and added stress.

• *Exhaustion.* The first two stages of GAS require a great deal of energy. If a stressor persists, or if several stressors occur in succession, general exhaustion sets in. This is not the sort of exhaustion you feel after a long, busy day. Rather, it's a life-threatening type of physiological exhaustion.

Allostatic Load

Although the GAS model is still viewed as a key conceptual contribution to the understanding of stress, some aspects of it are considered outdated. For example, increased susceptibility to disease after repeated or prolonged stress is now thought to be due to the effects of the stress response itself rather than to a depletion of resources (exhaustion state). In particular, long-term overexposure to stress hormones such as cortisol has been linked with health problems. Further, although physical stress reactions promote homeostasis (resistance stage), they also have negative effects on the body.

The long-term wear and tear of the stress response is called the **allostatic load.** A person's allostatic load depends on many factors, including genetics, life experiences, and emotional and behavioral responses to stressors. A high allostatic load may be due to frequent stressors, poor adaptation to common stressors, an inability to shut down the stress response, or imbalances in the stress response of different body systems. High allostatic load is linked to heart disease, hypertension, obesity, and reduced brain and immune system functioning. In other words, when your allostatic load exceeds your ability to cope, you are more likely to get sick.

Psychoneuroimmunology

One of the most fruitful areas of current research into the relationship between stress and disease is **psychoneuroimmunology (PNI).** PNI is the study of the interactions among the nervous system, the endocrine system, and the immune system. The underlying premise of PNI is that stress, through the actions of the nervous and endocrine systems, impairs the immune system and thereby affects health.

A complex network of nerve and chemical connections exists between the nervous, endocrine, and immune systems. In general, increased levels of cortisol are linked to a decreased number of immune system cells, or *lymphocytes* (see Chapter 13 for more about the immune system). Epinephrine appears to promote the release of lymphocytes but at the same time reduces their efficiency. Scientists have identified hormone-like substances called *neuropeptides* that appear to translate stressful emotions into biochemical events, some of which impact the immune system, providing a physical link between emotions and immune function.

Different types of stress may affect immunity in different ways. For instance, during **acute stress** (typically lasting between 5 and 100 minutes), white blood cells move into the skin, where they enhance the immune response. During a stressful event sequence, such as a personal trauma and the events that follow, however, there are typically no overall significant immune changes. Chronic (ongoing) stressors such as unemployment have negative effects on almost all functional measures of immunity. **Chronic stress** may cause prolonged secretion of cortisol and may accelerate the course of diseases that involve inflammation, including multiple sclerosis, heart disease, and type 2 diabetes.

Mood, personality, behavior, and immune functioning are intertwined. For example, people who are generally pessimistic may neglect the basics of health care, become passive when ill, and fail to engage in health-promoting behaviors. People who are depressed may reduce physical activity and social interaction, which may in turn affect the immune system and the cognitive appraisal of a stressor. Optimism, successful coping, and positive problem solving, on the other hand, may positively influence immunity.

Links between Stress and Specific Conditions

Although much remains to be learned, it is clear that people who have unresolved chronic stress in their lives or who handle stressors poorly are at risk for a wide range of health problems. In the short term, the problem might be just a cold, a stiff neck, or a stomachache. Over the long term, the problems can be more severe—cardiovascular disease (CVD), high blood pressure, impaired immune function, or a host of other problems.

Cardiovascular Disease   During the stress response, heart rate increases and blood vessels constrict, causing blood

Ask Yourself

QUESTIONS FOR CRITICAL THINKING AND REFLECTION

Have you ever been so stressed that you felt ill in some way? If so, what were your symptoms? How did you handle them? Did the experience affect the way you reacted to other stressful events?

TERMS

allostatic load   The long-term negative impact of the stress response on the body.

psychoneuroimmunology (PNI)   The study of the interactions among the nervous, endocrine, and immune systems.

acute stress   Stress immediately following a stressor; may last only minutes or may turn into chronic stress.

chronic stress   Stress that continues for days, weeks, or longer.

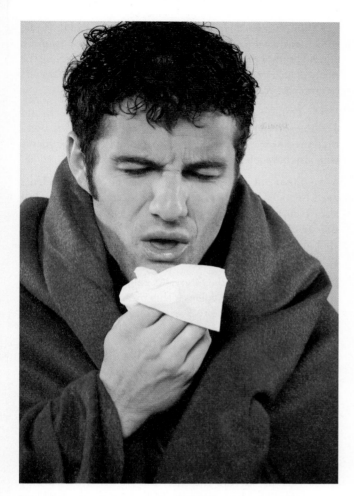

Ongoing stress has been shown to make people more vulnerable to everyday ailments, such as colds and allergies.

pressure to rise. Chronic high blood pressure is a major cause of *atherosclerosis*, a disease in which blood vessels become damaged and caked with fatty deposits. These deposits can block arteries, causing heart attacks and strokes. The stress response can precipitate a heart attack in someone with atherosclerosis. The stress response can also cause stress cardiomyopathy ("broken heart syndrome"), a condition that mimics a heart attack but doesn't damage the heart.

Certain emotional responses may increase a person's risk of CVD. As described earlier, people who tend to react to situations with anger and hostility are more likely to have heart attacks than are people with less explosive, more trusting personalities.

Psychological Problems The hormones and other chemicals released during the stress response cause emotional as well as physical changes. Stress also activates the enzyme PKC, which influences the brain's prefrontal cortex. Excess PKC can negatively affect focus, judgment, and the ability to think clearly. Moreover, many stressors are inherently anxiety-producing, depressing, or

both. Stress has been found to contribute to psychological problems such as depression, panic attacks, anxiety, eating disorders, and posttraumatic stress disorder (PTSD). PTSD, which afflicts war veterans, rape and child abuse survivors, and others who have suffered or witnessed severe trauma, is characterized by nightmares, flashbacks, and a diminished capacity to experience or express emotion.

Altered Immune Function PNI research helps explain how stress affects the immune system. Some of the health problems linked to stress-related changes in immune function include vulnerability to colds and other infections, asthma and allergy attacks, susceptibility to cancer, and flare-ups of chronic diseases such as genital herpes and HIV infection.

Headaches More than 45 million Americans suffer from chronic, recurrent headaches. Headaches come in various types but are often grouped into the three following categories:

- *Tension headaches.* Approximately 90% of all headaches are tension headaches, characterized by a dull, steady pain, usually on both sides of the head. It may feel as though a band of pressure is tightening around the head, and the pain may extend to the neck and shoulders. Acute tension headaches may last from hours to days, while chronic tension headaches may occur almost every day for months or even years. Psychological stress, poor posture, and immobility are the leading causes of tension headaches. There is no cure, but the pain can sometimes be relieved with over-the-counter painkillers and with therapies such as massage, acupuncture, relaxation, hot or cold showers, and rest.

- *Migraine headaches.* Migraines typically progress through a series of stages lasting from several minutes to several days. They may produce a variety of symptoms, including throbbing pain that starts on one side of the head and may spread, heightened sensitivity to light, visual disturbances such as flashing lights or temporary blindness, nausea, dizziness, and fatigue. About 70% of migraine sufferers are women, and migraine headaches may have a genetic component. Potential triggers include menstruation, stress, fatigue, atmospheric changes, bright light, specific sounds or odors, and certain foods. The frequency of attacks varies from a few in a lifetime to several per week. Aerobic exercise is frequently recommended to reduce the frequency and severity of migraines, but evidence for the effectiveness of exercise as a treatment is mixed. For some people, exercise can trigger a migraine.

- *Cluster headaches.* Cluster headaches are extremely severe headaches that cause intense pain in and around one eye. They usually occur in clusters of one to three headaches each day over a period of weeks or months, alternating with periods of remission in which no headaches occur. About 90% of people with cluster headaches are male. There is no known cause or cure for cluster headaches, but a number of treatments are available. During cluster periods,

QUICK STATS

11% of adult Americans suffer serious psychological distress.

—SAMHSA, 2009

it is important to refrain from smoking cigarettes and drinking alcohol, because these activities can trigger attacks.

Other Health Problems   Many other health problems may be caused or worsened by excessive stress, including the following:

- Digestive problems such as stomachaches, diarrhea, constipation, irritable bowel syndrome, and ulcers
- Insomnia and fatigue
- Injuries, including on-the-job injuries caused by repetitive strain
- Menstrual irregularities, impotence, and pregnancy complications

COMMON SOURCES OF STRESS

Recognizing potential sources of stress is an important step in successfully managing the stress in your life.

Major Life Changes

Any major change in your life that requires adjustment and accommodation can be a source of stress. Early adulthood and the college years are associated with many significant changes, such as moving out of the family home. Even changes typically thought of as positive—graduation, job promotion, marriage—can be stressful.

Clusters of life changes, particularly those that are perceived negatively, may be linked to health problems in some people. Personality and coping skills, however, are important moderating influences. People with strong support networks and stress-resistant personalities are less likely to become ill in response to life changes than are people with fewer resources.

Daily Hassles

Although major life changes are stressful, they seldom occur regularly. Researchers have proposed that minor problems—life's daily hassles, such as losing your keys or wallet—can be an even greater source of stress because they occur much more often.

People who perceive hassles negatively are likely to experience a moderate stress response every time they face one. Over time, this can take a significant toll on health. Studies indicate that for some people, daily hassles contribute to a general decrease in overall wellness.

College Stressors

College is a time of major changes and minor hassles. For many students, college means being away from home and family for the first time. Nearly all students share stresses like the following:

- *Academic stress.* Exams, grades, and an endless workload await every college student but can be especially troublesome for students just out of high school.

- *Interpersonal stress.* Most students are more than just students; they are also friends, children, employees, spouses, parents, and so on. Managing relationships while juggling the rigors of college life can be daunting, especially if some friends or family members are less than supportive.

- *Time pressures.* Class schedules, assignments, and deadlines are an inescapable part of college life. But these time pressures can be drastically compounded for students who also have job or family responsibilities.

- *Financial concerns.* The majority of college students need financial aid not just to cover the cost of tuition but also to survive from day to day while in school. For many, college life isn't possible without a job, and the pressure to stay afloat financially competes with academic and other stressors.

- *Worries about the future.* As college comes to an end, students face life after college. This means thinking about a career, choosing a place to live, and leaving the friends and routines of school behind.

As mentioned earlier, test anxiety is a source of stress for many students. To learn some proven techniques for overcoming test anxiety, see the Behavior Change Strategy at the end of this chapter.

Job-Related Stressors

Americans rate their jobs as a key source of stress in their lives. Various surveys indicate that 40–50% of working Americans say they typically feel tense or stressed out while at work. Tight schedules and overtime leave less time to exercise, socialize, and engage in other stress-proofing activities. While daily work activities can be stressful enough on their own, stress can be even worse for people who are left out of important decisions relating to their jobs. When workers are given the opportunity to shape how their jobs are performed, job satisfaction goes up and stress levels go down.

If job-related (or college-related) stress is severe or chronic, the result can be **burnout**—a state of physical, mental, and emotional exhaustion. Burnout occurs most often in highly motivated and driven individuals who come to feel that their work is not recognized or that they are not accomplishing their goals. People in the helping professions—teachers, social workers, caregivers, police officers, and so on—are also prone to burnout. For some people who suffer from burnout, a vacation or leave of absence may be appropriate. For others, a reduced work schedule, better communication with superiors, or a change in job goals may be necessary. Improving time management skills can also help.

burnout   A state of physical, mental, and emotional exhaustion.

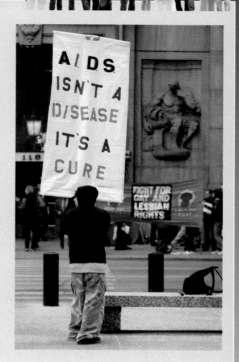

Stress is universal, but an individual's response to stress can vary depending on gender, cultural background, prior experience, and genetic factors. In diverse multiethnic and multicultural nations such as the United States, some groups face special stressors and have higher-than-average rates of stress-related physical and emotional problems. These groups include ethnic minorities, the poor, those with physical or mental disabilities, and those with atypical sexual orientations.

Discrimination occurs when people speak or act according to their prejudices—biased, negative beliefs or attitudes toward some group. A blatant example is painting a swastika on a Jewish studies house. A more subtle example is when an African American student notices that white shopkeepers in a mostly white college town tend to keep a close eye on him.

Recent immigrants to the United States have to learn to live in a new society. This requires a balance between assimilating and changing to be like the majority, on the one hand, and maintaining a connection to their own culture, language, and religion, on the other. The process of acculturation is generally stressful, especially when the person's background is radically different from that of the people he or she is now living among.

Both immigrants and minorities that have lived for generations in the United States can face job- and school-related stressors because of stereotypes and discrimination. They may make less money in comparable jobs with comparable levels of education and may find it more difficult to achieve leadership positions.

On a positive note, however, many who experience hardship, disability, or prejudice develop effective goal-directed coping skills and are successful at overcoming obstacles and managing the stress they face.

Social Stressors

Social networks can be real or virtual. Both types can help improve your ability to deal with stress, but any social network can also become a stressor in itself.

Real Social Networks Although social support is a key buffer against stress, your interactions with others can themselves be a source of stress. The college years, in particular, can be a time of great change in interpersonal relationships. The larger community where you live can also act as a stressor.

Social stressors include prejudice and discrimination. You may feel stress as you try to relate to people of other ethnic or socioeconomic groups. If you are a member of a minority ethnic group, you may feel pressure to assimilate into mainstream society or to spend as much time as possible with others who share your ethnicity or background. If English is not your first language, you may face the added burden of conducting daily activities in a language with which you are not comfortable. All these pressures can become significant sources of stress. (See the box "Diverse Populations, Discrimination, and Stress.")

Virtual Social Networks Technology can help you save time, but it can also increase stress. Being electronically connected to work, family, and friends all the time can impinge on your personal space, waste time, and distract you from your current real situation. If you are "always on"—that is, always available by voice or text messaging—some friends or colleagues may think it's all right to contact you anytime, even if you're in class or trying to work, and they may expect an immediate reponse. The convenience of staying electronically connected comes at a price.

Other Stressors

Have you tried to eat at a restaurant where the food was great, but the atmosphere was so noisy that it put you on edge? This is an example of an environmental stressor—a condition or event in the physical environment that causes stress.

Like the noisy atmosphere of some restaurants, many environmental stressors are mere inconveniences that are easy to avoid. Others, such as pollen or construction noise, may be unavoidable daily sources of stress. For those who live in poor or violent neighborhoods or in a war-torn country, the environment can contain major stressors (see the box "Coping with News of Traumatic Events").

Some stressors are found not in our environment but within ourselves. We pressure ourselves to reach goals and continually evaluate our progress and performance. Striving to reach goals can enhance self-esteem if the goals are reasonable. Unrealistic expectations, however, can be a significant source of stress and can damage self-esteem. Other internal stressors are physical and emotional states such as illness and exhaustion; these can be both a cause and an effect of unmanaged stress.

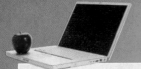
Natural disasters, terrorist attacks, and acts of violence are traumatic events that we seem to hear about almost daily. Both experiencing trauma and observing it can result in extreme stress, requiring time and effort to recover. Such events can weaken your sense of security and create uncertainty about how the future may unfold. People react to such news in different ways, depending on their proximity to the event and its recency. People far from the site may suffer emotional reactions simply from watching endless coverage on television.

Responses to trauma include disbelief, shock, fear, anger, resentment, anxiety, mood swings, irritability, sadness, depression, panic, guilt, apathy, feelings of isolation or powerlessness, and many of the symptoms of excess stress. Some people affected by such violence develop posttraumatic stress disorder (PTSD), a more serious condition.

In the case of the 2007 shooting rampage at Virginia Polytechnic Institute and State University (Virginia Tech) that left 32 students and teachers dead, the school and community mobilized quickly to respond to the expected surge in behavioral health needs generated by the attack. Hotline calls and emergency room visits increased dramatically, especially during the second

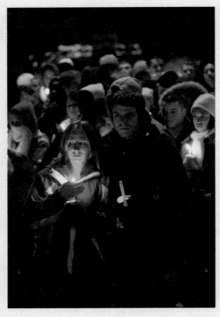

and third weeks following the shootings. Information sources and support groups were established for people grieving the loss of friends, family, neighbors, or colleagues. Volunteers contacted each family that was directly affected by the shootings to offer help in making arrangements and to provide other services.

If you are affected by a disastrous event such as a school shooting or terrorist attack, take these steps:

- Be sure you have the best information about what happened, whether a continuing risk is present, and what you can do to avoid it. That information may be posted on websites or on local radio or TV stations.

- Don't expose yourself to so much media coverage that it overwhelms you.

- Take care of yourself. Use the stress relief techniques discussed in this chapter.

- Share your feelings and concerns with others. Be a supportive listener.

- If you feel able, help others in any way you can, such as by volunteering to work with victims.

- If you feel emotionally distressed days or weeks after the event, consider asking for professional help.

MANAGING STRESS

You can control the stress in your life by taking the following steps:

- Shore up your support system.
- Improve your communication skills.
- Develop healthy exercise, eating, and sleeping habits.
- Learn to identify and moderate individual stressors.

The effort required is well worth the time. People who manage stress effectively not only are healthier but have more time to enjoy life and accomplish goals.

Social Support

Having the support of friends and family members seems to contribute to the well-being of body and mind. Research supports this conclusion, as the following examples demonstrate:

- Among college students living in overcrowded apartments, a study revealed that those students with a strong social support system were less distressed by their cramped quarters than were the loners who navigated life's challenges on their own.

- Young adults who have strong relationships with their parents tend to cope with stress better than peers with poor parental relationships.

- Many studies show that married people live longer than single people (including those who are divorced, widowed, or never married) and have lower death rates from practically all causes.

Social support can provide a critical counterbalance to the stress in our lives. Give yourself time to develop and maintain a network of people you can count on for emotional support, feedback, and nurturing. If you don't have enough social support, consider becoming a volunteer to help build your network of friends and to enhance your spiritual wellness. (See the box "Altruism: Is Doing Good Good for Your Health?")

Communication

Communicating in an assertive way that respects the rights of others—while protecting your own rights—can prevent

Ethics and religion have long told us that it is more blessed to give than to receive. Now scientists from many disciplines are finding empirical support for the notion that altruism—unselfish love and giving—benefits the giver at least as much as the receiver. These benefits come in the form of better psychological health, better physical health, and longer life.

What is the chain of events leading from altruism to health benefits, from volunteering to improved well-being, better health, and longer life? Scientists have proposed several mechanisms:

• **Better immune system functioning.** Altruistic love may block or reduce the stress response, which is known to suppress the immune system. A healthier immune system is more effective at fighting off infection and illness.

• **Better cardiovascular health.** The stress response also affects the cardiovascular system, increasing heart rate and raising blood pressure. Altruistic love may protect the heart and blood vessels from the damaging effects of stress.

• **Activation of the relaxation response.** Altruistic love may activate the relaxation response—the opposite of the stress response, inducing feelings of warmth, calm, and happiness.

• **Pain relief.** Altruistic love may reduce sensations of pain by inducing the release of endorphins, which are brain chemicals that block pain and produce feelings of euphoria.

• **Increase in the frequency and depth of positive emotions,** such as happiness and calmness. Positive emotions may reduce the burden of psychological and physiological stress and thereby provide benefits for health-related physiological processes.

• **Increased self-esteem** and positive beliefs about self-efficacy and self-worth.

• **Better overall mental health.** The combination of positive feelings and increased self-esteem is conducive to improved mental health. Part of the effect may come from reducing self-absorption, taking an outward focus, and shifting attention away from the individual's perceived problems.

• **Better social integration, more social support.** Volunteering provides people with meaningful social roles and a sense of purpose, as well as opportunities for social contact.

• **Improved spiritual health.** Altruism provides an avenue for putting deeply felt values into practice.

Studies show that not all giving is the same—for example, donating money does not have the same beneficial health effects as volunteering that involves personal contact. A few simple guidelines can help you get the most out of giving:

• Choose a volunteer activity that puts you in contact with people.

• Make helping voluntary. Obligatory helping can actually increase stress levels.

• Volunteer with a group. Sharing your interests with other volunteers increases social support. Volunteering seems to have the most benefits for people who also have other close relationships and social interests.

• Know your limits. Helping that goes beyond what you can handle depletes your own resources and is detrimental to your health.

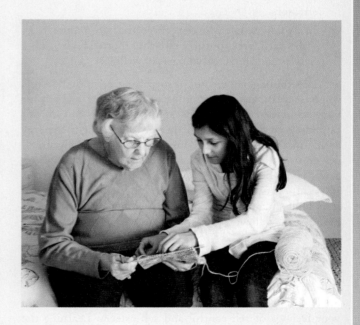

SOURCES: Sternberg, E. M. 2001. Approaches to defining mechanisms by which altruistic love affects health. Research Topic White Paper #3, Institute for Research on Unlimited Love, Altruism, Compassion, Service (http://www.altruists.org/f72); Pembroke, G. 2007. Compassion Rx: The many health benefits of altruism (http://epages.wordpress.com/2007/10/26/compassion-rx-the-many-health-benefits-of-altruism).

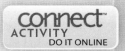

stressful situations from getting out of control. Better communication skills can help everyone form and maintain healthy relationships. If you typically suppress your feelings, you might want to take an assertiveness training course that can help you identify and change your patterns of communication. If you have trouble controlling your anger, you may benefit from learning anger management strategies.

Exercise

Exercise helps maintain a healthy body and mind and even stimulates the birth of new brain cells. Regular physical activity can also reduce many of the negative effects of stress. Consider the following examples:

- Taking a long walk can help decrease anxiety and blood pressure.
- A brisk 10-minute walk can leave you feeling more relaxed and energetic for up to two hours.
- People who exercise regularly react with milder physical stress responses before, during, and after exposure to stressors.
- In a study, people who took three brisk 45-minute walks each week for three months reported fewer daily hassles and an increased sense of wellness.

These findings should not be surprising, because the stress response mobilizes energy resources and readies the body for physical emergencies. If you experience stress and do not physically exert yourself, you are not completing the energy cycle. You may not be able to exercise while your daily stressors occur—during class, for example, or while sitting in a traffic jam—but you can be active at other times of the day. Physical activity allows you to expend the nervous energy you have built up and trains your body to more readily achieve homeostasis following stressful situations.

Nutrition

A healthful diet gives you an energy bank to draw from whenever you experience stress. Eating wisely also can enhance your feelings of self-control and self-esteem. Learning the principles of sound nutrition is easy, and sensible eating habits rapidly become second nature when practiced regularly.

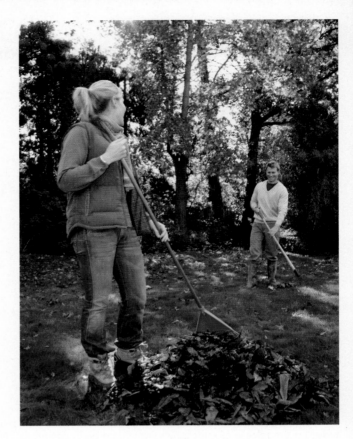

Exercise—even light activity—can be an effective antidote to stress.

While your diet has an effect on the way your body handles stress, the reverse is also true. Excess stress can negatively affect the way you eat. Many people, for example, respond to stress by overeating; other people skip meals or stop eating altogether during stressful periods. Both responses are not only ineffective (they don't address the causes of stress) but potentially unhealthy.

Sleep

Most adults need seven to nine hours of sleep every night to stay healthy and perform their best. Getting enough sleep isn't just good for you physically. Adequate sleep also improves mood, fosters feelings of competence and self-worth, enhances mental functioning, and supports emotional functioning.

How Sleep Works Sleep occurs in two phases: **rapid eye movement (REM) sleep** and **non–rapid eye movement (NREM) sleep**. A sleeper goes through several cycles of non-REM and REM sleep each night.

Ask Yourself

QUESTIONS FOR CRITICAL THINKING AND REFLECTION

What are the top two or three stressors in your life right now? Are they new to your life—as part of your college experience—or are they stressors you've experienced in the past? Do they include both positive and negative experiences (eustress and distress)?

TERMS

rapid eye movement (REM) sleep The portion of the sleep cycle during which dreaming occurs.

non–rapid eye movement (non-REM) sleep The portion of the sleep cycle that involves deep sleep; non-REM sleep includes four states of successively deeper sleep.

NREM sleep actually includes four stages of successively deeper sleep. As you move through these stages of sleep, a variety of physiological changes occur:

- Blood pressure drops.
- Respiration and heart rates slow.
- Body temperature declines.
- Growth hormone is released.
- Brain wave patterns become slow and even.

During REM sleep, dreams occur. REM sleep is characterized by the rapid movement of the eyes under closed eyelids. Heart rate, blood pressure, and breathing rate rise, and brain activity increases to levels equal to or greater than those during waking hours. Muscles in the limbs relax completely, resulting in a temporary paralysis. (This total relaxation may prevent you from acting out your dreams while you're asleep.)

Sleep and Stress Stress hormone levels in the bloodstream vary throughout the day and are related to sleep patterns. Peak concentrations occur in the early morning, followed by a slow decline during the day and evening. Concentrations return to peak levels during the final stages of sleep and in the early morning hours. Stress hormone levels are low during non-REM sleep and increase during REM sleep. With each successive sleep cycle during the night, REM sleep lasts a little longer. This increase in REM sleep duration with each sleep cycle may underlie the progressive increase in circulating stress hormones during the final stages of sleep.

Even though stress hormones are released during sleep, it is the *lack* of sleep that has the greatest impact on stress. In someone who is suffering from **sleep deprivation** (not getting enough sleep over time), mental and physical processes steadily deteriorate. A sleep-deprived person experiences headaches, feels irritable, is unable to concentrate, and is more prone to forgetfulness. Poor-quality sleep has long been associated with stress and depression. A small 2008 study of female college students further associated sleep deprivation with an increased risk of suicide.

Acute sleep deprivation slows the daytime decline in stress hormones, so evening levels are higher than normal. A decrease in total sleep time also causes an increase in the level of stress hormones. Together these changes may cause an increase in stress hormone levels throughout the day and may contribute to physical and mental exhaustion. Extreme sleep deprivation can lead to hallucinations and other psychotic symptoms, as well as to a significant increase in heart attack risk.

Sleep Problems According to the National Sleep Foundation's 2011 Sleep in America Poll, 14% of American adults sleep an average of less than six hours per night. (Compare this to the recommended seven to nine hours per night.) Although many of us can attribute the lack of sleep to long

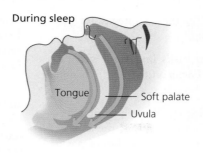 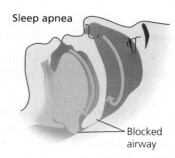

During sleep

Sleep apnea

Tongue — Soft palate — Uvula — Blocked airway

FIGURE 2.4 Sleep apnea. Sleep apnea occurs when soft tissues surrounding the airway relax, "collapsing" the airway and restricting airflow.

workdays and family responsibilities, as many as 70 million Americans suffer from chronic sleep disorders—medical conditions that prevent them from sleeping well.

According to National Sleep Foundation polls, more than 50% of adults report having trouble falling asleep or staying asleep—a condition called **insomnia.** The most common causes of insomnia are lifestyle factors, such as high caffeine or alcohol intake before bedtime; medical problems, such as a breathing disorder; and stress. About 75% of people who suffer from chronic insomnia report some stressful life event at the onset of their sleeping problems.

Another type of chronic sleep problem, called **sleep apnea,** occurs when a person stops breathing while asleep. Apnea can be caused by a number of factors, but it typically results when the soft tissue at the back of the mouth (such as the tongue or soft palate) "collapses" during sleep, blocking the airway (Figure 2.4). When breathing is interrupted, so is sleep, because the sleeper awakens repeatedly throughout the night to begin breathing again. In most cases, this occurs without the sleeper's even being aware of it. However, the disruption to sleep can be significant, and over time acute sleep deprivation can result from apnea. There are several treatments for apnea, including the use of medications, a special apparatus that helps keep the airway open during sleep, and surgery.

Time Management

Learning to manage your time can be crucial to coping with everyday stressors. Overcommitment, procrastination, and even boredom are significant stressors for many people. Along with gaining control of nutrition and exercise to maintain a healthy energy balance, time management is an important

> Most adults need **seven to nine hours of sleep every night** to stay healthy and perform their best.

TERMS

sleep deprivation A lack of sleep over a period of time.

insomnia A sleep problem involving the inability to fall or stay asleep.

sleep apnea The interruption of normal breathing during sleep.

element in a wellness program. Try these strategies for improving your time management skills:

- **Set priorities.** Divide your tasks into three groups: essential, important, and trivial. Focus on the first two, and ignore the third.

- **Schedule tasks for peak efficiency.** You've probably noticed you're most productive at certain times of the day (or night). Schedule as many of your tasks for those hours as you can, and stick to your schedule.

- **Set realistic goals and write them down.** Attainable goals spur you on. Impossible goals, by definition, cause frustration and failure. Fully commit yourself to achieving your goals by putting them in writing.

- **Budget enough time.** For each project you undertake, calculate how long it will take to complete. Then tack on another 10–15%, or even 25%, as a buffer.

- **Break up long-term goals into short-term ones.** Instead of waiting for large blocks of time, use short amounts of time to start a project or keep it moving.

- **Visualize the achievement of your goals.** By mentally rehearsing your performance of a task, you will be able to reach your goal more smoothly.

- **Keep track of the tasks you put off.** Analyze why you procrastinate. If the task is difficult or unpleasant, look for ways to make it easier or more fun.

- **Consider doing your least favorite tasks first.** Once you have the most unpleasant ones out of the way, you can work on the tasks you enjoy more.

- **Consolidate tasks when possible.** For example, try walking to the store so that you run your errands and exercise in the same block of time.

- **Identify quick transitional tasks.** Keep a list of 5- to 10-minute tasks you can do while waiting or between other tasks, such as watering your plants, doing the dishes, or checking a homework assignment.

- **Delegate responsibility.** Asking for help when you have too much to do is no cop-out; it's good time management. Just don't delegate the jobs you know you should do yourself.

- **Say no when necessary.** If the demands made on you don't seem reasonable, say no—tactfully, but without guilt or apology.

- **Give yourself a break.** Allow time for play—free, unstructured time when you can ignore the clock. Don't consider this a waste of time. Play renews you and enables you to work more efficiently.

- **Avoid your personal "time sinks."** You can probably identify your own time sinks—activities like watching television, surfing the Internet, or talking on the phone that consistently use up more time than you anticipate and put you behind schedule. Some days, it may be best to avoid problematic

activities altogether; for example, if you have a big paper due, don't sit down for a five-minute TV break if that's likely to turn into a two-hour break. Try a five-minute walk if you need to clear your head.

- **Stop thinking or talking about what you're going to do, and just do it!** Sometimes the best solution for procrastination is to stop waiting for the right moment and just get started. You will probably find that things are not as bad as you feared, and your momentum will keep you going.

Striving for Spiritual Wellness

Spiritual wellness is associated with greater coping skills and higher levels of overall wellness. It is a very personal wellness component, and there are many ways to develop it. Researchers have linked spiritual wellness to longer life expectancy, reduced risk of disease, faster recovery, and improved emotional health. Although spirituality is difficult to study, and researchers aren't sure how or why spirituality seems to improve health, several explanations have been offered:

- **Social support.** Attending religious services or participating in volunteer organizations helps people feel that they are part of a community with similar values and promotes social connectedness and caring.

- **Healthy habits.** Some of the paths to spiritual wellness may encourage healthy behaviors, such as eating a vegetarian diet or consuming less meat and alcohol, and may discourage harmful habits like smoking.

- **Positive attitude.** Spirituality can give a person a sense of meaning and purpose in life, and these qualities create a more positive attitude in the person, which in turn helps her or him cope with life's challenges.

- **Moments of relaxation.** Spiritual practices such as prayer, meditation, and immersion in artistic activities can reduce stress by eliciting the relaxation response.

Spiritual wellness does not require participation in organized religion. Many people find meaning and purpose in other ways. By spending time in nature or working on environmental issues, people can experience continuity with the natural world. Spiritual wellness can come through helping others in one's community or by promoting human rights, peace and harmony among people, and opportunities for human development on a global level. Other people develop spiritual wellness through art or through their personal relationships.

Spirituality provides an ethical path to personal fulfillment that includes connectedness with self, others, and a higher power or larger reality. Spiritual wellness can make you more aware of your personal values and can help clarify them. Without an awareness of personal values, you might be driven by immediate desires and the passing demands of others. Living according to values means considering your options carefully before making a choice, choosing between options without succumbing to outside pressures that oppose your values, and making a choice and acting on it rather than doing nothing.

Confiding in Yourself through Writing

Keeping a diary is analogous to confiding in others, except that you are confiding in yourself. This form of coping with severe stress may be especially helpful for those who are shy or introverted and find it difficult to open up to others. Although writing about traumatic and stressful events may have a short-term negative effect on mood, over the long term, stress is reduced and positive changes in health occur. A key to promoting health and well-being through journaling is to write about your emotional responses to stressful events. Set aside a special time each day or week to write down your feelings about stressful events in your life.

Cognitive Techniques

Some stressors arise in our own minds. Ideas, beliefs, perceptions, and patterns of thinking can add to our stress level. Each of the following techniques can help you change unhealthy thought patterns to ones that will help you cope with stress. As with any skill, mastering these techniques takes practice and patience.

Think and Act Constructively   Think back to the worries you had last week. How many of them were needless? Think about things you *can* control. Try to stand aside from the problem, consider the positive steps you can take to solve it, and then carry them out. Remember, if you can successfully predict that a stressor will occur, you can better control your response to it. In the evening, try to predict stressful events you might encounter the following day. Then decide how to handle them constructively. This may mean dealing positively with an unpleasant person or figuring out how to stay focused during a boring class. By taking a constructive approach, you can prevent stressors from becoming negative events and perhaps even turn them into positive experiences.

> Problem-solving skills can **improve your motivation, stress level, and grades**.

Take Control   A situation often feels more stressful if you feel you're not in control of it. Time may seem to be slipping away before a big exam, for example. Unexpected obstacles may appear in your path, throwing you off course. When you feel your environment is controlling you instead of the other way around, take charge! Concentrate on what is possible to control, and set realistic goals. Be confident of your ability to succeed.

Problem-Solve   Students with greater problem-solving abilities report easier adjustment to university life, higher motivation levels, lower stress levels, and higher grades. When you find yourself stewing over a problem, sit down with a piece of paper and do some problem solving. Try this approach:

1. Define the problem in one or two sentences.
2. Identify the causes of the problem.
3. Consider alternative solutions. Don't just stop with the most obvious one.
4. Weigh positive and negative consequences for each alternative.
5. Make a decision—choose a solution.
6. Make a list of tasks you must perform to act on your decision.
7. Begin to carry out the tasks on your list.
8. Evaluate the outcome and revise your approach if necessary.

Modify Your Expectations   Expectations are exhausting and restricting. The fewer expectations you have, the more you can live spontaneously and joyfully. The more you expect from others, the more often you will feel let down. And trying to meet the expectations others have of you is often futile.

Stay Positive   If you beat up on yourself—"Late for class again! You can't even cope with college! How do you expect to ever hold down a real job?"—try changing your inner dialogue. Talk to yourself as you would to a child you love: "You're a smart, capable person. You've solved other problems; you'll handle this one. Tomorrow you'll simply schedule things so you get to class with a few minutes to spare."

Practice Affirmations   One way of cultivating the positive is to systematically repeat positive thoughts, or *affirmations*, to yourself. For example, if you react to stress with low self-esteem, you might repeat sentences such as "I approve and accept myself completely" and "It matters not what others say, but what I believe." Saying affirmations to yourself every day may make them automatic and help you change the way you react.

Cultivate Your Sense of Humor   When it comes to stress, laughter may be the best medicine. Even a fleeting smile produces changes in your autonomic nervous system that can lift your spirits. And a few minutes of belly laughing can be as invigorating as brisk exercise. Hearty laughter elevates your heart rate, aids digestion, eases pain, and triggers the release of endorphins and other pleasurable and stimulating chemicals in the brain. After a good laugh, your muscles go slack; your pulse and blood pressure dip below normal. You are relaxed. Cultivate the ability to laugh at yourself, and you'll have a handy and instantly effective stress reliever.

Focus on What's Important   A major source of stress is trying to store too much data. Forget unimportant details (they will usually be self-evident) and organize important information. One technique you can try is to "chunk" important material into categories. If your next exam covers three chapters from your textbook, consider each chapter a chunk

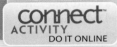

Here is a simple technique for eliciting the relaxation response.

The Basic Technique

1. Pick a word, phrase, or object to focus on. If you like, you can choose a word or phrase that has a deep meaning for you, but any word or phrase will work. Some meditators prefer to focus on their breathing.

2. Take a comfortable position in a quiet environment, and close your eyes if you aren't focusing on an object.

3. Relax your muscles.

4. Breathe slowly and naturally. If you're using a focus word or phrase, silently repeat it each time you exhale. If you're using an object, focus on it as you breathe.

5. Keep a passive attitude. Disregard thoughts that drift in.

6. Continue for 10–20 minutes, once or twice a day.

7. When you're finished, sit quietly for a few minutes with your eyes first closed and then open. Then stand up.

Suggestions

• Allow relaxation to occur at its own pace; don't try to force it. Don't be surprised if you can't quiet your mind for more than a few seconds at a time; it's not a reason for anger or frustration. The more you ignore the intrusions, the easier doing so will become.

• If you want to time your session, peek at a watch or clock occasionally, but don't set a jarring alarm.

• The technique works best on an empty stomach, before a meal or about two hours after eating. Avoid times of day when you're tired—unless you want to fall asleep.

• Although you'll feel refreshed even after the first session, it may take a month or more to get noticeable results. Be patient. Eventually the relaxation response will become so natural that it will occur spontaneously, or on demand, when you sit quietly for a few moments.

connect
ACTIVITY
DO IT ONLINE

---

of information. Then break down each chunk into its three or four most important features. Create a mental outline that allows you to trace your way from the most general category down to the most specific details. This technique can be applied to managing daily responsibilities as well.

Relaxation Techniques

The **relaxation response** is a physiological state characterized by a feeling of warmth and quiet mental alertness. This is the opposite of the fight-or-flight reaction. When you call upon a relaxation technique to trigger the relaxation response, your heart rate, breathing, and metabolism slow down, and your blood pressure and oxygen consumption decrease. At the same time, blood flow to the brain and skin increases, and brain waves shift from an alert beta rhythm to a relaxed alpha rhythm. Practiced regularly, relaxation techniques can counteract the debilitating effects of stress.

Progressive Relaxation   Unlike most of the other methods of relaxation, progressive relaxation requires no imagination, willpower, or self-suggestion. You simply tense and relax the muscles in your body, group by group. The technique, also known as deep muscle relaxation, helps you become aware of the muscle tension that occurs when you're under stress. When you consciously relax those muscles, other systems of the body get the message and ease up on the stress response.

Start, for example, with your right fist. Inhale as you tense it. Exhale as you relax it. Repeat. Next, contract and relax your right upper arm. Repeat. Do the same with your left arm. Then, beginning at your forehead and ending at your feet, contract and relax your other muscle groups. Repeat each contraction at least once, breathing in as you tense, breathing out as you relax. To speed up the process, tense and relax more muscles at one time—both arms simultaneously, for instance. With practice, you'll be able to relax very quickly and effectively by clenching and releasing only your fists.

Visualization   Also known as *imagery*, **visualization** lets you daydream without guilt. Next time you feel stressed, close your eyes. Imagine yourself floating on a cloud, sitting on a mountaintop, or lying in a meadow. Involve all your senses; imagine the sounds, the smells, and the other sensations that would be part of the scene. Your body will respond as if the imagery were real. An alternative: Close your eyes and imagine a deep purple light filling your body. Now change the color into a soothing gold. As the color lightens, so should your distress.

You can also use visualization to rehearse for an upcoming event and enhance performance. By experiencing an event

> **relaxation response**   A physiological state characterized by a feeling of warmth and quiet mental alertness.
>
> **visualization**   A technique for promoting relaxation or improving performance that involves creating or re-creating vivid mental pictures of a place or an experience; also called *imagery*.
>
> **TERMS**

ahead of time in your mind, you can practice coping with any difficulties that may arise. Think positively, and you can "psych yourself up" for a successful experience.

Meditation

The need to periodically stop our incessant mental chatter is so great that, from ancient times, hundreds of forms of **meditation** have developed in cultures all over the world. Meditation is a way of telling the mind to be quiet for a while. Because meditation has been at the core of many Eastern religions and philosophies, it has acquired an "Eastern" mystique that causes some people to shy away from it. Yet meditation requires no special knowledge or background. Whatever philosophical, religious, or emotional reasons may be given for meditation, it is potentially useful for reducing stress. According to a 2008 study, college students who learned how to use meditation for stress management were able to significantly reduce their daily stress levels. Further, those students found it easier to forgive others for perceived wrongdoings and spent less time focusing on negative thoughts.

Meditation helps you tune out the world temporarily, removing you from both internal and external sources of stress. The "thinker" takes time out to become the "observer"—calmly attentive, without analyzing, judging, comparing, or rationalizing. Regular practice of this quiet awareness will subtly carry over into your daily life, encouraging physical and emotional balance no matter what confronts you. For a step-by-step description of a basic meditation technique, see the box "Meditation and the Relaxation Response."

Another form of meditation, known as *mindfulness meditation*, involves paying attention to physical sensations, perceptions, thoughts, and imagery. Instead of focusing on a word or object to quiet the mind, you observe thoughts that occur without evaluating or judging them. Development of this ability requires regular practice but may eventually result in a more objective view of one's perceptions. It is believed that a greater understanding of one's moment-to-moment thought processes (mindful awareness) provides a richer and more vital sense of life and improves coping. Studies also suggest that people who rate high in mindfulness are less anxious and better able to deal with stress; among people with specific health problems, mindfulness can provide substantial benefits.

Deep Breathing

Your breathing pattern is closely tied to your stress level. Deep, slow breathing is associated with relaxation. Rapid, shallow, often irregular breathing occurs during the stress response. With practice, you can learn to slow and quiet your breathing pattern, thereby also quieting your mind and relaxing your body. Breathing techniques can be used for on-the-spot tension relief as well as for long-term stress reduction.

The primary goal of many breathing exercises is to change your breathing pattern from chest breathing to diaphragmatic ("belly") breathing. (The diaphragm is a sheet of muscle and connective tissue that divides the chest and abdominal cavities.) Except when sleeping, most adults breathe by expanding their chest and raising their shoulders rather than by expanding their abdomen. Diaphragmatic breathing is slower and deeper than chest breathing. To practice diaphragmatic breathing, lie on your back and place one hand on your chest and one hand on your abdomen to monitor your breathing. Take a slow, deep breath through your nose and into your belly. Your abdomen should rise significantly and your chest only slightly. Think of filling your belly with air. Exhale gently through your mouth. Once you become familiar with belly breathing, you can use it anywhere, any time, to dispel tension and stress.

Yoga

Hatha yoga, the most common yoga style practiced in the United States, emphasizes physical balance and breath control. It integrates components of flexibility, muscular strength and endurance, and muscle relaxation; it also sometimes serves as a preliminary to meditation. A session of yoga typically involves a series of postures, each held for a few seconds to several minutes, which involve stretching and balance and coordinated breathing. Yoga can induce the relaxation response and promote body awareness and flexibility. If you are interested in trying yoga, it's best to take a class from an experienced instructor.

Tai Chi

This martial art (in Chinese, *taijiquan*) is a system of self-defense that incorporates philosophical concepts from Taoism and Confucianism. In addition to self-defense, tai chi aims to bring the body into balance and harmony to promote health and spiritual growth. It teaches practitioners to remain calm and centered, to conserve and concentrate energy, and to manipulate force by becoming part of it—by "going with the flow." Tai chi is considered the gentlest of the martial arts. Instead of quick and powerful movements, tai chi consists of a series of slow, fluid, elegant movements, which reinforce the idea of moving *with* rather than *against* the stressors of everyday life. As with yoga, it's best to start tai chi with a class led by an experienced instructor.

Listening to Music

Listening to music is another method of inducing relaxation. It can influence pulse, blood pressure, and the electrical activity of muscles. Studies of newborns and hospitalized stroke patients have shown that listening to soothing, lyrical music can lessen depression, anxiety, and stress levels. Researchers have found that exposure to soothing music leads to reduced levels of the stress

QUICK STATS

1 in 10 Americans practices yoga in one form or another.
—Yoga Business Academy, 2011

TERMS

meditation A technique for quieting the mind by focusing on a particular word, object (such as a candle flame), or process (such as breathing).

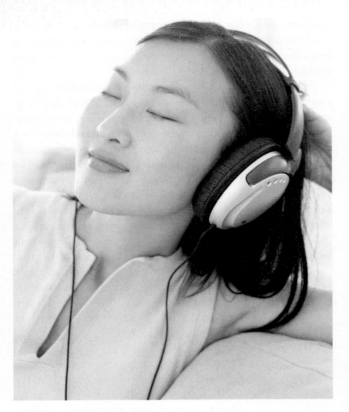

Listening to soothing music leads to reduced levels of stress hormones and can induce the relaxation response.

hormone cortisol and causes changes in the electrical activity in the brain.

To experience the stress management benefits of music yourself, set aside a time to listen. Choose music that you enjoy and that makes you feel relaxed.

Other relaxation techniques include biofeedback, massage, hypnosis and self-hypnosis, and autogenic training. To learn more about these and other techniques for inducing the relaxation response, refer to the "For More Information" section at the end of the chapter.

Counterproductive Coping Strategies

College is a time when you'll learn to adapt to new and challenging situations and gain skills that will last a lifetime. It is also a time when many people develop counterproductive and unhealthy habits in response to stress. Such habits can last well beyond graduation.

Tobacco Use   Cigarettes and other tobacco products contain *nicotine*, a chemical that enhances the actions of neurotransmitters. Nicotine can make you feel relaxed and even increase your ability to concentrate, but it is highly addictive. In fact, nicotine dependence itself is considered a psychological disorder. Cigarette smoke also contains substances that cause heart disease, stroke, lung cancer, and emphysema.

These negative consequences far outweigh any beneficial effects, and tobacco use should be avoided. The easiest thing to do is to not start.

Use of Alcohol and Other Drugs   Having a few drinks might make you feel temporarily at ease, and drinking until you're intoxicated may help you forget your current stressors. However, using alcohol to deal with stress places you at risk for all the short- and long-term problems associated with alcohol abuse. It also does nothing to address the actual causes of stress in your life. Although limited alcohol consumption may have potential health benefits for some people, many college students have patterns of drinking that detract from wellness.

Using other psychoactive drugs to cope with stress is also usually counterproductive:

- Caffeine raises cortisol levels and blood pressure and can make you feel more stressed; caffeine also disrupts sleep. Other stimulants, such as amphetamines, can activate the stress response. They also affect the same areas of the brain that are involved in regulating the stress response.

- Use of marijuana causes a brief period of euphoria and decreased short-term memory and attentional abilities. Physiological effects clearly show that marijuana use doesn't cause relaxation; in fact, some neurochemicals in marijuana act to enhance the stress response, and getting high on a regular basis can elicit panic attacks. To compound this, withdrawal from marijuana may also be associated with an increase in circulating stress hormones.

- Opioids such as morphine and heroin can mimic the effects of your body's natural painkillers and act to reduce anxiety. However, tolerance to opioids develops quickly, and many users become dependent.

Unhealthy Eating Habits   Eating is psychologically rewarding. The feelings of satiation and sedation that follow eating produce a relaxed state. However, regular use of eating as a means of coping with stress may lead to unhealthy eating habits. In fact, a survey by the American Psychological Association revealed that about 25% of Americans use food as a means of coping with stress or anxiety. These "comfort eaters" are twice as likely to be obese as average Americans.

CREATING A PERSONAL PLAN FOR MANAGING STRESS

What are the most important sources of stress in your life? Are you coping successfully with these stressors? No single strategy or program for managing stress will work for everyone, but you can use the principles of behavior management described in Chapter 1 to tailor a plan specifically to your needs.

> QUICK STATS
>
> **41%** of college-age Americans binge-drink.
> —National Survey on Drug Use and Health, 2010

STRESS JOURNAL		DATE _1-21-13_
TIME	**STRESSOR**	**REACTION/ COPING STRATEGY**
7:45 AM	Tara wouldn't get out of the shower	Yelled at her, started an argument
8:35 AM	Late for class	Slouched in back of room; chewed my nails
11:55 AM	Dad called to discuss credit card debt	Cried, skipped lunch and went out to smoke with Greg
5:30 PM	Power outage at dorm, couldn't study	Took a walk with Tara, made up for arguing this morning, then went to library to study
7:45 PM	Ed called, asked to borrow money	Stayed calm, put down phone and counted to 10, then explained that he already owes me $50.
8:30 PM	Ed called, angry, said he wanted to break up	Argued on phone, then went out with Tara for a drink

FIGURE 2.5   A sample stress journal. Tracking stressful events and reactions can help you understand how you normally cope with stress.

Identifying Stressors

Before you can learn to manage the stressors in your life, you have to identify them. Many experts recommend keeping a stress journal for a week or two (Figure 2.5). Each time you feel or express a stress response, record the time and the circumstances in your journal. Note what you were doing at the time, what you were thinking or feeling, and the outcome of your response.

After keeping your journal for a few weeks, you should be able to identify your key stressors and spot patterns in how you respond to them. Take note of the people, places, events, and patterns of thought and behavior that cause you the most stress. You may notice, for example, that mornings are usually the most stressful part of your day. Or you may discover that when you're angry at your roommate, you're apt to respond with behaviors that only make matters worse. Keeping a journal allows you to analyze what produces the most stress in your life and fills in where your conscious memory fails you.

Designing Your Plan

Once you have identified the key stressors in your life, choose the stress reduction techniques that will work best for you and create an action plan for change. Finding a buddy to work with you can make the process more fun and increase your chances of success. Some experts recommend drawing up a formal contract with yourself.

Whether or not you complete a contract, it's important to design rewards into your plan. You might treat yourself to a special breakfast in a favorite restaurant on the weekend (as long as you eat a nutritious breakfast every weekday morning). It's also important to evaluate your plan regularly and redesign it as your needs change. Under times of increased stress, for example, you might want to focus on good eating, exercise, and relaxation habits. Over time, your new stress management skills will become almost automatic. You'll feel better, accomplish more, and reduce your risk of disease.

Getting Help

If the techniques discussed so far don't provide you with enough relief from the stress in your life, you might want to learn more about specific areas to work on. Excellent self-help guides can be found in bookstores or the library. Additional resources are listed in the "For More Information" section at the end of the chapter.

Your student health center or student affairs office can tell you whether your campus has a peer counseling program. Such programs are usually staffed by volunteer students with special training that emphasizes maintaining confidentiality. Peer counselors can guide you to other campus or community resources or can simply provide understanding.

Support groups and short-term psychotherapy can also be tremendously helpful in dealing with stress-related problems.

connect™

Connect to Your Choices

Have you ever thought about why you handle stress the way you do? Many factors can influence the choices we make about stress management—some not as obvious as others. Do you try to do too much and then take your frustration out on other people because that's how stress was handled in your family? Do you blow off steam with alcohol on weekends because that's what your friends are doing? Do you dismiss relaxation techniques like yoga, meditation, or deep breathing because you think they're only for a certain type of person?

What are the external factors that influence your choices about stress management? What are your inner motivations and core values, and how do they affect your choices? Based on what you learned in this chapter, will you make some different choices in the future? If so, what will they be?

Go online to Connect to complete this activity: www.mcgraw-hillconnect.com

SUMMARY

- When confronted with a stressor, the body undergoes a set of physical changes known as the fight-or-flight reaction. The sympathetic nervous system and endocrine system act on many targets in the body to prepare it for action.

- Emotional and behavioral responses to stressors vary among individuals. Ineffective responses increase stress but can be moderated or changed.

- Factors that influence emotional and behavioral responses to stressors include personality, cultural background, gender, and past experiences.

- The general adaptation syndrome (GAS) has three stages: alarm, resistance, and exhaustion.

- A high allostatic load characterized by prolonged or repeated exposure to stress hormones can increase a person's risk of health problems.

- Psychoneuroimmunology (PNI) looks at how the physiological changes of the stress response affect the immune system and thereby increase the risk of illness.

- Health problems linked to stress include cardiovascular disease, colds and other infections, asthma and allergies, cancer, flare-ups of chronic diseases, psychological problems, digestive problems, headaches, insomnia, and injuries.

- A cluster of major life events that require adjustment and accommodation can lead to increased stress and an increased risk of health problems. Minor daily hassles increase stress if they are perceived negatively.

- Sources of stress associated with college may be academic, interpersonal, time-related, or financial pressures.

- Job-related stress is common, particularly for employees who have little control over decisions relating to their jobs. If stress is severe or prolonged, burnout may occur.

- New and changing relationships, prejudice, and discrimination are examples of interpersonal and social stressors.

- Social support systems help buffer people against the effects of stress and make illness less likely. Good communication skills foster healthy relationships.

- Exercise, nutrition, sleep, and time management are wellness behaviors that reduce stress and increase energy.

- Cognitive techniques for managing stress involve developing new and healthy patterns of thinking, such as practicing problem solving, monitoring self-talk, and cultivating a sense of humor.

- The relaxation response is the opposite of the fight-or-flight reaction. Techniques that trigger it, including progressive relaxation, imagery, meditation, and deep breathing, counteract the effects of chronic stress. Counterproductive coping strategies include smoking, drinking, and unhealthy eating.

- A successful individualized plan for coping with stress begins with the use of a stress journal or log to identify and study stressors and inappropriate behavioral responses. Completing a contract and recruiting a buddy can help your stress management plan succeed.

- Additional help in dealing with stress is available from self-help books, peer counseling, support groups, and psychotherapy.

FOR MORE INFORMATION

BOOKS

Goelitz, J., and R. A. Rees. 2011. *The College De-Stress Handbook: Keeping Cool Under Pressure from the Inside Out.* Boulder Creek, CA: Institute of HeartMath. *A brief guide to managing college stress, with tips on recognizing stressors, reducing their intensity, and learning new ways to respond.*

Greenberg, J. 2010. *Comprehensive Stress Management.* 12th ed. New York: McGraw-Hill. *Provides a clear explanation of the physical, psychological, sociological, and spiritual aspects of stress and offers numerous stress management techniques.*

Kabat-Zinn, J. 2011. *Mindfulness for Beginners: Reclaiming the Present Moment—and Your Life.* Louisville, CO: Sounds True. *A distillation of the ideas, attitudes, and practices that constitute the basics of mindfulness and mindful living.*

Pennebaker, J. W. 2004. *Writing to Heal: A Guided Journal for Recovering from Trauma and Emotional Upheaval.* Oakland, CA: New Harbinger Press. *Provides information about using journaling to cope with stress.*

ORGANIZATIONS AND WEBSITES

American Headache Society. Provides information for consumers and clinicians about different types of headaches, their causes, and their treatment.

http://www.americanheadachesociety.org

American Psychiatric Association: Healthy Minds, Healthy Lives. Provides information about mental wellness developed especially for college students.

http://www.healthyminds.org

American Psychological Association. Provides information about stress management and psychological disorders.

http://www.apa.org

http://www.apa.org/helpcenter

Association for Applied Psychophysiology and Biofeedback. Provides information about biofeedback and referrals to certified biofeedback practitioners.

http://www.aapb.org

Benson-Henry Institute for Mind Body Medicine. Provides information about stress management and relaxation techniques.

http://www.massgeneral.org/bhi

National Institute of Mental Health (NIMH). Publishes informative brochures about stress and stress management as well as other aspects of mental health.

http://www.nimh.nih.gov

National Sleep Foundation. Provides information about sleep and how to overcome sleep problems such as insomnia and jet lag.

http://www.sleepfoundation.org

The American Institute of Stress. A resource of in-depth information on stress, its causes, and its treatments.

http://www.stress.org

SELECTED BIBLIOGRAPHY

American College Health Association. 2011. *American College Health Association–National College Health Assessment II Reference Group Executive Summary, Spring 2011.* Hanover, MD: American College Health Association.

American Psychological Association. 2010. *Stress in America 2010.* Washington, DC: American Psychological Association.

American Psychological Association. 2012. *Mind/Body Health: Stress* (http://www.apa.org/helpcenter/stress.aspx).

Bartolomucci, A., and R. Leopardi. 2009. Stress and depression: Preclinical research and clinical implications. *PLoS One* 4(1): e4265.

Busch, V. 2008. Exercise in migraine therapy—is there any evidence for efficacy? A critical review. *Headache* 48(6): 890–899.

Caldwell, K., et al. 2010. Developing mindfulness in college students through movement-based courses: Effects on self-regulatory self-efficacy, mood, stress, and sleep quality. *Journal of American College Health* 58(5): 433–442.

Centers for Disease Control. 2012. *Coping with a Disaster or Traumatic Event: Information for Individuals and Families* (http://emergency.cdc.gov/mental-health/general.asp).

Dallman, M. 2010. Stress-induced obesity and the emotional nervous system. *Trends in Endocrinology and Metabolism* 21(3): 159–165.

Darabaneanu, S. 2011. Aerobic exercise as a therapy option for migraine: A pilot study. *International Journal of Sports Medicine* 32(6): 455–460.

Hefner, J., and D. Eisenberg. 2009. Social support and mental health among college students. *American Journal of Orthopsychiatry* 79(4): 491–499.

Flugel Colle, K. F., et al. 2010. Measurement of quality of life and participant experience with the mindfulness-based stress reduction program. *Complementary Therapies in Clinical Practice* 16(1): 36–40.

Freedman, N. 2010. Treatment of obstructive sleep apnea syndrome. *Clinics in Chest Medicine* 31(2): 187–201.

Hook, J. N., et al. 2010. Empirically supported religious and spiritual therapies. *Journal of Clinical Psychology* 66(1): 46–72.

Institute of Medicine Committee on Sleep Medicine and Research. 2006. *Sleep Disorders and Sleep Deprivation: An Unmet Public Health Problem,* ed. H. R. Colton and B. M. Altevogt. Washington, DC: National Academies Press.

National Sleep Foundation. 2011. *2011 Sleep in America Poll.* Washington, DC: National Sleep Foundation.

Nordboe, D. J., et al. 2007. Immediate behavioral health response to the Virginia Tech shootings. *Disaster Medicine and Public Health Preparedness* 1 (Suppl. 1.): S31–S32.

Roddenberry, A., and K. Renk. 2010. Locus of control and self-efficacy: Potential mediators of stress, illness, and utilization of health services in college students. *Child Psychiatry and Human Development* 41(4): 353–370.

Sirri, L., et al. 2012. Type A behavior: A reappraisal of its characteristics in cardiovascular disease. *International Journal of Clinical Practice* 66(9): 854–861.

Telles, S., et al. 2009. Effect of a yoga practice session and a yoga theory session on state anxiety. *Perceptual and Motor Skills* 109(3): 924–930.

U.S. Department of Health and Human Services, National Institutes of Health. 2012. *Stress* (http://www.nlm.nih.gov/medlineplus/stress.html).

BEHAVIOR CHANGE STRATEGY
Dealing with Test Anxiety

Do you perform as well as you should on tests? Does anxiety interfere with your ability to study effectively before a test and to think clearly in the test situation? If so, you may be experiencing test anxiety, an inefficient response to a stressful situation that can be replaced with a more effective one. Try some of these strategies for overcoming anxiety and succeeding in test situations:

- Before the test, find out everything you can about it—its format, the material to be covered, the grading criteria. Ask the instructor for practice materials. Study in advance; don't just cram the night before. Avoid all-nighters.

- Devise a study plan. This might include forming a study group with one or more classmates or outlining what you will study, when, where, and for how long. Generate your own questions and answer them.

- In the actual test situation, sit away from possible distractions, listen

carefully to instructions, and ask for clarification if you don't understand a direction.

- During the test, answer the easiest questions first. If you don't know an answer and there is no penalty for incorrect answers, guess. If there are several questions you have difficulty answering, review the ones you have already handled. Figure out approximately how much time you have to cover each question.

- For true-false questions, look for qualifiers such as *always* and *never*. Such questions are likely to be false.

- For essay questions, look for key words in the question that indicate what the instructor is looking for in the answer. Develop a brief outline of your answer, sketching out what you will cover, and keep track of the time you're spending on your answer. Don't get caught with unanswered questions when the time is up.

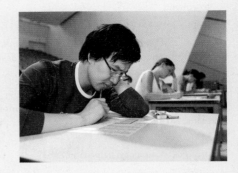

- Avoid worrying about past performance. If you start to become nervous, take some deep breaths and relax your muscles completely for a minute or so.

The best way to counter test anxiety is with successful test-taking experiences. If you find that these methods aren't sufficient to get your anxiety under control, you may want to seek professional help.

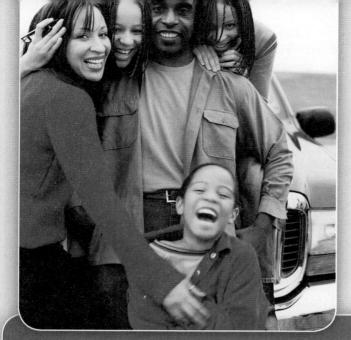

LOOKING AHEAD...

After reading this chapter, you should be able to

- **Describe what it means to be psychologically healthy**
- **Explain how to develop and maintain a positive self-concept and healthy self-esteem**
- **Discuss the importance of an optimistic outlook, good communication skills, and constructive approaches to dealing with loneliness and anger**
- **Describe common psychological disorders**
- **List the warning signs of suicide**
- **Describe the different types of help available for psychological problems**

Psychological Health

3

P sychological health contributes to every dimension of wellness. It can be difficult to maintain emotional, social, or even physical wellness if you are not psychologically healthy.

Psychological health, however, is a broad concept—one that is as difficult to define as it is important to understand. That is why the first section of this chapter is devoted to explaining what psychological health is and is not. The rest of the chapter discusses a number of common psychological problems, their symptoms, and their treatments.

DEFINING PSYCHOLOGICAL HEALTH

Psychological health (or *mental health*) can be defined either negatively as the absence of sickness or positively as the presence of wellness. The narrow, negative definition has two advantages: It concentrates attention on the worst problems and on the people most in need, and it avoids value judgments about the best way to lead our lives. If we think of everyone who is not severely mentally disturbed as being mentally healthy, however, we end up ignoring common problems that can be addressed. Finally, freedom from disorders is only one factor in psychological wellness.

Positive Psychology

A positive definition—psychological health as the presence of wellness—is a more ambitious goal.

During the 1960s Abraham Maslow adopted a perspective that he called "positive psychology" in his book *Toward a Psychology of Being*. Maslow defined a *hierarchy of needs* (Figure 3.1), listed here in order of decreasing importance:

- Physiological needs
- Safety
- Being loved
- Maintaining self-esteem
- Self-actualization

When urgent (life-sustaining) needs—such as the need for food and water—are satisfied, less basic needs take priority. Maslow's conclusions were based on his study of a group of visibly successful people who seemed to have lived, or to be living, at their fullest. He said that these people had achieved **self-actualization;** they had fulfilled a good measure of their human potential. Maslow suggested that self-actualized people all share certain qualities:

• *Realism.* Self-actualized people know the difference between what is real and what they want. As a result, they can cope with the world as it exists without demanding that it be

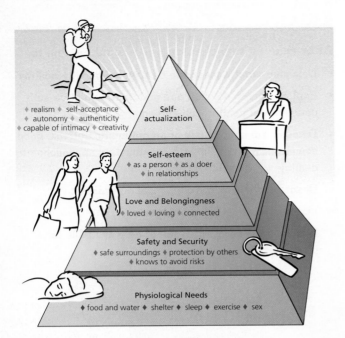

FIGURE 3.1 Maslow's hierarchy of needs.

SOURCE: Maslow, A. 1970. *Motivation and Personality,* 2nd ed. New York: Harper & Row.

• **Authenticity.** Autonomous people are not afraid to be themselves. Sometimes, in fact, their capacity for being "real" may give them a certain childlike quality. They respond in a genuine, or authentic, spontaneous way to whatever happens, without pretense or self-consciousness.

• **Capacity for intimacy.** Psychologically healthy people can share their feelings and thoughts without fear of rejection. A psychologically healthy person is open to the pleasure of physical contact and the satisfaction of being close to others—but without being afraid of the risks involved in intimacy, such as the risk of having one's feelings hurt. (Chapters 4 and 5 discuss intimacy in more detail.)

• **Creativity.** Psychologically healthy people continually look at the world with renewed appreciation. Such appreciation can inform one's creativity, which helps explain why so many mentally healthy people are creative.

Self-actualization is an ideal to strive for rather than something most people can reasonably hope to achieve. Maslow himself believed it was achieved quite rarely. Still, fulfilling one's own potential is a goal that everyone can work toward.

Positive psychology more recently has focused on clearly defining positive goals and on concrete, measurable ways of achieving them. According to psychologist Martin Seligman, we can achieve happiness by traveling three quite different but equally valid roads:

• **The pleasant life.** This life is dedicated to maximizing positive **emotions** about the past, present, and future, and to minimizing pain and negative emotions. Your feelings about the past should be of contentment, satisfaction, and serenity. Those about the present should include both immediate bodily pleasure and learned pleasures, such as the enjoyment of music. About the future, you should cultivate optimism and hopefulness.

• **The engaged life.** This life involves cultivating a strong character and exercising your talents. Most cultures admire personality traits such as courage, leadership,

different; they know what they can and cannot change. Just as important, realistic people accept evidence that contradicts what they want to believe.

• **Acceptance.** Psychologically healthy people have a **self-concept,** or *self-image,* that is positive but realistic. Such a person typically feels satisfaction and confidence in himself or herself, and so is said to have healthy **self-esteem.** Self-acceptance also means being tolerant of one's own imperfections—an ability that makes it easier to accept the imperfections of others.

• **Autonomy.** **P**sychologically healthy people are *autonomous,* meaning they can direct themselves, acting independently of their social environment. **Autonomy** is more than physical independence. It is social, emotional, and intellectual independence, as well.

> Emotional intelligence is not only a positive personality trait but also a **key to being engaged and successful in life**.

Ask Yourself

?

QUESTIONS FOR CRITICAL THINKING AND REFLECTION

Have you ever had a reason to feel concerned about your own psychological health? If so, what was the reason? Did your concern lead you to talk to someone about the issue or to seek professional help? If you did, what was the outcome, and how do you feel about it now?

TERMS

psychological health   Mental health, defined negatively as the absence of illness or positively as the presence of wellness.

self-actualization   The highest level of growth in Maslow's hierarchy of needs.

self-concept   The ideas, feelings, and perceptions a person has about himself or herself; also called *self-image.*

self-esteem   Satisfaction and confidence in oneself; the valuing of oneself as a person.

autonomy   Independence; the sense of being self-directed.

emotion   A feeling state involving some combination of thoughts, physiological changes, and an outward expression or behavior.

kindness, integrity, and originality along with the capacity to love and be loved. In this life, you become engaged and absorbed in what you do. You experience "flow" with complete immersion in what you do. Time stops, you are concentrated, and you feel completely at home.

Emotional intelligence is a positive personality trait and a key to being engaged and successful in life. An emotionally intelligent person can identify and manage his or her own emotions and the emotions of others. People with higher emotional intelligence can perceive their own emotions and also can harness them to reach their intended goals. They can read and understand the emotions of others and use that understanding to get along with people. Psychologists and educators believe that emotional intelligence is less fixed than abstract intelligence and can be taught.

- *The meaningful life.* Another road to happiness is to belong to and serve institutions that enable the best in human nature. Examples are institutions that educate and that cultivate strong families, democracy, or a free press. Many people find meaning in a connection to families, friends, religious institutions, and their work. Ultimately, meaning derives from belonging to and serving something larger than ourselves. It is strongest when meaning comes from more than one source.

Seligman and his colleagues are developing methods of assessing these three ways of life and of teaching people how to become happier by adopting one or more of them. They need not be mutually exclusive.

Not everyone accepts the ideas of positive psychology—or even the concept of psychological health—because they involve value judgments that are inconsistent with psychology's claim to be a science. Defining psychological health requires making assumptions and value judgments about what human goals are desirable, and some think these are matters for religion or philosophy. Positive psychology has also been criticized as promoting a short-sighted denial of reality and unwarranted optimism. In particular, therapists informed by existential philosophy believe that psychological health comes from acknowledging and accepting the painful realities of life.

What Psychological Health Is Not

Psychological health is not the same as psychological normality. Being mentally normal simply means being close to average. We can define normal body temperature because a few degrees above or below this temperature means physical sickness. But your ideas and attitudes can vary tremendously without your losing efficiency or feeling emotional distress. In fact, psychological diversity—with its wide range of ideas, lifestyles, and attitudes—is a valuable asset to society.

emotional intelligence   The capacity to identify and manage your own emotions and the emotions of others.

Never seeking help for personal problems does not prove you are psychologically healthy, any more than seeking help proves you are mentally ill. Unhappy people may avoid seeking help for many reasons, and severely disturbed people may not even realize they need help.

Further, we can't say people are "mentally ill" or "mentally healthy" based solely on the presence or absence of symptoms. Consider the symptom of anxiety, for example. Anxiety can help you face a problem and solve it before it becomes too big. Someone who shows no anxiety may be refusing to recognize problems or to do anything about them. A person who is anxious for good reason is likely to be judged more psychologically healthy in the long run than someone who is inappropriately calm.

Finally, we cannot judge psychological health from the way people look. All too often, a person who seems to be OK and even happy suddenly takes his or her own life. Usually such people lack close friends who might have known their desperation. At an early age, we learn to conceal our feelings and even to lie about them. We may believe that our complaints put unfair demands on others. While suffering in silence may sometimes be a virtue, it can also prevent us from getting help.

MEETING LIFE'S CHALLENGES

Life is full of challenges—large and small. Everyone, regardless of heredity and family influences, must learn to cope successfully with new situations and new people.

Growing Up Psychologically

Our responses to life's challenges influence the development of our personality and identity.

Developing an Adult Identity   A primary task beginning in adolescence is the development of an adult identity: a unified sense of self, characterized by attitudes, beliefs, and ways of acting that are genuinely our own. People with adult identities know who they are, what they are capable of, what roles they play, and their place among their peers. They have a sense of their own uniqueness but also appreciate what they have in common with others. They view themselves realistically and can assess their strengths and weaknesses without relying on the opinions of others. Achieving an identity also means that we can form intimate relationships with others while maintaining a strong sense of self.

Our identities evolve as we interact with the world and make choices about what we'd like to do and whom we'd like to model ourselves after. Developing an adult identity is particularly challenging in a heterogeneous, secular, and relatively affluent society like ours, in which many roles are possible, many choices are tolerated, and ample time is allowed for experimenting and making up one's mind.

Early identities are often modeled after parents—or the opposite of parents, in rebellion against what they represent. Over time, peers, rock stars, sports heroes, and religious figures are added to the list of possible role models. In high school and college, people often join cliques that assert a certain identity, such as the "jocks," the "brains," or the "slackers." Although much of our identity is internal—a way of viewing ourselves and the world—certain aspects of it can be external, such as styles of talking and dressing, body art, and hairstyles.

Early identities are rarely permanent. A student who works for good grades and approval one year can turn into a dropout devoted to hard rock and wild parties a year later. At some point, however, most of us adopt a more stable, individual identity that ties together the experiences of childhood and the expectations and aspirations of adulthood. However, we don't suddenly assume our final identity and never change after that. Life is more interesting for people who continue evolving into more distinct individuals, rather than being rigidly controlled by their pasts. Identity reflects a lifelong process, and it changes as a person develops new relationships and roles.

Developing an adult identity is an important part of psychological wellness. Without a personal identity, we begin to feel confused about who we are; this situation is called an **identity crisis.** Until we have "found ourselves," we cannot have much self-esteem because a self is not firmly in place.

Developing Intimacy Learning to live intimately with others and finding a productive role for yourself in society are other tasks of adulthood—to be able to love and work.

People with established identities can form intimate relationships and sexual unions characterized by sharing, open communication, long-term commitment, and love. Those who lack a firm sense of self may have difficulty establishing relationships because they feel overwhelmed by closeness and the needs of another person. As a result, they experience only short-term, superficial relationships with others and may remain isolated.

Developing Values and Purpose in Your Life **Values** are criteria for judging what is good and bad, and they underlie our moral decisions and behavior. The first morality of the young child is to consider "good" to mean what brings immediate and tangible rewards, and "bad" to mean whatever results in punishment. An older child will explain right and wrong in terms of authority figures and rules. But the final stage of moral development, one that not everyone attains, is being able to conceive of right and wrong in more abstract terms such as justice and virtue.

Healthy self-esteem means regarding yourself as **good, competent, and worthy of love**.

As adults we need to assess how far we have evolved morally and what values we actually have adopted. Without an awareness of our personal values, our lives may be hurriedly driven forward by immediate desires and the passing demands of others. Living according to values means doing the following:

- Considering your options carefully before making a choice.
- Choosing between options without succumbing to outside pressures that conflict with your values.
  - Making a choice and acting on it rather than doing nothing.

Your actions and how you justify them proclaim to others what you stand for.

Achieving Healthy Self-Esteem

Having a healthy level of self-esteem means regarding your self—which includes all aspects of your identity—as good, competent, and worthy of love. It is a critical component of wellness.

Developing a Positive Self-Concept Ideally a positive self-concept begins in childhood, based on experiences both within the family and outside it. Children need to develop a sense of being loved and being able to give love and to accomplish their goals. If they feel rejected or neglected by their parents, they may fail to develop feelings of self-worth. They may grow to have a negative concept of themselves.

Another component of self-concept is *integration.* An integrated self-concept is one that you have made for yourself—not someone else's image of you or a mask that doesn't quite fit. Important building blocks of self-concept are the personality characteristics and mannerisms of parents, which children may adopt without realizing it. Later they may be surprised to find themselves acting like one of their parents. Eventually such building blocks should be reshaped and integrated into a new, individual personality.

A further aspect of self-concept is *stability.* Stability depends on the integration of the self and its freedom from contradictions. People who have gotten mixed messages about themselves from parents and friends may have contradictory self-images, which defy integration and make them vulnerable to shifting levels of self-esteem. At times they regard themselves as entirely good, capable, and lovable—an ideal self—and at other times they see themselves as entirely bad, incompetent, and unworthy of love. Neither of these extreme self-concepts allows people to see themselves or others realistically, and their relationships with other people are filled with misunderstandings and ultimately with conflict.

TERMS

identity crisis Internal confusion about who one is.

values Criteria for judging what is good and bad, which underlie an individual's moral decisions and behavior.

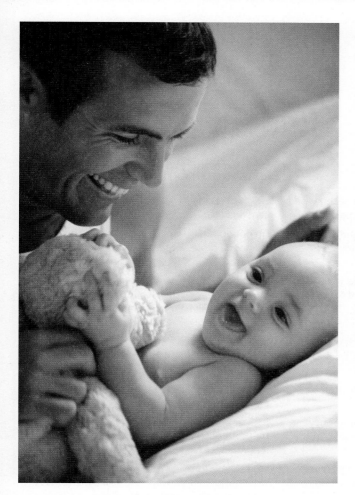

A positive self-concept begins in infancy. The knowledge that he's loved and valued by his parents gives this baby a solid basis for lifelong psychological health.

Meeting Challenges to Self-Esteem   As an adult, you sometimes run into situations that challenge your self-concept. People you care about may tell you they don't love you or feel loved by you, for example, or your attempts to accomplish a goal may end in failure.

You can react to such challenges in several ways. The best approach is to acknowledge that something has gone wrong and try again, adjusting your goals to your abilities without radically revising your self-concept. Less productive responses are denying that anything went wrong and blaming someone else. These attitudes may preserve your self-concept temporarily, but in the long run they keep you from meeting the challenge.

The worst reaction is to develop a lasting negative self-concept in which you feel bad, unloved, and ineffective—in other words, to become demoralized. Instead of coping, the demoralized person gives up (at least temporarily), reinforcing the negative self-concept and setting in motion a cycle of bad self-concept and failure. In people who are genetically predisposed to depression, demoralization can progress to additional symptoms, which are discussed later in the chapter.

One method for fighting demoralization is to recognize and test the negative thoughts and assumptions you may have about yourself and others. Try to note exactly when an unpleasant emotion—feeling worthless, wanting to give up, feeling depressed—occurs or gets worse, to identify the events or daydreams that trigger that emotion, and to observe whatever thoughts come into your head just before or during the emotional experience. It is helpful to keep a daily journal about such events.

People who are demoralized tend to use all-or-nothing thinking. They overgeneralize from negative events. They overlook the positive and jump to negative conclusions, minimizing their own successes and magnifying the successes of others. They take responsibility for unfortunate situations that are not their fault, then jump to more negative conclusions and more unfounded overgeneralizations. Patterns of thinking that make events seem worse than they are in reality are called **cognitive distortions.**

When you react to a situation, an important piece of that reaction is your **self-talk**—the statements you make to yourself inside your own mind. Rational thinking and self-talk will not only help get you through the situation without feeling upset, but also help you avoid damaging your own self-concept.

In your own fight against demoralization, it may be hard to think of a rational response until hours or days after the event that upset you. Responding rationally can be especially hard when you are having an argument with someone else, which is why people often say things they don't mean in the heat of the moment or develop hurt feelings even when the other person had no intention of hurting them.

Once you get used to noticing the way your mind works, however, you may be able to catch yourself thinking negatively and change the process before it goes too far. This approach to controlling your reactions is not the same as positive thinking—which means substituting a positive thought for a negative one. Instead you simply try to make your thoughts as logical and accurate as possible, based on the facts of the situation as you know them, and not on snap judgments or conclusions that may turn out to be false.

Demoralized people can be tenacious about their negative beliefs—so tenacious that they make their beliefs come true in a self-fulfilling prophesy. For example, if you conclude that you are so boring that no one will like you anyway, you may decide not to bother socializing. This behavior could make the negative belief become a reality because you limit your opportunities to meet people and develop new relationships.

For additional tips on changing distorted, negative ways of thinking, see the box "Realistic Self-Talk."

Being Less Defensive

Sometimes our wishes come into conflict with people in our lives or with our own conscience, and we become frustrated

> **cognitive distortion**   A pattern of negative thinking that makes events seem worse than they are.
>
> **self-talk**   The statements a person makes to himself or herself.
>
> TERMS

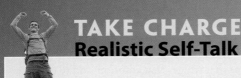

Do your patterns of thinking make events seem worse than they truly are? Do negative beliefs about yourself become self-fulfilling prophecies? Substituting realistic self-talk for negative self-talk can help you build and maintain self-esteem and cope better with the challenges in your life. Here are some examples of common types of distorted, negative self-talk, along with suggestions for more accurate and rational responses.

COGNITIVE DISTORTION	NEGATIVE SELF-TALK	REALISTIC SELF-TALK
Focusing on negatives	Babysitting is such a pain in the neck; I wish I didn't need the extra money so bad.	This is a tough job, but at least the money's decent and I can study once the kids go to bed.
Expecting the worst	I know I'm going to get an F in this course. I should just drop out of school now.	I'm not doing too well in this course. I should talk to my professor to see what kind of help I can get.
Overgeneralizing	My hair is a mess and I'm gaining weight. I'm so ugly. No one would ever want to date me.	I could use a haircut and should try to exercise more. This way I'll start feeling better about myself and will be more confident when I meet people.
Minimizing	It was nice of everyone to eat the dinner I cooked, even though I ruined it. I'm such a rotten cook.	Well, the roast was a little dry but they ate every bite. The veggies and rolls made up for it. I'm finally getting the hang of cooking!
Blaming others	Everyone I meet is such a jerk. Why aren't people more friendly?	I am going to make more of an effort to meet people who share my interests.
Expecting perfection	I cannot believe I flubbed that solo. They probably won't even let me audition for the orchestra next year.	It's a good thing I didn't stop playing when I hit that sour note. It didn't seem like anyone noticed it as much as I did.
Believing you're the cause of everything	Tom and Sara broke up and it's my fault. I shouldn't have insisted that Tom spend so much time with me and the guys.	It's a shame Tom and Sara broke up. I wish I knew what happened between them. Maybe Tom will tell me at soccer practice. At any rate, it isn't my fault; I've been a good friend to both of them.
Thinking in black and white	I thought that Mike was really cool, but after what he said today, I realize we have nothing in common.	I was really surprised that Mike disagreed with me today. I guess there are still things I don't know about him.
Magnifying events	I stuttered when I was giving my speech today in class. I must have sounded like a complete idiot. I'm sure everyone is talking about it.	My speech went really well, except for that one stutter. I bet most people didn't even notice it, though.

and anxious. If we cannot resolve the conflict by changing the external situation, we try to resolve the conflict internally by rearranging our thoughts and feelings. Table 3.1 lists some standard **defense mechanisms**. The drawback of many of these coping mechanisms is that they succeed temporarily, but make finding ultimate solutions much harder.

Recognizing your own defense mechanisms can be difficult because they've probably become habits, occurring unconsciously. But we all have some inkling about how our minds operate. By remembering the details of conflict situations you have been in, you may be able to figure out which defense mechanisms you used in successful or unsuccessful attempts to cope. Try to look at yourself as an objective, outside observer would and analyze your thoughts and behavior in a psychologically stressful situation from the past. Having insight into what strategies you typically use can lead to new, less defensive, and more effective ways of coping in the future.

Being Optimistic

Most of us have a predisposition toward optimism or pessimism. **Pessimism** is a tendency to focus on the negative and

> **TERMS**
>
> **defense mechanism** A mental mechanism for coping with conflict or anxiety.
>
> **pessimism** The tendency to expect an unfavorable outcome.

Table 3.1	Defense and Coping Mechanisms	
MECHANISM	DESCRIPTION	EXAMPLE
Projection	Reacting to unacceptable inner impulses as if they were from outside the self	A student who dislikes his roommate feels that the roommate dislikes him.
Repression	Expelling from awareness an unpleasant feeling, idea, or memory	The child of an alcoholic, neglectful father remembers only when his father showed consideration and love.
Denial	Refusing to acknowledge to yourself what you really know to be true	A person believes that smoking cigarettes won't harm her because she's young and healthy.
Displacement	Shifting your feelings about a person to another person	A student who is angry with one of his professors returns home and yells at one of his housemates.
Dissociation	Falling into a state of altered consciousness to avoid emotional distress	A woman who was raped experiences frightening images and confusion when something reminds her of the event.
Rationalization	Giving a false, acceptable reason when the real reason is unacceptable	A shy young man decides not to attend a dorm party, telling himself he'd be bored.
Reaction formation	Concealing emotions or impulses by exaggerating the opposite ones	A student struggling with homosexual impulses engages in gay-bashing.
Substitution	Replacing an unacceptable or unobtainable goal with an acceptable one	In love with an unavailable partner, a man throws himself into training for a marathon.
Passive-aggressive behavior	Expressing hostility toward someone by being covertly uncooperative or passive	A person tells a coworker, with whom she competes for assignments, that she'll help him with a project but then never follows through.
Humor	Finding something funny in unpleasant situations	A student whose bicycle has been stolen thinks how surprised the thief will be when he or she starts downhill and discovers the brakes don't work.

expect an unfavorable outcome; **optimism** is a tendency to dwell on the hopeful and expect a favorable outcome. Pessimists not only expect repeated failure and rejection but also accept it as deserved. They do not see themselves as capable of success and irrationally dismiss any evidence of their own accomplishments. This negative point of view is learned, typically at a young age from parents and other authority figures. Optimists, on the other hand, consider bad events to be more temporary than permanent, consider failure to be limited to the area of life in which it occurred rather than pervasive, hope that the causes of negative events are temporary, and ascribe negative events to other causes instead of blaming themselves.

You can learn to be optimistic by recording adverse events in a diary, along with the reactions and beliefs with which you met those events. By doing so, you learn to recognize and dispute the false, negative predictions you generate about yourself, like "The problem is going to last forever and ruin everything, and it's all my fault." Refuting such negative self-talk frees energy for realistic coping.

Maintaining Honest Communication

Another important area of psychological functioning is communicating honestly with others. It can be very frustrating for us and for people around us if we cannot express what we want and feel. Others can hardly respond to our needs if they

> Defense mechanisms may work right now, **but they can keep you from finding long-term solutions** to conflicts.

don't know what those needs are. We must recognize what we want to communicate and then express it clearly.

Some people know what they want others to do but don't state it clearly because they fear denial of the request, which they interpret as personal rejection. Such people might benefit from assertiveness training: learning to insist on their rights and to bargain for what they want. **Assertiveness** includes being able to say no or yes depending on the situation.

Dealing with Loneliness

It can be hard to strike the right balance between being alone and being with others. Some people are motivated to socialize by a fear of being alone—not the best reason to spend time with others. If you discover how to be happy by yourself, you'll be better able to cope with periods when you're forced to be alone—for example, when you've just broken off a romantic relationship or when your usual friends are away on vacation.

Unhappiness with being alone may come from interpreting it as a sign of rejection—that others are not interested in

optimism The tendency to expect a favorable outcome.

assertiveness Expression that is forceful but not hostile.

TERMS

spending time with you. Before you reach such a conclusion, be sure that you give others a real chance to get to know you. Examine your patterns of thinking: You may harbor unrealistic expectations about other people—for example, that everyone you meet must like you and, if they don't, you must be terribly flawed.

If you decide that you're not spending enough time with people, take action to change the situation. College life provides many opportunities to meet people. If you're shy, you may have to push yourself to join a group. Look for something you've enjoyed in the past or in which you have a genuine interest.

If your loneliness is the result of missing absent friends, remember that texting, e-mail, and cell phones are immediate and satisfying ways to keep up with friends.

Dealing with Anger

Common wisdom holds that expressing anger is beneficial for psychological and physical health. However, recent studies have questioned this idea by showing that overtly hostile people seem to be at higher risk for heart attacks. Angry words or actions don't contribute to psychological wellness if they damage relationships or produce feelings of guilt or loss of control. Perhaps the best way to resolve this contradiction is to distinguish between a gratuitous expression of anger and a reasonable level of self-assertiveness.

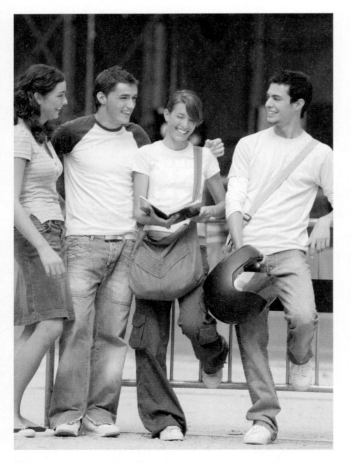

College offers many antidotes to loneliness in the forms of clubs, organized activities, sports, and just hanging out with friends.

At one extreme are people who never express anger or any opinion that might offend others, even when their own rights and needs are being jeopardized. If you have trouble expressing your anger, consider training in assertiveness and appropriate expressions of anger to help you learn to express yourself constructively.

At the other extreme are people whose anger is explosive or misdirected—a condition called *intermittent explosive disorder (IED)*. IED is often accompanied by depression or another disorder. Explosive anger or rage, like a child's tantrum, renders an individual temporarily unable to think straight or to act in his or her own best interest. During an IED episode, a person may lash out uncontrollably, hurting someone else or destroying property. Anyone who expresses anger this way should seek professional help.

Managing Your Own Anger   If you feel explosive anger coming on, consider the following two strategies to head it off.

First, try to *reframe* what you're thinking at that moment. You'll be less angry at another person if there is a possibility that his or her behavior was not intentionally directed against you. Imagine that another driver suddenly cuts in front of you. You would certainly be angry if you knew the other driver did it on purpose, but you probably would be less angry if you knew he simply did not see you. If you're angry because you've just been criticized, avoid mentally replaying scenes from the past when you received other unjust criticisms. Think about what is happening now, and try to act differently than in the past—less defensively and more analytically.

Second, until you're able to change your thinking, try to *distract* yourself. Use the old trick of counting to 10 before you respond, or start concentrating on your breathing. If necessary, cool off by leaving the situation until your anger has subsided. This does not mean that you should permanently avoid the issues and people who make you angry. Return to the matter after you've had a chance to think clearly about it.

Dealing with Anger in Other People   Anger can be infectious, and it disrupts cooperation and communication. If someone you're with becomes very angry, respond "asymmetrically" by reacting not with anger but with calm. Try to validate the other person by acknowledging that he or she has some reason to be angry. This does not mean apologizing if you don't think you're to blame or accepting verbal abuse, which is always inappropriate. Try to focus on solving the problem by allowing the person to explain why he or she is so angry and what can be done to alleviate the situation. Finally, if the person cannot be calmed, it may be best to disengage, at least temporarily. After a time-out, you may have better luck trying to solve the problem rationally.

PSYCHOLOGICAL DISORDERS

All of us feel anxious at times. In dealing with anxiety, we may avoid doing something that we want to do or should do. Most of us have periods of feeling down when we become

Psychological disorders differ in incidence and symptoms across cultures and ethnic groups around the world. This variability is usually attributable to cultural differences—factors such as how symptoms are interpreted and communicated, whether treatment is sought, and whether a social stigma is attached to a particular symptom or disorder.

Expression of Symptoms

People from different cultures or groups may manifest or describe symptoms differently. Consider the following examples:

• In Japan, people with social phobia may be more distressed about the imagined harm their social clumsiness causes to others than about their own embarrassment.

• Older African Americans may express depression in atypical ways—for example, denying depression by taking on a multitude of extra tasks.

• Somatization, the indirect reporting of psychological distress through nonspecific physical symptoms, is more prevalent among African Americans, Puerto Ricans, and Chinese Americans.

• Schizophrenia may manifest with different delusions depending on the local culture.

Differing Attitudes

It is relatively easy for Americans of northern European descent to regard an emotional problem as psychological in nature and to therefore accept a psychological treatment. For other groups, symptoms of psychological distress may be viewed as a spiritual problem, best dealt with by religious figures.

People from some groups may have little hesitation about communicating intimate, personal problems to professional care providers. However, for others, particularly men and members of certain ethnic groups, loss of emotional control may be seen as a weakness.

In addition, the use of mental health services is viewed negatively in many cultures; this stigma may partly account for the fact that African Americans and Asian Americans/Pacific Islanders are only about half as likely as whites to use any type of mental health service.

Assimilation

One of the largest immigrant groups in the United States is from Mexico. Surprisingly, surveys show that these immigrants are psychologically healthier than their own children born in the United States. Mexican, Cuban, and Puerto Rican Hispanics in this country come from a culture where family bonds are valued and divorce is rare. As they assimilate and begin using English exclusively, however, these family bonds tend to weaken, but less so for Cubans than for Puerto Ricans or Mexicans. With assimilation, the incidence of anxiety, depression, and substance abuse increases.

Biological Risk Factors

Biology can also play a role in the differences seen among patients of different ethnic groups. For example, psychotropic drugs are broken down in the body by a specific enzyme known as CYP2C19. Reduction of the activity of this enzyme is caused by two mutations, one of which appears to be found only in Asian populations. These "poor metabolizers" are very sensitive to medications that are broken down by this enzyme. The percentage of poor metabolizers among Asians is about 20%; among Latinos, about 5%; and among whites, 3%. Asian patients thus tend to have more adverse reactions to the doses of drugs standardized principally on white patients in the United States.

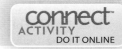

connect
ACTIVITY
DO IT ONLINE

---

pessimistic, less energetic, and less able to enjoy life. Many of us are bothered at times by irrational thoughts or odd feelings. Such feelings and thoughts can be normal responses to the ordinary challenges of life, but when emotions or irrational thoughts start to interfere with daily activities and rob us of our peace of mind, they can be considered symptoms of a psychological disorder.

Psychological disorders are generally the result of many factors. Genetic differences, which underlie differences in how the brain processes information and experiences, are known to play an important role, especially in certain disorders. However, exactly which genes are involved and how they alter the structure and chemistry of the brain are still under study. Learning and life events are important, too: Identical twins often don't have the same psychological disorders despite having identical genes. Some people have been exposed to more traumatic events than others, leading either to greater vulnerability to future traumas or, conversely, to the development of better coping skills. Further, what your parents, peers, and others have taught you strongly influences your level of self-esteem and how you deal with frightening or depressing life events (see the box "Ethnicity, Culture, and Psychological Disorders").

Ask Yourself

QUESTIONS FOR CRITICAL THINKING AND REFLECTION

Think about the last time you were truly angry. What triggered your anger? How did you express it? Do you typically handle your anger in the same manner? How appropriate does your anger management technique seem?

Anxiety Disorders

Fear is a basic and useful emotion. Its value for our ancestors' survival cannot be overestimated. For modern humans, fear motivates us to protect ourselves and to learn how to cope with new or potentially dangerous situations. We consider fear to be a problem only when it is out of proportion to real danger. **Anxiety** is another word for fear, especially a feeling of fear that is not in response to any definite threat. Anxiety is a disorder only when it occurs almost daily or in life situations that recur and cannot be avoided.

Specific Phobia   The most common and understandable anxiety disorder, called **specific phobia,** is a fear of something definite like lightning, a particular type of animal, or a place. Snakes, spiders, and dogs are commonly feared animals; frightening locations are often high places or enclosed spaces. Sometimes, but not always, these fears originate in bad experiences, such as being bitten by a snake.

Social Phobia   The 15 million Americans with **social phobia** fear humiliation or embarrassment while being observed by others. Fear of speaking in public is perhaps the most common phobia of this kind. Extremely shy people can have social fears that extend to almost all social situations.

Panic Disorder   People with **panic disorder** experience sudden unexpected surges in anxiety, accompanied by symptoms such as rapid and strong heartbeat, shortness of breath, loss of physical equilibrium, and a feeling of losing mental control. Such attacks usually begin in one's early twenties and can lead to a fear of being in crowds or closed places or of driving or flying. Sufferers fear that a panic attack will occur in a situation from which escape is difficult (such as while in an elevator), where the attack could be incapacitating and result in a dangerous or embarrassing loss of control (such as while driving a car or shopping), or where no medical help would be available if needed (such as when a person is alone away from home). Fears such as these lead to avoidance of situations that might cause trouble. The fears and avoidance may spread to a large variety of situations until a person is virtually housebound, a condition called **agoraphobia.**

Generalized Anxiety Disorder   A basic reaction to future threats is to worry about them. **Generalized anxiety disorder (GAD)** is a diagnosis given to people whose worries have taken on a life of their own, pushing out other thoughts and refusing banishment by any effort of will. For someone with GAD, ordinary concerns can become sources of overwhelming worries.

The GAD sufferer's worrying is not completely unjustified—after all, thinking about problems can result in solving them. But this kind of thinking seems to just go around in circles, and the more you try to stop it, the more you feel at its mercy. The end result is a persistent feeling of nervousness, often accompanied by depression.

Obsessive-Compulsive Disorder   Someone diagnosed with **obsessive-compulsive disorder (OCD)** contends with obsessions, compulsions, or both.

• **Obsessions** are recurrent, unwanted thoughts or impulses. Unlike the worries of GAD, they are not ordinary concerns but improbable fears such as of suddenly committing an antisocial act or of having been contaminated by germs.

• **Compulsions** are repetitive, difficult-to-resist actions usually associated with obsessions. A common compulsion is hand washing, associated with an obsessive fear of contamination by dirt. Other compulsions are counting and repeatedly checking whether something has been done—for example, whether a door has been locked or a stove turned off.

People with OCD feel anxious, out of control, and embarrassed. Their rituals can occupy much of their time and make them inefficient at work and difficult to live with.

Posttraumatic Stress Disorder   People who suffer from **posttraumatic stress disorder (PTSD)** are reacting to severely traumatic events (events that produce a sense of terror and helplessness) such as physical violence to themselves or their loved ones. Trauma occurs in personal assaults (rape, military combat), natural disasters (floods, hurricanes), and tragedies like fires and airplane or car crashes.

TERMS

anxiety   Fear that is not a response to any definite threat.

specific phobia   A persistent and excessive fear of a specific object, activity, or situation.

social phobia   An excessive fear of being observed by others; speaking in public is the most common example.

panic disorder   A syndrome of severe anxiety attacks accompanied by physical symptoms.

agoraphobia   An anxiety disorder characterized by fear of being alone away from help and by avoidance of many different places and situations; in extreme cases, a fear of leaving home.

generalized anxiety disorder (GAD)   An anxiety disorder characterized by excessive, uncontrollable worry about all kinds of things and anxiety in many situations.

obsessive-compulsive disorder (OCD)   An anxiety disorder characterized by uncontrollable, recurring thoughts and the performing of senseless rituals.

obsession   A recurrent, irrational, unwanted thought or impulse.

compulsion   An irrational, repetitive, forced action, usually associated with an obsession.

posttraumatic stress disorder (PTSD)   An anxiety disorder characterized by reliving traumatic events through dreams, flashbacks, and hallucinations.

Symptoms include reexperiencing the trauma in dreams and in intrusive memories, trying to avoid anything associated with the trauma, and numbing of feelings. Hyperarousal, sleep disturbances, and other symptoms of anxiety and depression also commonly occur. Such symptoms can last months or even years. PTSD symptoms often decrease substantially within three months, but up to one-third of PTSD sufferers do not fully recover. Recovery may be slower in those who have previously experienced trauma or who suffer from ongoing psychological problems.

The terrorist attacks on September 11, 2001, brought PTSD into the public spotlight. Among those affected were survivors, rescue workers, passersby, residents of Manhattan in general, and to some extent, television viewers around the world who saw countless repeated images of the devastation. An estimated 150,000 New Yorkers suffered PTSD following the attacks; some were still experiencing symptoms five years later. Hurricane Katrina had a similarly devastating effect; in one survey, 19% of police officers and 22% of firefighters in the Gulf Coast states reported symptoms of PTSD. Soldiers wounded in combat are also at risk for PTSD; among soldiers wounded in Iraq or Afghanistan, rates of PTSD increased during the first year after the injury, suggesting that the emotional impact deepens with time. When symptoms persist and daily functioning is disrupted, professional help is needed.

Treating Anxiety Disorders   Therapies for anxiety disorders range from medication to psychological interventions concentrating on a person's thoughts and behavior. Both drug treatments and cognitive-behavioral therapies are effective in panic disorder, OCD, and GAD. Specific phobias are best treated without drugs.

Mood Disorders

Daily, temporary mood changes typically don't affect our overall emotional state or level of wellness. A person with a **mood disorder,** however, experiences emotional disturbances that are intense and persistent enough to affect normal functioning. The two most common mood disorders are depression and bipolar disorder.

Depression   The National Institutes of Health estimates that **depression** strikes nearly 10% of Americans annually, making it the most common mood disorder. Depression affects the young as well as adults; about 9% of adolescents aged 12–17 suffer a major depressive episode each year, and nearly 50% of college students report depression severe enough to hinder their daily functioning. Depression tends to be more severe and persistent in blacks than in people of other races. Despite this, fewer than 50% of blacks affected by depression are treated for it.

> **QUICK STATS**
>
> **7.7 million adult Americans suffer from PTSD.**
>
> —National Institute of Mental Health, 2010

Almost twice as many women have serious depression as men. Why this is so is a matter of debate. Some experts think much of the difference is due to reporting bias: Women are more willing to admit experiencing negative emotions, being stressed, or having difficulty coping. Women may also be more likely to seek treatment. Other experts point to biologically based sex differences, particularly in the level and action of hormones. In addition, women's social roles and expectations are often different from those of men. Women may put more emphasis on relationships in determining self-esteem, so the deterioration of a relationship is a cause of depression that can hit women harder than men. In addition, culturally determined gender roles are more likely to place women in situations where they have less control over key life decisions, and lack of autonomy is associated with depression.

Depression takes different forms but usually involves demoralization and can include the following:

- A feeling of sadness and hopelessness
- Loss of pleasure in doing usual activities
- Poor appetite and weight loss
- Insomnia or disturbed sleep
- Restlessness or fatigue
- Thoughts of worthlessness and guilt
- Trouble concentrating or making decisions
- Thoughts of death or suicide

A person experiencing depression may not have all of these symptoms. Sometimes instead of poor appetite and insomnia, the opposite occurs—eating too much and sleeping too long. (Depression may contribute to weight gain in young women.) People can have multiple symptoms of depression without feeling depressed, although they usually experience a loss of interest or pleasure.

In major depression, symptoms are often severe; a diagnosis of *dysthymic disorder* may be applied to people who experience persistent symptoms of mild or moderate depression for two years or longer. In some cases, depression is a clear-cut reaction to specific events, such as the loss of a loved one or failing in school or work, whereas in other cases no trigger event is obvious.

One of the principal dangers of severe depression is suicide, which is discussed later in this chapter.

TERMS

mood disorder   An emotional disturbance that is intense and persistent enough to affect normal function; two common mood disorders are depression and bipolar disorder.

depression   A mood disorder characterized by loss of interest, sadness, hopelessness, loss of appetite, disturbed sleep, and other physical symptoms.

TREATING DEPRESSION   Although treatments are highly effective, only about 35% of people who suffer from depression currently seek treatment. Treatment for depression depends on its severity and on whether the depressed person is suicidal. The best initial treatment for moderate to severe depression is probably a combination of drug therapy and psychotherapy. Newer prescription antidepressants work well, although they may need several weeks to take effect, and patients may need to try multiple medications before finding one that works well. Therefore, when suicidal impulses are strong, hospitalization may be necessary.

Antidepressants work by affecting key neurotransmitters in the brain, including serotonin. The herbal supplement St. John's wort may also affect serotonin levels and may be effective in helping with mild to moderate symptoms of depression. However, it is not subject to the same testing and regulation as prescription medications, and it may interact with certain medications, reducing their effectiveness. These include oral contraceptives and some medications for heart disease, depression, HIV infection, and seizures. The safety of St. John's wort in pregnancy has not been established. Anyone who may be suffering from depression should seek a medical evaluation rather than self-treating with supplements.

When women take antidepressants, they may need a lower dose than men; at the same dosage, blood levels of medication tend to be higher in women. An issue for women who may become pregnant is whether antidepressants can harm a fetus or newborn. The best evidence indicates that the most frequently prescribed types of antidepressants do not cause birth defects, although some studies have reported withdrawal symptoms in some newborns whose mothers used certain antidepressants.

Electroconvulsive therapy (ECT) is effective for severe depression when other approaches have failed, including medications and other electronic therapies such as magnetic stimulation. In ECT, an epileptic-like seizure is induced by an electrical impulse transmitted through electrodes placed on the head. Patients are given an anesthetic and a muscle relaxant to reduce anxiety and prevent injuries associated with seizures. ECT usually includes three treatments per week for two to four weeks.

One type of depression is treated by having sufferers sit with eyes open in front of a bright light source every morning. These patients have **seasonal affective disorder (SAD)**; their depression worsens during winter months as daylight hours diminish, then improves with the spring and summer. The American Psychiatric Association estimates that 10–20% of Americans suffer symptoms that may be linked to SAD. SAD is more common among people who live at higher latitudes, where there are fewer hours of light in winter. Light therapy may work by extending the perceived length of the day and thus convincing the brain that it is summertime even during the winter months.

Mania and Bipolar Disorder   People who experience **mania,** a less common feature of mood disorders, are restless, have a lot of energy, need little sleep, and often talk nonstop. They may devote themselves to fantastic projects and spend more money than they can afford. Many manic people swing between manic and depressive states, a syndrome called **bipolar disorder** because of the two opposite poles of mood. Bipolar disorder affects men and women equally. Tranquilizers are used to treat individual manic episodes, while special drugs such as the salt lithium carbonate taken daily can prevent future mood swings. Anticonvulsants (used to prevent epileptic seizures) are also prescribed to stabilize moods; examples are Tegretol (carbamazepine) and Lamictal (lamotrigene).

> 1 in 100 Americans **has a schizophrenic episode** at least once in his or her lifetime.

Schizophrenia

Schizophrenia is a disorder that affects one's thinking and perceptions of reality. The disease can be severe and debilitating or so mild that it's hardly noticeable. Although people are capable of diagnosing their own depression, they usually don't diagnose their own schizophrenia because they often can't see that anything is wrong. This disorder is not rare; in fact, 1 in every 100 people has a schizophrenic episode sometime in his or her lifetime, most commonly starting in adolescence.

Scientists are uncertain about the exact causes of schizophrenia. Researchers have identified possible chemical and structural differences in the brains of people with the disorder

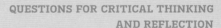

Ask Yourself

QUESTIONS FOR CRITICAL THINKING AND REFLECTION

Have you ever wondered if you were depressed? Try to recall your situation at the time. How did you feel, and what do you think brought about those feelings? What, if anything, did you do to bring about change and to feel better?

TERMS

electroconvulsive therapy (ECT)   The use of electric shock to induce brief, generalized seizures; used in the treatment of selected psychological disorders.

seasonal affective disorder (SAD)   A mood disorder characterized by seasonal depression, usually occurring in winter, when there is less daylight.

mania   A mood disorder characterized by excessive elation, irritability, talkativeness, inflated self-esteem, and expansiveness.

bipolar disorder   A mental illness characterized by alternating periods of depression and mania.

schizophrenia   A psychological disorder that involves a disturbance in thinking and in perceiving reality.

as well as several genes that appear to increase risk. Schizophrenia is likely caused by a combination of genes and environmental factors that occur during pregnancy and development. For example, children born to older fathers have higher rates of schizophrenia, as do children with prenatal exposure to certain infections or medications.

Some general characteristics of schizophrenia include the following:

- *Disorganized thoughts.* Thoughts may be expressed in a vague or confusing way.

- *Inappropriate emotions.* Emotions may be either absent or strong but inappropriate.

- *Delusions.* People with delusions—firmly held false beliefs—may think that their minds are controlled by outside forces, that people can read their minds, that they are great personages like Jesus Christ or the president of the United States, or that they are being persecuted by a group such as the CIA.

- *Auditory hallucinations.* Schizophrenic people may hear voices when no one is present.

- *Deteriorating social and work functioning.* Social withdrawal and increasingly poor performance at school or work may be so gradual that they are hardly noticed at first.

None of these characteristics is invariably present. Some schizophrenic people are quite logical except on the subject of their delusions. Others show disorganized thoughts but no delusions or hallucinations.

A schizophrenic person needs help from a mental health professional. Suicide is a risk in schizophrenia, and expert treatment can reduce that risk and minimize the social consequences of the illness by shortening the period when symptoms are active. The key element in treatment is regular medication. At times medication is like insulin for diabetes—it makes the difference between being able to function or not. Sometimes hospitalization is temporarily required to relieve family and friends.

SUICIDE

In the United States, suicide is the third leading cause of death for young people ages 15 to 24 and the 11th leading cause for people of all ages. About 15 attempts are made for every death. In this country, men have much higher suicide rates than women; white men over age 65 have the highest suicide rate (Figure 3.2). Whites and Native Americans have higher rates than most other groups, but rates among blacks have been rising. Women attempt three times as many suicides as men, yet men succeed at more than three times the rate of women. Suicide rates among adolescents and young adults and among adults over 65 have been falling for the last two decades.

Suicide rarely occurs without warning signs. About 60% of people who commit suicide are depressed. The more symptoms of depression a person has, the greater the risk. Other warning signs include the following:

- Expressing the wish to be dead or revealing contemplated methods.

- Increasing social withdrawal and isolation.

- A sudden, inexplicable lightening of mood (which can mean the person has decided to commit suicide).

QUICK STATS

52% of American suicides are committed with guns.

—National Center for Health Statistics, 2012

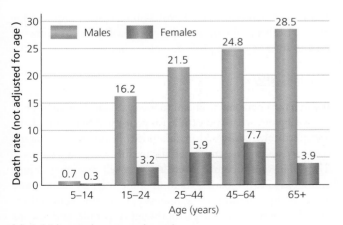

(a) Suicide rate by age and gender

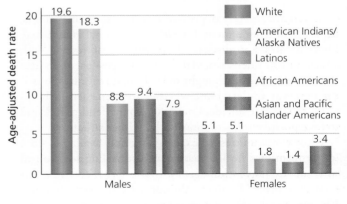

(b) Suicide rate by ethnicity and gender (all ages)

FIGURE 3.2 Rates of suicide per 100,000 people in the United States. The rate of suicide varies by gender, age, and ethnicity. Rates are higher among men than among women at all ages and are higher among whites compared to other groups. White men over age 65 have the highest rate of suicide. The age-adjusted national suicide rate is 10.0 per 100,000 people. These statistics are from 2006.

SOURCE: National Center for Health Statistics. 2009. *Health, United States, 2009.* Hyattsville, MD: National Center for Health Statistics.

In general, people want to be well and healthy, protect themselves from harm, and try to make use of the guidance that this book gives. But there are individuals—predominantly in their teens and early 20s—who deliberately harm themselves, although in a non-fatal way. One common method is to cut or burn their skin, leaving scars that may serve as visible representation of emotional pain that they shamefully hide beneath their clothes.

Self-cutting and other self-injurious behaviors are not aesthetically motivated. Many report seeking the physical sensations (including pain) produced by a self-inflicted injury, which may temporarily relieve feelings of tension, perhaps through a release of endorphins.

In 2011 a research group led by Alicia Meuret, an associate professor of psychology at Southern Methodist University, conducted surveys on more than 550 college students and found that over 20% had engaged in self-injury at some point, which is consistent with prevalence estimates in other studies on college populations.

In examining differences between self-injurers and non-injurers, researchers found that individuals who had recently engaged in self-harm were significantly more depressed, anxious, and disgusted with themselves. Compared to non-injurers, self-injurers were roughly 4 times more likely to report a history of physical abuse and 11 times more likely to report a history of sexual abuse.

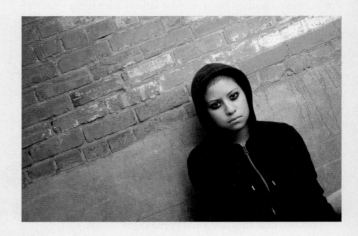

Self-injury is not the same as a suicide attempt, but individuals who repeatedly hurt themselves are more likely to commit suicide than the general population. In any case, self-injury should be taken seriously. If you do it, talk to a counselor. If someone you know does it, try to convince him or her to talk to a counselor.

Certain risk factors increase the likelihood of suicide:

- A history of previous attempts.
- A suicide by a family member or friend.
- Readily available means, such as guns or pills.
- A history of substance abuse or eating disorders.
- Serious medical problems.

If you are severely depressed or know someone who is, expert help from a mental health professional is essential. Don't be afraid to discuss the possibility of suicide with someone you fear is suicidal. You won't give them an idea they haven't already thought of. Asking direct questions is the best way to determine whether someone seriously intends to commit suicide. Encourage your friend to talk and to take positive steps to improve his or her situation.

Most communities have emergency help available, often in the form of a hotline telephone counseling service run by a suicide prevention agency. If you feel there is an immediate danger of suicide, do not leave the person alone. Call for help or take him or her to an emergency room.

Firearms are used in more suicides than homicides. Eighty-three percent of gun-related deaths in the home are the result of suicide, often by someone other than the gun owner. If you learn someone at high risk for suicide has access to a gun, try to convince him or her to put it in safe-keeping. Self-injury is not the same as a suicidal behavior, but someone who self-injures can benefit from professional help (see the box "Deliberate Self-Harm").

GETTING HELP

Knowing when self-help or professional help is required for mental health problems is usually not as difficult as knowing how to start or which professional to choose.

Self-Help

If you have a personal problem to solve, a smart way to begin is by finding out what you can do on your own. Some problems are specifically addressed in this book. Behavioral and some cognitive approaches are especially useful for helping yourself. They all involve becoming more aware of self-defeating actions and ideas and combating them in some way: by being more assertive; by communicating honestly; by raising your self-esteem by counteracting negative thoughts, people, and actions that undermine it; and by confronting, rather than avoiding, the things you fear. You can get more information from books in the psychology or self-help sections of libraries and bookstores, but be selective. Watch out for self-help books making fantastic claims or deviating from mainstream approaches.

Attention-deficit/hyperactivity disorder (ADHD)— characterized by impulsivity, hyperactivity, and/or an inability to stay focused— is the most commonly diagnosed mental disorder among American children and adolescents. Children with ADHD can struggle with conflict and aggression, peer rejection, and academic problems. Up to 7% of American children are affected by some form of ADHD, and about 4% of adults develop symptoms in any given year.

ADHD is commonly treated with the drug methylphenidate (Ritalin), a psychostimulant that has the seemingly paradoxical effect in people with ADHD of improving attention and decreasing distractibility. Although Ritalin is approved by the FDA for the treatment of ADHD, the long-term effects are not known.

In recent years, interest has grown in supplementing drug and behavioral therapy for children with ADHD by exposing them to natural environments. Researchers have found that when children spend time outdoors in natural settings, ADHD symptoms diminish. In one study, children with ADHD took 20-minute walks in a park, a residential neighborhood, and an urban downtown area, and their concentration was measured after each walk. After the nature walk, concentration improved significantly, comparable to the effects of medication. No one suggests that nature exposure should replace medication, and some believe that the positive effects are overstated, but researchers suggest that "doses of nature" may serve as safe, inexpensive complements to other ADHD treatments.

Some experts worry that almost all American children are missing out on nature these days, largely as a result of increased time spent on video games, computers, and TV. The term "nature deficit disorder" has been coined to describe this lack of exposure to the outside world, with associated childhood obesity and mental health problems like depression and anxiety. A grassroots movement called the No Child Left Inside Coalition has sprung up to get children outside and to teach them environmental responsibility. Many school districts participate in the program, incorporating environmental literacy into their curricula, beginning in elementary school. The U.S. government is also getting involved. In 2009 the No Child Left Inside Act was introduced in Congress, extending funding for environmental education programs in public schools. As part of the U.S. Department of Education's budget for fiscal year 2011, $1 billion was included specifically for environmental literacy programs.

Advocates say that, in addition to helping with ADHD, there are other good reasons for encouraging children to spend time outdoors. Today's children, they contend, may be losing their fundamental connection to nature, possibly resulting in an entire generation of Americans who feel less connected to—and less sympathetic toward—the environment. Given the urgency of global climate change, pollution, species endangerment and extinction, and other environmental issues, experts say, future generations must be environmentally literate and understand their role in protecting the planet—or risk causing more harm for themselves and their own children.

For a detailed discussion of environmental health—how the environment affects you and how you affect the environment—see Chapter 14.

SOURCES: Bennett, L. 2009. *Greening a K–12 Curriculum* (http://www.ecoliteracy.org/essays/greening-k-12-curriculum); Education.com. 2010. *Nature Deficit Disorder* (http://www.education.com/topic/nature-deficit-disorder); Faber, T. A., and F. E. Kuo. 2009. Children with attention deficits concentrate better after walk in the park. *Journal of Attention Disorders* 12(5): 402–409; Luov, R. 2005. *Last Child in the Woods.* Chapel Hill, NC: Algonquin.

Some people find it helpful to express their feelings in a journal. Grappling with a painful experience in this way provides an emotional release and can help you develop more constructive ways of dealing with similar situations in the future. Research indicates that using a journal this way can improve physical as well as emotional wellness.

For some people, religious belief and practice may promote psychological health. Religious organizations provide a social network and a supportive community, and religious practices, such as prayer and meditation, offer a path for personal change and transformation. Spending time in nature can have psychological benefits as well (see the box "ADHD and Exposure to Nature").

Peer Counseling and Support Groups

Sharing your concerns with others is another helpful way of dealing with psychological health challenges. Just being able to share what's troubling you with an accepting, empathetic person can bring relief. Comparing notes with people who have problems similar to yours can give you new ideas about coping.

Many colleges offer peer counseling through a health center or through the psychology or education department. Peer counseling is usually done by volunteer students who have special training that emphasizes confidentiality. Peer counselors may steer you toward an appropriate campus or community resource or simply offer a sympathetic ear.

Many self-help groups work on the principle of bringing together people with similar problems to share their experiences and support one another. Support groups are typically organized around a specific problem, such as eating disorders or substance abuse. Self-help groups may be listed in the campus newspaper or at the student health center.

QUICK STATS

22,690 psychiatrists and **100,700** psychologists were practicing in the United States in 2010.
—Bureau of Labor Statistics, 2011

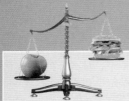

CRITICAL CONSUMER
Choosing and Evaluating Mental Health Professionals

College students are usually in a good position to find convenient, affordable mental health care. Larger schools typically have both health services that employ psychiatrists and psychologists and counseling centers staffed by professionals and student peer counselors. Resources in the community may include a school of medicine, a hospital, and a variety of professionals who work independently. It's a good idea to get recommendations from physicians, clergy, friends who have been in therapy, or community agencies if you decide to see an independent practitioner.

Financial considerations are also important. Find out how much different services will cost and what your health insurance will cover. If you're not adequately covered by a health plan, don't let that stop you from getting help; investigate low-cost alternatives. City, county, and state governments often support mental health clinics for those who can afford to pay little or nothing for treatment. Some on-campus services may be free or offered at very little cost.

The cost of treatment is linked to how many therapy sessions will be needed, which in turn depends on the type of therapy and the nature of the problem. Psychological therapies focusing on specific problems may require 8–10 sessions at weekly intervals. Therapies aiming for psychological awareness and personality change can last months or years.

Deciding whether a therapist is right for you will require meeting the therapist in person. Before or during your first meeting, find out about the therapist's background and training:

- Does she or he have a degree from an appropriate professional school and a state license to practice?

- Has she or he had experience treating people with problems similar to yours?

- How much will therapy cost?

You have a right to know the answers to these questions and should not hesitate to ask them. After your initial meeting, evaluate your impressions:

- Does the therapist seem like a warm, intelligent person who would be able to help you and seems interested in doing so?

- Are you comfortable with the personality, values, and beliefs of the therapist?

- Is he or she willing to talk about the techniques in use? Do these techniques make sense to you?

If you answer yes to these questions, this therapist may be satisfactory for you. If you feel uncomfortable—and you're not in need of emergency care—it's worthwhile to set up one-time consultations with one or two others before you make up your mind. Take the time to find someone who feels right for you.

Later in your treatment, evaluate your progress:

- Are you being helped by the treatment?

- If you are displeased, is it because you aren't making progress, or because therapy is raising difficult, painful issues you don't want to deal with?

- Can you express dissatisfaction to your therapist? Such feedback can improve your treatment.

If you're convinced your therapy isn't working or is harmful, thank your therapist for her or his efforts, and find another.

Professional Help

Sometimes self-help or talking to nonprofessionals is not enough. More objective, more expert, or more discreet help is needed. Many people have trouble accepting the need for professional help, and often those who most need help are the most unwilling to get it. You may someday find yourself having to overcome your own reluctance, or that of a friend, about seeking help.

Determining the Need for Professional Help   In some cases, professional help is optional. Some people are interested in improving their psychological health in a general way by going into individual or group therapy to learn more about themselves and how to interact with others. Seeking professional help for these reasons is a matter of individual choice. In some situations, such as friction among family members or between partners, professional help can mean the difference between a painful divorce and a satisfying relationship.

Professional help is appropriate in any of the following situations:

- Depression, anxiety, or other emotional problems interfere seriously with school or work performance or in getting along with others.
- Suicide is attempted or is seriously considered (see the warning signs listed earlier in the chapter).
- Symptoms such as hallucinations, delusions, incoherent speech, or loss of memory occur.
- Alcohol or drugs are used to the extent that they impair normal functioning during much of the week, finding or taking drugs occupies much of the week, or reducing their dosage leads to psychological or physiological withdrawal symptoms.

Choosing a Mental Health Professional   Mental health workers belong to several different professions and have different roles. Psychiatrists are medical doctors. They are experts in deciding whether a medical disease lies behind psychological symptoms, and they are usually involved in treatment if medication or hospitalization is required. Clinical psychologists typically hold a PhD degree; they are often experts in behavioral and cognitive therapies. Other mental health workers include social workers, licensed counselors, and clergy with special training in pastoral counseling. In hospitals and clinics, various mental health professionals may join together in treatment teams.

For more on finding appropriate help, see the box "Choosing and Evaluating Mental Health Professionals."

SUMMARY

- Psychological health encompasses more than a single particular state of normality. Psychological diversity is valuable among groups of people.

- Defining psychological health as the presence of wellness means that to be healthy you must strive to fulfill your potential.

- Maslow's definition of psychological health centers on self-actualization, the highest level in his hierarchy of needs. Self-actualized people have high self-esteem and are realistic, inner-directed, authentic, capable of emotional intimacy, and creative.

- Crucial parts of psychological wellness include developing an adult identity, establishing intimate relationships, and developing values and purpose in life.

- A sense of self-esteem develops during childhood as a result of giving and receiving love and learning to accomplish goals. Self-concept is challenged every day; healthy people adjust their goals to their abilities.

- Using defense mechanisms to cope with problems can make finding solutions harder. Analyzing thoughts and behavior can help people develop less defensive and more effective ways of coping.

- A pessimistic outlook can be damaging; it can be overcome by developing more realistic self-talk.

- Honest communication requires recognizing what needs to be said and saying it clearly. Assertiveness enables people to insist on their rights and to participate in the give-and-take of good communication.

- People may be lonely if they haven't developed ways to be happy on their own or if they interpret being alone as a sign of rejection. Lonely people can take action to expand their social contacts.

- Dealing successfully with anger involves distinguishing between a reasonable level of assertiveness and gratuitous expressions of anger, heading off rage by reframing thoughts and distracting oneself, and responding to the anger of others with an asymmetrical, problem-solving orientation.

- People with psychological disorders have symptoms severe enough to interfere with daily living.

- Anxiety is a fear that is not directed toward any definite threat. Anxiety disorders include simple phobias, social phobias, panic disorder, generalized anxiety disorder, obsessive-compulsive disorder, and posttraumatic stress disorder.

- Depression is a common mood disorder; loss of interest or pleasure in things seems to be its most universal symptom. Severe depression carries a high risk of suicide, and suicidally depressed people need professional help.

- Symptoms of mania include exalted moods with unrealistically high self-esteem, little need for sleep, and rapid speech. Mood swings between mania and depression characterize bipolar disorder.

- Schizophrenia is characterized by disorganized thoughts, inappropriate emotions, delusions, auditory hallucinations, and deteriorating social and work performance.

- Help is available in a variety of forms, including self-help, peer counseling, support groups, and therapy with a mental health professional. For serious problems, professional help may be the most appropriate.

FOR MORE INFORMATION

BOOKS

Antony, M. M., and R. P. Swinson. 2008. *The Shyness & Social Anxiety Workbook: Proven, Step-by-Step Techniques for Overcoming Your Fear*, 2nd ed. Oakland, CA: New Harbinger. *Practical suggestions for fears of interacting with people you don't know.*

Grieco, R., and L. Edwards. 2009. *The Other Depression: Bipolar Disorder*. New York: Routledge. *Provides a complete introduction to bipolar disorder, its symptoms, and its current treatments.*

Jenkins, J., D. Keltner, and K. Oatley. 2006. *Understanding Emotions*, 2nd ed. Oxford: Blackwell. *A comprehensive guide to emotions, including current research on the neuroscience of emotions, evolutionary and cultural approaches to emotion, and the expression and communication of emotions.*

Leahy, R. L. 2010. *Beating the Blues Before They Beat You: How to Overcome Depression*. New York: Hay House. *Describes strategies from cognitive behavioral therapy for changing thinking patterns that contribute to low self-esteem and depression; outlines symptoms, causes, and treatments, including therapy and medication.*

Nathan, P. E., and J. M. Gorman. 2007. *A Guide to Treatments That Work*, 3rd ed. New York: Oxford University Press. *A balanced and comprehensive report on various treatments for psychological disorders.*

Seligman, M. E. 2012. *Flourish: A Visionary New Understanding of Happiness and Well-Being*. New York: Free Press. *The author refines his ideas about learned optimism and happiness, identifying factors that contribute to a satisfying life: positive emotion, engagement, relationships, meaning, and accomplishment.*

ORGANIZATIONS, HOTLINES, AND WEBSITES

American Association of Suicidology. Provides information about suicide and resources for people in crisis.

http://www.suicidology.org

Anxiety Disorders Association of America (ADAA). Provides information and resources related to anxiety disorders.

http://www.adaa.org

Depression and Bipolar Support Alliance (DBSA). Provides educational materials and information about support groups.

http://www.dbsalliance.org

Cope, Care, Deal. Offers information on mental health issues specifically for teens.

http://www.copecaredeal.org

NAMI (National Alliance on Mental Illness). Provides information and support for people affected by mental illness.

800-950-NAMI (help line)

http://www.nami.org

National Hopeline Network. 24-hour hotline for people who are thinking about suicide or know someone who is; calls are routed to local crisis centers.

800-SUICIDE

http://www.hopeline.com

National Institute of Mental Health (NIMH). Provides helpful information about anxiety, depression, eating disorders, and other challenges to psychological health.

http://www.nimh.nih.gov

Mental Health America. Provides consumer information on a variety of issues, including how to find help.

http://www.nmha.org

Substance Abuse and Mental Health Services Administration. A one-stop source for information and resources relating to mental health.

http:// samhsa.gov

SELECTED BIBLIOGRAPHY

Agency for Healthcare Research and Quality. 2007. *Antidepressant Medicines: A Guide for Adults with Depression*. Rockville, MD: Agency for Healthcare Research and Quality Publication Number 07-EHC007-2A.

American Psychiatric Association. 2000. *Diagnostic and Statistical Manual of Mental Disorders*, 4th ed., Text Revision *(DSM-IV-TR)*. Washington, DC: American Psychiatric Association Press.

American Psychiatric Association. 2010. *Mental Health* (http://www.healthyminds.org/Main-Topic/Mental-Illness.aspx).

Banks, M. V., and K. Salmon. 2012. Reasoning about the self in positive and negative ways: Relationship to psychological functioning in young adulthood. *Memory*, Aug. 17 (Epub ahead of print).

Beard, C., et al. 2010. Health-related quality of life across the anxiety disorders: Findings from a sample of primary care patients. *Journal of Anxiety Disorders* 24(6): 559–564.

Carver, C. S., M. F. Scheier, and S. C. Segerstrom. 2010. Optimism. *Clinical Psychology Review* 30(7): 879–889.

Cawood, C. D., and S. K. Huprich. 2011. Late adolescent nonsuicidal self-injury: The roles of coping style, self-esteem, and personality pathology. *Journal of Personality Disorders* 25(6): 765–781.

Centers for Disease Control and Prevention. 2010. Attitudes toward Mental Illness—35 states, District of Columbia, and Puerto Rico, 2007. *Morbidity and Mortality Weekly Report* 59(20): 619–625.

Coryell, W. H. 2006. Clinical assessment of suicide risk in depressive disorder. *CNS Spectrums* 11(6): 455–461.

Dugas, E., et al. 2012. Early predictors of suicidal ideation in young adults. *Canadian Journal of Psychiatry* 57(7): 429–436.

Ferrier-Auerback, A. G., et al. 2010. Predictors of emotional distress reported by soldiers in the combat zone. *Journal of Psychiatric Research* 44(7): 470–476.

Forty, L., et al. 2009. Polarity at illness onset in bipolar I disorder and clinical course of illness. *Bipolar Disorders* 11(1): 82–88.

Greenhoot, A. F., et al. 2012. Making sense of traumatic memories: Memory qualities and psychological symptoms in emerging adults with and without abuse histories. *Memory*, Sept. 4 (epub ahead of print).

Heron, M., et al. 2010. Annual summary of vital statistics: 2007. *Pediatrics* 125(1): 4–15.

Jones, S. H., and G. Burrell-Hodgson. 2008. Cognitive-behavioral treatment of first diagnosis bipolar disorder. *Clinical Psychology & Psychotherapy* 15(6): 367–377.

Kasper, S., et al. 2006. Superior efficacy of St. John's wort extract WS(R) 5570 compared to placebo in patients with major depression: A randomized, double-blind, placebo-controlled, multi-center trial. *BMC Medicine* 4(1): 14.

Klein, D. N., et al. 2012. Predictors of first lifetime onset of major depressive disorder in young adulthood. *Journal of Abnormal Psychology*, Aug. 13 (Epub ahead of print).

Lin, Y. R., et al. 2008. Evaluation of assertiveness training for psychiatric patients. *Journal of Clinical Nursing* 17(21): 2875–2883.

National Institute of Mental Health. 2012. Social Phobia (Social Anxiety Disorder) (http://www.nimh.nih.gov/health/topics/social-phobia-social-anxiety-disorder/index.shtml).

National Institute of Mental Health. 2012. Depression (http://www.nimh.nih.gov/health/topics/depression/index.shtml).

Nemeroff, C. B. 2006. The burden of severe depression: A review of diagnostic challenges and treatment alternatives. *Journal of Psychiatric Research*, 25 July [Epub ahead of print].

Rickwood, D., and S. Bradford. 2012. The role of self-help in the treatment of mild anxiety disorders in young people: An evidence-based review. *Psychology Research and Behavior Management* 5:25–36.

Rosenthal, B. S., and W. C. Wilson. 2012 Race/ethnicity and mental health in the first decade of the 21st century. *Psychological Reports* 110(2): 645–662.

Rothwell, J. D. 2009. *In the Company of Others: An Introduction to Communication*, 3rd ed. New York: Oxford University Press.

Saewyc, E. M., and R. Tonkin. 2008. Surveying adolescents: Focusing on positive development. *Pediatrics & Child Health* 13(1): 43–47.

Schatzberg, A. F., J. O. Cole, and C. DeBattista. 2010. *Manual of Clinical Psychopharmacology*, 7th ed. Washington, D.C.: American Psychiatric Publishing.

Seligman, M. E. P., 2008. Positive health. *Applied Psychology: An International Review* 57, 3–18.

Simon, G. E., and J. Savarino. 2007. Suicide attempts among patients starting depression treatment with medications or psychotherapy. *American Journal of Psychiatry* 164(7): 1029–1034.

Simon, G. 2009. Collaborative care for mood disorders. *Current Opinion in Psychiatry*. 22(1): 37–41.

Singh, N. N., et al. 2007. Individuals with mental illness can control their aggressive behavior through mindfulness training. *Behavior Modification* 31(3): 313–328.

Soeteman, D., M. Miller, and J. J. Kim. 2012. Modeling the risks and benefits of depression treatment for children and young adults. *Value in Health* 15(5): 724–729.

Thurber, C. A., and E. A. Walton. 2012. Homesickness and adjustment in university students. *Journal of American College Health* 60(5): 415–419.

Turner, B. J., A. L. Chapman, and B. K. Layden. 2012. Intrapersonal and interpersonal functions of nonsuicidal self-injury: Associations with emotional and social functioning. *Suicide & Life-Threatening Behavior* 42(1): 366–355.

U.S. Food and Drug Administration. 2012. *Medication Guide for Antidepressant Drugs* (http://www.fda.gov/downloads/Drugs/DrugSafety/InformationbyDrugClass/ucm100211.pdf).

Verhaak, P. F., et al. 2009. Receiving treatment for common mental disorders. *General Hospital Psychiatry* 31(1): 46–55.

Williams, D., et al. 2007. Prevalence and distribution of major depressive disorder in African Americans, Caribbean blacks, and non-Hispanic whites. *Archives of General Psychiatry* 64: 305–315.

BEHAVIOR CHANGE STRATEGY
Dealing with Social Anxiety

Shyness is often the result of both high anxiety levels and lack of key social skills. To help overcome shyness, you need to learn to manage your fear of social situations and to develop social skills such as appropriate eye contact, initiating topics in conversations, and maintaining the flow of conversations by asking questions and making appropriate responses.

To reduce your anxiety in social situations, try some of the following strategies:

- Refocus your attention away from the stress reaction you're experiencing and toward the social task at hand. Your nervousness is much less visible than you think.

- Allow a warm-up period for new situations. Realize that you will feel more nervous at first, and take steps to relax and become more comfortable. Refer to the suggestions for deep breathing and other relaxation techniques in Chapter 2.

- If possible, take breaks during anxiety-producing situations. For example, if you're at a party, take a moment to visit the restroom or step outside. Alternate between speaking with good friends and striking up conversations with new acquaintances.

- Practice realistic self-talk. Replace your self-critical thoughts with more supportive ones: "No one else is perfect, and I don't have to be either." "It would have been good if I had a funny story to tell, but the conversation was interesting anyway."

Starting and maintaining conversations can be difficult for shy people, who may feel overwhelmed by their physical stress reaction. If small talk is a problem for you, try the following strategies:

- Introduce yourself early in the conversation. If you tend to forget names, repeat your new acquaintance's name to help fix it in your mind ("Nice to meet you, Amelia").

- Ask questions and look for shared topics of interest. Simple, open-ended questions like "How's your presentation coming along?" or "How do you know our host?" encourage others to carry the conversation for a while and help bring up a variety of subjects.

- Take turns talking, and elaborate on your answers. Simple yes and no answers don't move the conversation along. Try to relate something in your life—a course you're taking or a hobby you have—to something in the other person's life. Match self-disclosure with self-disclosure.

- Have something to say. Expand your mind and become knowledgeable about current events and local or campus news. If you have specialized knowledge about a topic, practice discussing it in ways that both beginners and experts can understand and appreciate.

- If you get stuck for something to say, try giving a compliment ("Great presentation!" or "I love your earrings.") or

performing a social grace (pass the chips or get someone a drink).

- Be an active listener. Reward the other person with your full attention and with regular responses. Make frequent eye contact and maintain a relaxed but alert posture.

At first, your new behaviors will likely make you anxious. Don't give up—things *will* get easier.

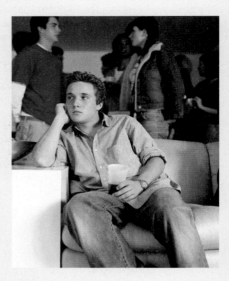

SOURCES: University of Texas at Dallas, Student Counseling Center. 2008 Update. *Self-Help: Overcoming Social Anxiety* (http://www.utdallas.edu/counseling/selfhelp/social-anxiety.html); Carducci, B. J. 2000. *Shyness: A Bold New Approach.* New York: Harper Paperbacks.

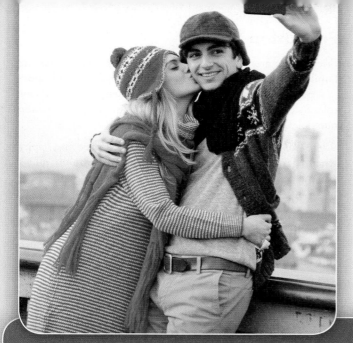

LOOKING AHEAD...

After reading this chapter, you should be able to

- Explain the qualities that help people develop intimate relationships
- Describe different types of love relationships and the stages they often go through
- Identify common challenges of forming and maintaining intimate relationships
- Explain some elements of healthy and productive communication
- List some characteristics of successful families and some potential problems families face

Intimate Relationships and Communication

4

Human beings need social relationships; we cannot thrive as solitary creatures. The human species could not survive if adults didn't cherish and support each other, if we didn't form strong mutual attachments with our infants, and if we didn't create families in which to raise children. Simply put, people need people.

Although people are held together in relationships by a variety of factors, the foundation of many relationships is the ability to both give and receive love. Love in its many forms—romantic, passionate, platonic, parental—is the wellspring from which much of life's meaning and delight flows. In our culture, it binds us together as partners, parents, children, and friends.

Just as important, we also need to develop a healthy relationship to ourselves, which includes the ability to self-soothe, to regulate our emotions, and to be alone with ourselves at times.

DEVELOPING INTIMATE RELATIONSHIPS

People who develop successful intimate relationships believe in themselves and in the people around them. They are willing to give of themselves—to share their ideas, feelings, time, and needs—and to accept what others want to give them.

Self-Concept, Self-Esteem, and Self-Acceptance

The principal element that we all bring to our relationships is our *selves*. To have successful relationships, we must first accept and feel good about ourselves. A positive self-concept and a healthy level of self-esteem help us love and respect others.

As discussed in Chapter 3, the roots of our identity and sense of self can be found in childhood, in the relationships we had with our parents and other family members. As adults, we are more likely to have a sense that we're basically lovable, worthwhile people and that we can trust others if we experienced the following as babies and children:

- We felt loved, valued, accepted, and respected.
- Adults responded to our needs in appropriate ways.
- Adults gave us the freedom to play, explore, and develop a sense of being separate individuals.

These conditions encourage us to develop the sense that we are acceptable and lovable and help us build a basic confidence that aids in navigating life's inevitable challenges. Successfully handling these challenges further bolsters self-acceptance, self-concept, and self-esteem.

Gender Role Another thing we learn in early childhood is *gender role*—the activities, abilities, and characteristics our culture deems appropriate for us based on our sex. In our society, men have traditionally been expected to provide for their families; to be aggressive, competitive, and power-oriented; and to solve problems logically. Women have been expected to take care of home and children; to be cooperative, supportive, and nurturing; and to approach life emotionally and intuitively. More egalitarian gender roles have emerged in our society, but the stereotypes we absorb in childhood can be deeply ingrained.

Attachment   Our ways of relating to others are also rooted in childhood. Some researchers have suggested that our adult styles of loving may be based on the type of **attachment** we established in infancy with our mother, father, siblings, or other primary caregivers. According to this view, people who are secure in their intimate relationships probably had a secure, trusting, mutually satisfying attachment to their mother, father, or other parenting figure. As adults, they find it relatively easy to get close to others. They don't worry about being abandoned or having someone get too close to them. They feel that other people like them and are generally well-intentioned.

People who are clinging and dependent in their relationships may have had an "anxious/ambivalent" attachment. Their parents' inconsistent responses made them unsure that their needs would be met. As adults, they worry whether their partners really love them and will stay with them. They tend to feel that others don't want to get as close as they do. They want to merge completely with another person, which can scare others away.

People who seem to run from relationships may have had an "anxious/avoidant" attachment, in which a parent's engulfing or abandoning responses made them want to escape from his or her sphere of influence. As adults, they feel uncomfortable being close to others. They're distrustful and fearful of becoming dependent. Their partners usually want more intimacy than they do.

Even if people's earliest experiences and relationships were less than ideal, however, they can still establish satisfying relationships in adulthood. In fact, relationships in adolescence and adulthood give us a golden opportunity to work on and through unresolved issues and conflicts from the past.

People can be resilient and flexible. They have the capacity to change their ideas, beliefs, and behaviors. They can learn ways to raise their self-esteem; they can become more trusting, accepting, and appreciative of others; and they can acquire the communication and conflict resolution skills required for maintaining successful relationships. Although it helps to have a good start in life, it may be even more important to begin again, right from where you are. Most important is to be accepting and kind to ourselves as we are in the present and do our best to grow and develop emotionally.

---

attachment   The emotional tie between an infant and his or her caregiver or between two people in an intimate relationship.

TERMS

Friendship

Friendships are the first relationships we form outside the family. The friendships we form in childhood are an important part of our development. Through them, we learn about tolerance, sharing, and trust. Friendships usually include most or all of the following characteristics:

- *Companionship.* Friends are usually relaxed and happy when they're together. They typically have common values and interests and plan to spend time together.

- *Respect.* Friends have a basic respect for each other's humanity and individuality. Good friends respect each other's feelings and opinions and work to resolve their differences without demeaning or insulting each other. They also show their respect by being honest.

- *Acceptance.* Friends accept each other, "warts and all." They feel free to be themselves and express their feelings without fear of ridicule or criticism.

- *Help.* Sharing time, energy, and even material goods is important to friendship. Friends know they can rely on each other in times of need.

- *Trust.* Friends are secure in the knowledge that they will not intentionally hurt each other.

- *Loyalty.* Friends can count on one another. They stand up for each other in both word and deed.

- *Mutuality.* Friends retain their individual identities, but close friendships are characterized by a sense of mutuality—"what affects you affects me." Friends share the ups and downs in each other's lives.

- *Reciprocity.* Friendships are reciprocal. There is give-and-take between friends and the feeling that both share joys and burdens more or less equally over time.

Intimate partnerships are like friendships in many ways, but friendships are usually considered both more stable and longer-lasting than intimate partnerships. Friends are often more accepting and less critical than lovers, probably because their expectations are different.

As important as friendships are, however, the average American's social circle is shrinking. In 2006 sociologists from Duke University and the University of Arizona released details of a study on this issue. According to the study, Americans have fewer close friends than ever before. Most have only two friends they consider close enough to discuss problems with. (Compare this number to 1985, when the average American had three confidants.) The study suggested several reasons for shrinking social circles but focused on the increasing use of technology as a means of communicating with one's friends. The growing use of the Internet, texting, and other electronic means of communication lets people share information quickly and at any time, but the study's authors worried that digital communications actually create distance between friends by allowing them to communicate without being in one another's presence.

A study released in 2009 by the Pew Internet and American Life Project verified this decline in the size of many Americans'

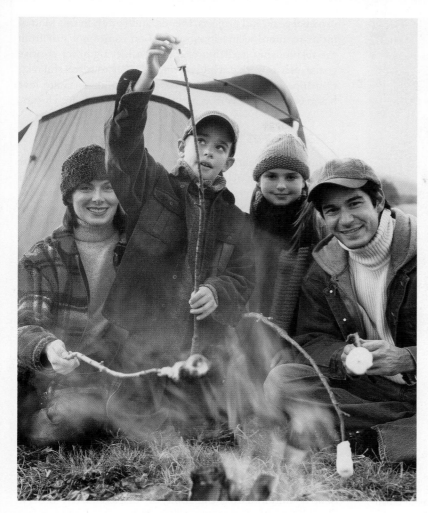

The type and strength of our attachment to our parents can affect other relationships throughout our lives.

For most people, love, sex, and commitment are closely linked ideals in intimate relationships. Love reflects the positive factors that draw people together and sustain them in a relationship. It includes trust, caring, respect, loyalty, interest in the other, and concern for the other's well-being. Sex brings excitement and passion to the relationship. It intensifies the relationship and adds fascination and pleasure.

Commitment, the determination to continue, reflects the stable factors that help maintain the relationship. Responsibility, reliability, and faithfulness are characteristics of commitment. Although love, sex, and commitment are related, they are not necessarily connected. One can exist without the others. Despite the various "faces" of love, sex, and commitment, most of us long for a special relationship that contains them all.

Other elements can be identified as features of love, such as euphoria, preoccupation with the loved one, idealization or devaluation of the loved one, and so on, but these tend to be temporary. These characteristics may include **infatuation,** which will fade or deepen into something more substantial. As relationships progress, the central aspects of love and commitment take on more importance.

Men and women tend to have different views of the relationship between love (intimacy) and sex (passion). Numerous studies have found that men can separate love from sex rather easily, although many men find that their most erotic sexual experiences occur in the context of a love relationship. Women generally view sex from the point of view of a relationship. Some people believe you can have satisfying sex without love—with friends, acquaintances, or strangers. Although sex with love is an important norm in our culture, it is frequently disregarded in practice, as the high incidence of extra-relational affairs attests.

The Pleasure and Pain of Love The experience of intense love has confused and tormented lovers throughout history. They live in a tumultuous state of excitement, subject to wildly fluctuating feelings of joy and despair. They lose their appetite, can't sleep, and can think of nothing but the loved one. Is this happiness? Misery? Both?

The contradictory nature of passionate love can be understood by recognizing that human emotions have two components: physiological arousal and an emotional explanation for

core networks, but it differed from the 2006 study in one important respect. That is, the Pew study refuted the assumption that our social circles are shrinking because of our increasing use of technology. The study showed that among demographically similar people, those who used technology to communicate did not have fewer close friends than those who didn't use the Internet or a cell phone. On the contrary, the study found that technology users had larger and more diverse core discussion networks and were just as involved in their communities as people who did not communicate via the Internet or a cell phone.

Love, Sex, and Intimacy

Love is one of the most basic and profound human emotions. It is a powerful force in all our intimate relationships. Love encompasses opposites: affection and anger, excitement and boredom, stability and change, bonds and freedom. Love does not give us perfect happiness, but it does give our lives meaning.

> QUICK STATS
>
> **6%** of Americans feel that they have no one "especially significant" in their lives.
>
> —Pew Internet & American Life Project, 2009

infatuation An idealizing, obsessive attraction, characterized by a high degree of physical arousal.

TERMS

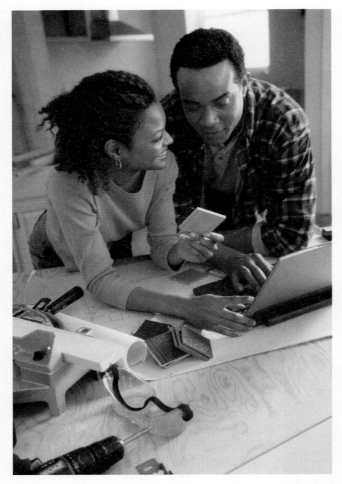

Although passion and physical intimacy often decline with time, other aspects of a relationship—such as commitment—tend to grow as the relationship matures.

the arousal. Love is just one of many emotions accompanied by physiological arousal. Many unpleasant emotions can also generate arousal, such as fear, rejection, frustration, and challenge. Although experiences like attraction and sexual desire are pleasant, extreme excitement is similar to fear and can be unpleasant. For this reason, passionate love may be too intense for some people to enjoy. Over time, the physical intensity and excitement tend to diminish. When this happens, pleasure may actually increase.

The Transformation of Love   All human relationships change over time, and love relationships are no exception. At first love is likely to be characterized by high levels of passion and rapidly increasing intimacy. After a while passion decreases as we become habituated to it and to the person. The diminishing of romance or passionate love is often experienced as a crisis in a relationship. If a more lasting love fails to emerge, the relationship will likely break up.

Unlike passion, however, commitment does not necessarily diminish over time. When intensity diminishes, partners often discover a more enduring love. They can now move from absorption in each other to a relationship that includes

external goals and projects, friends, and family. In this kind of intimate, more secure love, satisfaction comes not just from the relationship itself but also from achieving other creative goals, such as work or child rearing. The key to successful relationships is in transforming passion into an intimate love based on closeness, caring, and the promise of a shared future.

Challenges in Relationships

Many people believe that love naturally makes an intimate relationship easy to begin and maintain, but in fact obstacles arise and challenges occur. Even in the best of circumstances, a loving relationship will be tested. Partners enter a relationship with diverse needs and wants, some of which emerge only at times of change or stress.

Honesty and Openness   It's usually best to be yourself from the start to give both you and your potential partner a chance to find out if you are comfortable with each other's beliefs, interests, and lifestyles. Getting close to another person by sharing thoughts and feelings is emotionally risky, but it is necessary for a relationship to deepen. Take your time, and self-disclose at a slow but steady rate—one that doesn't make you feel too vulnerable or your partner too uncomfortable. Over time, you and your partner will learn more about each other and feel more comfortable sharing.

Emotional Intelligence   An emotionally intelligent person is more able to both give and receive the type of emotional support that many long for in a romantic partner. The key to developing emotional intelligence lies in cultivating the overarching skill of mindfulness—the ability to dispassionately observe thoughts and feelings as they occur. When we are able to note and observe emotions without judging them or immediately acting on them, we can make more measured, wise, and skillful responses to the situation at hand. These skills can be particularly helpful when we are involved in an argument or a conflict with someone with whom we have a close personal relationship.

Mindfulness can be cultivated by paying more attention to the operation of our minds, slowing down our lives enough to make more detailed observations, and staying in the moment as we go about our day-to-day activities. Although we often have limited control over external events, we have a great deal of ability to discipline, focus, and train our minds. Practicing mindfulness and developing emotional intelligence will improve your sense of self and the quality of your relationships.

Unequal or Premature Commitment   Sometimes one person in an intimate partnership becomes more serious about the relationship than the other partner. In this situation, it can be difficult to maintain the partnership without hurting the more serious partner. Sometimes a couple makes a premature commitment, and then one of the partners has second thoughts and wants to break off the relationship. Sometimes both partners begin to realize that something is wrong, but each is afraid to tell the other. Such problems usually can be resolved only by honest and sensitive communication.

Unrealistic Expectations Each partner brings hopes and expectations to a relationship, some of which may be unrealistic, unfair, and ultimately damaging to the relationship. For example, if you believe that love will eliminate all of your problems, you may start to blame your partner for anything that goes wrong in your life. Other unrealistic expectations include the following:

- Expecting your partner to change

- Assuming that your partner has all the same opinions, priorities, interests, and goals as you

- Believing that a relationship will fulfill all of your personal, financial, intellectual, and social needs

Competitiveness If one partner always feels compelled to compete and win, it can detract from the sense of connectedness, interdependence, equality, and mutuality between partners. The same can be said for a perfectionistic need to be right in every instance—to "win" every argument.

If competitiveness is a problem for you, ask yourself if your need to win is more important than your partner's feelings or the future of your relationship. Try noncompetitive activities or an activity where you are a beginner and your partner excels. Accept that your partner's views may be just as valid and important to your partner as your own views are to you.

Balancing Time Together and Apart You may enjoy time together with your partner, but you may also want to spend time alone or with other friends. If you or your partner interpret time apart as rejection or lack of commitment, it can damage the relationship. Talk with your partner about what time apart means and share your feelings about what you expect from the relationship in terms of time together. Consider your partner's feelings carefully, and try to reach a compromise that satisfies both of you.

Differences in expectations about time spent together can mirror differences in ideas about emotional closeness. Any romantic relationship involves giving up some degree of autonomy in order to develop an identity as a couple. But remember that every person is unique and has different needs for distance and closeness in a relationship.

Jealousy Jealousy is the angry, painful response to a partner's real, imagined, or likely involvement with a third person. Some people think that the existence of jealousy proves the existence of love, but jealousy is actually a sign of insecurity or possessiveness.

In its irrational and extreme forms, jealousy can destroy a relationship by its insistent demands and attempts at control. Jealousy is a factor in precipitating violence in dating relationships among both high school and college students, and abusive spouses often use jealousy to justify their violence.

People with a healthy level of self-esteem are less likely to feel jealous. When jealousy occurs in a relationship, it's important for the partners to communicate clearly with each other about their feelings.

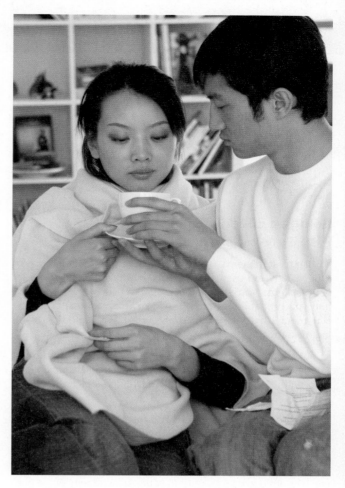

Supportiveness is a sign of commitment and compassion and is an important part of any healthy relationship.

Supportiveness Another key to successful relationships is the ability to ask for and give support. Partners need to know that they can count on each other during difficult times.

Unhealthy Relationships

Everyone should be able to recognize when a relationship is unhealthy. Relatively extreme examples of unhealthy relationships are those that are physically or emotionally abusive or that involve codependency.

Even relationships that are not abusive or codependent can still be unhealthy. If your relationship lacks love and respect and places little value on the time you and your partner have spent together, it may be time to get professional help or to end the partnership. Further, if your relationship is characterized by communication styles that include criticism, contempt, defensiveness, and withdrawal—despite real efforts to repair these destructive patterns—the relationship may not be salvageable.

Spiritual leaders suggest that relationships are unhealthy when you feel that your sense of spontaneity, your potential for inner growth and joy, and your connection to your spiritual life is deadened. There are negative physical and mental

TAKE CHARGE
Guidelines for Effective Communication

Getting Started

- When you want to have a serious discussion with your partner, choose a private place and a time when you won't be interrupted or rushed.

- Face your partner and maintain eye contact. Use nonverbal feedback to show that you are interested and involved.

Being an Effective Speaker

- State your concern or issue as clearly as you can.

- Use "I" statements rather than statements beginning with "you." When you use "I" statements, you take responsibility for your feelings. "You" statements are often blaming or accusatory and will probably get a defensive or resentful response. The statement "I feel unloved," for example, sends a clearer, less blaming message than the statement "You don't love me."

- Focus on a behavior, not the whole person. Be specific about the behavior you like or don't like. Avoid generalizations beginning with "you always" or "you never." Such statements make people feel defensive.

- Make constructive requests. Opening your request with "I would like" keeps the focus on your needs rather than your partner's supposed deficiencies.

- Avoid blaming, accusing, and belittling. Even if you are right, you have little to gain by putting your partner down. When people feel criticized or attacked, they are less able to think rationally or solve problems constructively.

- Ask for action ahead of time, not after the fact. Tell your partner what you would like to have happen in the future; don't wait for him or her to blow it and then express anger or disappointment.

Being an Effective Listener

- Provide appropriate nonverbal feedback (nodding, smiling, making eye contact, and so on).

- Don't interrupt.

- Listen reflectively. Don't judge, evaluate, analyze, or offer solutions (unless asked to do so). Your partner may just need to sort out his or her feelings. By jumping in to "fix" the problem, you may cut off communication.

- Don't give unsolicited advice. Giving advice implies that you know more about what a person needs to do than he or she does; therefore, it often evokes anger or resentment.

- Clarify your understanding of what your partner is saying by restating it in your own words and asking if your understanding is correct. "I think you're saying that you would feel uncomfortable having dinner with my parents and that you'd prefer to meet them in a more casual setting. Is that right?" This type of specific feedback prevents misunderstandings and helps validate the speaker's feelings and message.

- Be sure you are really listening, not off somewhere in your mind rehearsing your reply. Try to tune in to your partner's feelings as well as the words. Accurately reflecting the other person's feelings is often a more powerful way of connecting than just reframing his or her thoughts.

- Let your partner know that you value what he or she is saying and want to understand. Respect for the other person is the cornerstone of effective communication.

---

consequences of being in an unhappy relationship. Although breaking up is painful and difficult, it is ultimately better than living in a toxic relationship.

Ending a Relationship

Even when a couple starts out with the best of intentions, an intimate relationship may not last. Some breakups occur quickly following direct action by one or both partners, but many others occur over an extended period as the couple goes through a cycle of separating and reconciling.

Ending an intimate relationship is usually difficult and painful. Both partners may feel attacked and abandoned, but feelings of distress are likely to be more acute for the rejected partner. If you are involved in a breakup, the following suggestions may help make the ending easier:

- **Give the relationship a fair chance before breaking up**

- **Be fair and honest**

- **Be tactful and compassionate**

- **If you are the rejected person, give yourself time to resolve your anger and pain**

- **Recognize the value in the experience**

Use the recovery period following a breakup for self-renewal. Redirect more of your attention to yourself, and reconnect with people and areas of your life that may have been neglected as a result of the relationship. Time will help heal the pain of the loss of the relationship.

Finally, be aware of the tendency or impulse to "rebound" quickly into another relationship. Although a new relationship may mute the pain of a breakup, forming a relationship in order to avoid feeling pain is not a good strategy. Too often, rebound relationships fail because they were designed to be "life boats" or because one or both of the partners is not truly ready to be close to someone else again.

COMMUNICATION

The key to developing and maintaining any type of intimate relationship is good communication. Miscommunication creates frustration and distances us from our friends and partners.

Nonverbal Communication

Even when we're silent, we're communicating. We send messages when we look at someone or look away, lean forward or sit back, smile or frown. Especially important forms of nonverbal communication are touch, eye contact, and proximity. If someone we're talking to touches our hand or arm, looks into our eyes, and leans toward us when we talk, we get the message that the person is interested in us and cares about what we're saying. If a person keeps looking around the room while we're talking or takes a step backward, we get the impression the person is uninterested or wants to end the conversation.

The ability to interpret nonverbal messages correctly is important to the success of relationships. It's also important, when sending messages, to make sure our body language agrees with our words. When our verbal and nonverbal messages don't correspond, we send a mixed message.

Digital Communication

Recent years have brought about an enormous surge in digital communication—through texting, tweeting, social networking websites, Skype, e-mail, mobile phones, blogging, and instant messaging. These communication channels enable us to communicate more rapidly, but some experts question whether this capability is affecting interpersonal relations and possibly even affecting our ability to relate to others in person. But researchers disagree on the effect that these means of communication have on human relationships as a whole. While some worry that an increase in digital communication means a corresponding decrease in face-to-face contact, others are fascinated by the possibilities for making connections with people whom we might never have an opportunity to meet face-to-face.

> ### QUICK STATS
>
> **32.2%** of college students say their intimate relationships have been traumatic or hard to handle at least once in the past year.
>
> —American College Health Association, 2011

Communication Skills

Three keys to good communication in relationships are self-disclosure, listening, and feedback:

- *Self-disclosure* involves revealing personal information that we ordinarily wouldn't reveal because of the risk involved. It usually increases feelings of closeness and moves the relationship to a deeper level of intimacy. Friends often disclose the most to each other, sharing feelings, experiences, hopes, and disappointments. Married couples sometimes share less because they think they already know everything about each other.

- *Listening* requires that we spend more time and energy trying to fully understand another person's "story" and less time judging, evaluating, blaming, advising, analyzing, or trying to control. Empathy, warmth, respect, and genuineness are qualities of skillful listeners. Attentive listening encourages friends or partners to share more and, in turn, to be attentive listeners. To connect with other people and develop real emotional intimacy, listening is essential.

- *Feedback*, a constructive response to another's self-disclosure, is the third key to good communication. Giving positive feedback means acknowledging that the friend's or partner's feelings are valid—no matter how upsetting or troubling—and offering self-disclosure in response. If, for example, your partner discloses unhappiness about your relationship, it is more constructive to say that you're concerned or saddened by that and want to hear more about it than to get angry, to blame, to try to inflict pain, or to withdraw. Self-disclosure and feedback can open the door to change, whereas other responses block communication and change. (For tips on improving your skills, see the box "Guidelines for Effective Communication.")

Gender and Communication

Some of the difficulties people encounter in relationships can be traced to common gender differences in communication. In part because of the way we've been socialized, men and women generally approach conversation and communication differently. Men tend to use conversation in a *competitive* way, perhaps hoping to establish dominance in relationships. When male conversations are over, men often find themselves in a one-up or a one-down position. Women tend to use conversation in a more *affiliative* way, perhaps

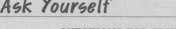

Ask Yourself

QUESTIONS FOR CRITICAL THINKING AND REFLECTION

Have you ever ended an intimate relationship? If so, how did you handle it? How did you feel after the breakup? How did the breakup affect your former partner? Did the experience help you in other relationships?

hoping to establish friendships. They negotiate various degrees of closeness, seeking to give and receive support. Men tend to talk more—though without disclosing more—and listen less. Women tend to use good listening skills such as eye contact, frequent nodding, focused attention, and asking relevant questions.

Although these are generalized patterns, they can translate into problems in specific conversations. Even when a man and a woman are talking about the same subject, their unconscious goals may be very different. The woman may be looking for understanding and closeness, while the man may be trying to demonstrate his competence by giving advice and solving problems. Both styles are valid; the problem comes when differences in style result in poor communication and misunderstanding.

Sometimes communication is not the problem in a relationship—the partners understand each other all too well. The problem is that they're unable or unwilling to change or compromise. Although good communication can't salvage a bad relationship, it does enable couples to see their differences and make more informed decisions.

> Although **good communication can't salvage a bad relationship**, it enables couples to see their differences and make more informed decisions.

Conflict and Conflict Resolution

Conflict is natural in intimate relationships. No matter how close two people become, they still remain separate individuals with their own needs, desires, past experiences, and ways of seeing the world. In fact, the closer the relationship, the more differences and the more opportunities for conflict there will be.

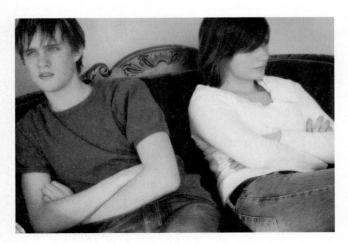

Conflict is an inevitable part of any intimate relationship. Couples need to develop constructive ways of resolving conflicts in order to maintain a healthy relationship.

Conflict itself isn't dangerous to a relationship. In fact, it may indicate that the relationship is growing. But if it isn't handled constructively, conflict can damage—and ultimately destroy—the relationship.

Conflict is often accompanied by anger—a natural emotion, but one that can be difficult to handle. If we express anger aggressively, we risk creating distrust, fear, and distance. If we act it out without thinking things through, we can cause the conflict to escalate. If we suppress anger, it turns into resentment and hostility. The best way to handle anger in a relationship is to recognize it as a symptom of something that requires attention and needs to be changed. When angry, partners should exercise restraint so as not to become abusive. It is important to express anger skillfully and not in a way that is out of proportion to the issue at hand.

The sources of conflict for couples change over time but primarily revolve around the basic tasks of living together: dividing the housework, handling money, spending time together, and so on. Sexual interaction is also a source of disagreement for many couples.

The following strategies can be helpful when negotiating with a partner:

1. *Clarify the issue.* Take responsibility for thinking through your feelings and discovering what's really bothering you. Agree that one partner will speak first and have the chance to speak fully while the other listens. Then reverse the roles. Try to understand your partner's position fully by repeating what you've heard and asking questions to clarify or elicit more information. Agree to talk only about the topic at hand and not get distracted by other issues. Sum up what your partner has said.

2. *Find out what each person wants.* Ask your partner to express his or her desires. Don't assume you know what your partner wants, and don't speak for him or her.

3. *Determine how you both can get what you want.* Brainstorm to come up with a variety of options.

4. *Decide how to negotiate.* Work out a plan for change. For example, one partner will do one task and the other will do another task. Be willing to compromise, and avoid trying to "win."

5. *Solidify the agreements.* Go over the plan and write it down, if necessary, to ensure that you both understand and agree to it.

6. *Review and renegotiate.* Decide on a time frame for trying out your plan, and set a time to discuss how it's working. Make adjustments as needed.

To resolve conflicts, partners have to feel safe in voicing disagreements. They have to trust that the discussion won't get out of control, that they won't be abandoned by the other, and that the partner won't take advantage of their vulnerability. Partners should follow some basic ground rules when they argue, such as avoiding ultimatums, resisting the urge to give the silent treatment, refusing to "hit below the belt," and not using sex to smooth over disagreements.

When you argue, maintain a spirit of goodwill and avoid being harshly critical or contemptuous. If you and your partner find that you argue again and again over the same issue, it may be better to stop trying to resolve that problem and instead come to accept the differences between you.

PAIRING AND SINGLEHOOD

Although most people eventually marry or commit to a partner, everyone spends some time as a single person, and nearly all people make some attempt, consciously or unconsciously, to find a partner. Intimate relationships are as important for singles as for couples.

Choosing a Partner

Most men and women select partners for long-term relationships through a fairly predictable process, although they may not be consciously aware of it. First attraction is based on easily observable characteristics: looks, dress, social status, and reciprocated interest. Most people pair with someone who

- Lives in the same geographic area
- Is from a similar ethnic and socioeconomic background

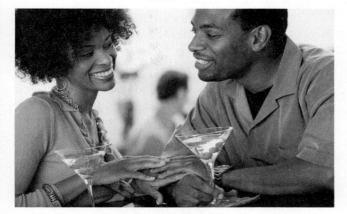

Regardless of an individual's intentions, physical attraction usually plays a strong role in the initial choosing of a partner. People tend to gravitate toward others who share similar characteristics, such as appearance, ethnicity, education, and socioeconomic background.

- Has similar educational attainment
- Lives a similar lifestyle
- Is like them in terms of physical attractiveness

Once the euphoria of romantic love winds down, personality traits and behaviors become more significant factors in how the partners view each other. The emphasis shifts to basic values and future aspirations regarding career, family, and children. At some point, they decide whether the relationship feels viable and is worthy of their continued commitment.

Perhaps the most important question for potential mates to ask is, "How much do we have in common?" Although differences add interest to a relationship, similarities increase the chances of a relationship's success. Differences can affect a relationship in the areas of values, religion, ethnicity, attitudes toward sexuality and gender roles, socioeconomic status, familiarity with each other's culture, and interactions with the extended family. But acceptance and communication skills go a long way toward making a relationship work, no matter how different the partners.

> The most important question for potential mates to ask is, **"How much do we have in common?"**

Dating

Many people find romantic partners through some form of dating. They narrow the field through a process of getting to know each other. Dating often revolves around a mutually enjoyable activity, such as seeing a movie or having dinner. Casual dating may then evolve into steady or exclusive dating, then engagement, and finally marriage.

In recent years, traditional dating has given way to a more casual form of getting together in groups. Two people may begin to spend more time together, but often in the group context. If sexual involvement develops, it is more likely to be based on friendship, respect, and common interests than on expectations related to gender roles. In this model, mate selection may progress from getting together to living together to marriage.

Among some teenagers and young adults, dating has been all but supplanted by hooking up—casual sexual activity without any relationship commitment. For more about this trend, see the box "Hooking Up."

Online Relationships

Online dating sites like Match.com and eHarmony have become incredibly popular in recent years, especially among young adults seeking an intimate partner or new friends. Connecting with people online has advantages and drawbacks. It allows people to communicate in a relaxed way, to try out different personas, and to share things they might not share when face-to-face with family or friends. It's easier to

Relationship sites also remove an important and powerful source of information from the process: chemistry and in-person intuition. Much of our communication is transmitted through body language and tone, which aren't obvious in text messages and can't be fully captured even by web cams and microphones. Trust your feelings about the process of the relationship. Are you revealing more than the other person? Is there a balance in the amount of time spent talking by each of you? Is the other person respecting your boundaries? Just as in real-life dating, online relationships require you to use common sense and to trust your instincts.

If you pursue an online relationship, the following strategies can help you have a positive experience and stay safe:

• To improve your chances of meeting people interested in you as a person, avoid sexually oriented websites. Some sites that seem like dating sites are actually used for "hooking up"—that is, arranging meetings for casual sex—rather than for building relationships. Inspect each site thoroughly before registering or providing any information about yourself. If you aren't comfortable with a site's content or purpose, close your web browser and clear out its cache and its store of cookies. (If you don't know how to do this, check your browser's help system for instructions.)

• Know what you are looking for as well as what you can offer someone else. If you are looking for a relationship, make that fact clear. Find out the other person's intentions.

• Dating sites let users upload photos, but your photo can be downloaded by anyone, distributed to other individuals or sites, and even altered. Don't post photos unless you are completely comfortable with the potential consequences.

• Don't give out personal information, including your real full name, school, or place of employment, until you feel sure that you are giving the information to someone who is trustworthy. Do not give out your contact information over the Internet.

• Set up a second e-mail account for sending and receiving dating-related e-mails. Don't use your primary e-mail account for dealing with relationship websites.

• If someone does not respond to a message, don't take it personally. There are many reasons why a person may not pursue the connection. Don't send messages to an unresponsive person; doing so could lead to an accusation of stalking. If someone stops responding, drop the interaction completely.

• Before deciding whether to meet an online friend in person, arrange to talk over the phone a few times.

• Don't agree to meet someone face-to-face unless you feel completely comfortable about it. Always meet initially in a very public place—a museum, a coffee shop, or a restaurant—not in private, and especially not at your home. Bring along a friend to increase your safety, and let others know where you will be.

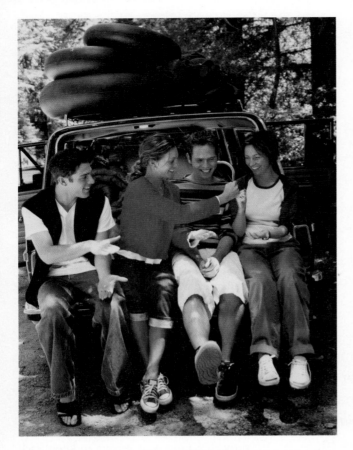

For many college students today, group activities have replaced dating as a way to meet and get to know potential partners.

put yourself out there without too much investment; you can get to know someone from the comfort of your own home, set your own pace, and start and end relationships at any time. With millions of singles using dating sites that let them describe exactly what they are seeking, the Internet can increase a person's chance of finding a good match.

There are drawbacks, however, to meeting people online. Too often participants misrepresent themselves, pretending to be very different—older or younger or even of a different sex—than they really are. Investing time and emotional resources in such relationships can be painful. In rare cases, online romances become dangerous or even deadly (see Chapter 16 for information on cyberstalking).

Because people have greater freedom to reveal only what they want to, users should also be aware of a greater tendency to idealize online partners—setting themselves up for later disappointment. If your online friend seems perfect, take that as a warning sign. Conversely, looking for partners online can be like shopping—all the choices may increase your tendency to search for perfection or find fault quickly and prevent you from giving people a chance. Keep your expectations realistic.

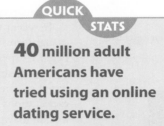

QUICK STATS

40 million adult Americans have tried using an online dating service.
—Statistic Brain, 2012

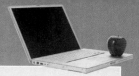

A current trend among teenagers, young adults, and college students is *hooking up*—having casual sexual encounters with acquaintances or strangers with no commitment or invest- ment in a relationship. The sexual activity can be anything from kissing to intercourse, but the key element is the lack of emotional intimacy. Although casual sex is not new, the differ- ence today is that hooking up seems to be the main form of sexual activity for many people, as opposed to sexual activity within a relationship. Some data indicate that more than 80% of college students have had at least one hookup experience. If dating occurs at all, it happens after people have had sex and become a couple.

Hooking up most likely has its roots in the changing social and sexual patterns of the 1960s. Since then, changes in college policies have contributed to the shift, such as the move away from colleges acting *in loco parentis* (in the place of parents), the trend toward coed dorms, and the increase in the percentage of women in student populations and the decreased availability of men. This behavior addresses the desire for "instant intimacy," but also protects the participants from the risk or responsibility of emotional involvement.

Because hooking up is often fueled by alcohol, it is associated with sexual risk taking and negative health effects, including the risk of acquiring a sexually transmitted disease. In 2007, for ex- ample, young adults aged 15 to 24 had rates of chlamydia that were 4 to 5.5 times the overall incidence rate for the general population, according to the CDC. Hooking up can also have emotional and mental health consequences, including sexual re- gret, negative emotional reactions, psychological distress, de- pression, and anxiety. Women are more likely to suffer these reactions after hooking up, but men experience them too. Bio- logical anthropologists suggest that having sex—even casual sex—sets off hormones that cause feelings of bonding and at- tachment, which are inevitably thwarted in a hookup.

On some campuses, a backlash against hooking up has taken place. In some cases, individuals are deciding they don't want to be part of the hookup culture. In other cases, groups and organi- zations have formed to call for a return to traditional dating or at least some middle ground between dating and hooking up that doesn't have the potential to cause physical and emotional harm. The existence of alternative social and sexual norms can help students think twice about their sexual activities.

SOURCES: Downing-Matibag, T. M., and Geisenger, B. 2009. Hooking up and sexual risk taking among college students: A health belief model perspective. *Qualitative Health Research* 19(9): 1196–1209; Bachtel, M. 2009 Is dating really dead? Emerging evidence on the college hookup culture and health issues. *Action Newsletter, American College Health Association* 49(2): 16–18; Chen, S. 2010. No hooking up, no sex for some coeds (http://www.cnn.com/2010/LIVING/04/19/college.anti.hookup.culture/index.html?hpt=Sbin).

If you pursue online relationships, don't let them interfere with your other personal relationships and social activities. Online dating can become addictive. To protect your emotional and personal wellness, use the Internet to widen your circle of friends, not shrink it.

Living Together

According to the U.S. Census Bureau, about 5.4 million opposite-sex couples and 700,000 same-sex couples live together in the United States. The Human Rights Campaign, however, estimates that the number of same-sex couples in the United States is closer to 1.6 million. Living together, or **cohabita- tion,** is one of the most rapid and dramatic social changes that has ever occurred in our society. It seems to be gaining acceptance as part of the normal mate selection process. By age 30, about half of all men and women will have cohabited. Cohabitation provides many of the benefits of marriage:

> **QUICK STATS**
>
> **Cohabitating couples have a 51% chance of marrying after three years together.**
>
> —CDC, 2010

companionship; a setting for an enjoyable and meaningful relationship; a chance to de- velop greater intimacy through learning, compromising, and sharing; a satisfying sex life; and a way to save on living costs.

Living together has certain advantages over marriage. For one thing, it can give the partners a greater sense of autonomy. Not bound by the social rules and expectations that are part of the institution of marriage, partners may find it easier to keep their identities and more of their independence. Cohabitation doesn't incur the same obliga- tions as marriage. If things don't work out, the partners may find it easier to leave a relationship that hasn't been legally sanctioned.

But living together has some drawbacks, too. In most cases, the legal protections of marriage are absent, such as health insurance benefits and property and inheritance rights. These considerations can be particularly serious if the couple has children. Couples may feel social or family pressure to marry or otherwise change their living arrangements, espe- cially if they have young children. The general trend, however, is toward legitimizing nonmarital partnerships; for example, some employers, communities, and states now extend bene- fits to unmarried domestic partners.

> **cohabitation** Living together in a sexual relationship without being married.   **TERMS**

Although many people choose cohabitation as a kind of trial marriage, unmarried partnerships tend to be less stable than marriages. A 2010 survey conducted by the National Center for Health Statistics revealed that cohabitation is much less likely than marriage to survive the one-, three-, and five-year milestones. There is little evidence that cohabitation before marriage leads to happier or longer-lasting marriages. In fact, some studies have found slightly less marital satisfaction and slightly higher divorce rates among couples who cohabited before marrying.

Same-Sex Partnerships

Regardless of **sexual orientation,** most people look for love in a committed relationship. A person whose sexual orientation is lesbian, gay, or bisexual (LGB) may be involved in a same-sex (**homosexual**) relationship. Same-sex couples have many similarities with **heterosexual** couples (those who seek members of the opposite sex). According to one study, most gay men and lesbians have experienced at least one long-term relationship with a single partner. Like any intimate relationship, same-sex partnerships provide intimacy, passion, and security.

Same-sex partnerships tend to be more egalitarian (equal) and less organized around traditional gender roles. Same-sex couples put greater emphasis on partnership than on role assignment. Domestic tasks are shared or split, and both partners usually support themselves financially.

Another difference between heterosexual and homosexual relationships is that same-sex partners often have to deal with societal hostility or ambivalence toward their relationship, in contrast to the societal approval and rights given to heterosexual couples (see the box "Same-Sex Marriage and Civil Unions"). *Homophobia,* which is fear or hatred of homosexuals, can be obvious, as in the case of violence or discrimination, or subtle, such as how same-sex couples are portrayed in the media. Because of societal disapproval, community resources and support may be more important for same-sex couples than for heterosexuals as a source of identity and social support.

People with diverse sexual orientations and gender identities are often grouped together in the category "LGBT," "LGBTQ," or "LGBTQI," where T is for transgender, Q is for questioning or queer, and I is for intersex. Transgender individuals—people whose biological sex doesn't match their gender identity—and intersex individuals—people born with ambiguous genitals—may be heterosexual, homosexual, or bisexual, or they may feel that current definitions of sexual orientation and gender are too narrow to apply to them.

Singlehood

Despite the popularity of marriage, a significant and growing number of adults in our society have never been married— more than 116 million single individuals. The largest group of unmarried adults have never been married (Figure 4.1).

Several factors contribute to the growing number of single people. One is the changing view of singlehood, which is increasingly being viewed as a legitimate alternative to marriage. Education and careers are delaying the age at which young people are marrying. The median age for marriage is now 28.2 years for men and 26.1 years for women. More young people are living with their parents as they complete their education, seek jobs, or strive for financial independence. Many other single people live together without being married. Gay people who would marry their partners if they were legally permitted to do so are counted among the single population. High divorce rates mean more singles, and people who have experienced divorce may have more negative attitudes about marriage and more positive attitudes about singlehood.

Being single, however, does not mean living without the benefit of close relationships. Single people date, enjoy active and fulfilling social lives, and have a variety of sexual experiences

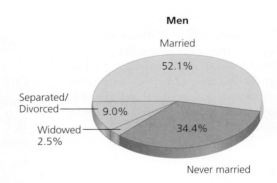

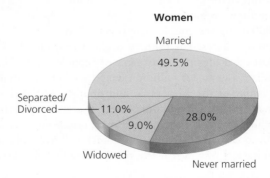

FIGURE 4.1   Marital status of the U.S. population aged 15 years and older, 2011.

SOURCE: U.S. Census Bureau. 2012. *America's Families and Living Arrangements, 2011* (http://www.census.gov/population/www/socdemo/hh-fam/cps2011.html).

sexual orientation   A consistent pattern of emotional and sexual attraction based on biological sex; it exists along a continuum that ranges from exclusive heterosexuality (attraction to people of the other sex) through bisexuality (attraction to people of both sexes) to exclusive homosexuality (attraction to people of one's own sex).

homosexual   Emotional and sexual attraction to people of one's own sex.

heterosexual   Emotional and sexual attraction to people of the other sex.

TERMS

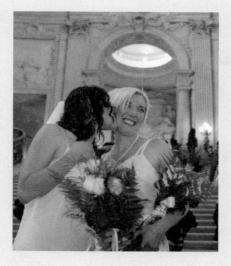

Marriage is an institution defined by state and federal statutes that confer legal and economic rights and responsibilities on every married couple. The U.S. General Accountability Office says more than 1000 federal laws make distinctions based on marriage. Marital status affects many aspects of life, such as Social Security benefits, federal tax status, inheritance, and medical decision making.

The push for legal recognition of same-sex partnerships has gone on for decades. Supporters of same-sex marriage rights, however, have met opposition at the local, state, and federal levels, in both the public and private sectors.

The majority of states and the federal government have passed laws and amendments that effectively ban same-sex marriage. The federal Defense of Marriage Act (DOMA), enacted in 1996, defines marriage as the legal union between one man and one woman and refuses federal recognition of same-sex marriages. It also allows states to refuse to recognize same-sex marriages and civil unions performed in other states or countries. (Such action might otherwise be in violation of the Constitution's provision that each state give "full faith and credit" to the laws of other states.)

In 2009, a bill called the Respect for Marriage Act was introduced in the U.S. House of Representatives. This bill would have repealed the Defense of Marriage Act and entitled legally married same-sex couples to the same benefits of marriage enjoyed by heterosexual couples. It would also have assured married same-sex couples that their federal rights would follow them if they moved to another state where same-sex marriage was not approved. The bill failed to make it through Congress in 2009, and it met the same fate again when reintroduced in 2011. However, efforts to repeal the Defense of Marriage Act continue in both houses of Congress.

Another proposed piece of federal legislation, called the Domestic Partnership Benefits and Obligations act, would extend the same benefits to domestic partners of federal civilian employees as those offered to employees' spouses. These benefits would include participa-

tion in retirement programs, compensation for work-related injuries, and life and health insurance benefits. Such benefits would be available to both same- and opposite-sex domestic partners of federal employees. As with the Respect for Marriage Act, this piece of legislation was reintroduced in the 111th Congress and is still pending.

As of early 2012, the status of same-sex marriage and civil union laws was as follows in the United States:

• Most states had enacted their own DOMAs and/or passed state constitutional amendments that ban same-sex marriages and/or civil unions. Most of these states further refuse to recognize same-sex marriages from other states.

• New York, Connecticut, Iowa, Massachusetts, New Hampshire, Vermont, and the District of Columbia issue marriage licenses to same-sex couples.

• Bills legalizing same-sex marriages had been passed or put forward in Washington, New Jersey, Maryland, and California. Each of those bills, however, was the subject of a court battle or a public referendum and so had not gone into effect.

• Several states now provide some or all state-level spousal rights to same-sex couples. The type of union and scope of rights vary from state to state.

• A growing number of municipalities and private corporations now extend

health insurance coverage and other benefits to the same-sex spouses and domestic partners of their gay and lesbian employees.

Opponents of civil unions and same-sex marriage offer several arguments against such unions. For example, opponents claim that the purpose of marriage is to procreate, that the Bible forbids same-sex unions, that homosexuals are seeking special rights, that same-sex unions are bad for children and families, and that most Americans oppose such unions. (Many recent polls show that most Americans oppose legalizing same-sex marriage, but a growing number support civil unions.) The primary argument, however, is that same-sex marriage undermines the sanctity and validity of marriage as it is traditionally understood and thus undermines society. Rules and restrictions on who can marry preserve the value of the institution of marriage, according to this view. The underlying assumption of this position is that homosexual behavior is a choice and that people can change their orientation, though the process may be difficult.

Proponents of civil unions and same-sex marriage believe that sexual orientation is outside the control of the individual and results from genetic and environmental factors that create an unchangeable orientation. The issue of same-sex union is then seen as one of basic civil rights, in which a group is being denied rights—to publicly express their commitment to one another, to provide security for their children, and to receive the legal and economic benefits afforded to married heterosexual couples—on the basis of something as unalterable as skin color.

Opponents and proponents of same-sex marriage agree that marriage is healthy for both men and women and is the main social institution promoting family values; both sides see this assertion as supportive of their position. What remains to be seen is how society in general is going to view same-sex marriage in the future—as a furthering of American values or as an attack on them.

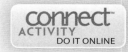

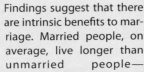
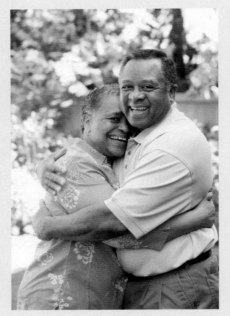

Findings suggest that there are intrinsic benefits to marriage. Married people, on average, live longer than unmarried people—whether single, divorced, or widowed—and they score higher on measures of mental health. They have a lower prevalence of headaches, low-back pain, inactivity, and psychological distress. Married people consistently report being happier than unmarried people.

The benefits of intimate relationships have been demonstrated for a range of conditions: People with strong social support are less likely to catch colds. They recover better from heart attacks, live longer with heart disease, and have higher survival rates for certain cancers. Married men with prostate cancer live significantly longer than those who are single, divorced, or widowed. Women in satisfying marriages are less likely to develop risk factors for cardiovascular diseases than unmarried or unhappily married women. People who never marry have a higher chance of dying prematurely than people who have been divorced, separated, or widowed.

What is it about marriage that supports wellness? Some studies suggest that partners may encourage and reinforce healthy habits, such as exercising, eating right, and seeing a physician when needed. In times of illness, a loving partner can give practical help and emotional support. Feeling loved, esteemed, and valued brings comfort in times of vulnerability, reduces anxiety, and mitigates the damaging effects of stress and social isolation.

Although good relationships may help people stay well, bad relationships may have the opposite effect. The impact of relationship quality on health may be partly explained by its effects on the immune system: A study of married couples whose fighting escalated to criticism and name-calling found them to have weaker immune responses than couples whose arguments were more civil. Hostile couples need more time for injuries to heal; their systems tend to contain higher levels of inflammatory agents (such as cortisol), which have been linked to long-term illness. High marital stress is linked with risky lifestyle choices and nonadherence to medical regimens. Unhappy marriages are associated with risk factors for heart disease, such as depression, hostility, and anger.

Marriage, of course, isn't the only support system available. If you have supportive people in your life, you are likely to enjoy better physical and emotional health than if you feel isolated and alone. So when you start planning lifestyle changes to improve your health and well-being, don't forget to nurture your relationships with family and friends. Strong relationships are powerful medicine.

connect
ACTIVITY
DO IT ONLINE

---

and relationships. Other advantages of being single include more opportunities for personal and career development without concern for family obligations and more freedom and control in making life choices. Disadvantages include loneliness and a lack of companionship, as well as economic hardships (mainly for single women). Single men and women alike experience some discrimination and often are pressured to get married.

Nearly everyone has at least one episode of being single in adult life, whether prior to marriage, between marriages, following divorce or the death of a spouse, or for one's entire life. How enjoyable and valuable this single time is depends on several factors, including how deliberately the person has chosen it; how satisfied the person is with his or her social relationships, standard of living, and job; how comfortable the person feels when alone; and how resourceful and energetic the person is about creating an interesting and fulfilling life.

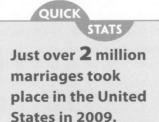

QUICK STATS

Just over 2 million marriages took place in the United States in 2009.

—National Center for Health Statistics, 2010

MARRIAGE

The majority of Americans marry at some time in their lives. Marriage continues to remain popular because it satisfies several basic needs. There are many important social, moral, economic, and political aspects of marriage, all of which have changed over the years. In the past people married mainly for practical reasons, such as raising children or forming an economic unit. Today people marry more for personal, emotional reasons.

The Benefits of Marriage

The primary functions and benefits of marriage are those of any intimate relationship: affection, personal affirmation, companionship, sexual fulfillment, and emotional growth. Marriage also provides a setting in which to raise children, although an increasing number of couples choose to remain childless, and people can also choose to raise children without being married. Marriage is also important for providing for the future. By committing themselves to the relationship, people establish themselves with lifelong companions as well as some insurance for their later years.

Research shows that good marriages have myriad positive effects on individuals' health. (See the box "Are Intimate Relationships Good for Your Health?")

Issues in Marriage

Although we might like to believe otherwise, love is not enough to make a successful marriage. Couples have to be strong and successful in their relationship before getting married, because relationship problems will be magnified rather than solved by marriage. The following relationship characteristics appear to be the best predictors of a happy marriage:

- The partners have realistic expectations about their relationship.
- Each feels good about the personality of the other.
- They communicate well.
- They have effective ways of resolving conflicts.
- They agree on religious/ethical values.
- They have an egalitarian role relationship.
- They have a good balance of individual versus joint interests and leisure activities.

Once married, couples must provide each other with emotional support, negotiate and establish marital roles, establish domestic and career priorities, handle their finances, make sexual adjustments, manage boundaries and relationships with their extended family, and participate in the larger community.

Marital roles and responsibilities have undergone profound changes over time. Many couples no longer accept traditional role assumptions, such as that the husband is solely responsible for supporting the family and the wife is solely responsible for domestic work. Many husbands share domestic tasks, and many wives work outside the home. In fact, over 50% of married women are in the labor force, including women with babies under one year of age. Although women still take most of the responsibility for home and children even when they work and although men still suffer more job-related stress and health problems than women do, the trend is toward an equalization of responsibilities in the home.

The Role of Commitment

Coping with all these challenges requires that couples be committed to remaining in their relationships through the inevitable ups and downs. They need to be tolerant of each other's imperfections and keep their perspective and sense of

> To many people, **commitment is a more important goal** than living together or marriage.

humor. Commitment is based on conscious choice rather than on feelings, which, by their very nature, are transitory. Commitment is a promise of a shared future—a promise to be together, come what may. Committed partners put effort and energy into the relationship, no matter how they feel. They take time to attend to their partners, give compliments, and deal with conflict when necessary. Commitment has become an important concept in recent years. To many people, commitment is a more important goal than living together or marriage.

Separation and Divorce

Divorce is fairly common in the United States (Figure 4.2). Those who have never experienced divorce personally—either their own or that of their parents—almost certainly have friends or relatives who have. The high rate of divorce in the United States may reflect our extremely high expectations

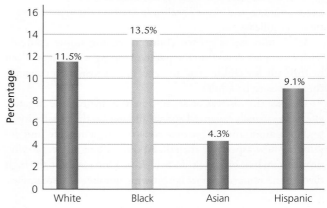

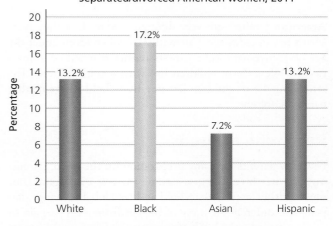

FIGURE 4.2 Percentage of separated and divorced Americans, 2011.

SOURCE: U.S. Census Bureau. 2012. *America's Families and Living Arrangements, 2011* (http://www.census.gov/population/www/socdemo/hh-fam/cps2011.html).

for emotional fulfillment and satisfaction in marriage. It may also indicate that our culture no longer embraces the permanence of marriage.

The process of divorce usually begins with an emotional separation. Often one partner is unhappy and looks beyond the relationship for other forms of validation. Dissatisfaction increases until the unhappy partner decides he or she can no longer stay. Physical separation follows, although it may take some time for the relationship to be over emotionally.

Except for the death of a spouse or family member, divorce is the greatest stress-producing event in life. Research shows that divorced women are more likely to develop heart disease than married, remarried, or widowed women. Both men and women experience turmoil, depression, and lowered self-esteem during and after divorce. People experience separation distress and loneliness for about a year and then begin a recovery period of one to three years. During this time they gradually construct a postdivorce identity, along with a new pattern of life. Most people are surprised by how long it takes to recover from divorce.

Children are especially vulnerable to the trauma of divorce, and sometimes counseling is appropriate to help them adjust to the changes in their lives. However, research has found that children who spend substantial time with both parents are usually better adjusted than those in sole custody arrangements and are as well-adjusted as their peers from intact families.

In certain cases, grown children leaving home coincide with a couple's decision to separate. Coping with divorce can be difficult for children at any age, even those who consider themselves to be adults.

Despite the distress of separation and divorce, the negative effects are usually balanced sooner or later by the possibility of finding a more suitable partner, constructing a new life, and developing new aspects of the self. About 75% of all people who divorce remarry, often within five years. One result of the high divorce and remarriage rate is a growing number of stepfamilies.

FAMILY LIFE

American families are very different today than they were even a few decades ago. Currently 69% of children under the age of 18 live with both parents (either married or unmarried), while 27% of children live with a single parent. The remaining 4% of children live in a household where neither parent is present.

Becoming a Parent

Few new parents have any preparation for the job of parenting, yet they literally must assume the role overnight. They must quickly learn how to hold and feed a baby, change diapers, and differentiate a cry of hunger from a cry of pain or fear. No wonder the birth of the first child is one of the most stressful transitions for any couple.

Even couples with an egalitarian relationship before their first child is born find that their marital roles become more traditional with the arrival of the new baby. The father typically becomes the primary provider and protector, and the mother typically becomes the primary nurturer. Most research indicates that mothers have to make greater changes in their lives than fathers do. Although men today spend more time caring for their infants than ever before, women still take the ultimate responsibility for the baby. Women are usually the ones who make job changes, either quitting work or reducing work hours in order to stay home with the baby for several months or more. Many mothers juggle the multiple roles of mother, homemaker, and employer/employee and feel guilty that they never have enough time to do justice to any of these roles.

Parenting

Sometimes being a parent is a source of unparalleled pleasure and pride—the first smile at you, the first word, the first home run. But at other times parenting can seem like an overwhelming responsibility.

Most parents worry about their ability to raise a healthy, responsible, and well-adjusted child. Parents may wonder about the long-term impact of each decision they make on their child's well-being and personality. According to parenting experts, no one action or decision (within limits) will determine a child's personality or development. Instead the *parenting style*, or overall approach to parenting, is most important. Parenting styles vary according to the levels of two characteristics of the parents:

- *Demandingness* encompasses the use of discipline and supervision, the expectation that children act responsibly and maturely, and the direct reaction to disobedience.

- *Responsiveness* refers to a parent's warmth and intent to facilitate independence and self-confidence in a child by being supportive, connected, and understanding of the child's needs.

Several parenting styles have been identified. Each style emerges according to the parents' balance of demandingness and responsiveness. Here are some examples:

- *Authoritarian* parents are high in demandingness and low in responsiveness. They give orders and expect obedience, giving very little warmth or consideration to their children's special needs.

Ask Yourself

QUESTIONS FOR CRITICAL THINKING AND REFLECTION

How do you define "commitment" in a relationship? Is it simply a matter of staying faithful to a partner, or is there more? In your own relationships, what signs of commitment do you look for from your partner? What signs of commitment does your partner see in you?

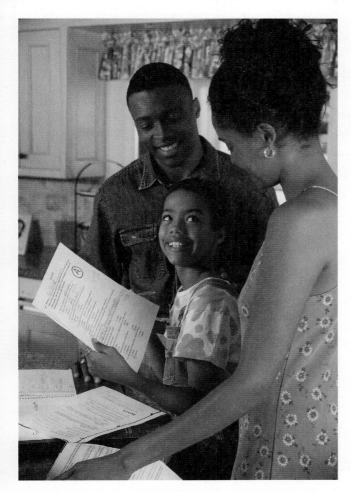

Setting clear boundaries, holding children to high expectations, and responding with warmth to children's needs are all positive parenting strategies.

- *Authoritative* parents are high in both demandingness and responsiveness. They set clear boundaries and expectations, but they are also loving, supportive, and attuned to their children's needs.

- *Permissive* parents are high in responsiveness and low in demandingness. They do not expect their children to act maturely but instead allow them to follow their own impulses. They are very warm, patient, and accepting, and they are focused on not stifling their child's innate creativity.

- *Uninvolved* parents are low in both demandingness and responsiveness. They require little from their children and respond with little attention, frequency, or effort. In extreme cases, this style of parenting might reach the level of child neglect.

Parenting and the Family Life Cycle   Parenting that is both responsive and demanding is the most beneficial for children. Providing a balance of firm limits and clear structure along with plenty of warmth, nurturing, and respect for the child's own special needs and temperament as well as her

or his growing independence is the best predictor for raising a healthy child.

At each stage of the family life cycle, the relationship between parents and children changes. And with those changes come new challenges. The parents' primary responsibility to a small, helpless baby is to ensure its physical well-being around the clock. As babies grow into toddlers and begin to walk and talk, they begin to be able to take care of some of their own physical needs. For parents, the challenge at this stage is to strike a balance between giving children the freedom to explore and setting limits that will keep the children safe and secure. As children grow toward adolescence, parents need to give them increasing independence and gradually be willing to let them risk success or failure on their own.

Marital satisfaction for most couples tends to decline while the children are in school. Reasons include the financial and emotional pressures of a growing family and the increased job and community responsibilities of parents in their thirties, forties, and fifties. Once the last child has left home, marital satisfaction usually increases because the couple have time to enjoy each other once more.

Single Parents

According to the U.S. Census Bureau, about 27% of all children under 18 live with only one parent. In some single-parent families, the traditional family life cycle is reversed and the baby comes before the marriage. In these families, the single parent is usually a teenage mother; she may very well be black or Hispanic, and she may never get married or may not marry for several years. In 2011 about 55% of all black children were living with a single parent, as were 29% of Hispanic children.

Economic difficulties are the primary problem for single mothers, especially for unmarried mothers who have not finished high school and have difficulty finding work. Divorced mothers usually experience a sharp drop in income the first few years on their own, but if they have job skills or education they usually can eventually support themselves and their children adequately. Other problems for single mothers are the often-conflicting demands of playing both father and mother and the difficulty of satisfying their own needs for adult companionship and affection.

Financial pressures are also a complaint of single fathers, but they do not experience them to the extent that single mothers do. Because they are likely to have less practice than mothers in juggling parental and professional roles, they may worry that they do not spend enough time with their children. Because single fatherhood is not as common as single motherhood, however, the men who choose it are likely to be stable, established, and strongly motivated to be with their children.

Research about the effect on children of growing up in a single-parent family is inconclusive. Evidence seems to indicate that these children tend to have less success in school and in their careers than children from two-parent families, but these effects may be associated more strongly with low educational attainment of the single parent than with the absence of the second parent. Two-parent families are not necessarily better if one of the parents spends little time relating to the children or is physically or emotionally abusive.

Stepfamilies

Single parenthood is usually a transitional stage: About three out of four divorced women and about four out of five divorced men will ultimately remarry. Rates are lower for widowed men and women, but overall, almost half the marriages in the United States are remarriages for the husband, the wife, or both. If either partner brings children from a previous marriage into the new family unit, a stepfamily (or "blended family") is formed.

Stepfamilies are significantly different from primary families and should not be expected to duplicate the emotions and relationships of a primary family. Research has shown that healthy stepfamilies are less cohesive and more adaptable than healthy primary families; they have a greater capacity to allow for individual differences and accept that biologically related family members will have emotionally closer relationships. Stepfamilies gradually gain more of a sense of being a family as they build a history of shared daily experiences and major life events.

Successful Families

Family life can be extremely challenging. A strong family is not a family without problems; it's a family that copes successfully with stress and crisis. Successful families are intentionally connected—members share experiences and meanings.

An excellent way to build strong family ties is to develop family rituals and routines—organized, repeated activities that have meaning for family members. Families with regular routines and rituals have healthier children, more satisfying marriages, and stronger family relationships. Some of the most common routines identified in research studies are dinner time, a regular bedtime, and household chores; common rituals include birthdays, holidays, and weekend activities. Family routines may even serve as protective factors, balancing out potential risk factors associated with single-parent families and families with divorce and remarriage. Incorpo-

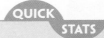

QUICK STATS

4% of American children live in a home where neither parent is present.
—U.S. Census Bureau, 2012

rating a regular family mealtime into a family's routine allows parents and children to develop closer relationships and leads to better parenting, healthier children, and better school performance.

Although there is tremendous variation in American families, researchers have proposed that six major qualities or themes appear in strong families:

1. *Commitment.* **The family is very important to its members. Sexual fidelity between partners is included in commitment.**

2. *Appreciation.* Family members care about one another and express their appreciation. The home is a positive place for family members.

3. *Communication.* Family members spend time listening to one another and enjoying one another's company. They talk about disagreements and attempt to solve problems.

4. *Time together.* Family members do things together—often simple activities that don't cost money.

5. *Spiritual wellness.* The family promotes sharing, love, and compassion for other human beings.

6. *Coping with stress and crisis.* When faced with illness, death, marital conflict, or other crises, family members pull together, seek help, and use other coping strategies to meet the challenge.

It may surprise some people that members of strong families are often seen at counseling centers. They know that the smartest thing to do in some situations is to get help.

connect™

Connect to Your Choices

Have you ever thought about why you handle your relationships the way you do? Many factors can influence the relationship choices we make—some not as obvious as others. Do you avoid intimate relationships because you don't want to replicate the patterns you saw in your parents' relationship? Are you frequently disappointed with your relationships because they aren't as blissful or as exciting as the relationships you see in movies or on TV? Do you go along with your partner's ideas because you're not sure what you want?

What are the external factors that influence your choices about relationships? What are your inner motivations and core values, and how do they affect your choices? Based on what you learned in this chapter, will you make some different choices in the future? If so, what will they be?

Go online to Connect to complete this activity: www.mcgraw-hillconnect.com

Ask Yourself

QUESTIONS FOR CRITICAL THINKING AND REFLECTION

Do you think of your own family as successful? Why or why not? Either way, what could you do to make your relationships in your family more successful? Are you comfortable talking to your family about these issues?

TIPS FOR TODAY AND THE FUTURE

A balanced life includes ample time for nourishing relationships with friends, family, and intimate partners.

RIGHT NOW YOU CAN:

- Seek out an acquaintance or a new friend and arrange a coffee date to get to know the person better.
- Call someone you love and tell him or her how important the relationship is to you. Don't wait for a crisis.

IN THE FUTURE YOU CAN:

- Think about the conflicts you have had in the past with your close friends or loved ones and consider how you handled them. Decide whether your conflict management methods were helpful. Using the suggestions in this chapter and Chapter 3, determine how you could better handle similar conflicts in the future.
- Think about your prospects as a parent. What kind of example have your parents set? How do you feel about having children in the future (if you don't have children already)? What can you do to prepare yourself to be a good parent?

SUMMARY

- Healthy intimate relationships are an important component of the well-being of both individuals and society. Many intimate relationships are held together by love.

- Characteristics of friendship include companionship, respect, acceptance, help, trust, loyalty, and reciprocity.

- Love, sex, and commitment are closely linked ideals in intimate relationships. Love includes trust, caring, respect, and loyalty. Sex brings excitement, fascination, and passion to the relationship.

- Common challenges in relationships relate to issues of self-disclosure, commitment, expectations, competitiveness, balancing time together and apart, and jealousy.

- Partners in successful relationships have strong communication skills and support each other in difficult times.

- The keys to good communication in relationships are self-disclosure, listening, and feedback.

- Conflict is inevitable in intimate relationships; partners need to find ways to negotiate their differences.

- People usually choose partners like themselves. If partners are very different, acceptance and good communication skills are especially necessary to maintain the relationship.

- Most Americans find partners through dating or getting together in groups. Cohabitation is a growing social pattern that allows partners to get to know each other intimately without being married.

- Gay and lesbian partnerships are similar to heterosexual partnerships, with some differences. Partners often don't conform to traditional gender roles, and they may experience societal hostility or ambivalence rather than approval of their partnerships.

- Singlehood is a growing option in our society. Advantages include greater variety in sex partners and more freedom in making life decisions; disadvantages include loneliness and possible economic hardship, especially for single women.

- Marriage fulfills many functions for individuals and society. It can provide people with affection, affirmation, and sexual fulfillment; a context for child rearing; and the promise of lifelong companionship.

- Love isn't enough to ensure a successful marriage. Partners must be realistic, feel good about each other, have communication and conflict resolution skills, share values, and balance their individual and joint interests.

- When problems can't be worked out, people often separate and divorce. Divorce is traumatic for all involved, especially children, but the negative effects are usually balanced in time by positive ones.

- At each stage of the family life cycle, relationships change. Marital satisfaction may be lower during the child-rearing years and higher later.

- Many families today are single-parent families. Problems for single parents include economic difficulties, conflicting demands, and time pressures.

- Stepfamilies are formed when single, divorced, or widowed people remarry and create new family units. Stepfamilies gradually gain more of a sense of being a family as they build a history of shared experiences.

- Important qualities of successful families include commitment to the family; appreciation of family members, communication, and time spent together; spiritual wellness; and effective methods of dealing with stress.

FOR MORE INFORMATION

For resources in your area, check your campus directory for a counseling center or peer counseling program, or search online.

BOOKS

Brooks, J. B. 2010. *The Process of Parenting*, 8th ed. New York: McGraw-Hill. *Demonstrates how parents and caregivers can translate their love and concern for children into effective parenting behavior.*

DeGenova, M. K., F. P. Rice., N. Stinnett, and N. Stinnett. 2010. *Intimate Relationships, Marriages, and Families*, 8th ed. New York: McGraw-Hill. *A comprehensive introduction to relationships.*

Lewis, T., F. Amni, and R. Lannon. 2000. *A General Theory of Love.* New York: Random House. *A lucid exploration of the biopsychosocial nature of love and interconnectedness of people.*

McKay, M., P. Fanning, and K. Paleg. 2006. *Couple Skills: Making Your Relationship Work*, 2nd rev. ed. New York: New Harbinger. *A comprehensive guide to improving communication, resolving conflict, and developing greater intimacy and commitment in relationships.*

Miller, R., 2011. *Intimate Relationships*, 6th ed. New York: McGraw-Hill. *A balanced presentation of both the positive and the problematic aspects of intimate relationships.*

Olson, D., J. DeFrain., and L. Skogrand. 2010 . *Marriages and Families: Intimacy, Diversity, and Strengths*, 7th ed. New York: McGraw-Hill. *A comprehensive introduction to relationships and families.*

ORGANIZATIONS AND WEBSITES

American Association for Marriage and Family Therapy. Provides information about a variety of relationship issues and referrals to therapists.

http://www.aamft.org

Association for Couples in Marriage Enrichment (ACME). An organization that promotes activities to strengthen marriage; a resource for books, tapes, and other materials.

http://www.bettermarriages.org

Conflict Resolution Information Source. Provides links to a broad range of Internet resources for conflict resolution. Information covers interpersonal, marriage, family, and other types of conflicts.

http://www.crinfo.org

Family Education Network. Provides information about education, safety, health, and other family-related issues.

http://www.familyeducation.com

The Gottman Relationship Institute. Includes tips and suggestions for relationships and parenting, including an online relationships quiz.

http://www.gottman.com

Parents without Partners (PWP). Provides educational programs, literature, and support groups for single parents and their children. Search the online directory for a referral to a local chapter.

http://www.parentswithoutpartners.org

United States Census Bureau. Provides current statistics on births, marriages, and living arrangements.

http://www.census.gov

See also the listings for Chapters 3 and 5.

SELECTED BIBLIOGRAPHY

American College Health Association. 2011. *American College Health Association–National College Health Assessment II Reference Group Executive Summary, Spring 2011.* Hanover, MD: American College Health Association.

Centers for Disease Control and Prevention, National Center for Health Statistics. 2010. Births, marriages, divorces, and deaths: Provisional data for 2009. *National Vital Statistics Reports* 58(25).

Centers for Disease Control and Prevention, National Center for Health Statistics. 2010. Marriage and cohabitation in the United States: A statistical portrait based on cycle 6 (2002) of the National Survey of Family Growth. *Vital and Health Statistics* 23(28): 1–46.

Centers for Disease Control and Prevention, National Center for Health Statistics. 2011. *Health, United States, 2010.* Hyattsville, MD: National Center for Health Statistics.

Christakis, N. A., et al. 2006. Mortality after hospitalization of a spouse. *New England Journal of Medicine* 354(7): 719–730.

Federal Interagency Forum on Child and Family Statistics. 2011. *America's Children: Key National Indicators of Well-Being, 2011.* Washington, DC: U.S. Government Printing Office.

Hampton, K., et al. 2009. *Social Isolation and New Technology: How the Internet and Mobile Phones Impact Americans' Social Networks* (http://www.pewinternet.org/Reports/2009/18--Social-Isolation-and-New-Technology.aspx).

Human Rights Campaign. 2011. *Marriage Equality and Other Relationship Recognition Laws* (http://www.hrc.org/files/assets/resources/Relationship_Recognition_Laws_Map%281%29.pdf).

Human Rights Campaign. 2012. *Issues: Marriage* (http://www.hrc.org/issues/marriage).

McPherson, M., L. Smith-Lovin, and M. Brashears. 2006. Social isolation in America: Changes in core discussion networks over two decades. *American Sociological Review* 71: 353–375.

National Conference of State Legislatures. 2012. *Defining Marriage: Defense of Marriage Acts and Same-Sex Marriage Laws* (http://www.ncsl.org/issues-research/human-services/same-sex-marriage-overview.aspx).

National Public Radio. 2012. *State by State: The Battle over Gay Marriage* (http://www.npr.org/2009/12/15/112448663/state-by-state-the-legal-battle-over-gay-marriage).

Pleis, J. R., and M. Lethbridge-Cejku. 2007. Summary health statistics for U.S. adults: National Health Interview Survey, 2006. *Vital and Health Statistics* 10(235): 1–153.

Roisman, G. I., et al. 2008. Adult romantic relationships as contexts of human development: A multimethod comparison of same-sex couples with opposite-sex dating, engaged, and married dyads. *Developmental Psychology* 44(1): 91–101.

Schoen, R., et al. 2007. Family transitions in young adulthood. *Demography* 44(4): 807–820.

Yarber, W., B. Sayad, and B. Strong. 2010. *Human Sexuality: Diversity in Contemporary America*, 7th ed. New York: McGraw-Hill.

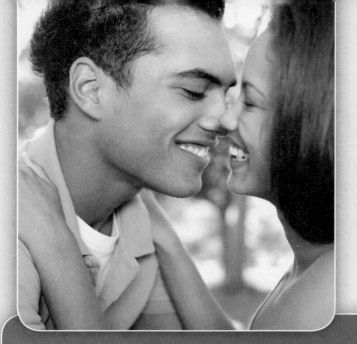

LOOKING AHEAD...

After reading this chapter, you should be able to

- Describe the structure and function of the female and male sex organs
- Explain the changes in sexual functioning that occur over the course of a person's life
- Describe the various ways human sexuality can be expressed
- Describe guidelines for safe, responsible sexual behavior
- Describe the physical and emotional changes a pregnant woman typically experiences
- Identify the stages of fetal development
- List the important components of good prenatal care
- Describe the process of labor and delivery

Sexuality, Pregnancy, and Childbirth

5

Humans are sexual beings. Sexual activity is the source of our most intense physical pleasures, a central ingredient in many of our intimate emotional relationships, and the key to reproduction. **Sexuality** is more than just sexual behavior. It is a complex, interacting group of biological characteristics and acquired behaviors people learn while growing up in a particular family, community, and society. Sexuality includes biological sex (being biologically male or female), gender (masculine and feminine behaviors), sexual anatomy and physiology, sexual functioning and practices, and social and sexual interactions with others. Our individual sense of identity is powerfully influenced by our sexuality. Most of us think of ourselves in fundamental ways as male or female; as heterosexual or homosexual; as single, attached, married, or divorced.

Basic information about the body, sexual functioning, and sexual behavior is vital to healthy adult life. Once we understand the facts, we have a better basis for evaluating the messages we get and for making informed, responsible choices about our sexual activities.

SEXUAL ANATOMY

Despite their different appearances, the sex organs of men and women arise from the same structures and fulfill sex-specific but parallel functions. Each person has a pair of **gonads:** ovaries in females and testes in males. The gonads produce **germ cells** and sex hormones. The germ cells are **ova** (eggs) in females and **sperm** in males. Ova and sperm are the basic units of reproduction; their union results in the creation of a new life.

Female Sex Organs

The external sex organs, or genitals, of the female are called the **vulva** (Figure 5.1). The *mons pubis*, a rounded mass of fatty tissue over the pubic bone, becomes covered with hair during puberty (biological maturation). Below it are two paired folds of skin called the *labia majora* (major lips) and the *labia minora* (minor lips). Enclosed within these folds are the clitoris, the opening of the urethra, and the opening of the vagina.

The **clitoris** is highly sensitive to touch and plays an important role in female sexual arousal and orgasm. The clitoris consists of a shaft, glans, and spongy tissue that fills with blood during sexual excitement. The glans is the most sensitive part of the clitoris and is covered by the clitoral hood, or **prepuce,** which is formed from the upper portion of the labia minora.

The female **urethra** is a duct that leads directly from the urinary bladder to its opening between the clitoris and the opening of the vagina. The urethra conducts urine from

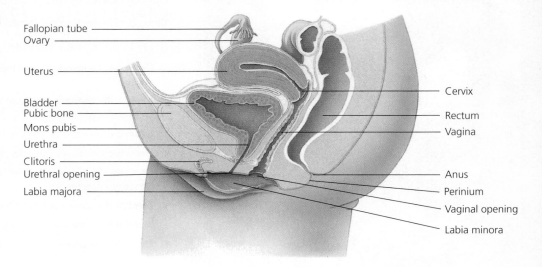

FIGURE 5.1 The female sex organs.

Fallopian tube
Ovary
Uterus
Bladder
Pubic bone
Mons pubis
Urethra
Clitoris
Urethral opening
Labia majora

Cervix
Rectum
Vagina
Anus
Perinium
Vaginal opening
Labia minora

the bladder to the outside of the body. The female urethra is not part of the reproductive tract.

The **vagina** is the passage that leads to the internal reproductive organs. It is the female structure for heterosexual sexual intercourse and serves as the birth canal. Projecting into the upper part of the vagina is the **cervix,** which is the opening of the **uterus**—or *womb*—where a fertilized egg is implanted and grows into a *fetus*.

A pair of **fallopian tubes** (or *oviducts*) extends from the top of the uterus. The end of each oviduct surrounds an **ovary** and guides the mature ovum down into the uterus after the egg exits the ovary.

Male Sex Organs

A man's external sex organs, or genitals, are the penis and the scrotum (Figure 5.2).

The **penis** consists of spongy tissue that becomes engorged with blood during sexual excitement, causing the organ to enlarge and become erect.

The **scrotum** is a pouch that contains a pair of sperm-producing male gonads, called **testes.** The scrotum maintains the testes at a temperature approximately 5°F below that of the rest of the body—that is, at about 93.6°F. The process of sperm production is extremely heat-sensitive. In hot temperatures, the muscles in the scrotum relax and the testes move away from the heat of the body.

The male urethra is a tube that runs through the entire length of the penis. The urethra carries both urine and **semen** (sperm-carrying fluid) to the opening at the tip of the penis. Although urine and semen share a common passage, they are prevented from mixing together by muscles that control their entry into the urethra.

During its brief lifetime, a sperm takes the following route:

1. Sperm are produced inside a maze of tiny, tightly packed tubules within the testes. As they begin to mature, sperm flow into a single storage tube called the **epididymis,** which lies on the surface of each testis.

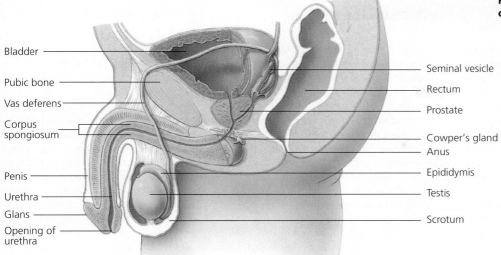

FIGURE 5.2 **The male sex organs.**

Bladder

Pubic bone

Vas deferens

Corpus spongiosum

Penis

Urethra

Glans

Opening of urethra

Seminal vesicle

Rectum

Prostate

Cowper's gland

Anus

Epididymis

Testis

Scrotum

2. Sperm move from each epididymis into another tube—called the **vas deferens**—which carries them upward into the abdominal cavity and through an organ called the **prostate gland.** This gland produces some of the fluid in semen, which helps transport and nourish the sperm.

3. The two *vasa deferentia* eventually merge into a pair of **seminal vesicles,** whose secretions provide nutrients for the semen.

4. On the final stage of their journey, sperm flow into the **ejaculatory ducts,** which join the urethra.

The **Cowper's glands** are two small structures flanking the urethra. During sexual arousal, these glands secrete a clear, mucuslike fluid that appears at the tip of the penis. Preejaculatory fluid may contain sperm, so withdrawal of the penis before ejaculation is not a reliable form of contraception.

The smooth, rounded tip of the penis is the highly sensitive **glans,** an important component in sexual arousal. The glans is partially covered by the foreskin, or prepuce, a retractable fold of skin that is removed by **circumcision** in about 55% of newborn males in the United States. Circumcision is performed for cultural, religious, and hygienic reasons. Rates of circumcision vary widely among different groups (see the box "Genital Alteration").

HORMONES AND THE REPRODUCTIVE LIFE CYCLE

The sex hormones produced by the ovaries or testes have a major influence on the development and function of the reproductive system throughout life. In addition to their effects on the reproductive organs, sex hormones influence many other organs in the body, including the brain.

The male sex hormones, made by the testes, are called **androgens,** the most important of which is *testosterone.* The female sex hormones, produced by the ovaries, belong to two groups: **estrogens** and **progestagens,** the most important of which is *progesterone.* The ovaries also produce a small amount of testosterone. The **adrenal glands** also produce sex hormones in both males and females.

QUICK STATS

20 million or more sperm per milliliter of semen is considered a normal sperm count.

—Mayo Clinic (www.mayoclinic.com), 2010

TERMS

vas deferens A tube that carries sperm from the epididymis through the prostate gland to the seminal vesicles; plural, *vasa deferentia.*

prostate gland A male reproductive organ; produces some of the fluid in semen, which helps transport and nourish sperm.

seminal vesicle A tube leading from the vas deferens to the ejaculatory duct; secretes nutrients for the semen.

ejaculatory duct A tube that carries mature sperm to the urethra so they can exit the body upon ejaculation.

Cowper's gland In the male reproductive system, a small organ that produces preejaculatory fluid.

glans The rounded head of the penis or the clitoris.

circumcision Surgical removal of the foreskin of the penis.

androgens Male sex hormones, produced by the testes.

estrogens A class of female sex hormones, produced by the ovaries, that bring about sexual maturation at puberty and maintain reproductive functions.

progestagens A class of female sex hormones, produced by the ovaries, that sustain reproductive functions.

adrenal glands Endocrine glands, located over the kidneys, that produce sex hormones.

Many societies have a tradition of altering the appearance and function of their children's genitalia, either shortly after birth or as part of a puberty rite. Such cultural customs can seem strange, and sometimes even barbaric, to those who are not part of that particular culture. Male circumcision and female genital cutting are both examples of genital alternation, and both are subjects of considerable controversy.

The most common form of genital alteration worldwide is male circumcision—the removal of the foreskin of the penis. Circumcision is a relatively minor surgical procedure that is performed for a variety of cultural, religious, aesthetic, and medical reasons. Worldwide an estimated one-third of males are circumcised. In the United States a little more than one-half of male newborns are circumcised (from a high of nearly 90% in the 1960s); over time, fewer American parents are having their sons circumcised.

Currently no major medical group in the United States recommends the routine circumcision of male infants. The procedure, though minor, carries some medical risks, including bleeding, infection, and damage to the penis. Circumcision causes pain to the infant, although most pain can be alleviated with appropriate use of local anesthetic. Circumci-

sion may change the sensitivity of the penis, and some critics claim that it can diminish a man's sexual pleasure. Opponents of circumcision point to the fact that most of the world's men are uncircumcised; why perform surgery, they ask, when there is no clear need for it?

On the other side of the debate, there are a number of health benefits of circumcision. Citing research findings, proponents argue that it promotes cleanliness and reduces the risk of urinary tract infections in newborns and the risk of sexually transmitted diseases, including HIV, later in life, as well as the risk of penile cancer. Studies conducted in developing countries have shown that circumcision can reduce a man's risk of acquiring HIV through heterosexual contact by as much as 60%. However, STD education and the practice of abstinence or low-risk sexual behaviors have a far greater impact on the transmission of STDs than does circumcision.

Far more controversial is the practice of female genital cutting (FGC), also called female genital mutilation. There are no medical or health reasons to perform these procedures, which range from removal of the external genitalia (including the clitoris and labia) to narrowing of the vaginal opening with a surgically created seal to less drastic forms of harm to the

genitalia. These practices were probably originally developed to control a woman's sexuality and ensure that she remained a virgin before marriage.

Each year about 3 million female children undergo FGC, usually between infancy and age 15, and about 140 million women worldwide are estimated to have had some form of genital cutting. FGC is often performed under unsterile conditions and without adequate anesthesia. Serious complications are common and include severe pain, infection, bleeding, and death. Common long-term health issues include infertility, difficulties with childbirth, and problems with urinary and sexual function.

The World Health Organization has come out strongly against FGC, declaring it a violation of the human rights of girls and women. FGC is now illegal in many countries, but it is still performed on large numbers of girls where the cultural tradition persists.

SOURCE: Centers for Disease Control and Prevention. 2011. Trends in in-hospital newborn male circumcision—United States, 1999–2010. *Morbidity and Mortality Weekly Report* 60(34): 1167–1168; World Health Organization. 2012. *Female Genital Mutilation* (http://www.who.int/topics/female_genital_mutilation/en/).

Sex hormones are regulated by the hormones of the **pituitary gland,** located at the base of the brain. This gland in turn is controlled by hormones produced by the **hypothalamus** in the brain.

Substances that act like hormones and disrupt normal endocrine activity, particularly activity related to reproduction and development, are also found in the environment. The most studied endocrine-disrupting chemicals, or EDCs, are environmental estrogens, which mimic the female sex hormone estrogen and can duplicate or exaggerate its effects. Other EDCs can block estrogen, mimic or block androgens (male sex hormones), or otherwise alter hormonal responses in the body.

Differentiation of the Embryo

An individual's biological sex is determined by the fertilizing sperm at the time of conception. All human cells normally contain 23 pairs of chromosomes. In 22 of the pairs, the two partner chromosomes match. But in the 23rd pair, the **sex chromosomes,** two configurations are possible. Individuals

with two matching X chromosomes are female, and individuals with one X and one Y chromosome are male. Thus at the time of conception the genetic sex is established: females are XX and males are XY.

Abnormalities sometimes occur in the sex chromosomes; the two most common disorders of sex chromosomes are Klinefelter's syndrome and Turner's syndrome. Klinefelter's syndrome, a condition where a male carries two or more X

> **TERMS**
>
> **pituitary gland**   An endocrine gland at the base of the brain that produces hormones and regulates the release of hormones—including sex hormones—by other glands.
>
> **hypothalamus**   A region of the brain above the pituitary gland whose hormones control the secretions of the pituitary; also involved in the control of many bodily functions, including hunger, thirst, temperature regulation, and sexual functions.
>
> **sex chromosomes**   The X and Y chromosomes, which determine an individual's biological sex.

chromosomes in addition to the Y chromosome, occurs in about 1 in 1000 males and causes infertility and small genitalia. Turner's syndrome occurs in about 1 in 2500 females. Women with Turner's have only a single complete X chromosome. These women are usually not able to have children and can sometimes have other medical problems.

Genetic sex dictates whether the undifferentiated gonads become ovaries or testes. If a Y chromosome is present, the gonads become testes and produce the male hormone **testosterone.** Testosterone circulates throughout the body and causes the undifferentiated reproductive structures to develop into male sex organs (penis, scrotum, and others). If a Y chromosome is not present, there is no testosterone; the gonads become ovaries and the reproductive structures develop into female sex organs (clitoris, labia, and others). The entire process is known as *sexual differentiation.*

Female Sexual Maturation

Although humans are fully sexually differentiated at birth, the differences between males and females are accentuated at **puberty,** the period during which the reproductive system matures, secondary sex characteristics develop, and the bodies of males and females begin to appear more distinctive. The changes of puberty are induced by testosterone in the male and estrogen and **progesterone** in the female.

Puberty in Females   The first sign of puberty in girls is breast development, followed by a rounding of the hips and buttocks. As the breasts develop, hair appears in the pubic region and later in the underarms. Shortly after the onset of breast development, girls show an increase in growth rate. Breast development usually begins between ages 8 and 13, and the time of rapid body growth occurs between ages 9 and 15.

The Menstrual Cycle   A major landmark of puberty for young women is the onset of the **menstrual cycle,** the monthly ovarian cycle that leads to menstruation (loss of blood and tissue lining the uterus) in the absence of pregnancy. The timing of **menarche** (the first *menstrual period*) varies with several factors, including ethnicity, genetics, and nutritional status. The current average age of menarche in the United States is around 12 and a half years of age, but menstruation may also normally start several years earlier or later.

The day of the onset of bleeding is considered to be day 1 of the menstrual cycle. For the purposes of our discussion, a cycle of 28 days will be used; however, normal cycles vary in length from 21 to 35 days. The menstrual cycle consists of the following four phases.

1. **MENSES** During **menses,** characterized by the menstrual flow, blood levels of hormones from the ovaries and the pituitary gland are relatively low. This phase of the cycle usually lasts from day 1 to about day 5.

2. **ESTROGENIC PHASE** The estrogenic phase begins when the menstrual flow ceases and the pituitary gland begins to produce increasing amounts of follicle-stimulating hormone (FSH) and luteinizing hormone (LH). Under the influence of FSH, an egg-containing ovarian **follicle** begins to mature, producing increasingly higher amounts of estrogen. Stimulated by estrogen, the **endometrium** (the uterine lining) thickens with large numbers of blood vessels and uterine glands.

3. **OVULATION** A surge of a potent estrogen called *estradiol* from the follicle causes the pituitary to release a large burst of LH and a smaller amount of FSH. The high concentration of LH stimulates the developing follicle to release its ovum. This event is known as **ovulation.** After ovulation, the follicle is transformed into the **corpus luteum,** which produces progesterone and estrogen.

Ovulation theoretically occurs about 14 days prior to the onset of menstrual flow, with the window of greatest fertility occurring from a few days before ovulation to about one day after. This information has been used to attempt to predict the

Ask Yourself

QUESTIONS FOR CRITICAL THINKING AND REFLECTION

What are your personal views on circumcision? Who or what has influenced those opinions? Are the bases of your views primarily cultural, moral, or medical?

most fertile time during the menstrual cycle for fertility treatments and natural family planning methods. However, a recent study showed that even women with regular menstrual cycles often have unpredictable ovulation, and can actually be fertile on any day of the month, including during menstruation. The "window of fertility" is especially unpredictable in teenagers and women who are approaching menopause.

4. PROGESTATIONAL PHASE During the progestational phase of the cycle, the amount of progesterone secreted from the corpus luteum increases and remains high until the onset of the next menses. Under the influence of estrogen and progesterone, the endometrium continues to develop, readying itself to receive and nourish a fertilized ovum. When pregnancy occurs, the fertilized egg produces the hormone human chorionic gonadotropin (HCG), which maintains the corpus luteum. Thus levels of ovarian hormones remain high and the uterine lining is preserved, preventing menses.

If pregnancy does not occur, the corpus luteum degenerates, and estrogen and progesterone levels gradually fall. Below certain hormonal levels, the endometrium can no longer be maintained, and it begins to slough off, initiating menses. As the levels of ovarian hormones fall, a slight rise in LH and FSH occurs, and a new menstrual cycle begins.

Menstrual Problems Menstruation is a normal biological process, but physical and/or emotional symptoms associated with the menstrual cycle are very common. Many women experience menstrual cramps, the severity of which tends to vary from cycle to cycle. **Dysmenorrhea**, discomfort associated with menstruation, can include any combination of the following symptoms: lower abdominal cramps, backache, vomiting, nausea, bloating, diarrhea, headache, and fatigue. Many of these symptoms can be attributed to uterine muscular contractions caused by chemicals called *prostaglandins*. Nonsteroidal anti-inflammatory drugs (NSAIDs) such as ibuprofen (Motrin, Advil) block the effects of prostaglandins and are often effective in relieving dysmenorrhea. Oral contraceptives are also effective in reducing dysmenorrheal symptoms in most women.

Many women experience transient emotional symptoms prior to the onset of their menstrual flow. Depending on their severity, these symptoms may be categorized along a continuum: **premenstrual tension, premenstrual syndrome (PMS),** and **premenstrual dysphoric disorder (PMDD).** Premenstrual tension symptoms are mild and may include negative mood changes and physical symptoms such as abdominal cramping and backache. More severe symptoms are classified as PMS; very severe symptoms that impair normal daily and social functioning are classified as PMDD. All three conditions share a definite pattern. Symptoms appear prior to the onset of menses and disappear within a few days after the start of menstruation. Premenstrual tension is quite

common, PMS affects about 1 in 5 women, and PMDD affects fewer than 1 in 10 women.

Symptoms associated with PMS and PMDD can include breast tenderness, water retention (bloating), headache, fatigue, insomnia or excessive sleep, appetite changes, food cravings, irritability, anger, increased interpersonal conflict, depression, anxiety, tearfulness, inability to concentrate, social withdrawal, and the sense of being out of control or overwhelmed.

Despite many research studies, the causes of PMS and PMDD are still unknown, and it is unclear why some women are more vulnerable than others. Most researchers feel that PMS is probably caused by a combination of hormonal, neurological, genetic, dietary, and psychological factors.

The following strategies provide relief for many women with premenstrual symptoms, and all of them can contribute to a healthy lifestyle at any time:

- *Limit salt intake.* Salt promotes water retention and bloating.
- *Exercise.* Women who exercise may experience fewer symptoms before and after menstrual periods.
- *Don't use alcohol or tobacco.* Alcohol and tobacco may aggravate certain symptoms of PMS and PMDD.
- *Eat a nutritious diet.* Choose a low-fat diet rich in complex carbohydrates from vegetables, fruits, and whole-grain breads, cereals, and pasta. Get enough calcium from calcium-rich foods and, if needed, supplements. Minimize your intake of sugar and caffeine, and avoid chocolate, which is rich in both.
- *Relax.* Stress reduction is always beneficial, and stressful events can trigger PMS symptoms. Try relaxation techniques during the premenstrual time.

If you're a female with persistent premenstrual symptoms, keep a daily diary to track the types of symptoms, their severity, and how they correlate with your menstrual cycle. See your physician for an evaluation and to learn about treatments that are available only by prescription.

Selective serotonin reuptake inhibitors (SSRIs), such as Prozac and Zoloft, are often used to treat PMS and PMDD.

> QUICK STATS
>
> **75%** of women experience premenstrual symptoms during their childbearing years.
>
> —National Institutes of Health, 2012

> **TERMS**
>
> **dysmenorrhea** Painful or problematic menstruation.
>
> **premenstrual tension** Mild physical and emotional changes associated with the time before the onset of menses.
>
> **premenstrual syndrome (PMS)** A disorder characterized by physical discomfort, psychological distress, and behavioral changes that begin after ovulation and cease when menstruation begins.
>
> **premenstrual dysphoric disorder (PMDD)** A severe form of PMS, characterized by symptoms serious enough to interfere with daily activities and relationships.

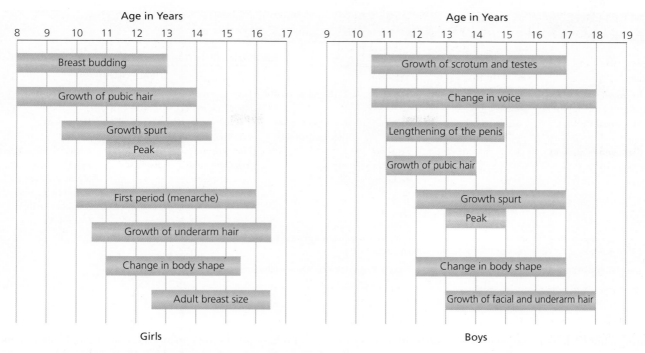

FIGURE 5.3 **Milestones in sexual maturation of girls and boys.**
Reprinted with permission from *The Merck Manual Home Health Handbook, Online Version*. © 2010–2011 Merck Sharp & Dohme Corp., a subsidiary of Merck & Co., Inc., Whitehouse Station, N.J., U.S.A. http://www.merckmanuals.com/home/childrens_health_issues/adolescents/physical_and_sexual_development.html

Until recently, women using SSRIs took the medication throughout the entire menstrual cycle, but taking the medication during just the progestational phase of the cycle is effective in some women.

Other drug treatments for PMS and PMDD include certain oral contraceptives, diuretics to minimize water retention, and NSAIDs such as ibuprofen. A number of vitamins, minerals, and other dietary supplements have also been studied for PMS relief. Only one supplement, calcium, has been shown to provide relief in rigorous clinical studies; several others show promise, but more research is needed.

Male Sexual Maturation

Reproductive maturation of boys occurs about two years later than that of girls; it usually begins at about age 10 or 11. Testicular growth is usually the first obvious sign of sexual maturity in boys. The penis also grows at this time, reaching adult size by about age 18. Pubic hair starts to develop after the genitals begin increasing in size, with underarm and facial hair gradually appearing. Hair on the chest, back, and abdomen increases later in development. Facial hair often continues to get thicker and darker for several years after puberty. The voice deepens as a result of the lengthening and thickening of the vocal cords.

Boys grow taller for about six years after the first signs of puberty, with a very rapid period of growth about two years after puberty starts. Largely because of the influence of testosterone, muscle development and bone density are much greater in males than in females. By adulthood, men on average have one and a half times the lean body mass of women, and only about half the body fat.

Aging and Human Sexuality

Hormone production and sexual functioning change as we age. Sexual "performance" may diminish, but sexuality and sensuality can continue to be a source of great pleasure and satisfaction. A study of sexuality in older Americans found that three-fourths of 57- to 64-year-olds were sexually active (defined as having had at least one sexual partner in the last year). Half of those ages 65–74 and about one-fourth of people ages 75–85 remained sexually active. People who remain healthy and active are much more likely to continue to be sexually active in their older years.

Menopause As a woman approaches age 50, her ovaries gradually cease to function and she enters **menopause,** the cessation of menstruation (Table 5.1). For some women, the associated drop in hormone production causes troublesome symptoms. The most common physical symptom of menopause is the hot flash, a sensation of warmth rising to the face from the upper chest, with or without perspiration and chills.

menopause The cessation of menstruation, occurring gradually around age 50.

TERMS

Table 5.1 — Reproductive Aging in Women

	REPRODUCTIVE YEARS			MENOPAUSAL TRANSITION			POSTMENOPAUSE
	FIRST PERIOD					FINAL PERIOD	
Average Age*	9–15	16–30	31–42	Early transition 40s	Late transition late 40s, early 50s	51	50s and beyond
Menstrual Cycles	Variable	Regular	Regular	Lengths of cycles vary increasingly	2 or more skipped periods	No period**	No periods
Signs and Symptoms			Fertility progressively declining		Hot flashes, irritability, and sleep disturbance; bone loss begins	Same as previous	Vaginal dryness, bone loss. Hot flashes can persist. For a few women, hot flashes continue into their 60s and 70s

*These are average ages. Women vary a great deal in the ages at which they go through these stages.
**Menopause is said to have occurred after 12 months without a period.

SOURCE: Copyright © 2007 by the American Society for Reproductive Medicine. Reproduced with permission.

During a hot flash, skin temperature can rise by more than 10 degrees. Other menopausal symptoms can include night sweats, insomnia, vaginal dryness, thinning of head hair, and mood changes. Osteoporosis—decreasing bone density—can develop, making older women more vulnerable to fractures.

As a result of decreased estrogen production during menopause, the vaginal walls become thin and lubrication in response to sexual arousal diminishes. Sexual intercourse may become painful. Hormonal treatment or the use of lubricants during intercourse can minimize these problems.

Doctors have known for decades that most of the symptoms of menopause can be relieved with the administration of estrogen. It became common for postmenopausal women to take estrogen for relief from hot flashes, vaginal dryness, bone loss, and a host of other symptoms. However, doctors discovered that giving estrogen alone to postmenopausal women resulted in higher rates of endometrial cancer. To alleviate this problem, it became customary to prescribe estrogen with a progestagen (called *hormone therapy*, or *HT*), since this combination reduced the risk for uterine cancer but still reduced menopausal symptoms. The medical community was taken by surprise in 2002 when a large study showed that women taking a common form of estrogen/progestagen therapy had higher rates of cardiovascular disease, blood clots, and breast cancer than postmenopausal women not taking hormones. Prescriptions for hormone therapy plummeted after this news. Breast cancer rates dropped over the next few years, but experts are not sure whether the decline in breast cancer was due to the decrease in hormone therapy or to other factors.

In the last several years, reanalysis of the data and information from newer studies has resulted in a more individualized approach to hormone therapy. It appears that younger women who have just become menopausal are more likely to benefit from hormone therapy and less likely to have serious side effects than older women. Current forms of hormone therapy include low-dose estrogen, sometimes in the form of a patch, cream, or vaginal ring, designed to treat specific symptoms of menopause but with a reduced risk of side effects.

Aging Male Syndrome Between the ages of 35 and 65, men experience a gradual decline in testosterone production, resulting in the aging male syndrome, sometimes referred to as *male menopause* or *andropause*. Some experts prefer the term *aging male syndrome* because the process is much more gradual than female menopause. Symptoms vary widely, but most men experience at least some of the following symptoms as they age: loss of muscle mass, increased fat mass, decreased sex drive, erectile problems, depressed mood, irritability, difficulties with concentration, increased urination, loss of bone mineral density, and sleep difficulties. In some cases, testosterone replacement therapy can help. Although taking testosterone can be harmful in young healthy men, older men with low testosterone levels may benefit from carefully prescribed testosterone treatment.

As men get older, they depend more on direct physical stimulation for sexual arousal. They take longer to achieve an erection and find it more difficult to maintain; orgasmic contractions are less intense. Older men with erectile dysfunction are often prescribed medications such as Viagra that increase blood flow to the penis, resulting in a firmer erection.

Unlike women, who are born with all the eggs they will ever have and stop being fertile at menopause, men continue to produce sperm throughout their lives and can sometimes father children well into their eighties and even nineties.

> Men over 40 are more likely to **produce children with health problems** such as autism, schizophrenia, and Down syndrome.

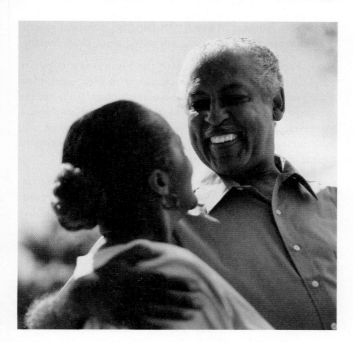

Although sexual physiology changes as people get older, many men and women readily adjust to these alterations.

Starting at about age 30, however, men become gradually less fertile. Regardless of the age of their female partners, couples in which the male is over age 35 have a 50% lower pregnancy rate than couples in which the man is 30 years old or younger. Men over age 40 are more likely to produce children with health problems such as autism, schizophrenia, and Down syndrome.

SEXUAL FUNCTIONING

Sexual activity is based on stimulus and response. Erotic stimulation leads to sexual arousal (excitement), which may culminate in the intensely pleasurable experience of orgasm. But sexual activity should not be thought of only in terms of the sex organs. Responses to sexual stimulation involve not just the genitals but the entire body and mind.

Sexual Stimulation

Sexual excitement can come from many sources, both physical and psychological. Although physical stimuli have an obvious and direct effect, some people believe psychological stimuli—thoughts, fantasies, desires, perceptions—are even more powerfully erotic.

Physical Stimulation   Physical stimulation comes through the senses: we are aroused by things we see, hear, taste, smell, and feel. The most obvious and effective physical stimulation is touching. Even though culturally defined practices vary and different people have different preferences, most sexual encounters eventually involve some form of touching with

hands, lips, and body surfaces. Kissing, caressing, fondling, and hugging are as much a part of sexual encounters as they are a part of expressing affection.

The most intense form of stimulation by touching involves the genitals. The clitoris and the glans of the penis are particularly sensitive to such stimulation. Other highly responsive areas include the vaginal opening, the nipples, the breasts, the insides of the thighs, the buttocks, the anal region, the scrotum, the lips, and the earlobes. Such sexually sensitive areas, or erogenous zones, are especially susceptible to sexual arousal for most people, most of the time. Often, though, what determines the response is not *what* is touched but how, for how long, and by whom. Under the right circumstances, touching any part of the body can cause sexual arousal.

Psychological Stimulation   Sexual arousal also has an important psychological component, regardless of the nature of the physical stimulation. Fantasies, ideas, memories of past experiences, and mood can all generate sexual excitement.

Arousal is also powerfully influenced by emotions. How you feel about a person and how the person feels about you matter tremendously in how sexually responsive you are likely to be. Even the most direct forms of physical stimulation carry emotional overtones. Kissing, caressing, and fondling express affection and caring. The emotional charge they give to a sexual interaction is at least as significant to sexual arousal as the purely physical stimulation achieved by touching.

The Sexual Response Cycle

Men and women respond physiologically with a predictable set of reactions, regardless of the nature of the stimulation. Two physiological mechanisms explain most genital and bodily reactions during sexual arousal and orgasm. These mechanisms are vasocongestion and muscular tension. **Vasocongestion** is the engorgement of tissues that results when more blood flows into an organ than is flowing out. Increased muscular tension culminates in rhythmical muscular contractions during orgasm.

vasocongestion   The accumulation of blood in tissues and organs.   **TERMS**

Four phases characterize the sexual response cycle:

1. In the *excitement phase*, in men, the penis becomes erect as its tissues become engorged with blood. The testes expand and are pulled upward within the scrotum. In women, the clitoris, labia, and vaginal walls are similarly engorged with blood. Tension increases in the vaginal muscles, and the vaginal walls become moist with lubricating fluid.

2. The *plateau phase* is an extension of the excitement phase. Reactions become more marked. In men, the penis becomes harder, and the testes become larger. In women, the lower part of the vagina swells, as its upper end expands and vaginal lubrication increases.

3. In the *orgasmic phase*, or **orgasm,** in men, rhythmic contractions occur along the man's penis, urethra, prostate gland, seminal vesicles, and muscles in the pelvic and anal regions. These involuntary muscular contractions lead to the ejaculation of semen, which consists of sperm cells from the testes and secretions from the prostate gland and seminal vesicles. In women, contractions occur in the lower part of the vagina and in the uterus, as well as in the pelvic region and the anus.

4. In the *resolution phase*, all the changes initiated during the excitement phase are reversed. Excess blood drains from tissues, the muscles in the region relax, and the genital structures return to their unstimulated state.

More general physical reactions accompany the genital changes in both men and women. Beginning with the excitement phase, nipples become erect, the woman's breasts begin to swell, and in both sexes the skin of the chest becomes flushed; these changes are more marked in women. The heart rate doubles by the plateau phase, and respiration becomes faster. During orgasm, breathing becomes irregular and the person may moan or cry out. A feeling of warmth leads to increased sweating during the resolution phase. Deep relaxation and a sense of well-being pervade the body and the mind.

Male orgasm is marked by the ejaculation of semen. After ejaculation, men enter a *refractory period*, during which they cannot be restimulated to orgasm. Women do not have a refractory period, and immediate restimulation to orgasm is possible for some women.

Sexual Problems

Both physical and psychological factors can interfere with sexual functioning. Many diseases specifically affect the sex organs. Any illness that affects your general health is likely to have some affect on your ability to function sexually. Disturbances in sexual desire, performance, or satisfaction are referred to as **sexual dysfunctions.** These problems may be due to psychological issues, physical problems, or both.

Common Sexual Health Problems   Medical conditions that affect women's sexual organs include the following:

• *Vaginitis* (inflammation of the vagina) is a common problem that can be caused by a variety of organisms: *Candida* (yeast infection), *Trichomonas* (trichomoniasis), and the overgrowth of a variety of bacteria (bacterial vaginosis). Symptoms include vaginal discharge, vaginal irritation, and pain during intercourse. Vaginitis is treated with a variety of topical and oral medications.

• *Endometriosis* is the growth of endometrial-like tissue outside the uterus. Endometriosis can cause serious problems if left untreated because endometrial tissue can scar and partially or completely block the oviducts, causing infertility (difficulty conceiving) or sterility (the inability to conceive).

• *Pelvic inflammatory disease (PID)* is an infection of the uterus, oviducts, or ovaries caused when microorganisms spread to these areas from the vagina. Approximately 50–75% of PID cases are caused by sexually transmitted organisms associated with diseases such as gonorrhea and chlamydia. PID can cause scarring of the oviducts, resulting in infertility or sterility.

Sexual health problems affecting men include the following:

• *Prostatitis* is an inflammation or infection of the prostate gland.

• *Testicular cancer* occurs most commonly in men in their twenties and thirties. A rare cancer, it has a very high cure rate if detected early. Every man should perform testicular self-exams regularly (see Chapter 12).

• *Epididymitis* is an inflammation of the epididymis (the coiled tube located on the top and back of each testicle). The most common cause of epididymitis is infection, often sexually transmitted. Symptoms include tenderness over the testicle, swelling, fever, and pain with ejaculation. The treatment is antibiotics.

• *Testicular torsion* occurs when the spermatic cord, which supplies blood to the testicle, becomes twisted. Decreased blood flow to the testicle causes severe, sudden pain, and if not treated quickly, it can cause permanent damage to the testicle. Testicular pain should be evaluated by a medical professional promptly; sudden, severe pain is a medical emergency.

> **QUICK STATS**
>
> **Sexually active women under 25 are at greatest risk of PID.**
>
> —CDC, 2012

---

orgasm   The discharge of accumulated sexual tension with characteristic genital and bodily manifestations and a subjective sensation of intense pleasure.   **TERMS**

sexual dysfunction   A disturbance in sexual desire, performance, or satisfaction.

Systemic diseases—illnesses that affect organs throughout the body—affect both men and women, and often affect sexual function. A common example is diabetes, which often results in sexual dysfunction because of poor blood flow to the sexual organs, along with impaired sensation and nerve function. Sexual difficulties are frequently the first sign of serious health problems because any disease that affects the cardiovascular, nervous, or endocrine system is likely to have an impact on sexual function.

Sexual Dysfunctions

The term *sexual dysfunction* encompasses disturbances in sexual desire, performance, or satisfaction. Many physical conditions and drugs can interfere with sexual functioning. Psychological causes and relationship problems can be important factors as well. Sexual satisfaction is highly individual, so no one should feel that it is necessary to live up to a particular standard of sexual performance or "normalcy." Only you can determine if some aspect of your sexuality is creating a problem for you or your partner.

COMMON SEXUAL DYSFUNCTIONS Three of the most common types of sexual difficulties in men are erectile dysfunction, premature ejaculation, and retarded ejaculation. **Erectile dysfunction** (previously called *impotence*) is the inability to achieve or maintain an erection sufficient for sexual intercourse. Erectile dysfunction occurs in men of all ages, but becomes much more common as men age. **Premature ejaculation** (ejaculation before or just after penetration of the vagina or anus) is also common, especially among younger men. If the problem is persistent and bothersome to the man and his partner, there are numerous treatments. **Retarded ejaculation** is the inability to ejaculate once an erection is achieved. Many men experience occasional difficulty achieving an erection or ejaculating because of excessive alcohol consumption, fatigue, or stress.

Female sexual problems generally involve a lack of desire to have sex, the failure to become physically aroused even when sex is desired, the failure to have an orgasm (**orgasmic dysfunction**), or pain during sexual contact. All of these problems can have physical and psychological components. Many medical problems can influence a woman's desire and ability to respond sexually. Hormonal factors, especially menopause, also have a major influence. Psychological and social issues such as relationship difficulties, family stresses, depression, and past sexual trauma are all frequent causes of sexual dysfunction.

Many women experience orgasm but not during intercourse, or they experience orgasm during intercourse only if the clitoris is directly stimulated at the same time. In general, the inability to experience orgasm under certain circumstances is a problem only if the woman considers it so.

Dyspareunia (painful intercourse) is a common symptom in women with many possible causes. Infection, lack of lubrication, endometriosis, past sexual trauma, and scarring due to childbirth are a few common reasons for pain during intercourse. In a small percentage of women, *vaginismus* (the involuntary contraction of pubic muscles) makes sexual penetration impossible.

TREATING SEXUAL DYSFUNCTION Most forms of sexual dysfunction are treatable. The first step is to have a physical examination to find a possible medical cause. Heart disease, diabetes, smoking, the use of alcohol or recreational drugs, and certain over-the-counter and prescription medications can all inhibit sexual response. Obesity is also a common cause of erectile dysfunction. Being overweight makes a man more vulnerable to cardiovascular problems, and it also can affect his hormonal balance.

Many treatments are available for erectile dysfunction. Viagra (sildenafil citrate), Cialis (tadalafil), and Levitra (vardenafil) work by enhancing the effects of nitric oxide, a chemical that relaxes smooth muscles in the penis. This increases blood flow and allows a natural erection to occur in response to sexual stimulation. The medications are generally safe for healthy men, but they should not be used by men who have a high risk of heart attack or stroke. They are effective in about 70% of users, but there are potential side effects, including headaches, indigestion, facial flushing, back pain, visual and hearing disturbances, and changes in blood pressure.

Viagra use by men between the ages of 18 and 45 has risen dramatically—possibly due to use of the drug for recreational purposes. The drug may cut the refractory period in men who do not have erectile dysfunction; younger men may also be using it to cope with performance anxiety or the effects of other drugs, such as antidepressants.

Although Viagra is not approved by the FDA for use by women, a growing number of women are trying the drug. Research findings are mixed as to whether Viagra can increase sex drive and satisfaction levels in women. Recent studies have shown, however, that the drug can sometimes help women with sexual dysfunction caused by use of antidepressant drugs.

Even when there is a physical reason for sexual dysfunction, emotional and social factors frequently compound the problem. Many people with no obvious physical disorder have sexual problems because of psychological and social issues. Too often sexual difficulties are treated with drugs when

> Any disease affecting the cardiovascular, nervous, or endocrine systems **may also affect sexual function**.

TERMS

erectile dysfunction The inability to achieve or maintain an erection sufficient for sexual intercourse.

premature ejaculation Involuntary orgasm before or shortly after the penis enters the vagina or anus; ejaculation that takes place sooner than desired.

retarded ejaculation The inability to ejaculate when one wishes to during intercourse.

orgasmic dysfunction The inability to experience orgasm.

nondrug strategies may be more appropriate. Psychosocial causes of dysfunction include troubled relationships, a lack of sexual skills, irrational attitudes and beliefs, anxiety, and psychosexual trauma such as sexual abuse or rape. Many of these problems can be addressed by sex therapy.

Premature ejaculation is an example of a common sexual problem that often responds well to nondrug therapy. On average, men typically ejaculate between 2 and 10 minutes after intercourse begins, but most men periodically ejaculate more quickly. There are several nondrug techniques that are frequently helpful for men who habitually ejaculate sooner than they would like. Kegel exercises, which strengthen and improve control of the pelvic muscles, are often helpful, as are other techniques that, with practice, increase control of ejaculation. Certain antidepressants delay ejaculation and are sometimes prescribed for this purpose.

Women who seek treatment for orgasmic dysfunction often have not learned what types of stimulation will excite them and bring them to orgasm. Most sex therapists treat this problem with **masturbation** (genital self-stimulation). Women are taught about their own anatomy and sexual responses and then are encouraged to experiment with masturbation until they experience orgasm.

Substances being tested for the treatment of female sexual dysfunction include prostaglandin creams and testosterone patches. A prostaglandin cream that improves blood flow to the clitoris is currently being developed and may be available to treat female sexual arousal disorder in the future. Another option is a device that creates suction over the clitoris to increase blood flow and sensitivity.

Dyspareunia and vaginismus are treated first by diagnosing and treating any underlying physical cause of the problem. The use of generous amounts of lubricant during sexual activity is important. Sexual therapy for vaginismus often involves gradual desensitization techniques. Recently Botox (a chemical that paralyzes muscles) injections have been used successfully in relaxing the pubic muscles in some women with vaginismus.

SEXUAL BEHAVIOR

Many behaviors stem from sexual impulses, and sexual expression takes a variety of forms. Probably the most basic aspect of sexuality is reproduction. But sexual excitement and satisfaction are aspects of sexual behavior separate from reproduction. The intensely pleasurable sensations of arousal and orgasm are probably the strongest motivators for human sexual behavior. People are infinitely varied in the ways they seek to experience erotic pleasure (see the box "Questions to Ask Before Getting Involved in a Sexual Relationship").

> **masturbation** Self-stimulation for the purpose of sexual arousal and orgasm.
> **TERMS**

Sexual Orientation

Sexual orientation is a consistent pattern of emotional, romantic, and sexual attraction to men, women, or both sexes. It exists along a continuum that ranges from exclusive heterosexuality (attraction to people of the other sex) through bisexuality (attraction to people of both sexes) to exclusive homosexuality (attraction to people of one's own sex). The terms *straight* and *gay* are often used to refer to heterosexuals and homosexuals, respectively, and female homosexuals are also referred to as *lesbians*. In recent years, the term *queer* has been reclaimed as a self-identifier by some elements of the gay community.

Sexual orientation involves feelings and self-concept, and individuals may or may not express their sexual orientation in their behavior. In national surveys, about 2–6% of men identify themselves as homosexuals and about 2% of women identify themselves as lesbians. Many theories try to account for the development of sexual orientation. At this time, most experts agree that sexual orientation results from multiple genetic, hormonal, cultural, social, and psychological factors. In addition, people's expressed sexual identities may be quite

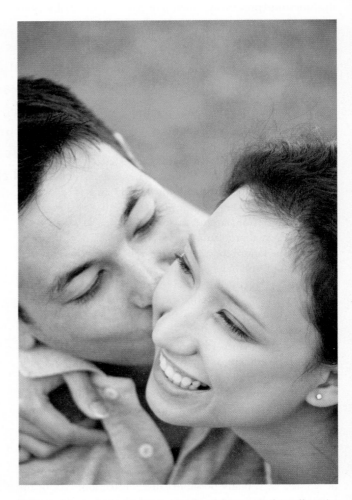

This couple's physical experiences together will be powerfully affected by their emotions, ideas, values, and the quality of their relationship.

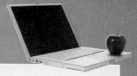
Whom am I sexually attracted to?

- What are the characteristics that usually attract me to someone in a physical way?

- How comfortable am I with the people I find sexually attractive? What would I change if I could?

- Are the people I am usually sexually attracted to the same types of people that I could envision having a long-term, stable relationship with? Why or why not?

What sexual behaviors are comfortable for me right now?

- What has influenced my comfort level with these behaviors?

- What am I not entirely comfortable with, but would be willing to experiment with in order to please a partner? What level of trust would I need to establish with that partner in order to proceed? What would we need to talk about ahead of time?

- What exactly do I say in order to make my comfort level clear to my partner? What do I do if my partner tries to push me beyond my comfort level?

How can I express my sexual needs, desires, and concerns to a potential sexual partner?

- When would be the best time to talk about these needs, desires, and concerns?

- How do I start the conversation?

- What will I do if my needs are not being met and/or my concerns are not taken seriously?

What preparations do I need to make in order to engage in the safest sex possible?

- If I am engaging in heterosexual sexual activity, I need to obtain birth control. Have I consulted a health professional to figure out the best method of birth control for myself and my partner? Do I know how to employ this method correctly? Have my partner and I discussed what we plan to do if a pregnancy occurs?

- If I am engaging in any type of sexual activity with a partner, I need protection from STDs. Have I consulted a health professional to figure out the best method of STD protection for myself and my partner? Do I know how to employ this method correctly? Have I discussed with my partner his or her sexual history, including information about risky behavior and STDs?

- What do I need from my partner in order to ensure that I feel emotionally safe before, during, and after our sexual behavior together?

- Do I engage in any behaviors that cause me to participate in sexual activity that I wouldn't otherwise be comfortable with, such as excessive drinking or drug use? What do I need to do in order to reduce or eliminate these behaviors?

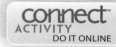

connect ACTIVITY DO IT ONLINE

---

different from their actual sexual practices. For example, some people identify as heterosexual, but most of their sexual partners may be of their own sex.

So far, most studies on the origin of sexual orientation have focused on males. The factors that determine sexual orientation in women may be even more complex. Perhaps the most important message is that sexual orientation is most likely the result of the complex interaction of biological, psychological, and social factors, possibly different in the case of each individual.

Varieties of Human Sexual Behavior

Some sexual behaviors are aimed at self-stimulation only, whereas other practices involve interaction with a partner. Some people choose not to express their sexuality at all.

Celibacy Continuous abstention from sexual activities, termed **celibacy,** can be a conscious and deliberate choice, or it can be necessitated by circumstances. Health considerations and religious and moral beliefs may lead some people to celibacy, particularly until marriage or until an acceptable partner appears. Many people use the related term *abstinence* to refer to avoidance of just one sexual activity—intercourse.

Autoeroticism and Masturbation The most common form of **autoeroticism** is **erotic fantasy**—creating imaginary experiences that range from fleeting thoughts to elaborate scenarios. Masturbation involves manually stimulating the genitals, rubbing them against objects, or using stimulating devices such as vibrators. It may be used as a substitute for sexual intercourse or as part of sexual activity with a partner.

Touching and Foreplay Touching is integral to sexual experiences, whether in the form of massage, kissing, fondling, or holding. Our entire body surface is a sensory organ, and touching almost anywhere can enhance intimacy and sexual arousal. Touching can convey a variety of messages, including affection, comfort, and a desire for further sexual contact.

During arousal, many men and women manually and orally stimulate each other by touching, stroking, and caressing

TERMS
celibacy Continuous abstention from sexual activity.
autoeroticism Behavior aimed at sexual self-stimulation.
erotic fantasy Sexually arousing thoughts and daydreams.

their partner's genitals. Men and women vary greatly in their preferences for the type, pacing, and vigor of such **foreplay.** Working out the details to accommodate each other's pleasure is a key to enjoying these activities. Direct communication about preferences can enhance sexual pleasure and protect both partners from physical and psychological discomfort.

Oral-Genital Stimulation Cunnilingus (the stimulation of the female genitals with the lips and tongue) and **fellatio** (the stimulation of the penis with the mouth) are common practices. Oral sex may be practiced either as part of foreplay or as a sex act culminating in orgasm. Although prevalence varies in different populations, 90% of men, 88% of women, and more than 50% of teens report that they have engaged in oral sex. Like all acts of sexual expression between two people, oral sex requires the cooperation and consent of both partners.

Anal Intercourse About 10% of heterosexuals and 50% of homosexual males regularly practice anal stimulation and penetration by the penis or a finger. Because the anus is composed of delicate tissues that tear easily under such pressure, anal intercourse is one of the riskiest of sexual behaviors for the transmission of HIV and all other sexually transmitted infections. Anal intercourse is also associated with increased risk of anal cancer, hemorrhoids, anal fissures, prolapsed rectum, and fecal incontinence. The use of condoms is highly recommended for anyone engaging in anal sex.

Sexual Intercourse For most adults, most of the time, **sexual intercourse** (*coitus*) is the ultimate sexual experience. The most common heterosexual practice is the man inserting his erect penis into the woman's dilated and lubricated vagina after sufficient arousal. Men and women engage in vaginal intercourse to fulfill sexual and psychological needs, as well as to reproduce. In a 2006 study by the National Center for Health Statistics, 87% of men aged 15–44 and 98% of women in the same age group reported having had vaginal intercourse. Among both men and women, one of the most popular reasons to have sex was to express emotional attachment to their partner.

Atypical and Problematic Sexual Behaviors

In American culture, many kinds of sexual behavior are accepted. However, some types of sexual expression are considered harmful; they may be illegal, classified as mental disorders, or both. Because sexual behavior occurs on a continuum, it is sometimes difficult to differentiate a behavior that is simply atypical from one that is harmful. When attempting to evaluate an unusual sexual behavior, experts consider the issues of consent between partners and whether physical or psychological harm is done to the individual or to others.

The use of force and coercion in sexual relationships is one of the most serious problems in human interactions. The most extreme manifestation of **sexual coercion**—forcing a person to submit to another's sexual desires—is rape, but sexual coercion occurs in many subtler forms, such as sexual harassment.

Commercial Sex

Conflicting feelings about sexuality are apparent in the attitudes of Americans toward commercial sex: prostitution and sexually oriented materials in a variety of formats. Our society supposedly disapproves of prostitution, but it also provides prostitutes with their customers. Pornography is readily available and widely viewed in our society, although many people are concerned about its ubiquitous nature and the blurring of pornography with popular culture.

Pornography Derived from the Greek word meaning "the writing of prostitutes," **pornography** (*porn*) is now often defined as obscene literature, art, or movies. A major problem in identifying pornographic material is that different people and communities have different opinions about what is obscene. Differing definitions of obscenity have led to many legal battles over potentially pornographic materials. Currently the sale and rental of pornographic materials is restricted so that only adults can legally obtain them; materials depicting children in sexual contexts are illegal in any format or setting.

Much of the debate about pornography focuses on whether it is harmful. Some people argue that adults who want to view pornographic materials in the privacy of their own homes should be allowed to do so. Others feel that the exposure to explicit sexual material can lead to delinquent or criminal behavior, such as rape or the sexual abuse of children. Currently there is no reliable evidence that pornography by itself leads to violence or harmful behavior, and debate is likely to continue.

> One of the commonly stated reasons for having sex is **to express emotional attachment to one's partner**.

TERMS

foreplay Kissing, touching, and any form of oral or genital contact that stimulates people toward intercourse.

cunnilingus Oral stimulation of the female genitals.

fellatio Oral stimulation of the penis.

sexual intercourse Sexual relations involving genital union; also called coitus, and also known as making love.

sexual coercion The use of physical or psychological force or intimidation to make a person submit to sexual demands.

pornography The explicit or obscene depiction of sexual activities in pictures, writing, or other material.

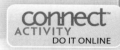

To talk with your partner about sexuality, follow the general suggestions for effective communication in Chapter 4. Getting started may be the most difficult part. Some people feel more comfortable if they begin by talking about talking—that is, initiating a discussion about why people are so uncomfortable talking about sexuality. Talking about sexual histories—how partners first learned about sex or how family and cultural background influenced sexual values and attitudes—is another way to get started. Reading about sex can also be a good beginning: partners can read an article or book and then discuss their reactions.

Be honest about what you feel and what you want from your partner. Cultural and personal obstacles to discussing sexual subjects can be difficult to overcome, but self-disclosure is important for successful relationships. Research indicates that when one partner openly discusses attitudes and feelings, the other partner is more likely to do the same. If your partner seems hesitant to open up, try asking open-ended or either/or questions: "Where do you like to be touched?" or "Would you like to talk about this now or wait until later?"

If something is bothering you about your sexual relationship, choose a good time to initiate a discussion with your partner. Be specific and direct but also tactful. Focus on what you actually observe rather than on what you think the behavior means. Try focusing on a specific behavior that concerns you rather than on the person as a whole—your partner can change behaviors but not his or her entire personality. For example, you could say "I'd like you to take a few minutes away from studying to kiss me" instead of "You're so caught up in your work, you never have time for me."

If you are going to make a statement that your partner may interpret as criticism, try mixing it with something positive: "I love being with you, but I feel annoyed when you. . . ." Similarly, if your partner says something that upsets you, don't lash back. An aggressive response may make you feel better in the short run, but it will not help the communication process or the quality of the relationship.

If you want to say no to some sexual activity, say no unequivocally. Don't send mixed messages. If you are afraid of hurting your partner's feelings, offer an alternative if it's appropriate: "I am uncomfortable with that. How about . . .?"

If you're in love, you may think that the sexual aspects of a relationship will work out magically without discussion. However, partners who never talk about sex deny themselves the opportunity to increase their closeness and improve their relationship.

connect ACTIVITY DO IT ONLINE

Online Porn and Cybersex   The appearance of thousands of sexually oriented websites has expanded the number of people with access to pornography and has made it more difficult for authorities to enforce laws regarding porn. Of special concern is the increased availability of child pornography, which previously could be acquired only with great difficulty and at great legal risk. Online porn is now a multibillion-dollar industry.

Hundreds of thousands of people also use the Internet to engage in **cybersex,** or *virtual sex*. Cybersex is erotic interaction between people who are communicating over the Internet. Although many people view cybersex as a safe form of sexual expression, it is not without problems. It can be addictive, and some cybersex addicts report spending more than 50 hours a week online for sexual purposes. People who become addicted to cybersex or viewing online porn may become isolated and perform poorly at work or school. Their addiction may also have a negative impact on their interpersonal relationships.

"Sexting," sending provocative photos from cell phone to cell phone, has become popular, sometimes with serious consequences. Images can end up traveling from person to person by cell phone and from there onto social networking websites like Facebook. These images can haunt individuals years later when they are viewed by potential employers or partners. Some teens have found themselves charged with child pornography and have even faced jail time as a result of forwarding a sexually explicit photo of an underaged person to a friend.

Prostitution   The exchange of sexual services for money is **prostitution.** Prostitutes may be men, women, or children, and the buyer of a prostitute's services is nearly always a man. Except in parts of Nevada, prostitution is illegal in the United States. Most customers are white, middle-class, middle-aged, and married. Although they come from a wide variety of backgrounds, prostitutes are usually motivated to join the profession because of money.

AIDS and other STDs are major concerns for prostitutes and their customers. Many prostitutes are injection drug users or are involved with men who are. The rate of HIV infection among prostitutes varies widely, but in some parts of the country it is as high as 25–50%. Unfortunately many prostitutes are children. The majority of prostitutes, both female and male, began working as prostitutes before they were 16 years of age. A majority of prostitutes report that they were sexually abused as children. Many prostitutes start out as child runaways, escaping abusive homes and turning to prostitution as a way to survive.

	TERMS
cybersex Erotic interaction between people over the Internet; also called virtual sex.	
prostitution The exchange of sexual services for money.	

Responsible Sexual Behavior

Healthy sexuality is an important part of adult life. It can be a source of pleasurable experiences and emotions and an important part of intimate partnerships. But sexual behavior also carries many responsibilities, as well as potential consequences such as pregnancy, STDs, and emotional changes in the relationship.

Open, Honest Communication   Each partner needs to clearly indicate what sexual involvement means to him or her. Does it mean love, fun, a permanent commitment, or something else? The intentions of both partners should be clear. For strategies on talking about sexual issues with your partner, see the box "Communicating about Sexuality."

Agreed-On Sexual Activities   No one should pressure or coerce a partner. Sexual behaviors should be consistent with the sexual values, preferences, and comfort level of both partners. Everyone has the right to refuse sexual activity at any time.

Sexual Privacy   Intimate relationships involving sexual activity are based on trust, and that trust can be violated if partners reveal private information about the relationship to others. Sexual privacy also involves respecting other people—not engaging in activities in the presence of others that would make them uncomfortable.

Using Contraception   If pregnancy is not desired, contraception should be used during sexual intercourse. Both partners need to take responsibility for protecting against unwanted pregnancy. Partners should discuss contraception before sexual involvement begins.

Safe Sex   Both partners should be aware of and practice safe sex to guard against STDs. Many sexual behaviors carry the risk of STDs, including HIV infection. Partners should be honest about their health and any medical conditions and work out a plan for protection.

Sober Sex   The use of alcohol or drugs in sexual situations increases the risk of unplanned, unprotected sexual activity. This is particularly true for young adults, many of whom binge-drink during social events. Alcohol and drugs impair judgment and should not be used in association with sexual activity. Be honest with yourself; if you need to drink in order to engage in sexual activities, maybe it's time to rethink your social life and relationships.

UNDERSTANDING FERTILITY

Conception is a complex process. Although many couples conceive easily, others face a variety of difficulties.

Conception

The process of conception involves the **fertilization** of a woman's ovum (egg) by a man's sperm. Every month during a woman's fertile years, her body prepares itself for conception and pregnancy. In one of her ovaries, an egg matures and is released from its follicle. The egg, about the size of a pinpoint, travels through an oviduct, or fallopian tube, to the uterus in three to four days. The endometrium, or lining of the uterus, has already thickened for the implantation of a **fertilized egg,** or *zygote.* If the egg is not fertilized, it lasts about 24 hours and then disintegrates. The woman's body then expels the egg's remains and the uterine lining during menstruation.

Fertilization   Sperm cells are produced in the man's testes and ejaculated from his penis into the woman's vagina during sexual intercourse. Sperm cells are much smaller than eggs. The typical ejaculate contains millions of sperm, but only a few complete the journey through the uterus and up the fallopian tube to the egg.

Of those that reach the egg, only one will penetrate its hard outer layer. As sperm approach the egg, they release enzymes that soften this outer layer. Enzymes from hundreds of sperm must be released in order for the egg's outer layer to soften enough to allow one sperm cell to penetrate. The first sperm cell that bumps into a spot that is soft enough can swim into the egg cell. It then merges with the nucleus of the egg, and fertilization occurs. The sperm's tail, its means of locomotion, gets stuck in the egg's outer membrane and drops off, leaving the sperm's head inside the egg. The egg then releases a chemical that makes it impenetrable by other sperm.

The ovum carries the hereditary characteristics of the mother and her ancestors; sperm cells carry the hereditary characteristics of the father and his ancestors. Each parent cell—egg or sperm—contains 23 chromosomes, each of which contains **genes,** which are packages of chemical instructions for the developing baby. Genes provide the blueprint for a

TERMS

fertilization   The initiation of biological reproduction: the union of the nucleus of an egg cell with the nucleus of a sperm cell.

fertilized egg   The egg after penetration by a sperm; a *zygote.*

gene   The basic unit of heredity; a section of a chromosome containing chemical instructions for making a particular protein.

unique individual based on the functional and health characteristics of his or her ancestors.

Twins   In the usual course of events, one egg and one sperm unite to produce one fertilized egg and one baby. But if the ovaries release two or more eggs during ovulation and if both eggs are fertilized, twins develop. The development of two or more fetuses in the same pregnancy is called *multiple gestation* and leads to a *multiple birth*. These twins will be no more alike than siblings from different pregnancies because each will have come from a different fertilized egg. Twins who develop this way are referred to as **fraternal twins;** they may be the same sex or different sexes. About 70% of twins are fraternal.

Twins can also develop from the division of a single fertilized egg into two cells that develop separately. Because these babies share all genetic material, they will be **identical twins.**

The most serious complication of multiple births is preterm delivery (delivery before the fetuses are adequately mature). The higher the number of fetuses that a woman carries, the earlier in gestation she will deliver.

Infertility

About 2 million American couples have difficulty conceiving. **Infertility** is defined as the inability to conceive after trying for a year or more. Infertility affected about 7.4% of reproductive-aged American women (15–44 years) in the United States in 2002 (the most recent year for which reliable statistics are available). Over 1 million women seek treatment for infertility each year. Although the focus is often on women (where the cause of infertility is found in 50% of cases), 26% of the factors contributing to infertility are male, and in 35% of infertile couples, both partners have problems. Therefore, it is important that both partners be evaluated.

Female Infertility   Female infertility usually results from one of two key causes—tubal blockage (14%) or failure to ovulate (21%). An additional 37% of cases of infertility are due to anatomical abnormalities, benign growths in the uterus, thyroid disease, and other uncommon conditions; the remaining 28% of cases are unexplained.

Blocked fallopian tubes are most commonly the result of *pelvic inflammatory disease (PID),* a serious complication of several sexually transmitted diseases especially untreated chlamydia and gonorrhea. One study found that out of 100,000 women aged 20–24 who were diagnosed with PID, 16,800 went on to have problems with infertility. More than 2.5 million cases of PID are treated each year, but physicians estimate that just as many may go untreated because of an absence of symptoms. Tubal blockages can also be caused by prior surgery or by *endometriosis,* which is typically treated with hormonal therapy and surgery.

Age also impacts fertility. Beginning around age 30, a woman's fertility naturally begins to decline. Age is probably the main factor in ovulation failure. Exposure to toxic chemicals or radiation also appears to reduce fertility, as does cigarette smoking.

Male Infertility   The leading causes of male infertility can be divided into four main categories: hypothalamic pituitary disease (1–2%), testicular disease (30–40%), disorders of sperm transport or posttesticular disorders (10–20%), and unexplained (40–50%). Some acquired disorders of the testes can lead to infertility, such as damage from drug use (including marijuana), smoking, infection, or environmental toxins.

Treating Infertility   The cause of infertility can be determined for about 85% of infertile couples. Most cases of infertility are treated with conventional medical therapies. Surgery can repair oviducts, remove endometriosis, and correct anatomical problems in men and women. Fertility drugs can help women ovulate but may cause multiple births. If these conventional treatments don't work, couples can turn to **assisted reproductive technology (ART)** techniques, as described in the following sections. According to 2010 estimates from the CDC, about 1–3% of births in the United States and Europe are the result of ART treatments.

Most infertility treatments are expensive and emotionally draining, and their success is hard to predict. Some infertile couples choose not to try to have children, whereas others turn to adoption. One measure you can take to avoid infertility is to protect yourself against STDs and get prompt treatment for any disease you contract. Couples who are ready should consider trying to conceive prior to the woman's late 30s to decrease the probability of age-related infertility.

INTRAUTERINE INSEMINATION   Male infertility can sometimes be overcome by collecting and concentrating the man's sperm and introducing it by syringe into a woman's vagina or uterus, a procedure known as **artificial (intrauterine) insemination.** To increase the probability of success, the woman is often given fertility drugs to induce ovulation prior to the insemination procedure. The success rate is about 5–20%. The wide range is due to age-related influences.

IVF, GIFT, AND ZIFT   Three related techniques for overcoming infertility involve surgically removing mature eggs from a woman's ovary:

- In **in vitro fertilization (IVF),** the harvested eggs are mixed with sperm in a laboratory dish. If eggs

---

TERMS

fraternal twins   Twins who develop from separate fertilized eggs; such twins are not genetically identical.

identical twins   Twins who develop from the division of a single zygote; such twins are genetically identical.

infertility   The inability to conceive after trying for a year or more.

assisted reproductive technology (ART)   Advanced medical techniques used to treat infertility.

artificial (intrauterine) insemination   The introduction of semen into the vagina by artificial means.

in vitro fertilization (IVF)   Combining eggs and sperm outside the body and inserting one or more fertilized eggs into the uterus.

are successfully fertilized, one or more of the resulting embryos are inserted into the woman's uterus. IVF is often used by women with blocked oviducts.

- In **gamete intrafallopian transfer (GIFT)**, eggs and sperm are surgically placed into the fallopian tubes prior to fertilization.

- In **zygote intrafallopian transfer (ZIFT)**, eggs are fertilized outside the woman's body and surgically introduced into the oviducts after they begin to divide.

GIFT and ZIFT can be used by women who have at least one open fallopian tube.

There are disadvantages to IVF. Success rates determined by live birth rates vary from about 5.1% to 41.1% depending on age. It costs more than $10,000 per procedure and may require five or more attempts to produce one live birth. It also increases the chance of multiple births, which in turn increases the risk of premature birth and maternal complications, including pregnancy-related hypertension and diabetes.

GESTATIONAL CARRIER (FORMERLY KNOWN AS SURROGACY) A gestational carrier (GC) is a fertile woman who agrees to carry a fetus for an infertile couple. The GC agrees to be artificially inseminated by the father's sperm or to undergo IVF with the couple's embryo, to carry the baby to term, and to give it to the couple at birth. In return, the couple pays her for her services (typically around $50,000). There are thought to be approximately 1000 gestational carrier pregnancies each year in the United States.

PREGNANCY

Pregnancy is usually discussed in terms of **trimesters**—three periods of about three months (or 13 weeks) each. During the first trimester, the mother experiences a few physical changes and some fairly common symptoms (see the box "Home Pregnancy Tests"). During the second trimester, often the most peaceful time of pregnancy, the mother gains weight, looks noticeably pregnant, and may experience a general sense of well-being if she is happy about having a child. The third trimester is the hardest for the mother because she must breathe, digest, excrete, and circulate blood for herself and the growing fetus.

> **QUICK STATS**
>
> **146,244 ART procedures were performed in the United States in 2009, resulting in more than 45,870 babies.**
>
> —CDC, 2011

Changes in the Woman's Body

Hormonal changes begin as soon as the egg is fertilized, and for the next nine months the woman's body nourishes the fetus and adjusts to its growth (Figure 5.4).

Early Signs and Symptoms   Early recognition of pregnancy is important, especially for women with physical problems and nutritional deficiencies. The following symptoms are not absolute indications of pregnancy, but they are reasons to visit a gynecologist:

- *A missed menstrual period.* When a fertilized egg implants in the uterine wall, the endometrium is retained to nourish the embryo.

- *Slight bleeding.* Slight bleeding follows implantation of the fertilized egg in about 14% of pregnant women. Because this happens about when a period is expected, the bleeding is sometimes mistaken for menstrual flow. It usually lasts only a few days.

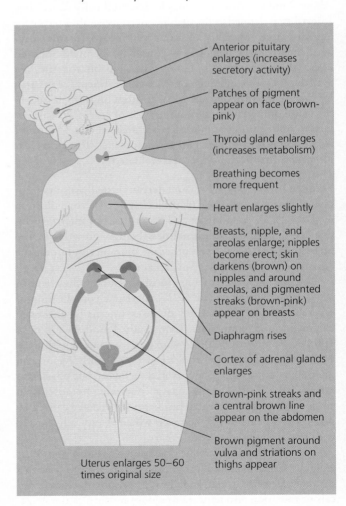

Anterior pituitary enlarges (increases secretory activity)

Patches of pigment appear on face (brown-pink)

Thyroid gland enlarges (increases metabolism)

Breathing becomes more frequent

Heart enlarges slightly

Breasts, nipple, and areolas enlarge; nipples become erect; skin darkens (brown) on nipples and around areolas, and pigmented streaks (brown-pink) appear on breasts

Diaphragm rises

Cortex of adrenal glands enlarges

Brown-pink streaks and a central brown line appear on the abdomen

Brown pigment around vulva and striations on thighs appear

Uterus enlarges 50–60 times original size

FIGURE 5.4   Physiological changes during pregnancy.

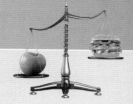

Women have access to a variety of over-the-counter home pregnancy tests today, but in general they all work the same way—by detecting the presence of the hormone *human chorionic gonadotropin (HCG)* in the woman's urine or blood. HGC is released by the implanted fertilized egg and can be detected within about two weeks of ovulation. Home pregnancy tests vary in such minor details as how the woman uses the test strips and how the strips display results.

Home pregnancy tests have become extremely accurate since their introduction in 1975, typically providing accurate results 99% of the time. However, there is variation among women in the time it takes a fertilized egg to implant in the uterus and begin releasing HGC. The earliest that implantation can occur is about seven days after ovulation, but ten to twelve days is more common. HGC levels double every two to three days. Many women who are pregnant won't have a positive test until the first day of a missed period or even a few days later.

A clinical blood test is more accurate but not necessarily more sensitive than a home pregnancy test. That is, it cannot detect pregnancy sooner than a urine test.

If you use a home pregnancy test, be aware of the limitations. If you're comfortable waiting, a sensitive test taken a week after your period is due will almost certainly give you accurate results. If you elect to take the test as early as the day after you've missed your period, remember that a negative result isn't 100% certain. A positive result may mean either a viable pregnancy or a pregnancy destined to end shortly after it began. With either of those results, you should plan on testing again a week later, just to be sure. For that reason, it's a good idea to buy tests in pairs; most commercially available home testing products come in multiple-test kits.

- *Nausea.* About 50–90% of pregnant women feel some level of nausea, probably as a reaction to increased levels of progesterone and other hormones. Although this nausea is often called *morning sickness,* some women have it all day long. It frequently begins during the 6th week and disappears by the 12th week. In some cases it lasts throughout the pregnancy.

- *Breast tenderness.* Some women experience breast tenderness, swelling, and tingling, usually described as different from the tenderness experienced before menstruation.

- *Increased urination.* Increased frequency of urination can occur soon after the missed period.

- *Sleepiness, fatigue, and emotional upset.* These symptoms result from hormonal changes. Fatigue can be surprisingly overwhelming in the first trimester but usually improves significantly around the third month of pregnancy.

The first reliable physical signs of pregnancy can be distinguished about four weeks after a woman misses her menstrual period. A softening of the uterus just above the cervix, called *Hegar's sign,* and other changes in the cervix and pelvis are apparent during a pelvic examination. The labia minora and the cervix may take on a purple color rather than their usual pink hue.

Continuing Changes in the Woman's Body   The most obvious changes during pregnancy occur in the reproductive organs. During the first three months, the uterus enlarges to about three times its nonpregnant size, but it still cannot be felt in the abdomen. By the fourth month, it is large enough to

make the abdomen protrude. By the seventh or eighth month, the uterus pushes up into the rib cage, which makes breathing slightly more difficult. The breasts enlarge and are sensitive; by week 8, they may tingle or throb. The pigmented area around the nipple, called the *areola,* darkens and broadens.

Other changes are going on as well. Early in pregnancy, the muscles and ligaments attached to bones begin to soften and stretch. The joints between the pelvic bones loosen and spread, making it easier to have a baby but harder to walk. The circulatory system becomes more efficient to accommodate higher blood volume, which increases by 50%, and the heart pumps it more rapidly. The mother's lungs also become more efficient, and her rib cage widens to permit her to inhale up to 40% more air.

The average weight gain during a healthy pregnancy is 27.5 pounds, although actual weight change varies with the individual. About 60% of the weight gain is directly related to the baby (such as the fetus and placenta); the rest accumulates over the woman's body as fluid and fat.

Changes during the Later Stages of Pregnancy   By the end of the sixth month, the increased needs of the fetus place a burden on the mother's lungs, heart, and kidneys. Her back may ache from the pressure of the baby's weight and from having to throw her shoulders back to keep her balance while standing. Her body retains more water, perhaps up to three extra quarts of fluid. Her legs, hands, ankles, or feet may swell, and she may be bothered by leg cramps, heartburn, or constipation. Despite discomfort, both her digestion and her metabolism are working at top efficiency.

The uterus prepares for childbirth with preliminary contractions, called *Braxton Hicks contractions.* Unlike true labor contractions, these are usually short, irregular, and painless.

FIGURE 5.5   A chronology of milestones in prenatal development.

The mother may only be aware that at times her abdomen is hard to the touch. These contractions become more frequent and intense as the delivery date approaches.

In the ninth month, the baby settles into the pelvic bones, usually head down, fitting snugly. This process, called **lightening,** allows the uterus to sink down about two inches, producing a visible change in the mother's profile. Pelvic pressure increases, and pressure on the diaphragm lightens. Breathing becomes easier; urination becomes more frequent. Sometimes, after a first pregnancy, the baby doesn't settle down into the pelvis until labor begins.

Fetal Development

Now that we've seen what happens to the mother's body during pregnancy, let's consider the development of the fetus (Figure 5.5).

The First Trimester   About 30 hours after an egg is fertilized, the cell divides, and this process of cell division repeats many times. As the cluster of cells drifts along the oviduct, several different kinds of cells emerge. The entire set of genetic instructions is passed to every cell, but each cell follows only certain instructions; if this were not the case, there would be no different organs or body parts. For example, all cells carry genes for hair color and eye color, but only the cells of the hair follicles and irises (of the eye) respond to that information.

On about the fourth day after fertilization, the cluster, now about 32–128 cells and hollow, arrives in the uterus; this is a **blastocyst.** On about the sixth or seventh day, the blastocyst attaches to the uterine wall, usually along the upper curve. Over the next few days, it becomes firmly implanted and begins to draw nourishment from the endometrium, the uterine lining.

The blastocyst becomes an **embryo** by about the end of the second week after fertilization. The inner cells of the blastocyst separate into three layers. One layer becomes inner body parts—the digestive and respiratory systems; the middle layer becomes muscle, bone, blood, kidneys, and sex glands; and the third layer becomes the skin, hair, and nervous tissue.

TERMS

lightening   A process in which the uterus sinks down because the baby's head settles into the pelvic area.

blastocyst   A stage of development, days 6–14, before the cell cluster becomes the embryo and placenta.

embryo   The stage of development between blastocyst and fetus; about weeks 2–8.

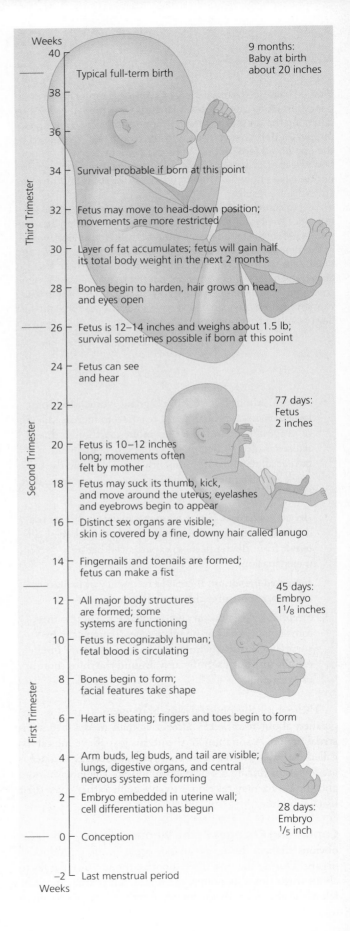

Weeks
40 — Typical full-term birth

9 months: Baby at birth about 20 inches

Third Trimester

38

36

34 — Survival probable if born at this point

32 — Fetus may move to head-down position; movements are more restricted

30 — Layer of fat accumulates; fetus will gain half its total body weight in the next 2 months

28 — Bones begin to harden, hair grows on head, and eyes open

26 — Fetus is 12–14 inches and weighs about 1.5 lb; survival sometimes possible if born at this point

24 — Fetus can see and hear

Second Trimester

22

77 days: Fetus 2 inches

20 — Fetus is 10–12 inches long; movements often felt by mother

18 — Fetus may suck its thumb, kick, and move around the uterus; eyelashes and eyebrows begin to appear

16 — Distinct sex organs are visible; skin is covered by a fine, downy hair called lanugo

14 — Fingernails and toenails are formed; fetus can make a fist

45 days: Embryo 1 1/8 inches

12 — All major body structures are formed; some systems are functioning

10 — Fetus is recognizably human; fetal blood is circulating

8 — Bones begin to form; facial features take shape

First Trimester

6 — Heart is beating; fingers and toes begin to form

4 — Arm buds, leg buds, and tail are visible; lungs, digestive organs, and central nervous system are forming

2 — Embryo embedded in uterine wall; cell differentiation has begun

28 days: Embryo 1/5 inch

0 — Conception

–2 — Last menstrual period
Weeks

The outermost shell of cells becomes the **placenta, umbilical cord,** and **amniotic sac**. A network of blood vessels called *chorionic villi* eventually forms the placenta. The human placenta allows a two-way exchange of nutrients and waste materials between the mother and the fetus. The placenta brings oxygen and nutrients to the fetus and transports waste products out. The placenta does not provide a perfect barrier between the fetal circulation and the maternal circulation, however. Some blood cells are exchanged, and certain substances, such as alcohol, pass freely from the maternal circulation through the placenta to the fetus.

The period between weeks 2 and 9 is a time of rapid differentiation and change. All the major body structures are formed during this time, including the heart, brain, liver, lungs, and sex organs. The eyes, nose, ears, arms, and legs also appear. Some organs begin to function, as well; the heart begins to beat, and the liver starts producing blood cells. Because body structures are forming, the developing organism is vulnerable to damage from environmental influences such as drugs and infections.

By the end of the second month, the brain sends out impulses that coordinate the functioning of other organs. The embryo is now a fetus, and most further changes will be in the size and refinement of working body parts. In the third month, the fetus becomes active. By the end of the first trimester, the fetus is about an inch long and weighs less than one ounce.

The Second Trimester

To grow during the second trimester, to about 14 inches and 1.5 pounds, the fetus must have large amounts of food, oxygen, and water, which come from the mother through the placenta. All body systems are operating, and the fetal heartbeat can be heard with a stethoscope. The mother can detect fetal movements beginning in the fourth or fifth month. Against great odds, a fetus born at 24–26 weeks (the end of the second trimester) has a 50–60% chance of survival.

The Third Trimester

The fetus gains most of its birth weight during the last three months of the pregnancy. Some of the weight is fat under the skin that insulates the fetus and supplies food. About 85% of the calcium and iron the mother consumes goes into the fetal bloodstream.

The fetus may live if it is born during the seventh month, but it needs the fat layer acquired in the eighth month and time for organs—especially the respiratory and digestive organs—to develop. It also needs the immunity supplied by the antibodies in the mother's blood during the final three months. The antibodies protect the fetus against many of the diseases to which the mother has acquired immunity.

Diagnosing Fetal Abnormalities

About 3% of babies are born with a major birth defect. Information about the health and sex of a fetus can be obtained prior to birth through prenatal testing.

Ultrasonography (also called *ultrasound*) uses high-frequency sound waves to create a **sonogram,** or visual image, of the fetus in the uterus. Sonograms show the fetus's position, size, and gestational age, and the presence of certain anatomical problems. Sonograms can sometimes be used to determine the sex of the fetus. Sonograms are considered safe for a pregnant woman and the fetus, but the FDA advises against "keepsake" sonograms performed for no medical purpose.

Amniocentesis involves the removal of fluid from the uterus with a long, thin needle inserted through the abdominal wall. It is usually performed between 16 and 18 weeks into the pregnancy. A genetic analysis of the fetal cells in the fluid can reveal the presence of chromosomal disorders, such as Down syndrome, and some genetic diseases, including Tay-Sachs disease. The sex of the fetus can also be determined.

Another prenatal test is **chorionic villus sampling (CVS),** which can be performed earlier in pregnancy than amniocentesis, between weeks 10 and 12. This procedure involves removal through the cervix (by catheter) or abdomen (by needle) of a tiny section of chorionic villi, which contain fetal cells that can be analyzed.

The **quadruple marker screen (QMS)** is a maternal blood test that can be used to help identify fetuses with neural tube defects, Down syndrome, and other anomalies. Blood is taken from the mother at 16–19 weeks of pregnancy and analyzed for four hormone levels—human chorionic gonadotropin (HCG), unconjugated estriol, alpha-fetoprotein (AFP), and inhibin-A. The hormone levels are compared to appropriate standards, and the results are used to estimate the probability that the fetus has particular anomalies. QMS is a screening test rather than a diagnostic test; in the case of abnormal QMS results, parents may choose further testing such as ultrasonography or amniocentesis.

> Against great odds, **a fetus born at the end of the second trimester might survive**.

TERMS

placenta   The organ through which the fetus receives nourishment and empties waste via the mother's circulatory system; after birth, the placenta is expelled from the uterus.

umbilical cord   The cord connecting the placenta and fetus, through which nutrients pass.

amniotic sac   A membranous pouch enclosing and protecting the fetus; also holds amniotic fluid.

ultrasonography   The use of high-frequency sound waves to view the fetus in the uterus; also known as *ultrasound*.

sonogram   The visual image of the fetus produced by ultrasonography.

amniocentesis   A process in which amniotic fluid is removed and analyzed to detect possible birth defects.

chorionic villus sampling (CVS)   Surgical removal of a tiny section of chorionic villi to be analyzed for genetic defects.

quadruple marker screen (QMS)   A measurement of four hormones, used to assess the risk of fetal abnormalities.

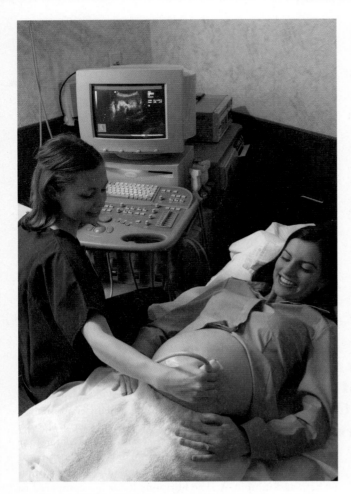

Ultrasonography provides information about the position, size, and physical condition of a fetus in the uterus.

First-trimester screening for Down syndrome combines ultrasound evaluation of nuchal translucency (the thickness of the back of the fetus's neck) with maternal blood testing. This test can be done between the 10th and 14th weeks of pregnancy. This can be combined with serum testing at 16 weeks for a sequential screen that has the highest sensitivity of all of the available tests. If results indicate an increased risk of abnormality, further diagnostic studies such as amniocentesis can be done for confirmation.

Researchers are developing new fetal screening techniques that are less invasive and that can be done earlier in pregnancy. One such test, MaterniT21, is a laboratory-developed test that analyzes maternal blood for fetal DNA as early as 10 weeks. It can detect increased levels of chromosome 21, which indicate a fetus with Down syndrome.

Fetal Programming   Amniocentesis, CVS, and QMS look for chromosomal, genetic, and other anomalies that typically cause immediate problems. A new area of study known as *fetal programming theory* focuses on how conditions in the womb may influence the risk of adult diseases. For example, researchers have linked low birth weight to an increased risk of heart disease, high blood pressure, obesity, diabetes, and schizophrenia. High birth weight in female infants, however, has been linked to an increased risk of breast cancer in later life.

Although fetal programming theory is not yet embraced by all scientists, these studies emphasize that everything that occurs during pregnancy can have an impact on the developing fetus. In the future, people may be able to use information about their birth weight and other indicators of gestational conditions just as they can now use family history and genetic information—to alert them to special health risks and to help them improve their health.

The Importance of Prenatal Care

Adequate prenatal care—as described in the following sections—is essential to the health of both mother and baby. All physicians recommend that women start getting regular prenatal checkups as soon as they become pregnant. Typically this means one checkup per month during the first eight months, then one checkup per week during the final month. About 84% of pregnant women begin receiving adequate prenatal care during the first trimester; about 3.5% wait until the last trimester or receive no prenatal care at all.

Regular Checkups   In the woman's first visit to her obstetrician, she will be asked for a detailed medical history of herself and her family. The physician or midwife will note any hereditary conditions that may assume increased significance during pregnancy. The tendency to develop gestational diabetes (diabetes during pregnancy only), for example, can be inherited; appropriate treatment during pregnancy reduces the risk of serious harm.

The woman is given a complete physical exam and is informed about appropriate diet. She returns for regular checkups throughout the pregnancy, during which her blood pressure and weight gain are measured, her urine is analyzed, and the fetus's size and position are monitored.

Blood Tests   A blood sample is taken during the initial prenatal visit to determine blood type and detect possible anemia or Rh incompatibilities. The **Rh factor** is a blood protein. If an Rh-positive father and an Rh-negative mother conceive an Rh-positive baby, the baby's blood will be incompatible with the mother's blood. This condition is completely treatable with a serum called *Rh-immune globulin*, which destroys Rh-positive cells as they enter the mother's body and prevents her from forming antibodies to them. Blood may also be tested for evidence of hepatitis B, syphilis, rubella immunity, thyroid problems, and, with the mother's permission, HIV infection.

Prenatal Nutrition   A nutritious diet throughout pregnancy is essential for both the mother and her unborn baby.

> **Rh factor**   A protein found in blood; Rh incompatibility between a mother and fetus can jeopardize the fetus's health.
>
> **TERMS**

Not only does the baby get all its nutrients from the mother, but it also competes with her for nutrients not sufficiently available to meet both their needs. When a woman's diet is low in iron or calcium, the fetus receives most of it, and the mother may become deficient in the mineral. To meet the increased nutritional demands of her body, a pregnant woman shouldn't just eat more; she should make sure that her diet is nutritionally adequate.

To maintain her own health and help the fetus grow, a pregnant woman typically needs to consume about 250–500 extra calories per day. Breastfeeding an infant requires even more energy—about 500 or more calories per day. To ensure that she's getting enough calories and nutrients, a pregnant woman should talk to her physician or a registered dietician about her dietary habits and determine what changes she should make.

Some physicians prescribe high-potency vitamin and mineral supplements to pregnant and lactating women. Supplements can help boost the levels of nutrients available to mother and child, helping with fetal development while ensuring that the mother doesn't become nutrient-deficient.

Pregnant and lactating women, however, should not take supplements without the advice of their physicians because some vitamins and minerals are harmful if taken in excess. Pregnant women also should not take herbal dietary supplements without consulting a physician.

Two vitamins—vitamin D and the B vitamin folate—are particularly important to pregnant women. Pregnant women who don't get enough vitamin D are more likely to deliver low-birth-weight babies. Chronic vitamin D deficiency has been linked to other health problems, including heart disease.

If a woman doesn't get the recommended daily amount of folate, both before and during pregnancy, her child has an increased risk of neural tube defects, including spina bifida. Any woman capable of becoming pregnant should get at least 400 µg (0.4 mg) of folic acid (the synthetic form of folate) daily from fortified foods and/or supplements, in addition to folate from a varied diet. Pregnant women should get 1000 µg every day.

Food safety is another special dietary concern for pregnant women because foodborne pathogens can be especially dangerous to them and their unborn children. Germs such as *Listeria monocytogenes* and *Toxoplasma gondii* are both particularly worrisome. Pregnant women should avoid eating undercooked and ready-to-eat meats and should be sure to thoroughly wash produce before eating it. Pregnant women should also follow the FDA's recommendations for consumption of fish and seafood. For complete information about nutrition and food safety, see Chapter 9.

Avoiding Drugs and Other Environmental Hazards

In addition to the food the mother eats, the drugs she takes and the chemicals she is exposed to affect the fetus. Everything the mother ingests may eventually reach the fetus in some proportion. Some drugs harm the fetus but not the mother because the fetus is in the process of developing and because the proper dose for the mother is a massive dose for the fetus.

During the first trimester, when the major body structures are rapidly forming, the fetus is extremely vulnerable to environmental factors such as viral infections, radiation, drugs, and other **teratogens,** any of which can cause **congenital malformations,** or birth defects. The most susceptible body parts are those growing most rapidly at the time of exposure. The rubella (German measles) virus, for example, can cause a congenital malformation of a delicate system such as the eyes or ears, leading to blindness or deafness, if exposure occurs during the first trimester, but it does no damage later in the

A woman's dietary needs change during pregnancy, so it's important to eat a nutritionally sound diet.

teratogen   An agent or influence that causes physical defects in a developing fetus.

congenital malformation   A physical defect existing at the time of birth, either inherited or caused during gestation.

TERMS

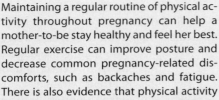
Maintaining a regular routine of physical activity throughout pregnancy can help a mother-to-be stay healthy and feel her best. Regular exercise can improve posture and decrease common pregnancy-related discomforts, such as backaches and fatigue. There is also evidence that physical activity may prevent gestational diabetes, relieve stress, and build stamina that can be helpful during labor and delivery.

A woman who was physically active before pregnancy should be able to continue her favorite activities in moderation, except for those that carry a risk of trauma, or unless there is a medical reason to reduce or stop exercise.

The American College of Obstetricians and Gynecologists (ACOG) offers advice regarding exercise during pregnancy. For example, pregnant women should avoid exercising in the supine position (lying on the back), especially after the first trimester. Women should avoid motionless standing and strenuous lifting throughout pregnancy. In general, experts encourage low-impact aerobic activities over high-impact exercise. Pregnant women should not let their heart rate exceed 140 beats per minute and should avoid getting overheated or dehydrated.

A woman who has never exercised regularly can safely start an exercise program during pregnancy after consulting with her health care provider. A routine of regular walking is considered a safe way to start exercising during pregnancy. The ACOG recommends that any pregnant woman who exercises should stop exercising if she experiences any of the following warning signs:

- Vaginal bleeding
- Shortness of breath before becoming exerted
- Dizziness
- Headache
- Pain in the chest or calves
- Weakness
- Preterm labor
- Decreased fetal movement
- Leakage of amniotic fluid

SOURCES: ACOG Committee on Obstetric Practice. 2002 (reaffirmed 2009). Committee opinion: Exercise during pregnancy and the postpartum period. *Obstetrics and Gynecology* 99(1): 171–173; Physical Activity Guidelines Advisory Committee. 2008. *Physical Activity Guidelines Advisory Committee Report,* 2008. Washington, DC: U.S. Department of Health and Human Services.

---

pregnancy. Similarly, retinoic acid exposure in the first trimester can lead to spontaneous abortion and fetal malformations such as microcephaly and cardiac anomalies. Another example is the class of medications known as anti-epileptics (such as valproic acid). The most common congenital malformations identified are open neural tube, congenital cardiac defects, urinary tract defects, skeletal abnormalities, and cleft palates.

ALCOHOL Alcohol is a potent teratogen. Getting drunk just one time during pregnancy may be enough to cause brain damage in a fetus. A high level of alcohol consumption during pregnancy is associated with spontaneous miscarriages and stillbirths. Fetuses born to mothers who have consumed alcohol are at risk for **fetal alcohol syndrome (FAS).** A baby born with FAS is likely to be characterized by a small head and body size, unusual facial features, congenital heart defects, defective joints, impaired vision, mental impairment, and abnormal behavior

> **QUICK STATS**
>
> **2.3** million **pregnant American women become infected with an STD every year.**
>
> —CDC, 2011

patterns. Researchers doubt that any level of alcohol consumption is safe, and they recommend total abstinence during pregnancy.

TOBACCO Smoking during pregnancy increases the risk of miscarriage, low birth weight, immune system impairment, and infant death; it may also cause genetic damage or physical deformations. If nicotine levels in a mother's bloodstream are high, fetal breathing rate and movement become more rapid; the fetus may also metabolize cancer-causing by-products of tobacco.

CAFFEINE Caffeine, a powerful stimulant, puts both mother and fetus under stress by raising the level of the hormone epinephrine. Caffeine also reduces the blood supply to the uterus. A pregnant woman should limit her caffeine intake to no more than the equivalent of two cups of coffee per day.

DRUGS Some prescription drugs, such as some blood pressure medications, can harm the fetus, so they should be used only under medical supervision. Many babies born to women who use antidepressants during pregnancy suffer withdrawal symptoms after birth. Recreational drugs, such as cocaine, are thought to increase the risk of major birth defects. Marijuana use may also interfere with fertility treatments, and methamphetamine use is associated with underweight babies.

> **TERMS**
>
> **fetal alcohol syndrome (FAS)** A combination of birth defects caused by excessive alcohol consumption by the mother during pregnancy.

STDS AND OTHER INFECTIONS Infections, including those that are sexually transmitted, are another serious problem for the fetus. Such infections can pose a threat before, during, and after birth. Rubella, syphilis, gonorrhea, hepatitis B, group B streptococcus, herpes, and HIV are among the most dangerous infections for the fetus. Treatment of the mother or immunization of the baby just after birth can help prevent problems from many infections. Women at risk for HIV infection should be tested before or during pregnancy because early treatment can dramatically reduce the chance that the virus will be passed to the fetus. Some experts advocate universal HIV screening for pregnant women.

Prenatal Activity and Exercise   Physical activity during pregnancy contributes to mental and physical wellness (see the box "Physical Activity during Pregnancy"). Women can continue working at their jobs until late in their pregnancy, provided the work isn't so physically demanding that it jeopardizes their health. At the same time, pregnant women need more rest and sleep to maintain their own well-being and that of the fetus.

Kegel exercises, to strengthen the pelvic floor muscles, are recommended for pregnant women. These exercises are performed by alternately contracting and releasing the muscles used to stop the flow of urine. Each contraction should be held for about five seconds. Kegel exercises should be done several times a day for a total of about 50 repetitions daily.

Preparing for Birth   Childbirth classes are almost a routine part of the prenatal experience for both mothers and fathers today. These classes typically teach the details of the birth process as well as relaxation techniques to help deal with the discomfort of labor and delivery. The mother learns and practices a variety of techniques so she will be able to choose what works best for her during labor when the time comes. The father typically acts as a coach, supporting his partner emotionally and helping her with her breathing and relaxing. He remains with her throughout labor and delivery, even when a cesarean section is performed.

Complications of Pregnancy and Pregnancy Loss

About 31% of mothers-to-be suffer complications during pregnancy. Some complications may prevent full-term development of the fetus or affect the health of the infant at birth. As discussed earlier in the chapter, exposure to harmful substances, such as alcohol or drugs, can harm the fetus. Other complications are caused by physiological problems or genetic abnormalities.

Ectopic Pregnancy   In an **ectopic pregnancy,** the fertilized egg implants and begins to develop outside of the uterus, usually in an oviduct (Figure 5.6).

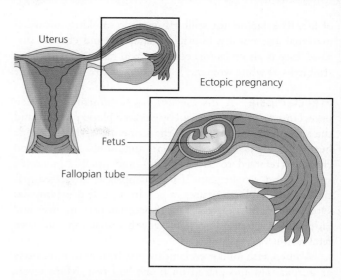

FIGURE 5.6   Ectopic pregnancy in a fallopian tube.

Ectopic pregnancies usually occur because the fallopian tube is blocked, most often as a result of pelvic inflammatory disease; smoking also increases a woman's risk for ectopic pregnancy. The embryo may spontaneously abort, or the embryo and placenta may continue to expand until they rupture the oviduct. Sharp pain on one side of the abdomen or in the lower back, usually in about the seventh or eighth week of pregnancy, may signal an ectopic pregnancy, and there may be irregular bleeding.

Surgical removal of the embryo and the oviduct may be necessary to save the mother's life, although microsurgery can sometimes be used to repair the damaged oviduct. If diagnosed early, before the oviduct ruptures, ectopic pregnancy can often be successfully treated without surgery with the drug methotrexate.

Spontaneous Abortion   A spontaneous abortion, or miscarriage, is the termination of pregnancy before the 20th week. Most miscarriages—about 60%—are due to chromosomal abnormalities in the fetus. Certain occupations that involve exposure to chemicals may increase the likelihood of a spontaneous abortion. One miscarriage doesn't mean that later pregnancies will be unsuccessful, and about 70–90% of women who miscarry eventually become pregnant again.

Stillbirth   The terms *fetal death, fetal demise, stillbirth,* and *stillborn* all refer to the delivery of a fetus that shows no signs

> A miscarriage doesn't mean future pregnancies will fail. **Up to 90% of women who miscarry get pregnant again**.

ectopic pregnancy   A pregnancy in which the embryo develops outside of the uterus, usually in an oviduct.

TERMS

of life. Risk factors for stillbirth include smoking, advanced maternal age, obesity, multiple gestations, and chronic disease. Race is also a factor; black women have twice as many stillbirths as white women.

Preeclampsia A disease unique to human pregnancy, **preeclampsia** is characterized by elevated blood pressure and the appearance of protein in the urine. Symptoms include headache, right upper-quadrant abdominal pain, vision changes (referred to as *scotomata*), and notable increased swelling and weight gain. If preeclampsia is untreated, patients can develop seizures, a condition called **eclampsia.** Other potential complications of preeclampsia are liver and kidney damage, bleeding, fetal growth restriction, and even fetal death.

Women with mild preeclampsia may be monitored closely as outpatients and placed on home bed rest. More severe cases may require hospitalization for close medical management and early delivery.

Placenta Previa In **placenta previa,** the placenta either completely or partially covers the cervical opening, preventing the mother from delivering the baby vaginally. As a result, the baby must be delivered by cesarean section. Risk factors include prior cesarean delivery, multiple pregnancies, intrauterine surgery, smoking, multiple gestations, and advanced maternal age.

Placental Abruption In **placental abruption,** a normally implanted placenta prematurely separates from the uterine wall. Patients experience abdominal pain, vaginal bleeding, and uterine tenderness. The condition increases the risk of fetal death. The risk factors for developing a placental abruption are maternal age, tobacco smoking, cocaine use, multiple gestation, trauma, preeclampsia, hypertension, and premature rupture of membranes.

Gestational Diabetes During gestation, about 4% of all pregnant women develop **gestational diabetes (GDM),** in which the body loses its ability to use insulin properly. In these women, diabetes occurs only during pregnancy. Women diagnosed with GDM have an increased risk of developing type 2 diabetes later in life. It is important to accurately diagnose and treat GDM because it can lead to preeclampsia, polyhydramnios (increased levels of amniotic fluid), large fetuses, birth trauma, operative deliveries, perinatal mortality, and neonatal metabolic complications.

Preterm Labor and Birth When a pregnant woman goes into labor before the 37th week of gestation, she is said to undergo *preterm labor.* About 30–50% of preterm labors resolve themselves, with the pregnancy continuing to full term. In other cases, interventions may be required to delay labor and allow gestation to continue.

If labor cannot be stopped, the baby may be **premature** (born before the 37th week of pregnancy).

In the United States, about 12.8% of babies are born prematurely. The rate has increased by 9% since 2000 and by 20% since 1990. Preterm birth rates vary widely among racial and ethnic groups.

Preterm birth is the leading direct cause of newborn death, accounting for about one-third of all infant deaths. Preterm birth is also the main risk factor for newborn illness and death from other causes, particularly infection. Babies born prematurely appear to be at a higher risk of long-term health and developmental problems, including delayed development and learning problems.

Risk factors for preterm birth include lack of prenatal care, smoking, drug use, stress, personal health history, infections or illness during pregnancy, obesity, exposure to environmental toxins, a previous preterm birth, and carrying multiple fetuses. However, only about half of the women who give birth prematurely have any known risk factors.

Labor Induction If pregnancy continues well beyond the baby's due date, it may be necessary to induce labor artificially. This is one of the most common obstetrical procedures and is typically offered to pregnant women who have not delivered and are 7–14 days past their due dates.

Low Birth Weight A **low-birth-weight (LBW)** baby is one that weighs less than 5.5 pounds at birth. LBW babies

Ask Yourself

QUESTIONS FOR CRITICAL THINKING AND REFLECTION

Do you know anyone who has lost a child to miscarriage, stillbirth, or a birth defect? If so, how did they cope with their loss? What would you do to help someone in this situation?

TERMS

preeclampsia A condition of pregnancy characterized by high blood pressure and protein in the urine.

eclampsia A severe, potentially life-threatening form of preeclampsia, characterized by seizures.

placenta previa A complication of pregnancy in which the placenta covers the cervical opening, preventing the mother from delivering the baby vaginally.

placental abruption A complication of pregnancy in which a normally implanted placenta prematurely separates from the uterine wall.

gestational diabetes (GDM) A form of diabetes that occurs during pregnancy.

premature Born before the 37th week of pregnancy.

low birth weight (LBW) Weighing less than 5.5 pounds at birth, often the result of prematurity.

may be premature or full-term. Babies who are born small even though they're full-term are referred to as *small-for-date* or *small-for-gestational-age* babies. Low birth weight affected 8.2% of babies born in 2008 in the United States. About half of all cases are related to teenage pregnancy, cigarette smoking, poor nutrition, and poor maternal health. Other maternal factors include drug use, stress, depression, and anxiety. Adequate prenatal care is the best way to prevent LBW. Full-term LBW babies tend to have fewer problems than premature infants.

Infant Mortality   The U.S. rate of **infant mortality,** the death of a child at less than 1 year of age, is near its lowest point ever; however, it remains far higher than rates in most of the developed world. Poverty and inadequate health care are key causes.

Other causes of infant death are congenital problems, infectious diseases, and injuries. In **sudden infant death syndrome (SIDS),** an apparently healthy infant dies suddenly while sleeping. About 2300 infant deaths are attributed to SIDS each year. Research suggests that abnormalities in the brainstem, the part of the brain that regulates breathing, heart rate, and other basic functions, underlie the risk for SIDS. Risk is greatly increased for infants with these innate differences if they are exposed to environmental risks, such as sleeping face down; being exposed to tobacco smoke, alcohol, or other drugs; or sleeping on a soft mattress or with fluffy bedding, pillows, or stuffed toys. Overbundling a baby or keeping a baby's room too warm also increases the risk of SIDS; because of this, SIDS deaths are more common in the colder months. Several studies have found that the use of a pacifier significantly reduces the risk of SIDS.

CHILDBIRTH

By the end of the ninth month of pregnancy, most women are tired of being pregnant; both parents are eager to start a new phase of their lives. Most couples find the actual process of birth to be an exciting and positive experience.

Choices in Childbirth

Many couples today can choose the type of practitioner and the environment they want for the birth of their child. A high-risk pregnancy is probably best handled by a specialist physician in a hospital with a nursery, but for low-risk births, many options are available.

Parents can choose to have their baby delivered by a physician (an obstetrician or family practitioner) or by a certified nurse-midwife. Certified nurse-midwives are registered nurses with special training in obstetrical techniques.

Most babies in the United States are delivered in hospitals. Many hospitals have introduced alternative birth centers in response to criticisms of traditional hospital routines. Alternative birth centers provide a comfortable, emotionally supportive environment in close proximity to up-to-date medical equipment.

A small number of American women elect to give birth at home or in birth facilities that offer low-technology care. Some organizations recommend against home births, but others support out-of-hospital births for healthy women with a low risk of complications. It's important for prospective parents to discuss all aspects of labor and delivery with their physician or midwife beforehand so they can learn what to expect and can state their preferences.

Labor and Delivery

The birth process occurs in three stages (Figure 5.7). **Labor** begins when hormonal changes in both the mother and the baby cause strong, rhythmic uterine **contractions** to begin. These contractions exert pressure on the cervix and cause the lengthwise muscles of the uterus to pull on the circular muscles around the cervix, causing effacement (thinning) and dilation (opening) of the cervix. The contractions also pressure the baby to descend into the mother's pelvis, if it hasn't already. The entire process of labor and delivery usually takes between 2 and 36 hours, depending on the size of the baby, the baby's position in the uterus, the size of the mother's pelvis, the strength of the uterine contractions, the number of prior deliveries, and other factors. The length of labor is generally shorter for second and subsequent births.

The First Stage of Labor   The first stage of labor averages 13 hours for a first birth, although there is a wide variation among women. It begins with cervical effacement and dilation and continues until the cervix is completely dilated. Contractions usually last about 30 seconds and occur every 15–20 minutes at first, more often later. The prepared mother relaxes as much as possible during these contractions to allow labor to proceed without being blocked by tension. Early in the first stage, a small amount of bleeding may occur as a plug of slightly bloody mucus that blocked the opening of the cervix during pregnancy is expelled. In some women, the

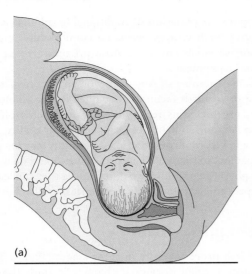

(a)

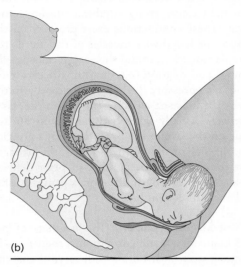

(b)

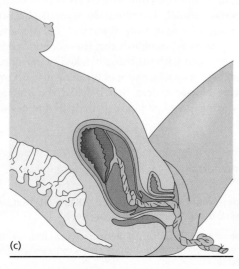

(c)

FIGURE 5.7 Birth: labor and delivery.
(a) The first stage of labor; (b) the second stage of labor: delivery of the baby; (c) the third stage of labor: expulsion of the placenta.

amniotic sac ruptures and the fluid rushes out; this is sometimes referred to as the "water breaking."

The last part of the first stage of labor, called **transition,** is characterized by strong and frequent contractions, much more intense than in the early stages of labor. Contractions may last 60–90 seconds and occur every 1–3 minutes. During transition the cervix opens completely, to a diameter of about 10 centimeters. The head of the fetus usually measures 9–10 centimeters; thus once the cervix has dilated completely, the head can pass through. Transition, which normally lasts about 30–60 minutes, is often the most difficult part of labor.

The Second Stage of Labor The second stage of labor begins with complete cervical dilation and ends with the delivery of the baby. The baby is slowly pushed down, through the bones of the pelvic ring, past the cervix, and into the vagina, which it stretches open. The mother bears down with the contractions to help push the baby down and out. Some women find this the most difficult part of labor; others find that the contractions and bearing down bring a sense of relief. The baby's back bends, the head turns to fit through the narrowest parts of the passageway, and the soft bones of the baby's skull move together and overlap as it is squeezed through the pelvis. When the top of the head appears at the vaginal opening, the baby is said to be *crowning*.

As the head of the baby emerges, the physician or midwife will remove any mucus from the mouth and nose, wipe the baby's face, and check to ensure that the umbilical cord is not around the neck. With a few more contractions, the baby's shoulders and body emerge. As the baby is squeezed through the pelvis, cervix, and vagina, the fluid in the lungs is forced out by the pressure on the baby's chest. Once this pressure is released as the baby emerges from the vagina, the chest expands and the lungs fill with air for the first time. The baby will still be connected to the mother via the umbilical cord, which is not cut until it stops pulsating. The baby will appear wet and often is covered with a cheesy substance. The baby's head may be oddly shaped at first, due to the molding of the soft plates of bone during birth, but it usually takes on a more rounded appearance within 24 hours.

The Third Stage of Labor In the third stage of labor, the uterus continues to contract until the placenta is expelled. This stage usually takes 5–30 minutes. It is important that the entire placenta be expelled; if part remains in the uterus, it may cause infection or bleeding. Breastfeeding soon after delivery helps control uterine bleeding because it stimulates the secretion of a hormone that makes the uterus contract.

The baby's physical condition is assessed with the **Apgar score,** a formalized system for assessing the baby's need for medical assistance. Heart rate, respiration, color, reflexes, and muscle tone are individually rated with a score of 0–2, and a total score between 0 and 10 is given at 1 and 5 minutes after birth. A score of 7–10 at 5 minutes is considered normal. Most newborns are also tested for 29 specific disorders, some of which are life-threatening. The American Academy of Pediatrics endorses these tests, but they are not routinely performed in every state.

Pain Relief during Labor and Delivery   Women vary in how much pain they experience in childbirth. It is recommended that women and their partners learn about labor and what kinds of choices are available for pain relief. Childbirth preparation courses are a good place to start, and communicating with one's obstetrician or midwife is essential to assessing pain relief options. Breathing and relaxation techniques such as Lamaze or Bradley have been used effectively.

The most commonly employed medical intervention for pain relief is the *epidural*. This procedure involves placing a thin plastic catheter between the vertebrae in the lower back. Medication that reduces the transmission of pain signals to the brain is given through this catheter. Local anesthetic drugs are given in low concentration to minimize weakening of the leg muscles so that the mother can effectively push during the birth. The amount of medication given is quite low and does not accumulate in the baby or interfere with the baby's transition after birth. The mother is awake and is an active participant in the birth.

Women can also elect to have narcotics, such as fentanyl or demerol, given for pain relief during labor, but these medications usually provide less pain relief than the epidural and, if given shortly before the birth, can cause the baby to be less vigorous at birth.

Cesarean Deliveries   In a **cesarean section,** the baby is removed through a surgical incision in the abdominal wall and uterus. Cesarean sections are necessary when a baby cannot be delivered vaginally—for example, if the baby's head is bigger than the mother's pelvic girdle or if the baby is in an unusual position. If the mother has a serious health condition such as high blood pressure, a cesarean may be safer for her than labor and a vaginal delivery. Cesareans are more common among women who are overweight or have diabetes. Other reasons for cesarean delivery include abnormal or difficult labor, fetal distress, and the presence of a dangerous infection like herpes that can be passed to the baby during delivery.

Repeat cesarean deliveries are also very common. About 90% of American women who have had one child by cesarean have subsequent children delivered the same way. Although the risk of complications from a vaginal delivery after a previous cesarean delivery is low, there is a small (1%) risk of serious complication to the mother and baby if the previous uterine scar opens during labor (uterine rupture). For this reason, women and their physicians may choose to deliver by elective repeat cesarean.

Like any major surgery, cesarean section carries some risk and should be performed only for valid medical reasons (not convenience). Women who have cesarean sections can remain conscious during the operation if they are given a regional anesthetic, and the father may be present.

The Postpartum Period

The **postpartum period,** a stage of about three months following childbirth, is a time of critical family adjustments. Parenthood begins literally overnight, and the transition can cause considerable stress.

Breastfeeding   Lactation, the production of milk, begins about three days after childbirth. Prior to that time (sometimes as early as the second trimester), **colostrum** is secreted by the nipples. Colostrum contains antibodies that help protect the newborn from infectious diseases and is also high in protein.

The American Academy of Pediatrics recommends breastfeeding exclusively for six months, then in combination with solid food until the baby is one year of age, and then for as long after that as a mother and baby desire. Currently only 11% of U.S. mothers breast-feed exclusively for six months. Human milk is perfectly suited to the baby's nutritional needs and digestive capabilities, and it supplies the baby with antibodies. Breastfeeding decreases the incidence of infant ear infections, allergies, anemia, diarrhea, and bacterial meningitis. Preschoolers who were breastfed as babies are less likely to be overweight, and school-age children who were breastfed are less anxious and better able to cope with stress. Breastfeeding even has a beneficial effect on blood pressure and cholesterol levels later in life.

Apgar score   A formalized system for assessing a newborn's need for medical assistance.

cesarean section   A surgical incision through the abdominal wall and uterus, performed to deliver a fetus.

postpartum period   The period of about three months after delivering a baby.

lactation   The production of milk.

colostrum   A yellowish fluid secreted by the mammary glands around the time of childbirth until milk comes in, about the third day.

TERMS

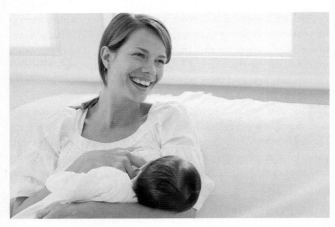
Breastfeeding can enhance the bond between mother and child. The American Academy of Pediatrics recommends breastfeeding exclusively for six months and then in combination with solid food until the baby is at least one year of age.

Breastfeeding is beneficial to the mother, as well. It stimulates contractions that help the uterus return to normal more rapidly, contributes to postpregnancy weight loss, and may reduce the risk of ovarian cancer, breast cancer, and postmenopausal hip fracture. For women who want to breastfeed but who have problems, help is available from support groups, books, or a lactation consultant. However, bottlefeeding can also provide adequate nutrition, and both breastfeeding and bottlefeeding can be part of loving, secure parent-child relationships.

When a mother doesn't nurse, menstruation usually begins within about 10 weeks. Breastfeeding can prevent the return of menstruation for six months or longer. However, ovulation—and pregnancy—can occur before menstruation returns, so breastfeeding is not a reliable contraceptive method.

Postpartum Depression   The majority of women experience fluctuating emotions during the postpartum period as hormone levels change. About 50–80% of new mothers experience "baby blues," characterized by episodes of sadness, weeping, anxiety, headache, sleep disturbances, and irritability. About 5–9% of new mothers experience **postpartum depression,** a more disabling syndrome characterized by despondency, mood swings, guilt, and occasional hostility. Rest, sharing feelings and concerns with others, and relying on supportive relatives and friends for assistance are usually helpful in dealing with mild cases of the baby blues or postpartum depression, which generally last only a few weeks. If the depression is serious, professional treatment may be needed.

Attachment   Another feature of the postpartum period is the development of attachment—the strong emotional tie that grows between the baby and the adult who cares for the baby. Parents can foster secure attachment relationships in the early weeks and months by responding sensitively to the baby's needs—for example, by responding appropriately to the baby's signals of gazing, looking away, smiling, and crying. A secure attachment relationship helps the child develop and function well socially, emotionally, and mentally.

For most people, the arrival of a child creates a deep sense of joy and accomplishment. However, adjusting to parenthood requires effort and energy. Talking with friends and relatives about their experiences during the first few weeks or months with a baby can help prepare new parents for the period when the baby's needs may require all the energy that both parents have to expend. But the pleasures of nurturing a new baby are substantial, and many parents look back on this time as one of the most significant and joyful of their lives.

TIPS FOR TODAY AND THE FUTURE

Wellness includes understanding your own sexuality and all its components. Preparation for being a parent begins long before pregnancy; it requires prospective parents to make responsible choices.

RIGHT NOW YOU CAN:

- Deal with any sexual question or problem you've been avoiding. Unless you're sure it isn't a physical problem, start by scheduling an appointment with your doctor.
- If you're in a sexual relationship, consider the information you and your partner have shared about sex. Are you comfortable that you and your partner know enough about each other to have a safe, healthy sexual relationship?
- Take some time to think about whether you really *want* to have children. Cut through the cultural, societal, family, and personal expectations that may stand in the way of making the decision you really want to make.
- Think of one thing your mother or father did as a parent that you particularly liked; if you become a parent, consider how you can be sure to do the same thing for your children.

IN THE FUTURE YOU CAN:

- If you're in a sexual relationship, or if you plan to begin one, open (or reopen) a dialogue with your partner about sex. Make time to talk at length about the responsibilities and consequences of a sexual relationship.
- Make behavioral changes that can improve your prospects as a parent. For example, you may need to adopt healthier eating habits or start exercising more consistently.
- If you want to be a parent someday, start looking at the many sources of information about pregnancy, childbirth, and parenting. This is a good idea for anyone—man or woman—who plans to have a family.

TERMS

postpartum depression   An emotional low that may be experienced by the mother following childbirth.

SUMMARY

- The female external sex organs are called the vulva; the clitoris plays an important role in sexual arousal and orgasm. The vagina leads to the internal female sex organs, including the uterus, oviducts, and ovaries.
- The male external sex organs are the penis and the scrotum; the glans of the penis is an important site of sexual arousal. Male internal sexual structures include the testes, vasa deferentia, seminal vesicles, and prostate gland.
- The menstrual cycle has four phases: menses, the estrogenic phase, ovulation, and the progestational phase.
- The ovaries gradually cease to function as women approach age 50 and enter menopause. The pattern of male sexual responses changes with age, and testosterone production gradually decreases.
- The sexual response cycle has four stages: excitement, plateau, orgasm, and resolution.
- Physical and psychological problems can both interfere with sexual functioning. Treatment for sexual dysfunction first addresses any underlying medical conditions and then looks at psychosocial problems.
- Human sexual behaviors include celibacy, erotic fantasy, masturbation, touching, cunnilingus, fellatio, anal intercourse, and coitus.
- Responsible sexuality includes open, honest communication; agreed-on sexual activities; sexual privacy; using contraception; safe sex practices; sober sex; and taking responsibility for consequences.
- Fertilization is a complex process culminating when a sperm penetrates the membrane of the egg released from the woman's ovary. Infertility affects about 15% of the reproductive-age population of the United States.
- During pregnancy, the uterus and breasts enlarges, muscles and ligaments soften and stretch, and other body functions become more efficient.
- The fetal anatomy is almost completely formed in the first trimester and is refined in the second; during the third trimester, the fetus grows and gains most of its weight.
- Prenatal tests include ultrasound, amniocentesis, chorionic villus sampling, and quadruple marker screening.
- Important elements of prenatal care include regular checkups, good nutrition, avoiding drugs and other harmful environmental agents, and talking childbirth classes.
- Pregnancy usually proceeds without major complications. Problems that can occur include ectopic pregnancy, spontaneous abortion, preeclampsia, and low birth weight.
- The first stage of labor begins with contractions that exert pressure on the cervix, causing effacement and dilation. The second stage begins with complete cervical dilation and ends when the baby emerges. The third stage of labor is expulsion of the placenta.
- During the postpartum period, the mother's body begins to return to its prepregnancy state, and she may begin to breast-feed. Both mother and father must adjust to their new roles as parents.

FOR MORE INFORMATION

BOOKS

American College of Obstetricians and Gynecologists. 2010. *Your Pregnancy and Childbirth: Month to Month,* 5th ed. Washington, DC: ACOG. *Advice on conception, pregnancy, prenatal care, and delivery options.*

American Dietetic Association. 2009. *Expect the Best: Your Guide to Healthy Eating Before, During, and After Pregnancy.* New York: Wiley. *Provides up-to-date dietary information and meal-planning guides for women who want to get pregnant, are pregnant, or have had a baby.*

Bogle, K. 2008. *Hooking Up: Sex, Dating and Relationships on Campus.* New York: New York University Press. *A sociologist looks at the "hookup" culture on college campuses today.*

Jones, S., and M. Jones. 2012. *Great Expectations: Your All-in-One Resource for Pregnancy & Childbirth.* New York: Sterling. *A comprehensive guide to pregnancy and early parenthood, written in an accessible style; illustrated.*

Kelly, G. F. 20011. *Sexuality Today,* 10th ed. New York: McGraw-Hill. *An accessible approach that highlights cross-cultural examples, popular topics and issues, and case studies featuring college-age individuals.*

Lees, C., et al. 2007. *Pregnancy and Birth: Your Questions Answered.* London: Dorling Kindersley. *Answers hundreds of common questions about conception, pregnancy, and delivery.*

McCarthy, B., and E. McCarthy. 2012. *Sexual Awareness: Your Guide to Healthy Couple Sexuality,* 5th Ed. New York: Routledge. *A guide to enriching couple relationships with improved sexual awareness and communication.*

Meston, C., and D. Buss. 2009. *Why Women Have Sex.* New York: Times Books. *Fascinating, readable, yet scholarly book about all aspects of female sexuality, especially sexual desire.*

Savage, D., and T. Miller, Eds. 2012. *It Gets Better: Coming Out, Overcoming Bullying, and Creating a Life Worth Living.* New York: Plume. *A collection of essays written to LGBT youth by celebrities, politicians, and ordinary people, conveying the message that a positive future is possible.*

Taverner, W. J. 2009. *Taking Sides: Clashing Views on Controversial Issues in Human Sexuality,* 11th ed. New York: McGraw-Hill. *Includes pro and con position statements on sexuality issues relating to biology, behavior, and legal and social issues.*

Wynbrandt, J. 2008. *Encyclopedia of Genetic Disorders and Birth Defects,* 3rd ed. New York: Facts on File, Inc. *A detailed overview of many types of birth defects, both inherited and noninherited.*

ORGANIZATIONS AND WEBSITES

American Association of Sex Educators, Counselors, and Therapists (AASECT). Certifies sex educators, counselors, and therapists and provides listings of local therapists dealing with sexual problems.

http://www.aasect.org

American College of Obstetricians and Gynecologists (ACOG). Provides written materials relating to many aspects of preconception care, pregnancy, and childbirth.

http://www.acog.org

American Psychological Association: Information about gender identity and sexual orientation. Question-and-answer format sections on transgender and homosexuality.

http://www.apa.org/topics/sexuality/transgender.aspx

The American Society for Reproductive Medicine. Provides up-to-date information about all aspects of infertility.

http://www.asrm.org

Centers for Disease Control and Prevention, National Center on Birth Defects and Developmental Disabilities. Provides information about a variety of topics related to birth defects, including fetal alcohol syndrome and the importance of folic acid.

http://www.cdc.gov/ncbddd

The Kinsey Institute for Research in Sex, Gender, and Reproduction. One of the oldest and most respected institutions doing research on sexuality.

http://www.kinseyinstitute.org

Sexuality Information and Education Council of the United States (SIECUS). Provides information about many aspects of sexuality and has an extensive library and numerous publications.

http://www.siecus.org

National Institute of Child Health and Human Development. Provides information about reproductive and genetic problems; sponsors the "Back to Sleep" campaign to fight SIDS.

http://www.nichd.nih.gov

SELECTED BIBLIOGRAPHY

American College Health Association. 2012. *American College Health Association—National College Health Assessment II: Reference Group Executive Summary Fall 2011.* Linthicum, MD: American College Health Association.

American Psychological Association. 2012. *Answers to Your Questions for a Better Understanding of Sexual Orientation and Homosexuality* (http://www.apa.org/topics/sexuality/orientation.aspx).

Bitzer, J., A. Giraldi, and J. Pfaus. 2012. Sexual desire and hypoactive sexual desire disorder in women. *Journal of Sexual Medicine,* September 13 (Epub ahead of print).

Blanchette, H. 2011. The rising cesarean delivery rate in America: What are the consequences? *Obstetrics & Gynecology* 118(3): 687–690.

Brown, R., and J. Harper. 2012. The clinical benefit and safety of current and future assisted reproductive technology. *Reproductive Biomedicine Online* 25(2): 108–117.

Centers for Disease Control and Prevention. 2009. *Assisted Reproductive Technology Report* (http://www.cdc.gov/art/ART2009/PDF/ART_2009_Full.pdf).

Centers for Disease Control and Prevention. 2012. *Breastfeeding Report Card—United States,* 2012 (http://www.cdc.gov/breastfeeding/data/reportcard.htm).

Centers for Disease Control and Prevention. 2012. *Sudden Infant Death Syndrome (SIDS) and Sudden Unexpected Infant Death (SUID)* (http://www.cdc.gov/SIDS/index.htm).

Chadwick, R., and R. Childs. 2012. Ethnical issues in the diagnosis and management of fetal disorders. Best Practice & Research: *Clinical Obstetrics & Gynaecology* 26(5): 541–550.

Clark, S. M., A. R. Carver, and G. D. Hankins. 2012. Vaginal birth after cesarean and trial of labor after cesarean: What should we be recommending relative to maternal risk:benefit? *Women's Health* 8(4): 371–383.

Doss, A. E., et al. 2012. Gestational age at delivery and perinatal outcomes of twin gestations. *American Journal of Obstetrics and Gynecology,* August 10 (Epub ahead of print).

Fleischman, A. R., et al. 2010. Rethinking the definition of "term pregnancy." *Obstetrics and Gynecology* 116(1): 136–139.

Freeman, Ellen. 2007. *Epidemiology and Etiology of Premenstrual Syndromes* (http://cme.medscape.com/viewarticle/553603).

Garcia-Falgueras, A., and D. Swaab. 2010. Sexual hormones and the brain: An essential alliance for sexual identity and sexual orientation. *Pediatric Endocrinology* 17:22–35.

Goyal, D., et al. 2010. How much does low socioeconomic status increase the risk of prenatal and postpartum depressive symptoms in first-time mothers? *Women's Health Issues* 20(2): 96–104.

Ismail, S., et al. 2010. Screening, diagnosing and prevention of fetal alcohol syndrome: Is this syndrome treatable? *Developmental Neuroscience* 32(2): 91–100.

Lavender, T., et al. 2006. Caesarean section for non-medical reasons at term. *Cochrane Database of Systematic Reviews* 19(3).

Leguizamon, G. F., and N. P. Zeff. 2006. Hypertension and the pregnancy complicated by diabetes. *Current Diabetes Reports* 6(4): 297–304.

Lewis, S. B. 2010. What is sexual addiction? *Journal of Sex and Marital Therapy* 36(3): 261–275.

Lindau, S. T., and N. Gavrilova. 2010. Sex, health, and years of sexually active life gained due to good health. *British Medical Journal* 340: c810.

Mayo Clinic. 20011. *Premenstrual Syndrome* (http://www.mayoclinic.com/health/premenstrual-syndrome/DS00134/DSECTION=lifestyle-and-home-remedies).

Mayo Clinic. 2011. *Erectile Dysfunction* (http://www.mayoclinic.com/health/erectile-dysfunction/DS00162).

McMahon, C. G., et al. 2012. Standard operating procedures in the disorders of orgasm and ejaculation. *Journal of Sexual Medicine,* September 12 (Epub ahead of print).

Merviel, P. et al. 2010. Predictive factors for pregnancy after intrauterine insemination (IUI): An analysis of 1038 cycles and a review of the literature. *Fertil Steril* 93(1): 79.

Meston, C., and D. Buss. 2007. Why humans have sex. *Archives of Sexual Behavior,* August.

Muglia, L. J., and M. Katz. 2010. The enigma of spontaneous preterm birth. *The New England Journal of Medicine* 362(6): 529–355.

National Center for Health Statistics. 2010. *Trends in Circumcision among Newborns* (http://www.cdc.gov/nchs/data/hestat/circumcisions/circumcisions.htm).

National Center for Health Statistics. 2011. Sexual Behavior, Sexual Attraction, and Sexual Identity in the United States: Data from the 2006–2008

National Survey of Family Growth. *National Health Statistics Reports*, No. 36, March 3.

National Center for Health Statistics. 2012. Fertility of Men and Women Aged 15-44 Years in the United States: National Survey of Family Growth, 2006–2010. *National Health Statistics Reports*, No. 51, April 12.

North American Menopause Society. 2010. *Estrogen and Progesterone Use in Post-Menopausal Women: 2010 Position Statement* (http://www.menopause.org/PSht10.pdf).

Reynolds, R. 2010. The effects of maternal labour analgesia on the fetus. *Best Practice & Research: Clinical Obstetrics & Gynaecology* 24(3): 289–302.

Sibai, B. M. 2011. Disparity in the rate of eclampsia and adverse pregnancy outcome from eclampsia: A tale of two countries. *Obstetrics & Gynecology* 118(5): 976–977.

Tournaye, H. J., and B. J. Cohlen. 2012. Management of male-factor infertility. *Best Practice & Research: Clinical Obstetrics & Gynaecology*, June 15 (Epub ahead of print).

U.S. Department of Health and Human Services. 2011. *Aging Male Syndrome* (http://womenshealth.gov/mens-health/teens-fathers-minorities-older-men/older-men.cfm#ams).

World Health Organization. 2010. *Female Genital Mutilation* (http://www.who.int/mediacentre/factsheets/fs241/en/).

World Health Organization. 2012. *Male Circumcision for HIV Prevention: Publications.* (http://www.who.int/hiv/pub/malecircumcision/en/).

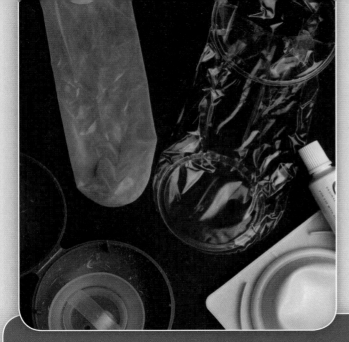

LOOKING AHEAD...

After reading this chapter, you should be able to

- Explain how contraceptives work and how to interpret information about a contraceptive method's effectiveness, risks, and benefits

- List the most popular contraceptives and discuss their advantages, disadvantages, and effectiveness

- Choose a method of contraception based on the needs of the user and the safety and effectiveness of the method

- Describe the history and current legal status of abortion in the United States

- Describe the methods of abortion available in the United States

Contraception and Abortion

6

People have always had a compelling interest in managing fertility and preventing unwanted pregnancies, a practice commonly known as **birth control.** Records dating to the fourth century BC describe the use of foods, herbs, drugs, douches, and sponges to prevent **conception,** which is the fusion of an ovum and sperm that creates a fertilized egg, or *zygote.* Early attempts at **contraception** (blocking conception through the use of a device, substance, or method) were based on the same principle as many modern birth control methods.

Today women and men can choose from many different types of **contraceptives** to avoid unwanted pregnancies. Modern contraceptive methods are much more predictable and effective than in the past. Still, about half of all pregnancies in the United States are unintended. Of these, about 40 percent end in **abortion**.

In addition to preventing pregnancy, many contraceptive products play an important role in protecting against **sexually transmitted diseases** or **STDs.** Being informed about the realities and risks and making responsible decisions about sexual and contraceptive behavior are crucial components of lifelong wellness.

PRINCIPLES OF CONTRACEPTION

There are many effective approaches to contraception, including the following:

- **Barrier methods** work by physically blocking the sperm from reaching the egg. Condoms are the most popular method based on this principle.

- **Hormonal methods,** such as oral contraceptives (birth control pills), alter the biochemistry of the woman's body, preventing ovulation (the release of the egg) and producing changes that make it more difficult for the sperm to reach the egg if ovulation does occur.

- **Natural methods** of contraception are based on the fact that the egg and the sperm have to be present at the same time if fertilization is to occur.

- **Surgical methods**—female and male sterilization—more or less permanently prevent transport of the sperm or eggs to the site of conception.

All contraceptive methods have advantages and disadvantages that make them appropriate for some people but not for others, and the best choice during one period of life may not be the best in another. Factors that affect the choice of method include effectiveness, convenience, cost, reversibility, side effects and risks, and protection against STDs. This chapter helps you sort through these factors to decide which contraceptive method is best for you (see the box "Contraception Use and Pregnancy among College Students").

Contraceptive effectiveness is partly determined by the reliability of the method itself—the failure rate if it were always used exactly as directed ("perfect use"). Effectiveness is also determined by characteristics of the user, including fertility of the individual, frequency of intercourse, and how consistently and correctly the method is used. This "typical use" **contraceptive failure rate** is based on studies that directly measure the percentage of women experiencing an unintended pregnancy in the first year of contraceptive use. For example, the 9% failure rate of oral contraceptives means 9 out of 100 typical users will become pregnant in the first year. This failure rate is likely to be lower for women who are consistently careful in following instructions and higher for those who are frequently careless; the "perfect use" failure rate is 0.3%.

Another measure of effectiveness is the **continuation rate**—the percentage of people who continue to use the method after a specified period of time. This measure is important because many unintended pregnancies occur when a method is stopped and not immediately replaced with another. Thus a contraceptive with a high continuation rate would be more effective at preventing pregnancy than one with a low continuation rate. A high continuation rate also gives an indication of user satisfaction with a particular method.

REVERSIBLE CONTRACEPTION

Reversibility is an extremely important consideration for young adults when they choose a contraceptive method because most people either plan to eventually have children or at least want to keep their options open until later in life.

Oral Contraceptives: The Pill

About a century ago, a researcher noted that ovulation does not occur during pregnancy. Further research revealed the hor-

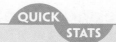

monal mechanism: during pregnancy, the corpus luteum secretes progesterone and estrogen in amounts high enough to suppress ovulation. **Oral contraceptives (OCs),** also known as *birth control pills* or "the pill," prevent ovulation by mimicking the hormonal activity of the corpus luteum. The active ingredients in OCs are estrogen and progestins, laboratory-made compounds that are closely related to progesterone. Today OCs are the most widely used form of contraception among unmarried women and are second only to sterilization among married women.

In addition to preventing ovulation, the birth control pill has other contraceptive effects. It inhibits the movement of sperm by thickening the cervical mucus, alters the rate of ovum transport by means of its hormonal effects on the fallopian tubes, and may prevent implantation by changing the lining of the uterus in the unlikely event that a fertilized ovum reaches that area.

TERMS

birth control The practice of managing fertility and preventing unwanted pregnancies.

conception The fusion of ovum and sperm, resulting in a fertilized egg, or *zygote*.

contraception The prevention of conception through the use of a device, substance, or method.

contraceptive Any agent or method that can prevent conception.

abortion The artificially induced expulsion of an embryo or fetus from the uterus.

sexually transmitted disease (STD) Any of several contagious diseases contracted through intimate sexual contact.

barrier method A contraceptive that acts as a physical barrier, blocking sperm from uniting with an egg.

hormonal method A contraceptive that alters the biochemistry of a woman's body, preventing ovulation and making it more difficult for sperm to reach an egg if ovulation does occur.

natural method An approach to contraception that does not use drugs or devices; requires avoiding intercourse during the phase of the woman's menstrual cycle when an egg is most likely to be present at the site of conception and the risk of pregnancy is greatest.

surgical method Sterilization of a male or female to permanently prevent the transport of sperm or eggs to the site of conception.

contraceptive failure rate The percentage of women using a particular contraceptive method who experience an unintended pregnancy in the first year of use.

continuation rate The percentage of people who continue to use a particular contraceptive after a specified period of time.

oral contraceptive (OC) Hormone compounds (made of estrogen and progestins) in pill form that prevent conception by preventing ovulation; also called the *birth control pill* or "the pill."

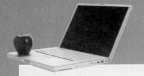
College tends to be a time of increased sexual activity for many young adults. Those who were sexually active in high school may have an increased number of partners or engage in riskier sexual behaviors once they enter college; those who abstained from intercourse during high school may begin to explore their sexuality once they enter this new environment. Surveys have shown that the majority of college students, up to 70%, engage in sexual activity, and some have more than one partner.

Though sexual activity significantly increases during the college years, a large percentage of students report not using contraception during their most recent sexual activity. The same study cited above found that only 56% of students used contraception during their most recent intercourse. Oral contraceptive pills were the most commonly used contraceptive, with about 60% of women utilizing a contraceptive selecting this method; males who utilized a contraceptive at last intercourse reported having used the male condom approximately 66% of the time. Of note, the withdrawal method was used by 27% of respondents; this method does not protect against STDs and has a high associated failure rate.

Black and white college students differ somewhat in contraceptive use. Black students were more likely to have used a condom the last time they had vaginal intercourse compared with white students (63% of blacks versus 58% of whites). On the other hand, white students were far more likely to use hormonal contraception than black students (66% versus 42%). About 6% of black students reported using no contraception the last time they had vaginal intercourse, compared with fewer than 3% of white students. Unintended pregnancies were nearly four times higher among black college students compared with white students.

While the oral contraceptive pill is a highly effective form of contraception when used as directed, and the male condom is effective at preventing the transmission of a wide variety of STDs, they must be used together to provide simultaneous protection against both pregnancy and STDs. This is particularly important for couples who are not in a long-term, mutually monogamous relationship. However, surveys show that college students use a male condom plus another form of contraception only about 45% of the time.

Around 2% of college women report having become pregnant in the prior year, many unintentionally. A disproportionate number of these pregnancies occur in students attending community colleges; a 2007 survey found that 5.3% of attendees at community colleges reported a pregnancy during the prior year, while only 1.8% of students at four-year universities reported the same.

The consequences of pregnancy among college students can be significant. For example, one study found that 61% of women who became pregnant while attending community college subsequently dropped out. Those who continue their education face added expenses and stress. Given the importance of education in achieving long-term career and financial goals, the implementation of effective contraception during the college years can have a significant impact on the lives of young women. Unfortunately only 42% of students report being provided any information about pregnancy prevention by their college.

SOURCES: U.S. Department of Education, National Center for Education Statistics. 2002. *Short-Term Enrollment in Postsecondary Education: Student Background and Institutional Differences in Reasons for Early Departure, 1996–98,* NCES 2003–2153. Washington, DC: U.S. Department of Education; American College Health Association. 2011. *National College Health Assessment: Reference Group Executive Summary Spring 2011* (http://www.acha-ncha.org/docs/ACHA-NCHA-II_ReferenceGroup_ExecutiveSummary_Spring2011.pdf).

The Combination Pill　The most common type of OC is the *combination pill,* which contains varying amounts of estrogen and progestin. Traditionally each one-month packet has contained a three-week supply of "active" pills that combine varying types and amounts of estrogen and progestin, as well as a one-week supply of "placebo" pills that do not contain hormones. Increasingly, however, combination pills are offering different schedules, including 24 active pills and 4 placebo pills, and 84 active pills and 7 placebo pills. During the time in which no hormones are taken, a light menstrual period occurs. The newer schedules allow a decreased frequency of menstrual periods. However, a side effect of these extended-cycle regimens is unpredictable light bleeding (known as *spotting*).

So far, altering the menstrual cycle has not been linked with any major health risks, but some experts are concerned that the suppression of menstruation for most of a woman's reproductive years could become commonplace and may result in unanticipated health problems in the future. Research is ongoing, but it may take many years to fully evaluate the consequences of suppressing menstruation for long periods of a woman's life.

The Minipill　A much less common type of OC is the *minipill,* a small dose of a synthetic progesterone taken every day of the month. Because the minipill contains no estrogen, it has fewer side effects and health risks, but it is associated with more irregular bleeding patterns. It is sometimes prescribed for women who are breastfeeding or have medical problems that make it unsafe for them to take estrogen.

How Oral Contraceptives Are Used　A woman is usually advised to start the first cycle of pills with a menstrual period to increase effectiveness and eliminate the possibility of unsuspected pregnancy. If pregnancy has been ruled out, the pill can be started immediately, but a backup contraceptive method, such as condoms, should also be used during the first week.

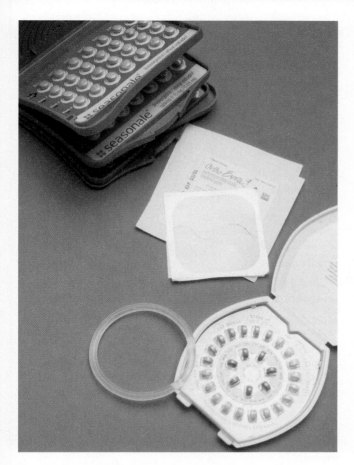

Reversible hormonal contraceptives are available in several forms. Shown here are the patch, the ring, and birth control pills.

Taking a few pills just prior to having sexual intercourse does not provide effective contraception. A backup method is recommended during the first week and any subsequent cycle in which the woman forgets to take any pills.

Advantages Oral contraceptives are very effective in preventing pregnancy. Nearly all unplanned pregnancies result because the pills were not taken as directed. The pill is relatively simple to use and does not hinder sexual spontaneity. Most women also appreciate the predictable regularity of periods, as well as the reduction in cramps and blood loss. Women who have significant problems associated with menstruation may benefit from menstrual suppression with extended-cycle OCs. For young women, the pill's reversibility is especially important; **fertility**—the ability to reproduce—returns after the pill is discontinued.

Medical advantages include a decreased incidence of benign breast disease, acne, iron-deficiency anemia, ectopic

pregnancy, colon and rectal cancer, endometrial cancer, and ovarian cancer. OC use reduces dysmenorrhea (painful periods), endometriosis, and polycystic ovary syndrome.

Disadvantages Although oral contraceptives are effective in preventing pregnancy, they do not protect against STDs. OCs have been associated with increased risk of cervical chlamydia in some studies but not in others.

The majority of women do not experience any side effects associated with OC use. Among women who experience problems with OCs, the most common issue is bleeding during midcycle (called *breakthrough bleeding*), which is usually slight and tends to disappear after a few cycles. Symptoms of early pregnancy—such as morning nausea and swollen breasts—may appear during the first few months of OC use, although these side effects are uncommon with the low-dose pills in current widespread use. Other side effects can include depression, nervousness, changes in sex drive, dizziness, headaches, migraine, and vaginal discharge.

Older OCs with high-dose hormones were sometimes associated with weight gain. However, research shows that currently used low-dose OCs do not, on average, cause weight gain. Most women experience no change in their weight, while a small percentage lose weight, and about an equal percentage gain weight while taking OCs. The myth that OCs cause women to gain weight is dangerous because many unintended pregnancies have resulted when women avoided taking OCs due to unfounded fear of weight gain.

Another myth about OCs is that they can cause cancer. Actually, taking the pill greatly reduces a woman's risk for endometrial and ovarian cancers. OC use is associated with little, if any, increase in breast cancer and a slight increase in cervical cancer, but earlier detection and other variables (such as a woman's number of sexual partners) may account for much of this increase.

Serious OC side effects have been reported in a small number of women. These include blood clots, stroke, and heart attack, concentrated mostly in older women who smoke or have a history of circulatory disease. Recent studies have shown no increased risk of stroke or heart attack for healthy, young, nonsmoking women on lower-dosage pills. OC users may be slightly more prone to high blood pressure, gallbladder disease, and, very rarely, benign liver tumors.

Birth control pills are not recommended for women with a history of blood clots (or a close family member with unexplained blood clots at an early age), heart disease or stroke, migraines with changes in vision, any form of cancer or liver tumor, or impaired liver function. Women with certain other health conditions or behaviors, including migraines without changes in vision, high blood pressure, cigarette smoking, and sickle-cell disease, require close monitoring when taking the pill.

When deciding whether to use OCs, each woman needs to weigh the benefits against the risks. To make an informed decision, she should begin by getting advice from a health

| **fertility** The ability to reproduce. | **TERMS** |

care professional. If you take the pill, you can take several steps to reduce the risks associated with OC use:

1. Request a low-dosage pill. (OCs recommended for most new users contain 20–35 micrograms of estrogen.)

2. Stop smoking.

3. Follow the directions carefully and consistently, making sure to take the pills at the same time every day.

4. Be alert to preliminary danger signals, which can be remembered by the word ACHES:

   Abdominal pain (severe).

   Chest pain (severe), cough, shortness of breath, or sharp pain on breathing in.

   Headaches (severe), dizziness, weakness, or numbness, especially if one-sided.

   Eye problems (vision loss or blurring) and/or speech problems.

   Severe leg pain (calf or thigh).

5. Make sure your health practitioner knows your personal and family medical history to help determine whether OCs may be unsafe for you.

6. Have regular **Pap tests,** pelvic exams, and breast exams as recommended by your health practitioner.

For the vast majority of young women, the known, directly associated risk of death from taking birth control pills is much, much lower than the risk of death from pregnancy (Table 6.1). Overall, OC risks are generally very small unless you are over 35, are a smoker, and/or have specific medical problems.

Effectiveness   Oral contraceptive effectiveness varies substantially because it depends so much on individual factors. If taken exactly as directed, its failure rate is extremely low (0.3%). Among average users, however, lapses such as forgetting to take a pill do occur, and the typical first-year failure rate is 9%. The continuation rate for OCs also varies; the average rate is 67% after one year. Besides forgetting to take the pill, another reason for OC failure is poor absorption of the drug due to vomiting or diarrhea, or to interactions with other medicines (including certain antibiotics, antiseizure medications, and the commonly used herb St. John's wort).

Contraceptive Skin Patch

The contraceptive skin patch, Ortho Evra, is a thin, 1¾-inch square patch that slowly releases an estrogen and a progestin into the bloodstream. The contraceptive patch prevents pregnancy in the same way as combination OCs. Each patch is worn continuously for one week and is replaced on the same day of the week for three consecutive weeks. The fourth

Table 6.1	Risks of Contraception, Pregnancy, and Abortion
CONTRACEPTION	**RISK OF DEATH**
Oral contraceptives	
Nonsmoker	
Age 15–34	1 in 1,667,000
Age 35–44	1 in 33,300
Smoker	
Age 15–34	1 in 57,800
Age 35–44	1 in 5,200
IUDs	1 in 10,000,000
Barrier methods, spermicides	None
Fertility awareness–based methods	None
Tubal ligation	1 in 66,700
PREGNANCY	**RISK OF DEATH**
Pregnancy	1 in 6,900
ABORTION	**RISK OF DEATH**
Spontaneous abortion	1 in 142,900
Medical abortion	1 in 200,000
Surgical abortion	1 in 142,900

SOURCE: Hatcher, R. A., et al. *Contraceptive Technology*, 20th revised edition. Copyright © 2011 Ardent Media. Reprinted with permission.

week is patch-free, allowing a woman to have her menstrual period.

The patch can be worn on the upper outer arm, abdomen, buttocks, or upper torso (excluding the breasts); it is designed to stick to skin even during bathing or swimming. If a patch should fall off for more than a day, the FDA advises starting a new four-week cycle of patches and using a backup method of contraception for the first week. Patches should be discarded according to the manufacturer's directions to avoid leakage of hormones into the environment.

Advantages   With both perfect and typical use, the patch is as effective as OCs in preventing pregnancy. Compliance seems to be higher with the patch than with OCs, probably because the patch requires weekly instead of daily action. Medical benefits are comparable to those of OCs.

Disadvantages   Like other hormonal contraceptives, the patch doesn't protect against STDs. Patch users should also use condoms for STD protection unless they are in a long-term monogamous relationship with an uninfected partner. Minor side effects are similar to those of OCs, although breast discomfort may be more common in patch users. Some women also experience skin irritation around the patch. More serious complications are thought to be similar to those of OCs, including an increased risk of side effects among women who smoke. However, because Ortho Evra exposes users to higher doses of estrogen than most OCs, patch use may further increase the risk of blood clots (venous thromboembolism). Recent studies show conflicting results regarding the

> **Pap test**   A scraping of cells from the cervix for examination under a microscope to detect cancer.
>
> TERMS

risk of blood clots, but it is possible that the risk is slightly higher with the patch compared to low-dose OCs.

Effectiveness   With perfect use, the patch's failure rate is very low (0.3%) in the first year of use. The typical failure rate is approximately 9%, similar to that of the oral contraceptive pill.

Vaginal Contraceptive Ring

The NuvaRing is a vaginal ring that is molded with a mixture of progestin and estrogen. The two-inch ring slowly releases hormones and maintains blood hormone levels comparable to those found with OC use. The ring prevents pregnancy in the same way as OCs. A woman inserts the ring anytime during the first five days of her menstrual period and leaves it in place for three weeks. During the fourth week, when the ring is removed, her next menstrual period occurs. A new ring is then inserted. Rings should be discarded according to the manufacturer's directions to avoid leakage of hormones into the environment. Backup contraception must be used for the first seven days of the first ring use or if the ring has been removed for more than three hours.

Advantages   The NuvaRing offers one month of protection with no daily or weekly action required. It does not require a fitting by a clinician, and exact placement in the vagina is not critical as it is with a diaphragm. Medical benefits are probably similar to those of OCs.

Disadvantages   The NuvaRing provides no protection against STDs. Side effects are roughly comparable to those seen with OC use, except for a lower incidence of nausea and vomiting. Other side effects may include vaginal discharge, vaginitis, and vaginal irritation. Medical risks also are similar to those found with OC use.

Effectiveness   As with the pill and patch, the perfect use failure rate is around 0.3%. The ring's typical use failure rate is similar to the pill's at 9%.

Contraceptive Implants

Contraceptive implants are placed under the skin of the upper arm and deliver a small but steady dose of progestin (a synthetic progesterone) over a period of years. One such implant, called Implanon, is a single implant that is effective for three years and is considered to be one of the most effective forms of contraception. Contraceptive implants are best suited for women who wish to have continuous, highly effective, and long-term protection against pregnancy.

Advantages   Contraceptive implants are highly effective. After insertion of the implants, no further action is required;

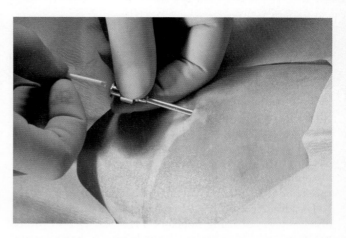

Only trained health professionals can insert a contraceptive implant.

contraceptive effects are quickly reversed upon removal. Because implants, unlike the combination pill, contain no estrogen, they carry a lower risk of certain side effects, such as blood clots and other cardiovascular complications. Women who are breastfeeding can use Implanon.

Disadvantages   Like the pill, an implant provides no protection against STDs. Although the implants are barely visible, their presence may bother some women. The costs associated with the implant can be significant; therefore, the device is only cost-effective for users desiring multiple years of contraception.

Common side effects of contraceptive implants are menstrual irregularities, including longer menstrual periods, spotting between periods, or having no bleeding at all. The menstrual cycle usually becomes more regular after one year of use. Less common side effects include headaches, weight gain, breast tenderness, nausea, acne, and mood swings.

Effectiveness   The overall failure rate for Implanon is estimated at about 0.05%. It is one of the most effective methods of contraception and also one of the most discreet.

Injectable Contraceptives

The first injectable contraceptive approved for use in the United States was Depo-Provera, which uses long-acting progestins. Injected into the arm or buttocks, Depo-Provera is usually given every 12 weeks, although it may provide effective contraception for a few weeks beyond that. The product prevents pregnancy in the same ways as implants.

Advantages   Injectable contraceptives are highly effective and require little action on the part of the user. Because the injections leave no trace and involve no ongoing supplies, injectable contraceptives allow women almost total privacy in their decision to use contraception. Depo-Provera

> It's important to remember that **hormonal contraceptives provide no protection from STDs.**

has no estrogen-related side effects. It requires only periodic injections.

Disadvantages Injectable contraceptives provide no protection against STDs. A woman must visit a health care facility every three months to receive the injections. The side effects of Depo-Provera are similar to those of implants; menstrual irregularities are the most common, and after one year of using Depo-Provera many women have no menstrual bleeding at all. Weight gain is a common side effect. After discontinuing the use of Depo-Provera, women may experience temporary infertility for up to 12 months.

Disadvantages of using Depo-Provera are similar to the disadvantages of using implants. However, Depo-Provera has a unique risk: it can cause a reduction in bone density, especially in women who use it for an extended period. Decreased bone density is a risk factor for osteoporosis and fractures. Women who use Depo-Provera are advised to do weight-bearing exercise and ensure an adequate intake of dietary calcium. The FDA cautions women not to use Depo-Provera for longer than two years due to risk of bone loss. However, many gynecologic associations believe the benefits of Depo-Povera outweigh its risks.

Effectiveness The perfect use failure rate is 0.2% for Depo-Provera. With typical use, the failure rate increases to 6% in the first year of use.

Intrauterine Devices (IUDs)

An **intrauterine device (IUD)** is a small device placed in the uterus as a contraceptive. Two types of IUDs are now available in the United States: the Copper T-380A (also known as the ParaGard), which provides protection for up to 10 years, and the Levonorgestrel IUD (Mirena), which releases small amounts of progestin and is effective for up to 5 years.

Researchers do not know exactly how IUDs prevent pregnancy. Current evidence suggests that ParaGard works primarily by preventing fertilization. The copper in this IUD may cause biochemical changes in the uterus and affect the movement of sperm and eggs. ParaGard may also interfere with implantation of fertilized eggs. Mirena slowly releases very small amounts of progestin, disrupting ovulation, fertilization, or implantation.

An IUD must be inserted and removed by a trained professional. The device is threaded into a sterile inserter, which is introduced through the cervix; a plunger pushes the IUD into the uterus. IUDs have two threads attached that protrude from the cervix into the vagina so a woman can feel them to make sure the device is in place. These threads are trimmed so that only 1–1½ inches remain in the upper vagina.

Advantages Intrauterine devices are highly reliable and are simple and convenient to use, requiring no attention except for a periodic check of the string position. They do not require the woman to anticipate or interrupt sexual activity. Multiple studies have also shown a reduction in endometrial cancer rates among Mirena IUD users. IUDs usually have only localized side effects, and in the absence of complications they are considered a fully reversible contraceptive. The long-term expense of using an IUD is low.

Disadvantages The IUD offers no protection against STDs. Heavy menstrual flow and increased menstrual cramping sometimes occur with ParaGard, while Mirena causes a reduction in bleeding and cramping. Spontaneous expulsion of the IUD happens to 4–6% of women within the first year, most commonly during the first months after insertion.

A serious but rare complication of IUD use is pelvic inflammatory disease (PID). Most pelvic infections among IUD users occur shortly after insertion, are relatively mild, and can be treated successfully with antibiotics. Early and adequate treatment is critical—a lingering infection can lead to tubal scarring and subsequent infertility. Early signs of a problem with an IUD are abdominal pain, fever, chills, foul-smelling vaginal discharge, and unusual vaginal bleeding.

The IUD is typically most cost-effective for women who desire contraception for many years.

Effectiveness The typical first-year failure rate of IUDs is 0.8% for the ParaGard and 0.2% for Mirena. Effectiveness can be increased by periodically making sure that the device is in place and by using a backup method for the first week of IUD use. If pregnancy occurs, the IUD may need to be removed to safeguard the woman's health and to maintain the pregnancy.

Male Condoms

The **male condom** is a thin sheath designed to cover the penis during sexual intercourse. Most brands available in the United States are made of latex, although condoms made of polyurethane and polyisoprene are also available. Condoms prevent sperm from entering the vagina and provide protection against STDs, including HIV. Many couples combine various contraceptives,

> **QUICK STATS**
>
> **Condom use among teens continues to rise. 8 out of 10 teens now report using a condom the first time they had sex.**
> —Center for Disease Control, 2011

TERMS

intrauterine device (IUD) A device inserted into the uterus as a contraceptive.

male condom A thin sheath that covers the penis during sexual intercourse; used for contraception and to prevent STD transmission.

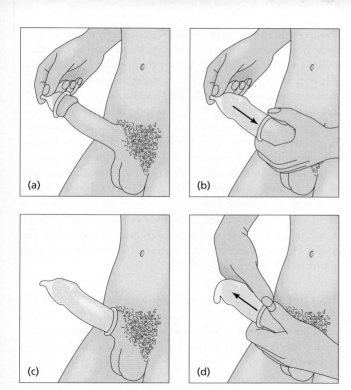

FIGURE 6.1 Use of the male condom. (a) Place the rolled-up condom over the head of the erect penis. Hold the top half-inch of the condom (with air squeezed out) to leave room for semen. (b) While holding the tip, unroll the condom onto the penis. Gently smooth out any air bubbles. (c) Unroll the condom down to the base of the penis. (d) To avoid spilling semen after ejaculation, hold the condom around the base of the penis as the penis is withdrawn. Remove the condom away from your partner, taking care not to spill any semen.

using condoms for STD protection and another contraceptive method for greater protection against pregnancy.

The man or his partner must put the condom on the penis before it is inserted into the vagina because the small amounts of fluid that may be secreted unnoticed prior to **ejaculation** often contain sperm capable of causing pregnancy. The rolled-up condom is placed over the head of the erect penis and unrolled down to the base of the penis, leaving a half-inch space (without air) at the tip to collect semen (Figure 6.1). Some brands of condoms have a reservoir tip designed for this purpose. Uncircumcised men must first pull back the foreskin of the penis. Partners must be careful not to damage the condom with fingernails, rings, or other rough objects.

Many condoms are prelubricated with water-based or silicone-based lubricants. These lubricants make the condom more comfortable and less likely to break. Many people find that using extra, non-oil-based lubricant can be helpful. Prelubricated condoms are also available containing the **spermicide**

nonoxynol-9, the same agent found in many of the contraceptive creams that women use. However, spermicidal condoms are no more effective than condoms without spermicide. They cost more and have a shorter shelf life than most other condoms. Further, condoms with nonoxynol-9 have been associated with urinary tract infections in women and, if they cause tissue irritation, an increased risk of HIV transmission. Planned Parenthood and many other public health agencies advise against the use of condoms lubricated with nonoxynol-9.

Water-based lubricants such as K-Y Jelly or Astroglide can be used as needed. Any products that contain mineral or vegetable oil—including baby oil, many lotions, regular petroleum jelly, cooking oils, and some vaginal lubricants and antifungal or anti-itch creams—should not be used with latex condoms. Such products can cause latex to start disintegrating within 60 seconds, thus greatly increasing the chance of condom breakage. (Polyurethane is not affected by oil-based products.)

Advantages Condoms are easy to purchase and are available without prescription or medical supervision. In addition to being free of medical side effects (other than occasional allergic reactions), latex condoms help protect against STDs. A recent study determined that condoms may also protect women from human papillomavirus (HPV), which causes cervical cancer. Condoms made of polyurethane are appropriate for people who are allergic to latex. However, they are more likely to slip or break than latex condoms, and therefore may give less protection against STDs and pregnancy. Polyurethane condoms are also more expensive than latex condoms. Polyisoprene condoms, marketed under the brand name SKYN, are safe for most people with latex allergies, stretchier, and less expensive than polyurethane condoms. Condoms made of lambskin are also available but permit the passage of HIV and other disease-causing organisms, so they can be used only for pregnancy prevention, not the prevention of STDs. Except for abstinence or intercourse within a monogamous relationship with an uninfected partner, the correct and consistent use of latex male condoms offers the most reliable available protection against the transmission of HIV.

Disadvantages The two most common complaints about condoms are that they diminish sensation and interfere with spontaneity. Although some people find these drawbacks serious, others consider them only minor distractions.

Effectiveness In actual use, the failure rate of condoms varies considerably. During the first year of typical condom use among 100 users, approximately 18 pregnancies will occur. With perfect use, the first-year failure rate is only about 2%. At least some pregnancies happen because the condom is carelessly removed after ejaculation. Some may also occur because of breakage or slippage, which may happen 1–2 times in every 100 instances of use for latex condoms and up to 10 times in every 100 instances for polyurethane condoms. Breakage is more common among inexperienced users. Other contributing factors include poorly fitting condoms, insufficient lubrication (which increases the risk of breakage), excessively vigorous sex, and improper storage. (Because heat destroys rubber, latex condoms should not be stored for long periods in a wallet or a car's glove compartment.) To help ensure quality, condoms should not be used past their expiration date or more than five years past their date of manufacture (two years for those with spermicide).

If a condom breaks or is carelessly removed, a woman can reduce the risk of pregnancy somewhat by immediately taking an emergency contraceptive (discussed later in the chapter).

Female Condoms

The female condom is a clear, stretchy, disposable pouch with two rings that can be inserted into a woman's vagina. It is about as effective in preventing pregnancy and the spread of STDs as the male condom.

The first version of the female condom was expensive and did not become very popular as a result. A new, more affordable female condom is now available. Called the FC2, it is a one-size-fits-all, disposable device that consists of a soft, loose-fitting, nonlatex rubber sheath with two flexible rings. The ring at the closed end is inserted into the vagina and placed at the cervix much like a diaphragm. The ring at the open end remains outside the vagina. The female condom protects the inside of the vagina and part of the external genitalia.

The directions that accompany the FC2 should be followed closely. The manufacturer strongly recommends practicing inserting the female condom several times before actually using it for intercourse. The FC2 comes prelubricated with a silicone lubricant, but extra lubricant or a spermicide can be used if desired. As with male condoms, users need to take care not to tear the condom during insertion or removal. Following intercourse, the woman should remove the condom before standing up. By twisting and squeezing the outer ring, she can prevent the spilling of semen.

Advantages Female condoms can be inserted up to eight hours before sexual activity and are thus less disruptive than male condoms. Because the outer part of the condom covers the area around the vaginal opening as well as the base of the penis during intercourse, it offers potentially better protection against genital warts or herpes. The synthetic rubber pouch can be used by people who are allergic to latex. Because the material is thin and pliable, there is little loss of sensation. The FC2 is generously lubricated and the material conducts heat well, increasing comfort and natural feel during intercourse.

When used correctly, the female condom should theoretically provide protection against HIV transmission and STDs comparable to that of the latex male condom. However, in research involving typical users, the female condom was slightly less effective in preventing both pregnancy and STDs. Effectiveness improves with careful practice and instruction.

Disadvantages The female condom is unfamiliar to most people and requires some practice to learn to use effectively. The outer ring of the female condom, which hangs visibly outside the vagina, may be bothersome to some couples during foreplay; if so, couples may choose to put the device in just before intercourse. During coitus, both partners must take care that the penis is inserted into the pouch, not outside it, and that the device does not slip inside the vagina. Female condoms, like male condoms, are made for one-time use. A single female condom costs about three to four times as much as a single male condom. Female condoms are harder to find than male condoms. Some pharmacies do not currently carry them, but this will change as the FC2 becomes more popular. You can buy the FC2 at Planned Parenthood and online. Go to the FC2 website (www.fcs.us.com) for more information about where you can buy the FC2.

Effectiveness The typical first-year failure rate of the female condom is 21%. For women who follow instructions carefully and consistently, the failure rate is considerably lower—about 5%. Having emergency contraception available is recommended.

The Diaphragm with Spermicide

The **diaphragm** is a dome-shaped cup of latex or silicone stretched over a collapsible metal ring. When correctly used with spermicidal cream or jelly, the diaphragm covers the cervix, blocking sperm from the uterus.

Diaphragms are available only by prescription. Because of individual anatomical differences among women, a diaphragm must be carefully fitted by a trained clinician to ensure both comfort and effectiveness. The fit should be checked with each routine annual medical examination, as well as after childbirth, abortion, abdominal or pelvic surgery, or a weight change of more than 10 pounds.

The woman spreads spermicidal jelly or cream on the diaphragm before inserting it and checking its placement (Figure 6.2). If more than six hours elapse between the time of insertion and the time of intercourse, additional spermicide must be applied. The diaphragm must be left in place for at least six hours after the last act of coitus to give the spermicide enough time to kill all the sperm. With repeated intercourse, a condom should be used for additional protection.

To remove the diaphragm, the woman hooks the front rim down from the pubic bone with one finger and pulls it out. After each use, a diaphragm should be washed with mild soap and water, rinsed, patted dry, and examined for holes or cracks. A diaphragm should be stored in its case.

> **diaphragm** A contraceptive device consisting of a flexible, dome-shaped cup that covers the cervix and prevents sperm from entering the uterus.
>
> **TERMS**

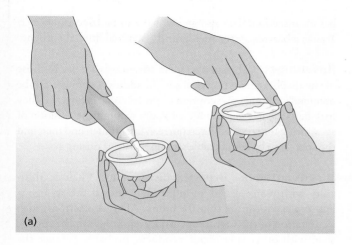

(a)

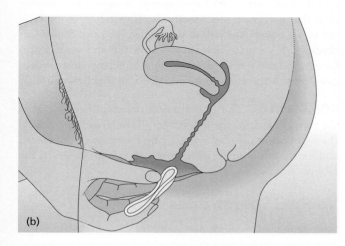

(b)

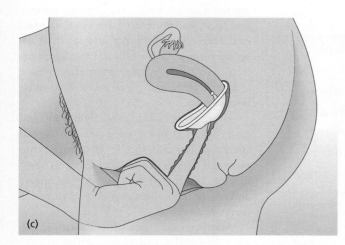

(c)

FIGURE 6.2 Use of the diaphragm. Wash your hands with soap and water before inserting the diaphragm. It can be inserted while squatting, lying down, or standing with one foot raised. (a) Place about a tablespoon of spermicidal jelly or cream in the concave side of the diaphragm, and spread it around the inside of the diaphragm and around the rim. (b) Squeeze the diaphragm into a long, narrow shape between the thumb and forefinger. Insert it into the vagina, and push it up along the back wall of the vagina as far as it will go. (c) Check its position to make sure the cervix is completely covered and that the front rim of the diaphragm is tucked behind the pubic bone.

Advantages   Diaphragm use is less intrusive than male condom use because a diaphragm can be inserted up to six hours before intercourse. Its use can be limited to times of sexual activity only, and it allows for immediate and total reversibility. The diaphragm is free of medical side effects (other than rare allergic reactions).

Disadvantages   Diaphragms must always be used with a spermicide, so a woman must keep both of these supplies with her whenever she anticipates sexual activity. Diaphragms require extra attention because they must be cleaned and stored with care to preserve their effectiveness. Some women cannot wear a diaphragm because of their vaginal or uterine anatomy or frequent bladder infections.

Diaphragms have also been associated with a slightly increased risk of **toxic shock syndrome (TSS),** an occasionally fatal bacterial infection. To reduce the risk of TSS, a woman should wash her hands carefully with soap and water before inserting or removing the diaphragm, should not use the diaphragm during menstruation or when abnormal vaginal discharge is present, and should never leave the device in place for more than 24 hours.

Effectiveness   With perfect use, the failure rate is about 6%. Typical failure rates are 12% during the first year of use. The main causes of failure are incorrect insertion, inconsistent use, and inaccurate fitting. If a diaphragm slips during intercourse, a woman may choose to use emergency contraception.

The Cervical Cap

The **cervical cap,** another barrier device, is a small flexible cup that fits snugly over the cervix and is held in place by suction. The cervical cap is a clear silicone cup with a brim around the dome to hold spermicide and trap sperm and a removal strap over the dome. It comes in three sizes and must be fitted by a trained clinician. It is used like a diaphragm, with a small amount of spermicide placed in the cup and on the brim before insertion. The cervical cap is reusable but must be replaced annually.

Advantages   Advantages of the cervical cap are similar to those associated with diaphragm use. It is an alternative for women who cannot use a diaphragm because of anatomical reasons or recurrent urinary tract infections. The cap fits tightly, so it does not require backup condom use with repeated intercourse. It may be left in place for up to 48 hours.

TERMS

toxic shock syndrome (TSS)   A bacterial disease usually associated with tampon use; symptoms include fever, rash, nausea, headache, dizziness, confusion, fainting, sore throat, cough, and abdominal pain.

cervical cap   A small flexible cup that fits over the cervix; used with spermicide.

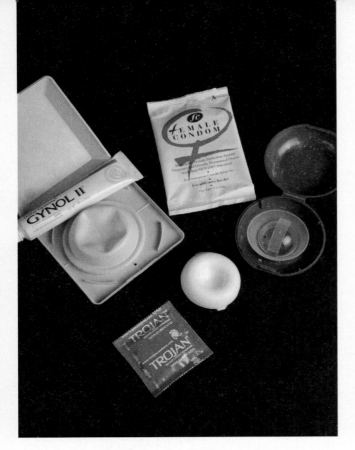

Many contraceptive methods work by blocking sperm from entering the cervix. Barrier methods pictured here are the diaphragm, the female condom, the male condom, the sponge, and the cervical cap.

before insertion. The sponge, which can be used only once, acts as a barrier, a spermicide, and a seminal fluid absorbent.

Advantages   The sponge offers advantages similar to those of the diaphragm and cervical cap. In addition, sponges can be obtained without a prescription or professional fitting, and they may be safely left in place for 24 hours without the addition of spermicide for repeated intercourse. Most women and men find the sponge to be comfortable and unobtrusive during sex.

Disadvantages   Reported disadvantages include difficulty with removal and an unpleasant odor if the sponge is left in place for more than 18 hours. Allergic reactions, such as irritation of the vagina, are more common with the sponge than with other spermicide products, probably because the overall dose contained in each sponge is significantly higher than that used with other methods. If irritation of the vaginal lining occurs, the risk of yeast infections and STDs (including HIV) may increase. Because the sponge has also been associated with toxic shock syndrome, the same precautions must be taken as those described for diaphragm use.

Effectiveness   The typical effectiveness of the sponge is the same as that of the diaphragm (12% failure rate during the first year of use) for women who have never experienced childbirth. For women who have had a child, however, the failure rate rises to 24%.

Vaginal Spermicides

Spermicidal compounds developed for use with a diaphragm have been adapted for use without a diaphragm by combining them with a bulky base. Foams, creams, and jellies must be placed deep in the vagina near the cervical entrance and must be inserted no more than 60 minutes before intercourse. After an hour, their effectiveness is drastically reduced, and a new dose must be inserted.

The spermicidal suppository is small and easily inserted like a tampon. The vaginal contraceptive film (VCF) is a paper-thin two-inch square of film that contains spermicide. It is folded over one or two fingers and placed high in the vagina, as close to the cervix as possible.

Another application of spermicide is also required before each repeated act of coitus. If the woman wants to **douche,** she should wait for at least six hours after

Disadvantages   Along with most of the disadvantages associated with the diaphragm, difficulty with insertion and removal is more common for cervical cap users. Because there may be a slightly increased risk of TSS with prolonged use, the cap should not be left in place for more than 48 hours.

Effectiveness   Studies indicate that the average failure rate for the cervical cap is 16% for women who have never had a child and 32% for women who have had a child. Failure rates drop significantly with perfect use.

The Contraceptive Sponge

The **contraceptive sponge** is a round, absorbent device about two inches in diameter with a polyester loop on one side (for removal) and a concave dimple on the other side, which helps it fit snugly over the cervix. The sponge is made of polyurethane and is presaturated with the same spermicide that is used in contraceptive creams and foams. The spermicide is activated when moistened with a small amount of water just

---

QUICK **STATS**

98.9% of American girls age 15–19 report using at least one form of contraceptive during intercourse.

—National Survey of Family Growth, 2011

TERMS

contraceptive sponge   A contraceptive device that fits over the cervix and acts as a barrier, spermicide, and seminal fluid absorbent.

douche   To apply a stream of water or other solution to a body part or cavity such as the vagina; not a contraceptive technique.

the last intercourse to make sure that there has been time for the spermicide to kill all the sperm; douching is not recommended, however, because it can irritate vaginal tissue and increase the risk of various infections.

Advantages   The use of vaginal spermicides is relatively simple and can be limited to times of sexual activity. They are readily available in most drugstores and do not require a prescription or a pelvic examination. Spermicides allow complete and immediate reversibility, and the only medical side effects are occasional allergic reactions.

Disadvantages   When used alone, vaginal spermicides must be inserted shortly before intercourse, so their use may be seen as an annoying disruption. Spermicides can alter the balance of bacteria in the vagina and may increase the occurrence of yeast infections and urinary tract infections. Also, this contraception method does not protect against gonorrhea, chlamydia, or HIV. Overuse of spermicides can irritate vaginal tissues; if this occurs, the risk of HIV transmission may increase.

Effectiveness   The typical failure rate is about 28% during the first year of use. Spermicide is generally recommended only in combination with other barrier methods or as a backup to other contraceptives. Emergency contraceptives provide a better backup than spermicides, however.

Abstinence, Fertility Awareness, and Withdrawal

Millions of people throughout the world do not use any of the contraceptive methods described earlier because of religious convictions, cultural prohibitions, poverty, or lack of information and supplies. If they use any method at all, they are likely to use one of the following relatively "natural" methods.

Abstinence   The decision not to engage in sexual intercourse for a chosen period of time, or **abstinence,** has been practiced throughout history for a variety of reasons. Until relatively recently, many people abstained because they had no other contraceptive measures. Concern about possible contraceptive side effects, STDs, and unwanted pregnancy may be factors. For others, the most important reason for choosing abstinence is a moral one, based on cultural or religious beliefs or personal values. Many people feel that sexual intercourse is appropriate only for married couples or for people in serious, committed relationships. Abstinence may also be considered the wisest choice in terms of one's emotional needs. A period of abstinence, for example, may be useful as a time to focus on other aspects of one's life.

Couples may choose abstinence to allow time for their relationship to grow. A period of abstinence allows partners to get to know each other better and to develop trust and respect for each other. Many couples who choose to abstain from sexual intercourse in the traditional sense turn to other mutually satisfying alternatives. These may include dancing, massage, hugging, kissing, petting, mutual masturbation, and oral-genital sex.

Fertility Awareness–Based Methods   Women who practice a **fertility awareness–based method** of contraception abstain from intercourse during the fertile phase of their menstrual cycle. Ordinarily only one egg is released by the ovaries each month, and it lives about 24 hours unless it is fertilized. Sperm deposited in the vagina may be capable of fertilizing an egg for up to six or seven days, so conception can theoretically occur only during six to eight days of any menstrual cycle. However, predicting which eight days is difficult.

Recent studies show that even in women who have regular menstrual cycles, it is possible to become pregnant at any time during the menstrual cycle. It is even more difficult to predict the fertile time of the cycle in women who have irregular menses—a situation that is very common, especially in teenagers and women who are approaching menopause.

Methods that attempt to predict the fertile times of a woman's cycle include calendar methods, temperature methods, and methods that rely on observation of the cyclical changes of the cervical mucus as well as other characteristics of the cervix. Some women use a combination of methods to determine the time of ovulation.

Calendar methods are based on the idea that the average woman releases an egg 14–16 days before her period begins. To avoid pregnancy, she should abstain from intercourse for about eight days during her cycle, beginning several days before and during the time that ovulation is most likely to occur. However, in one recent study only about 10% of women with regular 28-day cycles actually ovulated 14 days before the next period. The situation is further complicated by the fact that many women have somewhat or very irregular cycles; calendar methods are extremely unreliable for these women.

Temperature methods are based on the knowledge that a woman's body temperature drops slightly just before ovulation and rises slightly after ovulation. A woman using the temperature method records her basal (resting) body temperature (BBT) every morning before getting out of bed and before eating or drinking anything. Once the temperature

QUICK STATS

5.4% of women who practice some sort of contraception rely on withdrawal as their birth control method.

—National Survey on Family Growth, 2011

abstinence   Avoidance of sexual intercourse; a method of contraception.

fertility awareness–based method   A method of preventing conception based on avoiding intercourse during the fertile phase of a woman's cycle.

TERMS

Table 6.2   Contraceptive Methods and STD Protection

METHOD	LEVEL OF PROTECTION
Hormonal methods	Do not protect against HIV or STDs in lower reproductive tract; may increase risk of cervical chlamydia; provide some protection against PID.
IUD	Does not protect against STDs; mildly associated with PID in first month after insertion.
Latex, polyisoprene, or polyurethane male condom	Best method for protection against STDs (if used correctly); does not protect against infections from lesions that are not covered by the condom. (Lambskin condoms do not protect against STDs.)
Female condom	Reduction of STD risk similar to that of male condom; may provide extra protection for external genitalia.
Diaphragm, sponge, or cervical cap	Provides some protection against cervical infections and PID. Diaphragms, sponges, and cervical caps should not be relied on for protection against HIV.
Spermicide	Modestly reduces the risk of some vaginal and cervical STDs; does not reduce the risk of HIV, chlamydia, or gonorrhea. If vaginal irritation occurs, infection risk may increase.
Fertility awareness–based methods	Do not protect against STDs.
Sterilization	Does not protect against STDs.
Abstinence	Complete protection against STDs (as long as all activities that involve the exchange of body fluids are avoided).

pattern is apparent (usually after about three months), the unsafe period for intercourse can be calculated as the interval from day 5 (day 1 is the first day of the period) until three days after the rise in BBT. To arrive at a shorter unsafe period, some women combine the calendar and temperature methods, calculating the first unsafe day from the shortest cycle of the calendar chart and the last unsafe day as the third day after a rise in BBT.

The *mucus method* (or Billings method) is based on changes in the cervical secretions throughout the menstrual cycle. During the estrogenic phase, cervical mucus increases and is clear and slippery. At the time of ovulation, some women can detect a slight change in the texture of the mucus and find that it is more likely to form an elastic thread when stretched between thumb and finger. After ovulation, these secretions become cloudy and sticky and decrease in quantity. Infertile, safe days are likely to occur during the relatively dry days just before and after menstruation. These additional clues have been found to be helpful by some couples who rely on fertility awareness–based methods.

Fertility awareness–based methods are not recommended for women who have very irregular cycles—about 15% of all menstruating women. Any woman for whom pregnancy would be a serious problem should not rely on these methods alone because the failure rate is high—approximately 25% during the first year of use. Further, fertility awareness–based methods offer no protection against STDs. Some women use fertility awareness in combination with a barrier method to reduce their risk for unwanted pregnancy. Fertility awareness methods are recommended by the Catholic church because the church does not approve of other forms of contraception.

Withdrawal   In **withdrawal,** or *coitus interruptus*, the male removes his penis from the vagina just before he ejaculates. Withdrawal has a high failure rate because the male has to overcome a powerful biological urge. Further, because pre-ejaculatory fluid may contain viable sperm, pregnancy can oc-

cur even if the man withdraws prior to ejaculation. Sexual pleasure is often affected because the man must remain in control and the sexual experience of both partners is interrupted.

The failure rate for typical use is about 22% in the first year. Men who are less experienced with sexual intercourse and withdrawal or who have difficulty in foretelling when ejaculation will occur have higher failure rates. Withdrawal does not protect against STDs.

Combining Methods

Couples can choose to combine the preceding methods in a variety of ways, both to add STD protection and to increase contraceptive effectiveness. For example, condoms are strongly recommended along with OCs and other forms of hormonal contraception whenever there is a risk of STDs (Table 6.2). For many couples, and especially for women, the added benefits far outweigh the extra effort and expense of using multiple methods. Table 6.3 summarizes the effectiveness of available contraceptive methods.

EMERGENCY CONTRACEPTION

Emergency contraception (EC) refers to postcoital methods—those used after unprotected sexual intercourse. An emergency contraceptive may be appropriate if a regularly used method has failed (for example, if a condom breaks)

TERMS

withdrawal   A method of preventing conception in which the man withdraws his penis from the vagina prior to ejaculation; also called *coitus interruptus*.

emergency contraception (EC)   A birth control method used after unprotected sexual intercourse has occurred.

Table 6.3	Contraceptives: From Most Effective to Least (Percentage of Women Experiencing Unintended Pregnancy within the First Year of Use)	
METHOD	TYPICAL USE	PERFECT USE
REVERSIBLE METHODS		
Extremely effective:		
Complete abstinence		0.0%
Implant (Implanon)	0.05%	0.05%
Mirena IUD	0.2%	0.2%
ParaGard IUD	0.8%	0.6%
Injectable (3-month)	6.0%	0.2%
Very effective:		
Pill	9.0%	0.3%
Patch	9.0%	0.3%
Ring	9.0%	0.3%
Moderately effective:		
Male condom	18.0%	2.0%
Diaphragm	12.0%	6.0%
Sponge (if never had a child)	12.0%	9.0%
Cervical cap (if never had a child)	16.0%	9.0%
Female condom	21.0%	5.0%
Less effective:		
Periodic abstinence	24.0%	
Withdrawal	22.0%	4.0%
Spermicides	28.0%	18.0%
Sponge (if have had a child)	24.0%	20.0%
Cervical cap (if have had a child)	32.0%	26.0%
PERMANENT METHODS		
Vasectomy	0.15%	0.1%
Essure	0.2%	0.2%
Tubal sterilization	0.5%	0.5%
No method	85.0%	85.0%

SOURCE: Trussell J. Trussell J. "Contraceptive Efficacy." In Hatcher, R.A., J. Trussell, A.L. Nelson, W. Cates, F.H. Stewart, and D. Kowal. Contraceptive Technology, 20th Revised Edition. Copyright © 2011 Ardent Media. Reprinted with permission.

or if unprotected sex has occurred. Sometimes called the "morning-after pill," emergency contraceptives are designed only for emergency use and should not be relied on as a regular birth control method; other methods of birth control are more effective.

When emergency contraceptives were first approved by the FDA, opponents feared that they might act as an **abortifacient**—preventing implantation of a fertilized egg,

Emergency contraceptives **do not result in an abortion** and do not interfere with an existing pregnancy.

abortifacient   An agent or substance that induces abortion.

TERMS

theoretically causing abortion. However, recent evidence indicates that emergency contraceptives do not interrupt an established pregnancy. Postcoital pills work primarily by inhibiting or delaying ovulation and by altering the transport of sperm and eggs; they do not affect a fertilized egg already implanted in the uterus and thus do not cause abortion.

Until recently, the most frequently used emergency contraceptive was a two-dose regimen of oral contraceptives. Newer products—Plan B, Plan B One-Step, and Next Choice—are now in common use and are more effective, with fewer side effects, than older methods of EC. Plan B One-Step, which replaced Plan B in 2009, contains a single progestin-only pill, whereas Next Choice has two pills that are taken 12 hours apart. The pills should be taken as soon as possible after inadequately protected sex. If taken within 24 hours after intercourse, emergency contraceptives may prevent as many as 95% of expected pregnancies. Overall they reduce pregnancy risk by about 89%. They are most effective if initiated in the first 12 hours, but they can be taken up to 120 hours after unprotected intercourse. Possible side effects include nausea, stomach pain, headache, dizziness, and breast tenderness. If a woman is already pregnant, these pills will not interfere with the pregnancy. Current emergency contraceptives are considered very safe.

Plan B One-Step and Next Choice are available as over-the-counter (OTC) drugs (no prescription required) for women and men aged 17 and older. They remain prescription drugs for those under ages 17. To buy an emergency contraceptive, you need to ask for it at the pharmacy counter and show proof of age. It is recommended that you call ahead to make sure your pharmacy has EC on hand. The vast majority of pharmacies, especially the larger chains, currently carry emergency contraceptives.

Some clinicians advise women to keep a package of emergency contraceptives on hand in case their regular contraception method fails or they have unprotected intercourse. Research has found that ready access to emergency contraception improves the rate of use as well as decreasing the time to use. However, it does not lead to an increase in unprotected intercourse or STDs.

To find out more about emergency contraception and how to obtain it in your area, visit the Emergency Contraception website at http://ec.princeton.edu. Planned Parenthood is a good source of information, as are most pharmacies. You can also call the Emergency Contraception Hotline (888-NOT-2-LATE) for more information about access.

Intrauterine devices can also be used for emergency contraception. If inserted within five days of unprotected intercourse, the Copper T ParaGard IUD (discussed earlier) is even more effective than pills for emergency contraception. It has the added benefit of providing up to 10 years of contraception.

A new emergency contraceptive, ulipristal acetate, was approved for use by the Food and Drug Administration in 2010.

Sold under the name ella, this drug is effective if taken up to five days after unprotected intercourse. At the time of this writing, ella is available by prescription only.

PERMANENT CONTRACEPTION

Sterilization is permanent, and it is highly effective at preventing pregnancy. At present it is tied with the pill as the most commonly used contraceptive method in the United States and is by far the most common method used worldwide. It is especially popular among couples who have been married 10 or more years and have had all the children they intend to have. Sterilization does not protect against STDs.

An important consideration in choosing sterilization is that, in most cases, it cannot be reversed. Some couples choosing male sterilization store sperm to extend the option of childbearing.

Many studies indicate that male sterilization is preferable to female sterilization for a variety of reasons. The overall cost of a female procedure is about four times that of a male procedure, and women are much more likely than men to experience complications following the operation. Further, feelings of regret seem to be more prevalent in women than in men after sterilization.

Male Sterilization: Vasectomy

The procedure for male sterilization, **vasectomy,** involves severing the vasa deferentia, two tiny ducts that transport sperm from the testes to the seminal vesicles. The testes continue to produce sperm, but the sperm are absorbed into the body. Because the testes contribute only about 10% of the total seminal fluid, the actual quantity of ejaculate is only slightly reduced. Hormone production from the testes continues with very little change, and secondary sex characteristics are not altered.

Vasectomy is ordinarily performed in a physician's office and takes about 30 minutes. A local anesthetic is injected into the skin of the scrotum near the vasa. Small incisions are made at the upper end of the scrotum where it joins the body, and the vas deferens on each side is exposed, severed, and tied off or sealed by electrocautery. Some doctors seal each of the vasa with a plastic clamp, which is the size of a grain of rice.

The incisions are then closed with sutures, and a small dressing is applied. Pain and swelling are usually slight and can be relieved with ice compresses and a scrotal support. Bleeding and infection occasionally develop but are usually easily treated.

Men can have sex after vasectomy as soon as they feel no discomfort, usually after about a week. Another method of contraception must be used for at least three months after vasectomy, however, because sperm produced before the operation may still be present in the semen.

Vasectomy is highly effective. In a small number of cases, a severed vas rejoins itself, so some physicians advise yearly examination of a semen sample. The overall failure rate for vasectomy is 0.15%. About one-half of vasectomy reversals are successful, though this rate can vary significantly depending on the number of years since the initial surgery.

Female Sterilization

The most common method of female sterilization involves severing or blocking the oviducts, thereby preventing eggs from reaching the uterus and sperm from entering the fallopian tubes. Ovulation and menstruation continue, but the unfertilized eggs are released into the abdominal cavity and absorbed. Although progesterone levels in the blood may decline slightly, hormone production by the ovaries and secondary sex characteristics are generally not affected.

Tubal sterilization (also called *tubal ligation*) is most commonly performed by a method called **laparoscopy.** A laparoscope, a camera containing a small light, is inserted through a small abdominal incision, and the surgeon looks through it to locate the fallopian tubes. Instruments are passed either through the laparoscope or through a second small incision, and the two fallopian tubes are sealed off with ties or staples or by electrocautery. General anesthesia is usually used. The operation takes about 30 minutes, and women can usually leave the hospital two to four hours after surgery. Tubal sterilization can also be performed shortly after a vaginal delivery, or in the case of cesarean section, immediately after the uterine incision is repaired.

Although tubal sterilization is somewhat riskier than vasectomy, with a rate of minor complications of about 6–11%, it is the more common procedure (see the box "Contraceptive

TERMS

sterilization   Surgically altering the reproductive system to prevent pregnancy. Vasectomy is the procedure in males; tubal sterilization or hysterectomy is the procedure in females.

vasectomy   The surgical severing of the ducts that carry sperm to the ejaculatory duct.

tubal sterilization   Severing or blocking the oviducts to prevent eggs from reaching the uterus; also called *tubal ligation*.

laparoscopy   Examining the internal organs by inserting a small camera through an abdominal incision.

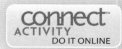

Nearly all American women use contraceptives at some time during their lives. According to the National Center for Health Statistics, 99% of all U.S. women who have ever had intercourse have used a contraceptive.

About 62 million women in the United States are in their childbearing years (15–44) and thus face decisions about contraception. About 62% of these women currently use some form of contraception. Most of the remaining 38% are sterile, pregnant, trying to become pregnant, or not sexually active.

Only about 7% of American women are fertile, sexually active, not seeking pregnancy, and not using contraceptives. This small group accounts for almost half of the 3 million unintended pregnancies that occur each year. The unintended pregnancies that occur among contraceptive users are usually the result of inconsistent or incorrect use of methods. For example, one-third of barrier method users report not using their method every time they have intercourse.

Oral contraceptives and female sterilization are the two most popular methods among American women (see the accompanying table). However, choice of contraceptive method and consistency of use vary with age, marital status, and other factors:

- **Age:** Sterilization is much more common among older women, particularly those who are over 35 years of age and/or who have had children. Young women in their teens and twenties are more likely to use the pill or condoms. Older women, however, are more likely to use reversible methods consistently. They are less likely to miss pills and more likely to use barrier methods during every act of intercourse.

- **Marital status:** Women who are or were married have much higher rates of sterilization than women who have never been married. Those who have never been married have high rates of OC and condom usage.

- **Ethnicity:** Overall rates of contraceptive use and use of OCs are highest among white women. Female sterilization, implants, and injectable contraceptives are more often used by African American women and Latinas, and IUD use is highest among Latinas. Condom use is highest among Asian American women and is similar across other ethnic groups. Male sterilization is much more common among white men than among men of other ethnic groups.

- **Socioeconomic status and educational attainment:** Low socioeconomic status and low educational attainment are associated with high rates of female sterilization and low rates of pill and condom use. However, women who are poor or have low educational attainment and who use OCs have higher rates of consistent use than women who are wealthier or have more education. About 20% of women ages 15–44 lack adequate health insurance, increasing the cost and difficulty of obtaining contraceptives.

- **New trends:** About 10% of American women have used emergency contraception at least once, up from 4% in 2002. The percentage of women who have ever used the patch rose from 1% to 10% in the last six years. Rates of IUD use, especially among women who have already had at least one child, have also risen dramatically.

Some trends in contraceptive use may also reflect the differing priorities and experiences of women and men. For example, female sterilization is more expensive and carries greater health risks than male sterilization—yet it is more than twice as common. (Worldwide, female sterilization is more than four times as common as male sterilization.) This pattern may reflect culturally defined gender roles and the fact that women are more directly affected by unintended pregnancy. In surveys, women rate pregnancy prevention as the single most important factor when choosing a contraceptive method; in contrast, men rate STD prevention as equally important.

Method	Percentage of Users
Pill	28.0
Tubal sterilization	27.1
Male condom	16.1
Vasectomy	9.9
IUD	5.5
Withdrawal	5.2
Three-month injectable (Depo-Provera)	3.2
Vaginal ring (Nuva-Ring)	2.4
Implant (Implanon), one month injectable (Lunelle), or patch (Ortho Evra)	1.1
Periodic abstinence (calendar method)	0.9
Other* (includes emergency contraception, sponge, cap, female condom)	0.4

SOURCES: Frost, L. J., et al. 2007. Factors associated with contraceptive use and nonuse, United States, 2004. *Perspectives on Sexual and Reproductive Health* 39(2): 90–99; Guttmacher Institute. 2010. *Facts in Brief: Facts on Contraceptive Use* (http:// www.guttmacher.org/pubs/fb_contr_use.html); Mosher, W. D., and J. Jones. 2010. Use of contraception in the U.S.: 1982–2008. National Center for Health Statistics. *Vital Health Statistics* 23(29).

connect ACTIVITY DO IT ONLINE

Use among American Women"). Potential problems include bowel injury, wound infection, and bleeding. Serious complications are rare, and the death rate is low.

The failure rate for tubal sterilization is about 0.5%. When pregnancies occur, an increased percentage of them are ectopic (occurring outside the uterus). Ectopic pregnancy is dangerous and can even cause death, so any woman who suspects she might be pregnant after having tubal sterilization should seek medical help. Because successful reversal rates are low and the procedure is costly, female sterilization should be considered permanent.

Two new forms of incision-free female sterilization have recently become available. Each of these procedures can be performed with local anesthetic in a doctor's office, and both have short recovery times. The first, called the Essure System, consists of tiny springlike metallic implants that are inserted through the vagina and into the fallopian tubes, using a special catheter. Within several months, scar tissue forms over the implants, blocking the tubes.

In 2009 the FDA approved a second, somewhat similar, method for blocking a woman's fallopian tubes without an incision. The procedure, marketed under the name Adiana, involves using low-frequency waves to create small lesions just inside the entrance to each fallopian tube. A small silicone insert, the size of a grain of rice, is then placed in each tube. As the lesions heal, healthy new tissue grows on and around the device, eventually blocking the fallopian tube. The three-year failure rate of the Adiana procedure is about 1.8%.

Hysterectomy, removal of the uterus, is the preferred method of sterilization for only a small number of women, usually those with preexisting menstrual or other uterine problems.

WHICH CONTRACEPTIVE METHOD IS RIGHT FOR YOU?

Each person must consider many variables in deciding which method is most acceptable and appropriate for her or him. Key considerations include those listed here:

1. *Health risks.* When considering any contraceptive method, determine whether it may pose a risk to your health. For example, hormonal methods should be used only after a clinical evaluation of your medical history. Other methods have only minor and local side effects. Talk with your health care provider about the potential health effects of different methods for you. Remember that pregnancy and abortion carry significant health risks that are generally much greater than the risks of any method of contraception.

2. *The implications of an unplanned pregnancy.* Many teens and young adults fail to consider how their lives would be affected by an unexpected pregnancy. When considering contraception (or deciding whether to have sex at all), think about the potential conse-quences of your choices.

3. *STD risk.* STDs are another potential consequence of sex. In fact, several activities besides vaginal intercourse (such as oral and anal sex) can put you at risk for an STD. Condom use is of critical importance whenever any risk of STDs is present, even if you are using another contraceptive method to prevent pregnancy. This is especially true whenever you are not in an exclusive, long-term relationship. Abstinence or activities that don't involve intercourse or any other exchange of body fluids can be a satisfactory alternative for some people.

4. *Convenience and comfort level.* The hormonal methods are generally ranked high in this category for most women. If forgetting to take pills is a problem for you, a vaginal ring, contraceptive patch, implant, or injectable method may be a good alternative to the pill. For those who choose a barrier method, the diaphragm, cervical cap, contraceptive sponge, female condom, and spermicides can be inserted before intercourse begins. Some people think condom use disrupts spontaneity, but creative approaches to condom use can decrease these concerns.

5. *Type of relationship.* Barrier methods require more motivation and sense of responsibility from *each* partner than hormonal methods do. When the method depends on the cooperation of one's partner, assertiveness is necessary, no matter how difficult (see the box "Talking with a Partner About Contraception"). This is especially true in new relationships, when condom use is most important. When sexual activity is infrequent, a barrier method may make more sense than an IUD or one of the hormonal methods.

6. *Ease and cost of obtaining and maintaining each method.* Investigate the costs of different methods. If you have insurance, find out if it covers any of the costs. Remember that your student health clinic probably provides family planning services, and most communities have low-cost family planning clinics, such as Planned Parenthood.

7. *Religious or philosophical beliefs.* For some people, abstinence and/or fertility awareness–based methods may be the only permissible contraceptive methods.

8. *Potential noncontraceptive benefits.* Women with dysmenorrhea, irregular periods, acne, endometriosis, severe PMS, and other medical problems may benefit from using a particular method of contraception. Be sure to discuss these issues with your health care provider so that you can take advantage of the noncontraceptive benefits associated with many methods of birth control.

hysterectomy Total or partial surgical removal of the uterus.

 TERMS

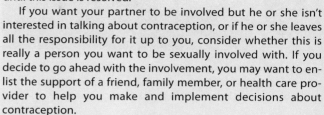

Many people have a difficult time talking about contraception with a potential sex partner. How should you bring it up? And whose responsibility is it? Talking about the subject may be embarrassing at first, but imagine the possible consequences of not talking about it. An unintended pregnancy or a sexually transmitted disease could profoundly affect you for the rest of your life. Talking about contraception is one way of showing that you care about yourself, your partner, and your future.

Before you talk with your partner, explore your own thoughts and feelings. Find out the facts about different methods of contraception, and decide which one you think would be most appropriate for you. If you're nervous about having this discussion with your partner, it may help to practice with a friend.

Pick a good time to bring up the subject. It makes sense to have this discussion before you start having sex, but even if you've already had intercourse with your partner, it's important to be on the same page about contraception. A time when you're both feeling comfortable and relaxed will improve your chances of having a good discussion. Tell your partner what you know about contraception and how you feel about using it, and talk about what steps you both need to take to get and use a method

you can live with. Listen to what your partner has to say, and try to understand his or her point of view. You may need to have more than one discussion, and it may take some time for both of you to feel comfortable with the subject. But don't have sex until this issue is resolved.

If you want your partner to be involved but he or she isn't interested in talking about contraception, or if he or she leaves all the responsibility for it up to you, consider whether this is really a person you want to be sexually involved with. If you decide to go ahead with the involvement, you may want to enlist the support of a friend, family member, or health care provider to help you make and implement decisions about contraception.

If you have been involved in hooking up with people you don't know well and are not having an ongoing relationship with, discussions about contraception may seem unrealistic. At a minimum, refuse to have sex with anyone who won't use a condom. If you are a woman, purchase emergency contraception ahead of time, and don't hesitate to use it.

Whatever your needs, circumstances, or beliefs, *do* make a choice about contraception. Not choosing anything is the one method known *not* to work. This is an area in which taking charge of your health has immediate and profound implications for your future.

THE ABORTION ISSUE

Few issues are as complex and emotionally charged as abortion. In the United States, public attention has focused on the legal definition of abortion and the issues of how and when its practice should be restricted. While this debate is important, the most difficult aspects of abortion are personal—especially for women who must decide whether to have an abortion.

The word *abortion*, by strict definition, means the expulsion of an embryo or fetus from the uterus before it is sufficiently developed to survive outside the uterus. As commonly used, however, the term *abortion* refers only to those expulsions that are artificially induced by mechanical means or drugs. The term **miscarriage** is generally used when referring to a *spontaneous abortion*—one that occurs naturally with no causal intervention. In this chapter, *abortion* refers to a deliberately induced expulsion.

Legal Status of Abortion

Abortion was relatively unregulated in the United States until the early 1800s, when an anti-abortion movement began. By the 1900s abortion was illegal in every state. These anti-

abortion laws stayed in effect until the 1960s, when courts began to invalidate them on the grounds of constitutional vagueness and violation of the right to privacy.

In 1973 the U.S. Supreme Court made abortion legal in the landmark case of *Roe v. Wade*. To replace the restrictions most states still imposed at that time, the justices devised new standards to govern abortion decisions. They divided pregnancy into three parts, or *trimesters*, giving a woman less choice about abortion as her pregnancy advances toward full term.

According to *Roe v. Wade*, in the first trimester, the abortion decision must be left to the judgment of the pregnant woman and her physician. During the second trimester, similar rights remain up to the point when the fetus becomes **viable**—that is, capable of surviving outside of the uterus. Today most clinicians define this point as 24 weeks of gestation. When the fetus is considered viable, a state may regulate and even bar all abortions except those considered necessary to preserve the mother's life or health.

Although abortion remains legal throughout the United States, subsequent rulings by the Supreme Court have allowed states to regulate abortion throughout pregnancy as long as no "undue burden" is imposed on women seeking the procedure. As a result, states have passed multiple laws every

> **TERMS**
>
> **miscarriage**   A naturally occurring spontaneous abortion.
>
> **viable**   apable of surviving outside of the uterus.

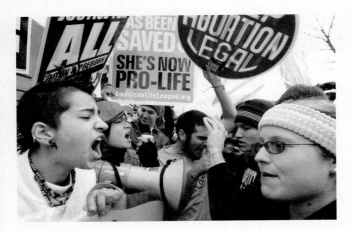

Pro-choice groups believe that the decision to end or continue a pregnancy is a personal matter. Pro-life groups oppose abortion on the basis of their belief that life begins at conception.

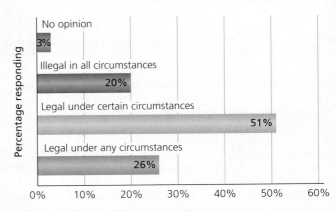

FIGURE 6.3 **Public opinion about abortion.**

SOURCE: Gallup, Inc. 2012. *Public Opinion about Abortion* (http://www.gallup.com/poll/1576/abortion.aspx). Reprinted by permission.

year that regulate access to abortions. Thus abortion laws vary widely from state to state.

Public Opinion

Along with the legal debates are ongoing arguments between pro-life and pro-choice groups regarding the ethics of abortion. Central to the pro-life position is the belief that the fertilized egg must be afforded the same rights as a human being from the moment of conception and that abortion at any time is equivalent to murder. In contrast, the pro-choice viewpoint holds that distinctions must be made between the stages of fetal development and that preserving the fetus early in pregnancy is not always the ultimate moral concern. Members of this group maintain that women have the right to decide whether and when to have children; they argue that pregnancy can result from contraceptive failure or other factors out of a woman's control.

Although the most vocal groups in the abortion debate tend to paint a black-and-white picture, most Americans view abortion as a complex issue without any easy answers. Many Americans approve of legal abortion as an option when destructive health or welfare consequences could result from continuing pregnancy. Overall, the majority of adults in the United States approve of legal abortion in certain instances (Figure 6.3).

Personal Considerations

For the pregnant woman who is considering abortion, the legal and moral arguments may sound meaningless as she attempts to weigh the many short- and long-term ramifications for all those who are directly concerned. If she chooses abortion, can she accept the decision in terms of her own religious and moral beliefs? What are her long-term feelings likely to be

> ### QUICK STATS
> **More than one in three** American women have an abortion before they turn 45.
> —Planned Parenthood, 2012

regarding this decision? What are her partner's feelings regarding abortion, and how will she deal with his response? Does she know supportive people who will help her through the emotional adjustment? Which medical facility offering abortions would be most suitable for her? What about transportation and costs?

For the woman who decides against abortion and chooses instead to continue the pregnancy, there are other questions. If she decides to raise the child herself, will she have the resources to do it well? Is a supportive, lasting relationship with her partner likely? If not, how does she feel about being a single parent?

If the pregnant woman considers adoption, she will have to try to predict her emotional responses throughout the full-term pregnancy and the adoption process. What are her long-term feelings likely to be? What is the best setting for her during pregnancy? What type of adoption would be most appropriate? (The box "The Adoption Option" addresses some of these questions.)

A Man's Rights Regarding Abortion

Discussions regarding abortion frequently focus on a woman's role in the decision and the effects on her mental and physical health. However, increasingly debated is the role the man should play in the decision to pursue an abortion. Multiple cases have been brought to the courts by men seeking the right to prevent an abortion. However, at this time, men do not have the legal right to prevent an abortion from occurring. The decision rests solely with the woman from a legal perspective. Nevertheless, men are often involved in the decision-making process with their partners and may experience a similar range of emotions as women. A small survey found that men felt guilt, grief, relief, and a sense of responsibility in the months following their partner's abortion.

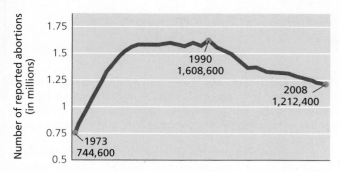

FIGURE 6.4 Number of reported abortions in the United States, 1973–2008.

SOURCE: Jones, R. K., et al. 2011. Abortion incidence and access to services in the United States, 2008. *Perspectives on Sexual and Reproductive Health* 43(1): 41–50.

Abortion Statistics

Abortions are fairly common in the United States. Among American women, about 50% of all pregnancies are unintended; about 40% of such pregnancies end in abortion. About 22% of all pregnancies—wanted and unwanted—end in abortion, not including those that end in miscarriage.

After the Supreme Court's ruling in *Roe v. Wade*, the number of abortions rapidly increased in the United States (Figure 6.4). According to the Guttmacher Institute (a private organization that tracks statistics on reproductive health issues, including contraception and abortion), nearly 750,000 abortions occurred in 1973; the number rose each year after that until hitting a peak of 1.6 million in 1990. The number reported has steadily declined since then to around 1.2 million abortions performed each year from 2001 through 2008.

The number of late-term abortions has dropped over time, as well. In 2006, 91% of abortions occurred during the first 13 weeks (the first trimester) of pregnancy; about 1.3% were performed after the 21st week (Figure 6.5).

Planned Parenthood estimates that about one out of three American women will have an abortion by age 45. Women who choose to have an abortion vary widely; they represent various ages, religions, races, and levels of education (see Figure 6.5). Therefore, it is impossible to paint a picture of a woman most likely to pursue an abortion of an unintended pregnancy. On average, however, American women who get abortions are under age 25, have previously

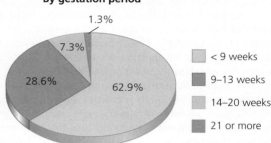

By woman's age

By gestation period

FIGURE 6.5 Distribution of abortions by the woman's age and by the weeks of gestation: 2008.

SOURCE: Jones, R. K., L. B. Finer, and S. Singh. 2010. *Characteristics of U.S. Abortion Patients, 2008.* New York: Guttmacher Institute; Centers for Disease Control and Prevention. 2012. Abortion surveillance—United States, 2008. *Morbidity and Mortality Weekly Report* 60 (SS15): 1–41.

given birth, have never been married, are poor, and live in a metropolitan area.

Methods of Abortion

Abortion methods can be divided into two categories: surgical and medical. Surgical abortion is by far the most common, accounting for about 85% of all abortions performed in the United States in 2008.

The most common method of abortion performed from the 6th to the 12th week of pregnancy is **suction curettage** (commonly known as *dilation and curettage*, or *D & C*). The procedure can be done quickly, usually on an outpatient basis, and the risk of complications is small.

A sedative may be given, either through an IV or orally, prior to beginning the procedure. A local anesthetic may then be injected into the cervix. The cervix is dilated, and a specially designed tube, called a *suction curette*, is inserted into the uterus. The curette is attached to the rubber tubing of an electric pump, and suction is applied. In 20–30 seconds, the uterus is emptied. Moderate cramping is common during evacuation. To ensure that no fragments of

Ask Yourself

QUESTIONS FOR CRITICAL THINKING AND REFLECTION

Suppose you are in the position of lending support to a friend who has gone through an abortion. What sort of physical or emotional signals would you look for? What kind of support would you be willing to offer?

suction curettage Removal of the embryo or fetus by means of suction. TERMS

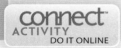

Every woman facing an unintended pregnancy has three options: to continue the pregnancy, to seek an abortion, or to place her child up for adoption. Before 1977, nearly 9% of unmarried pregnant women gave their children up for adoption. Today only 1% of women choose to place a child for adoption. This decline may be due to a variety of factors, including increased rates of contraceptive use and an easing of the social stigma of single parenthood. The drop in adoption rates in the 1970s probably reflected an increase in the abortion rate following the 1973 legalization of abortion. Since 1990, however, adoption rates have remained steady while the abortion rate has declined, indicating that women are not choosing abortion over adoption.

The decision to go through an unwanted pregnancy and then give the baby to another family is difficult. Adoption is permanent: the adoptive parents will raise the child and have legal authority for his or her welfare. Knowing this, the birth mother should think about her life now and in the future as she weighs alternatives.

Many people can help a pregnant woman consider her options, including her partner, friends, family members, a professional counselor, a crisis pregnancy center, a family planning clinic, or a family services, social services, or adoption agency. A counselor should always be respectful and willing to discuss all the options—keeping the baby, having an abortion, or arranging an adoption.

Adoptions can be confidential or open. In a confidential adoption, the birth parents and the adoptive parents never know each other. Adoptive parents receive any information they might need to take care of the child. A later meeting between the child and birth parents is possible in confidential adoption, however, if the birth parents leave information with the agency or lawyer who handles the adoption and/or in a national adoption registry.

In an open adoption, the birth parents and adoptive parents know something about each other. There are different levels of openness, ranging from reading a brief description of prospective adoptive parents to meeting them and sharing full information. Birth parents may also be able to stay in touch with the family by visiting, calling, or writing.

In all states, a mother can work with a licensed child placement (adoption) agency. It may also be possible to work directly with an adopting couple or their attorney; this is called a private or independent adoption.

A woman who gives a child up for adoption should also consider the reaction and rights of the birth father. A woman can choose to have an abortion without the consent or knowledge of the father, but once the baby is born, the father has certain rights. These rights vary from state to state, but at a minimum, most states require that the birth father be notified of the adoption. In some states, the birth father may be able to take the child even if the mother prefers that the child go to an adoptive family.

As with abortion, there are emotional and physical risks associated with pregnancy, childbirth, and adoption. Throughout the adoption process, the mother should make sure that she has the help she needs and that she carefully considers all her options.

SOURCES: Child Welfare Information Gateway. 2010 Update. *Are You Pregnant and Thinking about Adoption?* (http://www.childwelfare.gov/pubs/f_pregna/index.cfm); Child Welfare Information Gateway. 2010 Update. *Voluntary Relinquishment for Adoption: Numbers and Trends* (http://www.childwelfare.gov/pubs/s_place.cfm).

connect
ACTIVITY
DO IT ONLINE

---

tissue are left in the uterus, the doctor may scrape the uterine lining with a metal curette. The entire procedure takes 5–10 minutes. A follow-up exam is important to verify that the abortion was complete and that no signs of infection are present.

In **manual vacuum aspiration (MVA),** plastic tube attached to a handheld syringe is inserted through the cervix and into the uterus. The syringe provides gentle suction, which empties the uterus.

MVA has several advantages over suction curettage. Manual vacuum aspiration does not require an electric pump or additional equipment, and therefore it can be used in a wider variety of settings. It is also significantly cheaper than suction curettage, and it has been successfully used by midlevel providers such as midwives and nurses. For these reasons, MVA is ideal for low-resource settings. A number of recent studies have shown that the two techniques have equivalent safety profiles and low rates of complications when done up to 10 weeks of gestation.

Multi-fetal pregnancy reduction (MFPR) is a procedure that reduces the number of fetuses in a multiple pregnancy. It is usually performed during the first trimester. In the most common method of MFPR, the fetal heart is injected with potassium chloride. The dead fetus is then absorbed by the mother's body. Multi-fetal reduction reduces the risk of preterm delivery for the remaining fetus and improves maternal pregnancy outcomes.

Only about 1 in 10 abortions is performed after the 12th week of pregnancy. The method most commonly used for

> **TERMS**
>
> **manual vacuum aspiration (MVA)** The vacuum aspiration of uterine contents, performed manually with a handheld syringe.
>
> **multi-fetal pregnancy reduction (MFPR)** A method of abortion used to reduce the number of fetuses in a multiple-fetus pregnancy.

abortion from 13 to 24 weeks of pregnancy is **dilation and evacuation (D & E)**. Depending on the gestational age of the fetus at the time of the abortion, cervical dilators may be placed within the cervix the day prior to the procedure, which gradually expand within the cervix overnight while the woman is at home. The next day, the uterus is emptied using surgical instruments and an aspirating machine.

Intact dilation and extraction (known controversially as *partial birth abortion*) is a surgical abortion wherein an intact fetus is removed from the uterus. This procedure is performed only rarely, representing less than 1% of all abortions in the United States. Experts say that intact dilation and extraction can be useful when certain fetal anomalies are present, such as severe hydrocephalus (swelling of the fetus's head), and that the procedure may be the safest option for the mother in some circumstances. Intact dilation and extraction became illegal after the 2007 Supreme Court ruling in the case of *Gonzales v. Carhart*, even in situations where the mother's health may be in jeopardy.

Medical abortion is generally used in very early pregnancy, within 49 days of the last menstrual period. The combination of drugs that is given causes the embryo and products of conception to be passed out through the vagina, as in a natural miscarriage. Medical abortion is generally safer than surgical abortion because it doesn't involve anesthesia or surgical risks. Some women feel that medical abortion allows them to take more control of the procedure and gives them more privacy than a surgical abortion would. The major disadvantages of medical abortion are that the process can take days to complete and that bleeding after the procedure is often heavier and lasts longer than with surgical abortion. Medical abortion also generally requires more clinic visits than surgical abortion. The cost to the patient is generally about the same.

Complications of Abortion

Along with questions regarding the actual procedure of abortion, many people have concerns about possible aftereffects. More information is gradually being gathered about this important subject.

QUICK STATS

Only **11%** of U.S. abortion service providers offer abortions at 24 or more weeks of gestation.
—Guttmacher Institute, 2011

Abortion-related mortality rates have declined substantially since abortion was legalized in 1973.

Possible Physical Effects The incidence of immediate problems following an abortion (infection, bleeding, trauma to the cervix or uterus, and incomplete abortion requiring repeat curettage) varies widely. The potential for problems is significantly reduced by a woman's good health, early timing of the abortion, use of the suction method, performance by a well-trained clinician, and the availability and use of prompt follow-up care.

Problems related to infection can be minimized through preabortion testing and treatment for gonorrhea, chlamydia, and other infections. Postabortion danger signs are fever above 100°F, abdominal pain or swelling, cramping, backache, abdominal tenderness (to pressure), Prolonged or heavy bleeding, Foul-smelling vaginal discharge, Vomiting or fainting, or delay in resuming menstrual periods (six weeks or more).

Some cramping and bleeding are an expected part of ending a pregnancy. In rare cases, life-threatening bleeding, infections, or other problems can occur following a miscarriage, surgical abortion, or medical abortion. Prompt medical attention should be sought if heavy bleeding, severe abdominal pain, or fever occurs.

Possible Psychological Effects After an exhaustive review completed in 1988, the then–surgeon general, C. Everett Koop, concluded that the available evidence failed to demonstrate either a negative or a positive long-term impact of abortion on mental health. More recent research has resulted in the same general conclusion. The frequency of any psychiatric diagnoses in women who have undergone an abortion procedure is no higher than in women with no such history.

The psychological side effects of abortion, however, are less clearly defined than the physical ones. Responses vary and depend on the individual woman's psychological makeup, family background, current personal and social relationships, cultural attitudes, and many other factors. A woman who has specific goals with a somewhat structured life may be able to incorporate her decision to have an abortion as the unequivocally best and most acceptable course more easily than a woman who feels uncertain about her future.

Although many women experience relief after an abortion, some go through a period of sadness while making the decision to proceed with an abortion or shortly after it is performed. They may also feel guilt, regret, loss, or anger.

For a woman who experiences psychological or emotional effects after an abortion, talking with a close friend or family member can be helpful. Supportive people can help her feel positive about herself and her decision. If unresolved emotions persist, a woman should seek professional counseling.

TERMS

dilation and evacuation (D & E) The method of abortion most commonly used between 13 and 24 weeks of pregnancy. Following dilation of the cervix, both vacuum aspiration and curettage instruments are used as needed.

intact dilation and extraction A rarely used method of late-term abortion, wherein an intact fetus is removed from the uterus.

TIPS FOR TODAY AND THE FUTURE

Your decisions about contraception are among the most important you will make in your life. You may never have to face an unintended pregnancy, but you should know what choices you would have, as well as where you stand on the issue of abortion.

RIGHT NOW YOU CAN:

- If you're sexually active, consider whether you are confident that you're doing everything possible to prevent an unwanted pregnancy.
- If you're sexually active, discuss your contraceptive method with your partner. Make sure you are using the method that works best for you.
- Work with your partner to choose a backup contraceptive method to use in case your primary method isn't effective enough. Consider keeping an emergency contraceptive on hand in case of a slip-up.
- Examine your feelings about the possibility of becoming a parent, especially if it were to happen unintentionally.
- Consider your views on the morality of abortion, and whether it is acceptable under certain circumstances.

IN THE FUTURE YOU CAN:

- Talk to your physician about contraception and get his or her advice on choosing the best method.
- Occasionally discuss your contraceptive method with your partner to make sure it continues to meet your needs. A change in health status or lifestyle may make a different form of contraception preferable in the future.
- If you are sexually active or plan to become sexually active, talk to your partner about abortion. Do you share similar views and feelings, or are they different? How would you resolve conflicts about this issue?

SUMMARY

- The choice of contraceptive method depends on effectiveness, convenience, cost, reversibility, side effects and risk factors, protection against STDs, and noncontraceptive benefits.

- Hormonal methods may include a combination of estrogen and progestins or progestins alone. Hormones may be delivered via pills, patch, vaginal ring, implants, or injections. Hormonal methods prevent ovulation, inhibit the movement of sperm, and affect the uterine lining so that implantation is prevented.

- IUDs can provide very effective long-term (5–10 years) contraception and are especially useful for women who have already been pregnant and are in monogamous relationships.

- Male condoms are simple to use, are immediately reversible, and provide STD protection; female condoms can be inserted hours before intercourse.

connect™

Connect to Your Choices

Have you ever thought about why you choose the contraceptive methods you use—or choose not to use? Many factors can influence the contraceptive choices we make, some not as obvious as others. Do you choose what's readily available in pharmacies because you don't want to go to a clinic, even if another method might be more appropriate or effective for you? Do you use a method your health care provider recommended, even though you don't like it? Do you go along with your partner's preferences because it's easier than saying what you would like?

What are the external factors that influence your choices about contraception? What are your inner motivations and core values, and how do they affect your choices? Based on what you learned in this chapter, will you make some different choices in the future? If so, what will they be?

Go online to Connect to complete this activity: www.mcgraw-hillconnect.com

- The diaphragm, cervical cap, and contraceptive sponge cover the cervix and block sperm from entering; all are used with or contain spermicide.

- Vaginal spermicides come in the form of foams, creams, jellies, suppositories, and film.

- So-called natural methods include abstinence, withdrawal, and fertility awareness–based methods.

- Combining methods can increase contraceptive effectiveness and help protect against STDs. The most common combination is a hormonal method, such as the birth control pill, combined with condoms.

- The most commonly used emergency contraceptives are Plan B One-Step and Next Choice, which are available without a prescription to men and women 17 and older.

- Vasectomy—male sterilization—involves severing the vasa deferentia. Female sterilization involves severing or blocking the oviducts so that the egg cannot reach the uterus.

- Issues to be considered in choosing a contraceptive include the individual health risks of each method, the implications of an unplanned pregnancy, STD risk, convenience and comfort level, type of relationship, the cost and ease of obtaining and maintaining each method, and religious or philosophical beliefs.

- The 1973 *Roe v. Wade* Supreme Court case devised new standards to govern abortion decisions; based on the trimesters of pregnancy, it limited a woman's choices as her pregnancy advanced.

- Although the Supreme Court continued to uphold its 1973 decision, later rulings gave states further power to regulate abortion.

- The controversy between pro-life and pro-choice viewpoints focuses on the issue of when life begins. Overall public opinion in the

United States supports legal abortion in at least some circumstances and opposes overturning *Roe v. Wade.*

- Methods of surgical abortion include suction curettage, manual vacuum aspiration, dilation and evacuation, and intact dilation and extraction.

- Medical abortion is performed with a combination of drugs very early in pregnancy.

- Physical complications following abortion can be minimized by overall good patient health, early timing, use of the suction method, a well-trained physician, and follow-up care. Psychological aftereffects of abortion vary with the individual.

FOR MORE INFORMATION

BOOKS

Adamec, C. A., and L. C. Miller. 2006. *The Encyclopedia of Adoption* (Facts on File Library of Health and Living), 3rd ed. New York: Facts on File, Inc. *Covers a wide range of adoption-related issues, such as gay/lesbian adoptions, the rights of birth fathers, transracial adoptions, and international adoptions.*

Boston Women's Health Book Collective. 2011. *Our Bodies, Ourselves.* New York: Simon & Schuster. *Broad coverage of many women's health concerns, with extensive coverage of contraception.*

Davenport, D. 2006. *The Complete Book of International Adoption.* New York: Broadway Books. *A detailed look at the process of adopting children from different countries.*

Glasier, A., and B. Winikoff. 2009. *Fast Facts: Contraception,* 3rd ed. Oxford: Health Press. *Basic facts and figures related to contraceptive methods. Succinct and easy to read.*

Hatcher, R. A., et al. 2011. *Contraceptive Technology,* 20th ed. New York: Bridging the Gap Foundation. *A reliable source of up-to-date information on contraception.*

National Abortion and Reproductive Rights Action League Foundation. 2012. *Who Decides? The Status of Women's Reproductive Rights in the United States,* 21st ed. Washington, DC: NARAL Foundation. *An in-depth annual review of the legal status of reproductive rights in the United States..*

ORGANIZATIONS AND WEBSITES

Association of Reproductive Health Professionals. Offers educational materials about family planning, contraception, and other reproductive health issues; the website includes an interactive questionnaire to help people choose contraceptive methods.

http://www.arhp.org

Emergency Contraception website. Provides extensive information about emergency contraception; sponsored by the Office of Population Research at Princeton University.

http://ec.princeton.edu

Guttmacher Institute. A nonprofit institute for reproductive health research, policy analysis, and public education.

http://www.guttmacher.org

Managing Contraception. Provides brief descriptions and tips for using many forms of contraception. Features a detailed survey to help with contraceptive choices.

http://www.managingcontraception.com

MedlinePlus: Abortion. Managed by the National Library of Medicine and the National Institutes of Health, this site provides a list of informational resources about various aspects of abortion.

http://www.nlm.nih.gov/medlineplus/abortion.html

National Abortion and Reproductive Rights Action League. Provides information about the politics of the pro-choice movement. Also provides information about the abortion laws and politics in each state.

http://www.prochoiceamerica.org

National Abortion Federation. Provides information and resources on the medical and political issues relating to abortion; managed by health care providers.

http://www.prochoice.org

National Adoption Center. A national agency focused on finding adoptive homes for children with special needs or who are currently in foster care.

http://www.adopt.org

National Right to Life Committee. Provides information about alternatives to abortion and the politics of the pro-life movement.

http://www.nrlc.org

Planned Parenthood Federation of America. Provides information about family planning, contraception, and abortion and provides counseling services.

http://www.plannedparenthood.org

See also the listings for Chapters 5, 6, and 8.

SELECTED BIBLIOGRAPHY

American College of Obstetricians and Gynecologists. 2008. Depot medroxyprogesterone acetate and bone effects. *Obstetrics and Gynecology* 112(3): 727.

American College of Obstetricians and Gynecologists. 2010. Noncontraceptive uses of hormonal contraceptives. *Obstetrics and Gynecology* 115(1): 206–218.

American College of Obstetricians and Gynecologists. 2011. *Contraceptives* (http://www.acog.org/~/media/For%20Patients/faq021.pdf?dmc=1&ts=20120301T1336161249).

Bitzer, J., and J. A. Simon. 2011. Current issues and available options in hormonal contraception. *Contraception* 84(4): 342–356.

Boonstra, H., et al. 2006. *Abortion in Women's Lives.* New York: Guttmacher Institute.

Broen, A. N., et al. 2006. Predictors of anxiety and depression following pregnancy termination: a longitudinal five-year follow-up study. *Acta Obstetricia et Gynecologica Scandinavica* 85(3): 317–323.

Burke, A. E. 2011. The state of hormonal contraception today: Benefits and risks of hormonal contraceptives: Progestin-only contraceptives. *American Journal of Obstetrics and Gynecology* 205(4): S14–S17.

Centers for Disease Control and Prevention. 2012. Abortion surveillance—United States, 2008. *Morbidity and Mortality Weekly Report* 60 (SS15): 1–41.

Charles, V. E., et al. 2008. Abortion and long-term mental health outcomes: a systematic review of the evidence. *Contraception* 78(6): 436–450.

Cohen, A. L., et al. 2007. Toxic shock associated with *Clostridium sordellii* and *Clostridium perfringens* after medical and spontaneous abortion. *Obstetrics and Gynecology* 110(5): 1027–1033.

Cremer, M., and R. Masch. 2010. Emergency contraception: Past, present and future. *Minerva Ginecol* 62(4): 361–371.

Dehlendorf, C., et al. 2011. Race, ethnicity and differences in contraception among low-income women. *Perspectives on Sexual and Reproductive Health* 43(3): 181–187.

Diedrich, J., et al. 2010. Induction of fetal demise before abortion. *Contraception* 81(6): 462–473.

Ely, G. E., and C. N. Dulmus. 2010. Disparities in access to reproductive health options for female adolescents. *Social Work in Public Health* 25(3): 341–351.

Fiala, C., and K. Gemzel-Danielsson. 2006. Review of medical abortion using mifepristone in combination with a prostaglandin analogue. *Contraception* 74(1): 66–86.

Finer, L. B., and M. R. Zolna. 2011. Unintended pregnancy in the United States: incidence and disparities, 2006. *Contraception* 84(5): 478–485.

Guttmacher Institute. 2012. *State Policies in Brief: An Overview of Abortion Laws* (http://www.guttmacher.org/statecenter/spibs/spib_OAL.pdf).

Guttmacher Institute. 2012 Update. *U.S. Teenage Pregnancies, Births and Abortions: National and State Trends and Trends by Race and Ethnicity* (www.guttmacher.org/pubs/USTPtrends.pdf).

Jones, R. K., L. B. Finer, and S. Singh. 2010. *Characteristics of U.S. Abortion Patients, 2008*. New York: Guttmacher Institute.

Jones, R. K., and M. L. Kavanaugh. 2011. Changes in abortion rates between 2000 and 2008 and lifetime incidence of abortion. *Obstetrics and Gynecology* 117(6): 1358–1366.

Kero, A., and A. Lalos. 2004. Reactions and reflection in men, 4 and 12 months post-abortion. *Journal of Psychosomatic Obstetrics and Gynecology* 25: 135–143.

Kossler, K., et al. 2011. Perceived racial, socioeconomic and gender discrimination and its impact on contraceptive choice. *Contraception* 84(3): 273–279.

Kulier, R., et al. 2011. Medical methods for first trimester abortion. *Cochrane Database Systematic Review* 11:CD002885.

Lyus, R., et al. 2011. Use of the Mirena LNG-IUS and Paragard CuT380A intrauterine devices in nulliparous women. *Contraception* 81(5): 367–371.

Macaluso, M., et al. 2007. Efficacy of the male latex condom and of the female polyurethane condom as barriers to semen during intercourse: A randomized clinical trial. *American Journal of Epidemiology* 166(1): 88–96.

Mansour, D., et al. 2011. Fertility after discontinuation of contraception: A comprehensive review of the literature. *Contraception* 84(5): 465–477.

Michielsen, D., and R. Beerthuizen. 2010. State-of-the-art of non-hormonal methods of contraception: IV. Male sterilization. *European Journal of Contraception and Reproductive Health Care* 15(2): 136–149.

Mohamad, A. M., et al. 2011. Combined contraceptive ring versus combined oral contraceptive. *International Journal of Gynaecology and Obstetrics* 114(2): 145–148.

Raymond, E. G., and D. A. Grimes. 2012. The comparative safety of legal induced abortion and childbirth in the United States. *Obstetrics and Gynecology* 119(2.1): 215–219.

Richardson, A. R., and F. N. Maltz. 2011. Ulipristal acetate: review of the efficacy and safety of a newly approved agent for emergency contraception. *Clinical Therapy*, Dec. 7.

Sedgh, G., et al. 2012. Induced abortion: Incidence and trends worldwide from 1995 to 2008. *Lancet*, in press.Tips for todayand the future

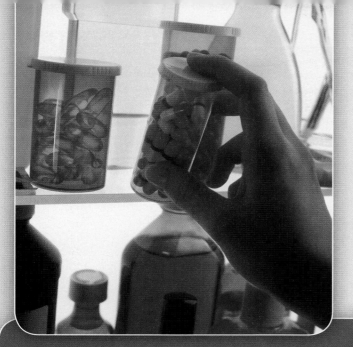

LOOKING AHEAD...

After reading this chapter, you should be able to

- Define and discuss the concepts of addictive behavior, substance abuse, and substance dependence
- Explain factors contributing to drug abuse and addiction
- List the major categories of psychoactive drugs and describe their effects, methods of use, and potential for abuse and addiction
- Discuss social issues related to drug abuse and its prevention and treatment
- Evaluate the role of drugs and other addictive behaviors in your life and identify your risk factors for abuse or addiction

7

Drug Abuse and Addiction

The use of **drugs** for both medical and social purposes is widespread in America (Table 7.1). Many Americans believe that every problem has or should have a chemical solution. For fatigue, many turn to caffeine; for insomnia, sleeping pills; for anxiety or boredom, prescription medication or alcohol or other recreational drugs. Advertisements, social pressures, and the human desire for quick solutions to difficult problems all contribute to the prevailing attitude that drugs can ease all pain. But benefits often come with the risk of harmful consequences, and drug use can—and in many cases does—pose serious or even life-threatening risks.

The most serious risks are abuse and addiction. The drugs most often associated with abuse are **psychoactive drugs**—those that alter a person's experiences or consciousness. In the short term, psychoactive drugs can cause **intoxication,** a state in which sometimes unpredictable physical and emotional changes occur. A person who is intoxicated may experience potentially serious changes in physical functioning. His or her emotions and judgment may be affected in ways that lead to uncharacteristic and unsafe behavior. In the long term, recurrent drug use can have profound physical, emotional, and social effects.

ADDICTIVE BEHAVIOR

Although addiction is most often associated with drug use, many experts now extend the concept of addiction to other behaviors. **Addictive behaviors** are habits that have gotten out of control, with resulting negative effects on a person's health. The American Society of Addiction Medicine defines **addiction** as a chronic disease that disrupts brain systems that regulate motivation and reward. The most characteristic feature of addiction is behavioral—a nearly uncontrollable pursuit of physical or psychological reward and/or relief through substance use or behaviors such as gambling. Addiction involves craving and the inability to recognize both significant risk and other problems with behaviors, interpersonal relationships, and emotional response. Like other chronic diseases, addiction often involves cycles of relapse and remission. Without treatment, addiction is progressive and can result in disabling or deadly health consequences.

What Is Addiction?

Historically the term *addiction* was applied only when the habitual use of a drug produced chemical changes in the user's body. Though experts now agree that addiction is

Table 7.1	Nonmedical Drug Use among Americans, 2010

	PERCENTAGE USING SUBSTANCE IN THE PAST 30 DAYS			
	ADULTS AGED 26 OR OLDER	YOUNG ADULTS AGED 18–25	YOUTHS AGED 12–17	ALL AMERICANS AGED 12 AND OLDER
ILLICIT DRUGS	6.6	21.5	10.1	8.9
Marijuana and hashish	4.8	18.5	7.4	6.9
Cocaine	0.5	1.5	0.2	0.6
Crack	0.2	0.2		0.1
Heroin	0.1	0.2		0.2
Methamphetamine	0.1	0.2		0.1
Hallucinogens	0.2	2.0	0.9	0.5
LSD	0.3	0.3		0.1
PCP	0.0	0.0		0.0
Ecstasy	1.3	0.6	0.5	0.3
Inhalants	0.1	0.2	1.1	0.7
Nonmedical use of psychotherapeutics	2.2	5.9	3.0	2.7
Pain relievers	4.8	4.4		2.0
Oxycontin	0.4	0.4		0.2
Tranquilizers	1.7	1.7		0.9
Stimulants	1.0	1.1		0.4
Sedatives	0.1	0.3		0.1
TOBACCO (ALL FORMS)	27.2	40.8	10.7	27.4
Cigarettes	33.5	34.2	8.3	23.0
Smokeless tobacco	5.8	6.4	2.3	3.5
Cigars	13.4	11.2		5.2
Pipe tobacco	1.9	1.8		0.8
ALCOHOL	48.7	69.5	13.6	51.8%
Binge alcohol use	33.7	40.6	7.8	23.3
Heavy alcohol use		13.6	1.7	

SOURCE: Substance Abuse and Mental Health Services Administration, *Results from the 2010 National Survey on Drug Use and Health: Summary of National Findings,* NSDUH Series H-41, HHS Publication No. (SMA) 11-4658. Rockville, MD: Substance Abuse and Mental Health Services Administration, 2011.

more fully defined by behavioral characteristics, they also agree that changes in the brain underlie addiction. One such change is **tolerance**, in which the body adapts to a drug so that the initial dose no longer produces the original emotional or psychological effects. This process means the user has to take larger and larger doses of a drug to achieve the same high. The concept of addiction as a disease process, one based in identifiable changes to brain cells and brain chemistry rather than a moral failing, has led to many advances in the understanding and treatment of drug addiction.

Some scientists think that other behaviors may share some of the chemistry of drug addiction. They suggest that activities like gambling, eating, exercising, and sex release brain chemicals that cause a pleasurable rush in much the same way that psychoactive drugs do. The brain's own chemicals thus become the "drug" that can cause addiction. These theorists suggest that all addictions—whether to drugs or to pleasurable activities—have a common mechanism in the brain. In this view, addiction is partly the result of our own natural wiring.

The view that addiction is based in our brain chemistry does *not* imply that people are not responsible for their

TERMS

drug   Any chemical other than food intended to affect the structure or function of the body.

psychoactive drug   A drug that can alter a person's consciousness or experience.

intoxication   The state of being mentally affected by a chemical (literally, a state of being poisoned).

addictive behavior   Compulsive behavior associated with craving and pursuit of physical or psychological reward that interferes with family, school, work, and recreational activities.

addiction   A chronic disease that disrupts the brain's system of motivation and reward, characterized by a compulsive desire and increasing need for a substance or behavior, and by harm to the individual and/or society.

tolerance   A physical state in which the body adapts to a drug so that the initial dose no longer produces the original physical or psychological effects.

addictive behavior. All addictions involve an initial voluntary step, and many people are able to overcome addictions.

Characteristics of Addiction

Experts have identified some general characteristics typically associated with addictive behaviors:

• *Reinforcement.* Addictive behaviors reinforce themselves. Reinforcement can be positive—the activity or situation reliably results in pleasure or reward. It can also be negative—avoiding the drug or activity results in stress, anxiety, discomfort, or depression.

• *Compulsion or craving.* The addict feels a strong compulsion—a nearly irresistible "hunger"—to engage in the behavior. Craving often is associated with environmental cues and accompanied by obsessive planning for the next opportunity to perform it.

• *Loss of control.* The addict loses control over the behavior and cannot block the impulse to do it.

• *Escalation.* Addiction often involves a pattern of escalation in response to tolerance. More and more of the substance or activity is required to produce its desired effects.

• *Negative consequences.* The behavior continues despite serious negative consequences, such as problems with academic or job performance, personal relationships, and health; legal or financial troubles are also typical.

The Development of Addiction

An addiction often starts when a person does something to bring pleasure or avoid pain. The activity may be drinking a beer, using the Internet, playing the lottery, or shopping. If it works, the person is likely to repeat it. Reinforcement leads to an increasing dependence on the behavior. Tolerance develops, and the person needs more of the substance or behavior to feel the expected effect. Eventually the behavior becomes a central focus of the person's life, and other areas such as school performance or relationships deteriorate. The behavior no longer brings pleasure, but repeating it is necessary to avoid **withdrawal**, the physical and mental pain that results from going without it. Something that started as a seemingly innocent way of feeling good has triggered physiological changes in the brain that create a behavioral prison.

Although many common behaviors are potentially addictive, most people who engage in them do not develop

problems. The reason lies in the combination of factors that are involved in the development of addiction, including personality, lifestyle, heredity, the social and physical environment, and the nature of the substance or behavior in question.

Characteristics of People with Addictions

The causes and course of an addiction are extremely varied, but people with addictions (commonly referred to as *addicts*) seem to share some characteristics. Many use a substance or activity as a substitute for healthier coping strategies. People vary in their ability to manage their lives, and those who have trouble dealing with stress and painful emotions may be susceptible to addiction.

Some people may have a genetic predisposition to addiction to a particular substance based on a variation in brain chemistry. People with addictive disorders usually have a distinct preference for a particular addictive behavior. They also often have problems with impulse control and self-regulation and tend to be risk takers.

Examples of Addictive Behaviors

Behaviors that are not related to drugs can become addictive for some people such as eating, shopping onlne, and playing video games. Any substance or activity that becomes the focus of a person's life at the expense of other needs and interests can be damaging to health.

Compulsive Gambling Compulsive gamblers cannot control the urge to gamble, even in the face of ruin. The consequences of compulsive gambling are not just financial; the suicide rate of compulsive gamblers is 20 times higher than that of the general population. About 1% of adult Americans are compulsive (pathological) gamblers, and another 2% are "problem gamblers." Some 42% of college students gamble at least once in a year, and about 3% gamble at least once a week.

The American Psychiatric Association (APA) recognizes pathological gambling as a mental disorder associated with 10 characteristic behaviors, including preoccupation with gambling, unsuccessful efforts to quit, and lying to family members to conceal the extent of gambling. Many compulsive gamblers also have drug and alcohol abuse problems.

Compulsive Exercising Compulsive exercising is now recognized as a serious departure from normal behavior. Compulsive exercising is often accompanied by more severe psychiatric disorders such as anorexia nervosa and bulimia. Traits often associated with compulsive exercising include an

withdrawal Physical and psychological symptoms that follow the interrupted use of a drug or behavior on which a user has become dependent.

TERMS

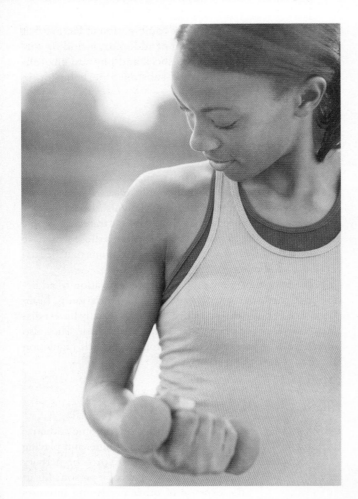

When taken to an extreme, even healthy activities such as exercise can become addictive.

excessive preoccupation and dissatisfaction with body image, use of laxatives or vomiting to lose weight, and development of other obsessive-compulsive symptoms.

Work Addiction   People who are excessively preoccupied with work are often called *workaholics*. Work addiction, however, is actually based on a set of specific symptoms, including an intense work schedule; the inability to limit one's own work schedule; the inability to relax, even when away from work; and failed attempts at curtailing the intensity of work (in some cases).

Work addiction typically coincides with a well-known risk factor for cardiovascular disease—the Type A personality. Traits associated with Type A personality include competitiveness, ambition, drive, time urgency, restlessness, hyperalertness, and hostility.

Sex and Love Addiction   Behaviors associated with sex addiction include an extreme preoccupation with sex, a compulsion to have sex repeatedly in a given period of time, spending a great deal of time and energy looking for partners or having sex, using sex as a means of relieving painful feelings, and suffering negative emotional, personal, and professional consequences as a result of sexual activities.

Even therapists who challenge the concept of sex addiction recognize that some people become overly preoccupied with sex, cannot seem to control their sex drive, and act in potentially harmful ways.

Compulsive Buying or Shopping   A compulsive buyer repeatedly gives in to the impulse to buy more than he or she needs or can afford. Compulsive spenders usually buy luxury items rather than daily necessities, even though they are usually distressed by their behavior and its social, personal, and financial consequences. Some experts link compulsive shopping with neglect or abuse during childhood; it also seems to be associated with eating disorders, depression, and bipolar disorder.

Internet Addiction   Millions of Americans have become compulsive Internet users—as much as 10% of the U.S. population by some estimates. To spend more time online, Internet addicts skip other important activities, including tasks at work and interpersonal relationships. Despite negative financial, social, or academic consequences, compulsive Internet users don't feel able to stop. As with other addictive behaviors, online addicts may be using their behavior to alleviate stress or avoid painful emotions.

DRUG USE, ABUSE, AND ADDICTION

Using drugs to alter consciousness is an ancient and universal pursuit. People have used alcohol for celebration and intoxication for thousands of years. People in all parts of the world have exploited the psychoactive properties of plants, such as the coca plant in South America and the opium poppy in the Far East. But many drugs have addictive properties and change the chemistry of the brain; their use can open the door to the problems of abuse and dependence.

Diagnosing Drug Abuse and Addiction

The American Psychiatric Association's (APA) *Diagnostic and Statistical Manual of Mental Disorders* is the authoritative reference for defining all sorts of behavioral disorders, including those related to drugs. The APA has chosen not to use the term *addiction*. Instead the APA's diagnostic manual refers to two forms of substance (drug) disorders: substance abuse

Ask Yourself

QUESTIONS FOR CRITICAL THINKING AND REFLECTION

Have you ever repeatedly or compulsively engaged in a behavior that had negative consequences? What was the behavior, and why did you continue? Did you ever worry that you were losing control? Were you able to bring the behavior under control?

and substance dependence. The APA uses the term **physical dependence** to describe tolerance and withdrawal.

Abuse The APA diagnostic criteria for abuse require that drug use involve at least one of the following four characteristics:

- Continued use despite social or interpersonal problems
- Repeated use resulting in failure to fulfill obligations at work, school, or home
- Repeated use resulting in physically hazardous situations
- Use resulting in legal problems

Dependence The APA definition of **substance dependence** incorporates what many people associate with the idea of addiction. To be considered addicted—or in the APA's language, dependent—one must experience a cluster of three or more of these symptoms during a 12-month period:

- Developing tolerance to the substance
- Experiencing withdrawal
- Taking the substance in larger amounts or over a longer period than was originally intended
- Expressing a persistent desire to cut down or regulate substance use
- Spending a great deal of time getting the substance, using it, or recovering from its effects
- Giving up or reducing important social, school, work, or recreational activities because of substance use
- Continuing to use the substance despite the knowledge that it is contributing to a psychological or physical problem

Who Abuses Drugs?

Drug abuse and addiction occur at all income and education levels, among all ethnic groups, and across all age groups (see the box "Drug Use among College Students"). Society is concerned with the casual or recreational use of illegal drugs because it is not possible to know when it will lead to addiction. Some casual users develop substance-related problems; others do not. Some drugs are more likely than others to lead to addiction, with nicotine, methamphetamine, crack cocaine, barbiturates, and heroin and the other opioids considered among the most addictive. However, even some heroin or cocaine users do not meet the APA's criteria for substance dependence.

It isn't possible to accurately predict who will abuse drugs or become addicted, but young people at a high risk of *trying* drugs—the first step toward abuse—share certain characteristics:

- *Being male.* Males are twice as likely as females to abuse drugs, a gender difference that holds over the entire lifespan (Table 7.2).
- *Being a troubled adolescent.* Teens are more likely to try drugs if they have poor self-image or self-control, use tobacco, or suffer from certain mental or emotional problems.
- *Being a thrill-seeker.* A sense of invincibility is a factor in drug experimentation.
- *Being in a dysfunctional family.* A chaotic home life or parental abuse increases the risk of drug use. The same is true for children from a single-parent home or whose parents didn't complete high school.
- *Being in a peer group that accepts drug use.* Young people who are uninterested in school and earn poor grades are more likely to try drugs.
- *Being poor.* Young people who live in disadvantaged areas are more likely to be around drugs at a young age.

QUICK STATS

In 2010 an estimated **22.6** million Americans aged 12 or older were current illicit drug users.
—National Survey on Drug Use and health, 2011

TERMS

physical dependence The result of physiological adaptation that occurs in response to the frequent presence of a drug; typically associated with tolerance and withdrawal.

substance dependence A cluster of cognitive, behavioral, and physiological symptoms that occur in someone who continues to use a substance despite suffering significant substance-related problems, leading to significant impairment or distress; also known as *addiction*.

Table 7.2	Gender and Drug Use	
	NATIONAL SURVEY RESULTS: PERCENTAGE REPORTING IN PAST YEAR	
	MALES	FEMALES
Illicit drug use*	16.4	12.2
Age 12–17	10.4	9.8
Age 18–25	36.9	29.9
Age 26 and older	12.3	8.5
Drove under the influence of an illicit drug	5.5	2.6
Illicit drug or alcohol abuse or dependence	11.5	6.4
Treatment for drug or alcohol dependence	2.2	1.0

*Illicit drugs include marijuana/hashish, cocaine, heroin, hallucinogens, inhalants, and prescription-type psychotherapeutics used nonmedically.

SOURCE: Substance Abuse and Mental Health Services Administration. 2011. *Results from the 2010 National Survey on Drug Use and Health: National Findings.* Rockville, MD: Office of Applied Studies, NSDUH Series H-36, HHS Publication No. SMA 11-4434.

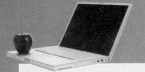
According to the most recent survey data from the Substance Abuse and Mental Health Services Administration (SAMHSA), 21.5% of young adults aged 18–25 reported using an illicit drug in the past 30 days (see Table 7.1). This number represents a slight increase from 2008, driven largely by an increase in marijuana use. Other surveys show that recreational drug use is fairly common among college students. According to the 2011 American College Health Association National College Health Assessment, 15.9% of college students reported using marijuana at least once in the past 30 days. Another 12.9% said they had used some other drug at least once in the past 30 days.

Family history, peer pressure, depression, anxiety, low self-esteem, and the dynamics of college life (for example, the drive to compete and a distorted perception of drug use among peers) have been suggested as potential explanations for college-age drug use.

Excessive alcohol use often accompanies illicit drug use, and the risk of combining drugs and alcohol increases with the number of drinks a young adult consumes during a single session. In 2010, among the 16.9 million heavy drinkers aged 12 or older, 31.8% were current illicit drug users as well. The combined use of alcohol and other drugs (AOD) is associated with anxiety and depression, although its is not clear whether these psychiatric conditions precede AOD use or precollege exposure to AOD use exacerbates these conditions by the time a student enters college. It may be that AOD use, depression, and anxiety share common causes such as genetic predisposition and/or family history.

However, one aspect of drug use among college students remains clear: AOD use has dramatic consequences for the educational, family, and community lives of students. Poor academic performance has been linked with AOD use. Further, driving while intoxicated remains one of the most dangerous outcomes associated with AOD use affecting families and communities.

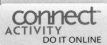

connect
ACTIVITY
DO IT ONLINE

- *Dating young.* Adolescent girls who date boys two or more years older than themselves are more likely to use drugs.

What about people who *don't* use drugs? As a group, nonusers also share some characteristics. Not surprisingly, people who perceive drug use as risky and who disapprove of it are less likely to use drugs than those who believe otherwise. Drug use is also less common among people who have positive self-esteem and self-concept and who are assertive, independent thinkers who are not controlled by peer pressure. Self-control, social competence, optimism, academic achievement, and regular church attendance are also linked to lower rates of drug use.

Home environments are also influential. Young people who communicate openly with and feel supported by their parents are less likely to use drugs.

Why Do People Use Drugs?

Young people may be drawn to drugs by the allure of the exciting and illegal. They may be curious, rebellious, or vulnerable to peer pressure. Young people may want to imitate adult models in their lives or in the movies. Most people who take illicit drugs do so experimentally, typically trying a drug one or more times but not continuing. The main factors in the initial choice of a drug are whether it is available and whether peers are using it.

Although some people use drugs because they have a desire to alter their mood or are seeking a spiritual experience, others are motivated by a desire to escape boredom, anxiety, depression, feelings of worthlessness, or other distressing symptoms of psychological problems. They use drugs as a way to cope with the difficulties they experience in life. For people living in poverty in the inner cities, many of these reasons for using drugs are magnified. The problems are more devastating, the need for escape more compelling. Further, the buying and selling of drugs provide access to an unofficial alternative economy that may seem like an opportunity for success.

Risk Factors for Abuse and Addiction

Research indicates that some people may be born with a brain chemistry or metabolism that makes them more vulnerable to addiction.

Psychological risk factors for drug abuse include difficulty in controlling impulses and a strong need for excitement, stimulation, and immediate gratification. Feelings of rejection, hostility, aggression, anxiety, or depression are also associated with drug abuse. People may turn to drugs to blot out their emotional pain. People with mental illnesses have a very high risk of substance dependence.

Other Risks of Drug Abuse

Addiction is not the only serious potential consequence of drug abuse. In 2009 over 2 million emergency department visits were related to drug misuse or abuse.

Intoxication People who are under the influence of drugs—intoxicated—may act in uncharacteristic and unsafe ways because both their physical and mental functioning are impaired. They are more likely to be injured from a variety of causes, to have unsafe sex, and to be involved in incidents of aggression and violence.

Unexpected Side Effects   Psychoactive drugs have many physical and psychological effects beyond the alteration of consciousness. These effects range from nausea and constipation to paranoia, depression, and heart failure. Some drugs also carry the risk of fatal overdose.

Unknown Drug Constituents   There is no quality control in the illegal drug market, so the composition, dosage, and toxicity of street drugs are highly variable. Studies indicate that half of all street drugs don't contain their promised primary ingredient. In some cases, a drug may be present in unsafe dosages or mixed with other drugs to boost its effects. Makers of street drugs aren't held to any safety standards, so illicit drugs can be contaminated or even poisonous.

Risks Associated with Injection Drug Use   Many injection drug users (IDUs) share or reuse needles, syringes, and other injection supplies, which can easily become contaminated with the user's blood. Small amounts of blood can carry enough human immunodeficiency virus (HIV) and hepatitis C virus (HCV) to be infectious. In 2008 injection drug use accounted for more than 10% of all new HIV/AIDS cases; many more were attributed to sexual contact with IDUs. Injection drug use also accounts for nearly half of new HCV infections.

The surest way to prevent diseases related to injection drug use is never to inject drugs. Syringe exchange programs (SEPs)—where IDUs can trade a used syringe for a new one—have been advocated to help slow the spread of HIV and reduce the rates and cost of other health problems associated with injection drug use. Getting people off drugs is clearly the best solution, but there are far more IDUs than treatment facilities can currently handle.

Legal Consequences   Many psychoactive drugs are illegal, so possessing them can result in large fines and imprisonment. According to the Federal Bureau of Investigation (FBI), the highest arrest counts for all types of crimes were for drug abuse violations (estimated at 1,663,582 out of 13,687,241 total arrests in 2009).

HOW DRUGS AFFECT THE BODY

The same drug may affect different people differently or the same person in different ways under different circumstances. Beyond a fairly predictable general change in brain chemistry, the effects of a drug may vary depending on drug factors, (characteristics of the drug), user factors, (physical and psychological characteristics of the user), and social factors.

Changes in Brain Chemistry

Once a psychoactive drug reaches the brain, it acts on one or more **neurotransmitters,** either increasing or decreasing their concentration and actions. Cocaine, for example, affects dopamine, a neurotransmitter thought to play a key role in the process of reinforcement—the brain's way of telling itself "That's good; do the same thing again." Heroin, nicotine, alcohol, and amphetamines also affect dopamine levels.

The duration of a drug's effect depends on many factors and may range from 5 minutes (crack cocaine) to 12 or more hours (LSD). As drugs circulate through the body, they are metabolized by the liver and eventually excreted by the kidneys in urine. Small amounts may also be eliminated in other ways, including in sweat, in breast milk, and via the lungs.

Drug Factors: Characteristics of the Drug

When different drugs or dosages produce different effects, the differences are usually caused by one or more of five different drug factors:

1. The **pharmacological properties** of a drug are its effects on a person's body chemistry, behavior, and psychology. Pharmacological properties also include the amount of a drug required to exert various effects, the time course of the effects, and other characteristics, such as a drug's chemical composition.

Psychoactive drugs work by **affecting one or more neurotransmitters in the brain.**

TERMS

neurotransmitter   A brain chemical that transmits nerve impulses.

pharmacological properties   The overall effects of a drug on a person's behavior, psychology, and chemistry.

Ask Yourself

QUESTIONS FOR CRITICAL THINKING AND REFLECTION

Have you ever tried a psychoactive drug for fun? What were your reasons for trying it? Whom were you with, and what were the circumstances? What was your experience like? What would you tell someone else who was thinking about trying a drug?

2. The **dose-response function** is the relationship between the amount of drug taken and the type and intensity of its effects. Many psychological effects of drugs reach a plateau in the dose-response function, so that increasing the dose does not increase the effect any further. With LSD, for example, the maximum changes in perception occur at a certain dose, and no further changes in perception take place if higher doses are taken. However, all drugs have more than one effect, and the dose-response functions usually are different for different effects. This means that increasing the dose of any drug may begin to result in additional effects, which are likely to be more unpleasant or dangerous at high doses.

3. The **time-action function** is the relationship between the time elapsed since a drug was taken and the intensity of its effect. A drug's effects are greatest when its concentrations in body tissues are changing fastest, especially if they are increasing.

4. The person's *drug use history* may influence the effects of a drug. A given amount of alcohol, for example, will generally affect a habitual drinker less than an occasional drinker. Tolerance to some drugs, such as LSD, builds rapidly. To experience the same effect, a user has to abstain from the drug for a period of time before that dosage will again exert its original effects.

5. The *method of use* (or *route of administration*) has a direct effect on how strong a response a drug produces. Methods of use include ingestion, inhalation, injection, and absorption through the skin or tissue linings. Drugs are usually injected in one of three ways: intravenously (IV, or mainlining), intramuscularly (IM), or subcutaneously (SC, or skin popping).

User Factors: Physical Characteristics

Certain physical characteristics help determine how a person will respond to a drug. Body mass is one variable: the effects of a certain dose of a drug on a 150-pound person will be greater than its effect on a 200-pound person. Other variables include general health and genetic factors. For example, some people have an inherited ability to rapidly metabolize a cough suppressant called dextromethorphan, which also has psychoactive properties. These people must take a higher-than-normal dose to get a given cough suppressant effect.

If a person's biochemical state is already altered by another drug, this too can make a difference. Some drugs intensify the effects of other drugs, as is the case with alcohol and sedatives. Some drugs block the effects of other drugs, such as when a tranquilizer is used to relieve anxiety caused by cocaine. Interactions between drugs, including many prescription and OTC medications, can be unpredictable and dangerous.

One physical condition that requires special precautions is pregnancy. It can be risky for a woman to use any drugs at all during pregnancy, including alcohol and common OTC products like cough medicine. The risks are greatest during the first trimester, when the fetus's body is rapidly forming and even small biochemical alterations in the mother can have a devastating effect on fetal development. Even later, the fetus is more susceptible than the mother to the adverse effects of any drugs she takes. The fetus may even become physically dependent on a drug being taken by the mother and suffer withdrawal symptoms after birth.

User Factors: Psychological Considerations

Sometimes a person's response to a drug is strongly influenced by the user's expectations about how he or she will react (the psychological *set*). With large doses, the drug's chemical properties seem to have the strongest effect on the user's response. But with small doses, psychological (and social) factors are often more important.

When people strongly believe that a given drug will affect them a certain way, they are likely to experience those effects regardless of the drug's pharmacological properties. In one study, regular users of marijuana reported a moderate level of intoxication (**high**) after using a cigarette that smelled and tasted like marijuana but contained no THC, the active ingredient in marijuana. This is an example of the **placebo effect**—when a person receives an inert substance yet responds as if it were an active drug. In other studies, subjects who smoked low doses of real marijuana that they believed to be a placebo experienced no effects from the drug. Clearly the user's expectations had a greater effect on the smokers than the drug itself.

Social Factors

The *setting* is the physical and social environment surrounding the drug use. If a person uses marijuana at home with trusted friends and pleasant music, the effects are likely to be different from the effects if the same dose is taken in an austere experimental laboratory with an impassive research technician. Similarly, a dose of alcohol that produces mild euphoria and stimulation at a noisy, active cocktail party might induce sleepiness and slight depression when taken at home while alone.

TERMS

dose-response function   The relationship between the amount of a drug taken and the intensity and type of the resulting effect.

time-action function   The relationship between the time elapsed since a drug was taken and the intensity of its effect.

high   The subjectively pleasing effects of a drug, usually felt quite soon after the drug is taken.

placebo effect   A response to an inert or innocuous substance given in place of an active drug.

Ask Yourself

QUESTIONS FOR CRITICAL THINKING AND REFLECTION

Has an over-the-counter medication (such as a decongestant) ever made you feel strange, drowsy, or even high? Did you expect to react to the medication that way? Do such reactions influence the way you use over-the-counter drugs?

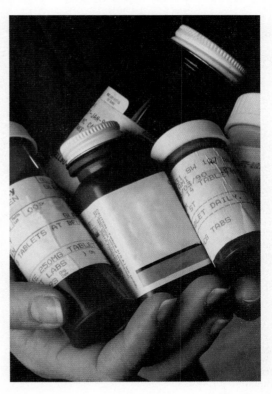

Prescription painkillers such as oxycodone and hydrocodone are opioids that can have serious consequences such as fatal respiratory depression.

REPRESENTATIVE PSYCHOACTIVE DRUGS

The following sections and Figure 7.1 introduce six representative groups of psychoactive drugs: opioids, central nervous system (CNS) depressants, central nervous system stimulants, marijuana and other cannabis products, hallucinogens, and inhalants. Some of these drugs are classified according to how they affect the body. Others—the opioids and the cannabis products—are classified according to their chemical makeup.

Opioids

Also called *narcotics*, **opioids** are natural or synthetic (laboratory-made) drugs that relieve pain, cause drowsiness, and induce **euphoria.** Opium, morphine, heroin, methadone, codeine, hydrocodone, oxycodone, meperidine, and fentanyl are opioids. When taken at prescribed doses, opioids have beneficial medical uses, including pain relief and cough suppression. Opioids tend to reduce anxiety and produce lethargy, apathy, and an inability to concentrate. Opioid users become less active and less responsive to frustration, hunger, and sexual stimulation. These effects are more pronounced in novice users; with repeated use, many effects diminish.

Opioids are typically injected. They can also be absorbed into the body through the stomach, intestines, nasal membranes (from snorting or sniffing), or lungs (from smoking). Effects depend on the method of administration. If brain levels of the drug change rapidly, more immediate effects result. Although the euphoria associated with opioids is an important factor in their abuse, many people experience a feeling of uneasiness when they first use these drugs. Users also often feel nauseated and vomit, and they may have other unpleasant sensations. Even so, the abuse of opioids often results in dependence. Tolerance can develop rapidly and be pronounced. Withdrawal symptoms include cramps, chills, sweating, nausea, tremors, irritability, and feelings of panic.

Rates of heroin use have always been low, and in 2010 they were around 0.2% of the population aged 12 and over. The potentially high but variable purity of street heroin poses a risk of unintentional overdose. Symptoms of overdose include respiratory depression, coma, and constriction of the pupils; death can result.

Nonmedical use of prescription pain relievers that contain oxycodone and hydrocodone, including Oxycontin and Vicodin, hovered at around 2% of the population aged 12 and over from 2002 to 2010. When taken as prescribed in tablet form, these drugs treat moderate to severe chronic pain and do not typically lead to abuse. However, as is the case with other opioids, use of prescription painkillers can lead to abuse and addiction. Oxycodone and hydrocodone can be abused orally; the long-acting form of oxycodone is also sometimes crushed and snorted or dissolved and injected, providing a powerful heroin-like high. When taken in large doses or combined with other drugs, oxycodone and hydrocodone can cause fatal respiratory depression.

Central Nervous System Depressants

Central nervous system **depressants,** also known as **sedative-hypnotics,** slow down the overall activity of the **central nervous system (CNS).** The result can range from mild

---

TERMS

opioid   Any of several natural or synthetic drugs that relieve pain and cause drowsiness and/or euphoria; examples are opium, morphine, and heroin; also called a *narcotic*.

euphoria   An exaggerated feeling of well-being.

depressant, or sedative-hypnotic   A drug that decreases nervous or muscular activity, causing drowsiness or sleep.

central nervous system (CNS)   The brain and spinal cord.

Category	Representative drugs	Street names	Appearance	Methods of use	Short-term effects
Opioids	Heroin	Dope, H, junk, brown sugar, smack	White/dark brown powder; dark tar or coal-like substance	Injected, smoked, snorted	Relief of anxiety and pain; euphoria; lethargy, apathy, drowsiness, confusion, inability to concentrate; nausea, constipation, respiratory depression
	Opium	Big O, black stuff, hop	Dark brown or black chunks	Swallowed, smoked	
	Morphine	M, Miss Emma, monkey, white stuff	White crystals, liquid solution	Injected, swallowed, smoked	
	Oxycodone, codeine, hydrocodone	Oxy, O.C., killer, Captain Cody, schoolboy, vike	Tablets, powder made from crushing tablets	Swallowed, injected, snorted	
Central nervous system depressants	Barbiturates	Barbs, reds, red birds, yellows, yellow jackets	Colored capsules	Swallowed, injected	Reduced anxiety, mood changes, lowered inhibitions, impaired muscle coordination, reduced pulse rate, drowsiness, loss of consciousness, respiratory depression
	Benzodiazepines (e.g., Valium, Xanax, Rohypnol)	Candy, downers, tranks, roofies, forget-me pill	Tablets	Swallowed, injected	
	Methaqualone	Ludes, quad, quay	Tablets	Injected, swallowed	
	Gamma hydroxy butyrate (GHB)	G, Georgia home boy, grievous bodily harm	Clear liquid, white powder	Swallowed	
Central nervous system stimulants	Amphetamine, methamphet-amine	Bennies, speed, black beauties, uppers, chalk, crank, crystal, ice, meth	Tablets, capsules, white powder, white crystals	Injected, swallowed, smoked, snorted	Increased heart rate, blood pressure, metabolism; increased mental alertness and energy; nervousness, insomnia, impulsive behavior; reduced appetite
	Cocaine, crack cocaine	Blow, C, candy, coke, flake, rock, toot	White powder, beige pellets or rocks	Injected, smoked, snorted	
	Ritalin	JIF, MPH, R-ball, Skippy	Tablets	Injected, swallowed, snorted	
Marijuana and other cannabis products	Marijuana	Dope, grass, joints, Mary Jane, reefer, skunk, weed	Dried leaves and stems	Smoked, swallowed	Euphoria, slowed thinking and reaction time, confusion, anxiety, impaired balance and coordination, increased heart rate
	Hashish	Hash, hemp, boom, gangster	Dark, resin-like compound formed into rocks or blocks	Smoked, swallowed	
Hallucinogens	LSD	Acid, boomers, blotter, yellow sunshines	Blotter paper, liquid, gelatin tabs, pills	Swallowed, absorbed through mouth tissues	Altered states of perception and feeling; nausea; increased heart rate, blood pressure; delirium; impaired motor function; numbness, weakness
	Mescaline (peyote)	Buttons, cactus, mesc	Brown buttons, liquid	Swallowed, smoked	
	Psilocybin	Shrooms, magic mushrooms	Dried mushrooms	Swallowed	
	Ketamine	K, special K, cat valium, vitamin K	Clear liquid, white or beige powder	Injected, snorted, smoked	
	PCP	Angel dust, hog, love boat, peace pill	White to brown powder, tablets	Injected, swallowed, smoked, snorted	
	MDMA (ecstasy)	X, peace, clarity, Adam	Tablets	Swallowed	
Inhalants	Solvents, aerosols, nitrites, anesthetics	Laughing gas, poppers, snappers, whippets	Household products, sprays, glues, paint thinner, petroleum products	Inhaled through nose or mouth	Stimulation, loss of inhibition, slurred speech, loss of motor coordination, loss of consciousness

FIGURE 7.1 Commonly abused drugs and their effects.

SOURCES: The Partnership for a Drug-Free America. 2010. *Drug Guide by Name* (http://www.drugfree.org/portal/drug_guide); U.S. Drug Enforcement Agency. 2006. *Photo Library* (http://www.usdoj.gov/dea/photo_library.html); U.S. Drug Enforcement Agency. 2010. *Drug Information* (http://www.justice.gov/dea/concern/concern.htm); National Institute on Drug Abuse. 2010. *Commonly Abused Drugs* (http://www.drugabuse.gov/DrugPages/DrugsofAbuse.html).

sedation to death, depending on the factors involved. CNS depressants include alcohol, barbiturates, and other sedatives.

Types   The various types of barbiturates are similar in chemical composition and action, but they differ in how quickly and how long they act. Drug users call barbiturates "downers" or "downs" and refer to specific brands by names that describe the color and design of the capsules. People usually take barbiturates in capsules, but may also inject them.

Antianxiety agents, also called sedatives or **tranquilizers,** include the benzodiazepines such as Xanax, Valium, Librium, clonazepam (Klonopin), and flunitrazepam (Rohypnol, also called roofies). Other CNS depressants include methaqualone (Quaalude), ethchlorvynol (Placidyl), chloral hydrate, and gamma hydroxybutyrate (GHB).

Effects   CNS depressants reduce anxiety and cause mood changes, impaired muscular coordination, slurring of speech, and drowsiness or sleep. Mental functioning is also affected, but the degree varies from person to person and also depends on the kind of task the person is trying to do. Most people become drowsy with small doses, although a few become more active.

From Use to Abuse   People are usually introduced to CNS depressants either through a medical prescription or through drug-using peers. The use of Rohypnol and GHB is often associated with dance clubs and raves. The abuse of CNS depressants by a medical patient may begin with repeated use for insomnia and progress to dependence through increasingly larger doses at night, coupled with doses during stressful times during the day.

Most CNS depressants, including alcohol, can lead to addiction. Tolerance, sometimes for up to 15 times the usual dose, can develop with repeated use. Tranquilizers can produce physical dependence even at ordinary prescribed doses. Withdrawal symptoms can be more severe than those accompanying opioid addiction. They may begin as anxiety, shaking, and weakness but may turn into convulsions and possibly cardiovascular collapse and death.

While intoxicated, people on depressants cannot function well. They are confused and are frequently obstinate, irritable, and abusive. Long-term use of depressants like alcohol can lead to serious physical effects including brain damage, with impaired ability to reason and make judgments.

Overdosing with CNS Depressants   Too much depression of the central nervous system slows respiration and may stop it entirely. CNS depressants are particularly dangerous in combination with another depressant, such as alcohol.

Club Drugs   Some people refer to club drugs as soft drugs because they see them as recreational—for the casual week-end user—rather than as addictive. But club drugs have many potential negative effects and are particularly potent and unpredictable when mixed with alcohol. Substitute drugs are often sold in place of club drugs, putting users at risk for taking dangerous combinations of unknown drugs.

Rohypnol (flunitrazepam) is a sedative that is 10 times more potent than Valium. Its effects, which are magnified by alcohol, include reduced blood pressure, dizziness, confusion, gastrointestinal disturbances, and loss of consciousness. Users of Rohypnol may develop physical and psychological dependence on the drug. Rohypnol and some other club drugs are used as "date rape drugs." Because they can be added to beverages surreptitiously, these drugs may be unknowingly consumed by intended rape victims. In addition to depressant effects, some drugs also cause *anterograde amnesia*—the loss of memory of things occurring while under the influence of the drug. Rohypnol can be fatal if combined with alcohol.

GHB (gamma hydroxybutyrate) can be produced in clear liquid, white powder, tablet, and capsule form. GHB is a central nervous system depressant that in large doses or when taken in combination with alcohol or other depressants can cause sedation, loss of consciousness, respiratory arrest, and death. GHB may cause prolonged and potentially life-threatening withdrawal symptoms. GHB is often produced clandestinely, resulting in widely varying degrees of purity; it has been responsible for many poisonings and deaths.

Central Nervous System Stimulants

Central nervous system **stimulants** speed up the activity of the nervous or muscular system. Under their influence, the heart rate accelerates, blood pressure rises, blood vessels constrict, the pupils and bronchial tubes dilate, and gastric and adrenal secretions increase. There is greater muscular tension and sometimes an increase in motor activity. Small doses usually make people feel more awake and alert, less fatigued and bored. The most common CNS stimulants are cocaine, amphetamines, nicotine, ephedrine, and caffeine.

Cocaine   Usually derived from the leaves of coca shrubs that grow high in the Andes in South America, cocaine is a potent CNS stimulant. It is usually snorted and absorbed through the nasal mucosa or injected intravenously, providing rapid increases of the drug's concentration in the blood

TERMS

sedation   The induction of a calm, relaxed, often sleepy state.

tranquilizer   A CNS depressant that reduces tension and anxiety.

stimulant   A drug that increases nervous or muscular activity.

and therefore fast, intense effects. Another method of use involves processing cocaine with baking soda and water, yielding the ready-to-smoke form of cocaine known as crack. Crack is typically available as small beads or pellets smokable in glass pipes.

EFFECTS The effects of cocaine are usually intense but short-lived. The euphoria lasts from 5 to 20 minutes and ends abruptly, to be replaced by irritability, anxiety, or slight depression. When cocaine is absorbed via the lungs by either smoking or inhalation, it reaches the brain in about 10 seconds, and the effects are particularly intense. This is part of the appeal of smoking crack. The effects from IV injections occur almost as quickly—in about 20 seconds. Since the mucous membranes in the nose briefly slow absorption, the onset of effects from snorting takes 2–3 minutes. Heavy users may inject cocaine intravenously every 10–20 minutes to maintain the effects.

The larger the cocaine dose and the more rapidly it is absorbed into the bloodstream, the greater the immediate—and sometimes lethal—effects. Sudden death from cocaine is most commonly the result of excessive CNS stimulation that causes convulsions and respiratory collapse, irregular heartbeat, extremely high blood pressure, blood clots, and possibly heart attack or stroke. Although rare, fatalities can occur in healthy young people; among people aged 18–59, cocaine users are seven times more likely than nonusers to have a heart attack. Chronic cocaine use produces inflammation of the nasal mucosa, which can lead to persistent bleeding and ulceration of the septum between the nostrils. The use of cocaine may also cause paranoia and aggressiveness. When steady cocaine users stop taking the drug, they experience a sudden "crash" characterized by depression, agitation, and fatigue, followed by a period of withdrawal.

COCAINE USE DURING PREGNANCY A woman who uses cocaine during pregnancy is at higher risk for miscarriage, premature labor, and stillbirth. She is more likely to deliver a low-birth-weight baby who has a small head circumference. Her infant may be at increased risk for defects of the genitourinary tract, cardiovascular system, central nervous system, and extremities. It is difficult to pinpoint the effects of cocaine because many women who use cocaine also use tobacco and/or alcohol.

Infants whose mothers use cocaine may also be born intoxicated. Cocaine also passes into breast milk and can intoxicate a breastfeeding infant.

Amphetamines
Amphetamines (uppers) are a group of synthetic chemicals that are potent CNS stimulants. Some common drugs in this family are amphetamine (Benzedrine), dextroamphetamine (Dexedrine), and methamphetamine (Methedrine). Crystal methamphetamine (also called ice) is a smokable, high-potency form of methamphetamine, or meth.

EFFECTS Small doses of amphetamines usually make people feel more alert. Amphetamines generally increase motor activity

but do not measurably alter a normal, rested person's ability to perform tasks calling for challenging motor skills or complex thinking. When amphetamines improve performance, it is primarily by counteracting fatigue and boredom. In small doses, amphetamines increase heart rate and blood pressure and change sleep patterns.

Amphetamines are sometimes used to curb appetite, but after a few weeks the user develops tolerance and higher doses are necessary. When people stop taking the drug, their appetite usually returns, and they gain back the weight they lost.

ABUSE AND ADDICTION Much amphetamine abuse begins as an attempt to cope with a temporary situation. A student cramming for an exam or an exhausted long-haul truck driver can go a little longer by taking amphetamines. The likelihood of making bad judgments significantly increases. The stimulating effects may also wear off suddenly, and the user may precipitously feel exhausted or fall asleep ("crash").

Another problem is **state dependence,** the phenomenon whereby information learned in a certain drug-induced state is difficult to recall when the person is not in that same physiological state. Performance may deteriorate when students use drugs to study and then take tests in their normal, non-drug state.

Repeated use of amphetamines, even in moderate doses, often leads to tolerance and the need for increasingly larger doses. The result can be severe disturbances in behavior, including delusions of persecution and episodes of unprovoked violence.

Methamphetamine is more addictive than other forms of amphetamine. It also is more dangerous because it is more toxic and its effects last longer. In the short term, meth can cause rapid breathing, increased body temperature, insomnia, tremors, anxiety, and convulsions. Meth use has been linked to high-risk sexual behavior and increased rates of STDs, including HIV infection. In the long term, the effects of meth can include weight loss, severe acne, hallucinations, paranoia, violence, and psychosis. Meth use causes extensive tooth decay and tooth loss, a condition referred to as "meth mouth." Meth takes a toll on the user's heart and can cause heart attack and stroke. Methamphetamine users have signs of brain damage similar to those seen in Parkinson's disease patients that appear to persist even after drug use ceases, causing impaired memory and motor coordination. Withdrawal from meth causes symptoms that may include muscle aches and tremors, profound fatigue, deep depression, despair, and apathy. Addiction to methamphetamine is associated with pronounced psychological cravings and obsessive drug-seeking behavior.

Women who use amphetamines during pregnancy risk premature birth, stillbirth, low birth weight, and early infant

---

TERMS

state dependence A situation in which information learned in a drug-induced state is difficult to recall when the effect of the drug wears off.

death. Babies born to amphetamine-using mothers have a higher incidence of cleft palate, cleft lip, and deformed limbs. They may also experience symptoms of withdrawal.

Ritalin A stimulant with amphetamine-like effects, Ritalin (methylphenidate) is used to treat attention-deficit/hyperactivity disorder (ADHD). When taken orally at prescribed levels, it has little potential for abuse. When injected or snorted, however, dependence and tolerance can rapidly result.

Caffeine Caffeine is probably the most popular psychoactive drug and also one of the most ancient. It is found in coffee, tea, cocoa, soft drinks, headache remedies, and OTC preparations like NōDōz. (Table 7.3 lists typical levels of caffeine in several popular beverages.) In ordinary doses, caffeine produces greater alertness and a sense of well-being. It also decreases feelings of fatigue or boredom, so using caffeine may enable a person to keep at physically tiring or repetitive tasks longer. Such use is usually followed, however, by a sudden letdown. Caffeine does not noticeably influence a person's ability to perform complex mental tasks unless fatigue, boredom, or other factors have already affected normal performance.

Caffeine mildly stimulates the heart and respiratory system, increases muscular tremor, and enhances gastric secretion. Higher doses may cause nervousness, anxiety, irritability, headache, disturbed sleep, and gastric irritation or peptic ulcers. In people with high blood pressure, caffeine can cause blood pressure to rise even further above normal; in people with type 2 diabetes, caffeine may cause glucose and insulin levels to rise after meals.

Drinks containing caffeine are rarely harmful for most people, but some tolerance develops, and withdrawal symptoms of irritability, headaches, and even mild depression occur.. People can usually avoid problems by simply decreasing their daily intake of caffeine.

ENERGY "SHOTS" The popularity of small (1.5–3 oz) energy drinks has increased dramatically in recent years. Worldwide sales of products such as 5-Hour Energy reached $9 billion in 2011. Because these products are sold as dietary supplements rather than food, their caffeine content is not regulated by the Food and Drug Administration. Each 2-oz "shot" typically contains the same amount (roughly 100 mg) of caffeine as a regular-size cup of coffee.

Marijuana and Other Cannabis Products

Marijuana is the most widely used illegal drug in the United States, with 17.4 million current users. Marijuana is usually smoked, but it can also be ingested.

Marijuana is a crude preparation of various parts of the Indian hemp plant *Cannabis sativa*, which grows in most parts of the world. THC (tetrahydrocannabinol) is the main active ingredient in marijuana. The potency of marijuana prepara-

| Table 7.3 | Caffeine Content of Popular Beverages |

	SERVING SIZE	TYPICAL CAFFEINE LEVEL (MG)*
COFFEE		
Regular coffee, brewed	8 oz.	95
Regular coffee, instant	8 oz.	93
Espresso	1 oz.	64
Decaffeinated coffee, brewed	8 oz.	5
Decaffeinated coffee, instant	8 oz.	2
TEA		
Regular tea, brewed	8 oz.	47
Decaffeinated tea, brewed	8 oz.	2
Green tea, brewed	8 oz.	Varies
SODA		
Code Red Mountain Dew	12 oz.	54
Mello Yello	12 oz.	53
Diet Coke	12 oz.	47
Dr. Pepper, Diet Dr. Pepper	12 oz.	41
Sunkist Orange Soda	12 oz.	41
Pepsi	12 oz.	38
Coca-Cola Classic, Diet Pepsi	12 oz.	35
ENERGY DRINKS		
No Name	8.4 oz.	280
SoBe No Fear	16 oz.	174
Monster Energy, Rockstar	16 oz.	160
SoBe Adrenaline Rush	16 oz.	152
Full Throttle, Full Throttle Fury	16 oz.	144
AMP Energy Drink	16 oz.	143
Red Bull	8.3 oz.	76
Vault	8 oz.	47

*Caffeine levels vary greatly by brand of product, manner of preparation, and amount consumed. The amounts shown here are averages based on tests conducted by a variety of organizations. The U.S. Food and Drug Administration limits the amount of caffeine in cola and pepper soft drinks to 71 milligrams per 12-ounce serving. To find the exact amount of caffeine in any product, check that product's label.

SOURCES: Center for Science in the Public Interest. 2007. *Caffeine Content of Food & Drugs* (http://www.cspinet.org/new/cafchart.htm); Mayo Clinic. 2008. *Caffeine Content in Tea, Soda, and More* (http://www.mayoclinic.com/health/caffeine/AN01211); U.S. Department of Agriculture, Agricultural Research Service. 2009. *USDA National Nutrient Database for Standard Reference, Release 22* (http://www.ars.usda.gov/ba/bhnrc/ndl).

tions depends on the THC content and varies widely. Marijuana plants that grow wild often have less than 1% THC in their leaves. When selected strains are cultivated by separation of male and female plants (*sinsemilla*), the bud leaves from the flowering tops may contain 7–8% THC. Hashish, a potent preparation made from the thick resin that exudes from the marijuana leaves, may contain up to 14% THC.

These various preparations have all been known and used for centuries, so the frequently heard claim that today's marijuana is more potent than the marijuana of the 1970s is not

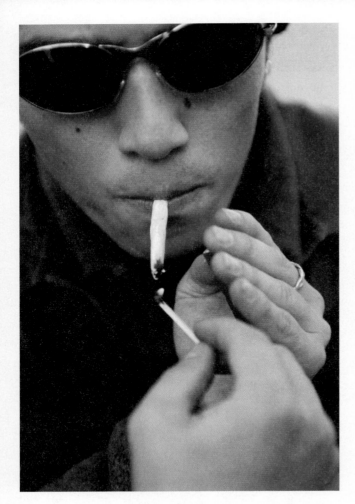

Marijuana is the most widely used illegal drug in the United States.

alcohol and marijuana significantly impairs driving performance and increases crash risk.

In 1999 the Institute of Medicine determined that some compounds in marijuana may have legitimate medical use. For example, marijuana has been shown to ease pain, reduce nausea, and increase appetite. These benefits led several states to approve the use of "medical marijuana" by extremely ill patients, with physician monitoring. However, because growing, selling, or possessing marijuana is a federal crime, the Supreme Court has held that state laws permitting medical marijuana use cannot supersede federal law. This means anyone who uses marijuana for medical reasons—even in a state that approves such use—can still be prosecuted under federal drug laws. Currently more than 30 states have medical marijuana laws on their books.

Long-Term Effects The most probable long-term effect of smoking marijuana is respiratory damage, including impaired lung function and chronic bronchial irritation. Although there is no evidence linking marijuana use to lung cancer, it may cause changes in lung tissue that promote cancer growth. Marijuana users may be at increased risk for emphysema and cancer of the head and neck, and among people with chronic conditions like cancer and AIDS, marijuana use is associated with increased risk of fatal lung infections. Heavy users may experience learning problems, as well as subtle impairments of attention and memory that may or may not be reversible following long-term abstinence. Long-term use may also decrease testosterone levels and sperm counts and increase sperm abnormalities.

Heavy marijuana use during pregnancy may cause impaired fetal growth and development, low birth weight, and increased risk of ectopic pregnancy. Marijuana may act synergistically with alcohol to increase the damaging effects of alcohol on the fetus. THC rapidly enters breast milk and may impair an infant's early motor development.

Dependence Regular users of marijuana can develop tolerance; some develop dependence, and researchers estimate that 1.5% of Americans meet the APA criteria for marijuana dependence. Withdrawal symptoms may occur in the majority of dependent or heavy users. Common symptoms include anger or aggression, irritability, nervousness or restlessness, sleep difficulties, and decreased appetite or weight loss.

Hallucinogens

Hallucinogens are a group of drugs whose predominant pharmacological effect is to alter the user's perceptions, feelings,

strictly true. However, because a greater proportion of the marijuana sold today is the higher-potency (and more expensive) sinsemilla, the average potency of street marijuana has increased.

Short-Term Effects and Uses At low doses, marijuana users typically experience euphoria, a heightening of subjective sensory experiences, a slowing down of the perception of passing time, and a relaxed attitude. With moderate doses, marijuana's effects become stronger, and the user can also expect to have impaired memory function, disturbed thought patterns, lapses of attention, and feelings of **depersonalization,** in which the mind seems to be separated from the body.

Very high doses produce feelings of depersonalization, marked sensory distortion, and changes in body image (such as a feeling that the body is very light). Inexperienced users sometimes think these sensations mean they are going crazy and become anxious or panicky.

Physiologically, marijuana increases heart rate and dilates certain blood vessels in the eyes, which creates the characteristic bloodshot eyes. Because THC affects parts of the brain controlling balance, coordination, and reaction time, marijuana use impairs driving performance. The combination of

> **TERMS**
>
> **depersonalization** A state in which a person loses the sense of his or her reality or perceives his or her body as unreal.
>
> **hallucinogen** Any of several drugs that alter perception, feelings, or thoughts; examples are LSD, mescaline, and PCP.

and thoughts. Hallucinogens include LSD (lysergic acid diethylamide), MDMA (methylenedioxymethamphetamine), mescaline, psilocybin, STP (4-methyl-2,5-dimethoxyamphetamine), DMT (dimethyltryptamine), ketamine, and PCP (phencyclidine). These drugs are most commonly ingested or smoked

Many hallucinogens induce tolerance so quickly that after only one or two doses their effects decrease substantially. The user must then stop taking the drug for several days before his or her system can be receptive to it again. These drugs cause little drug-seeking behavior and no physical dependence or withdrawal symptoms.

The immediate effects of low doses of hallucinogens are determined largely by expectations and setting. Many effects are hard to describe because they involve subjective and unusual dimensions of awareness—the **altered states of consciousness** for which these drugs are famous. For this reason, hallucinogens have acquired a certain aura not associated with other drugs.

LSD LSD is one of the most powerful psychoactive drugs. Tiny doses will produce noticeable effects in most people, such as an altered sense of time, visual disturbances, and an improved sense of hearing, mood changes, and distortions in how people perceive their bodies. Dilation of the pupils and slight dizziness, weakness, and nausea may also occur. With larger doses, users may experience a phenomenon known as **synesthesia,** feelings of depersonalization, and other alterations in the perceived relationship between the self and external reality.

A severe panic reaction can result from taking any dose of LSD. Even after the drug's chemical effects have worn off, spontaneous **flashbacks** and other psychological disturbances can occur.

MDMA MDMA (methylenedioxymethamphetamine), also known as Ecstasy, may be classified as a hallucinogen or a stimulant. Users may experience euphoria, increased energy, and a heightened sense of belonging. Using MDMA can produce dangerously high body temperature and potentially fatal dehydration. Some users experience confusion, depression, anxiety, paranoia, muscle tension, involuntary teeth clenching, blurred vision, nausea, and seizures. Even low doses can affect concentration, judgment, and driving ability. Tolerance can develop, leading users to take the drug more frequently, to use higher doses, or to combine MDMA with other drugs to enhance the drug's effects.

Other Hallucinogens Most other hallucinogens have the same general effects as LSD, but there are some variations. For example, a DMT or ketamine high does not last as long as an LSD high; an STP high lasts longer. MDMA has both hallucinogenic and amphetamine-like properties. Tolerance to MDMA develops quickly, and high doses can cause anxiety, delusions, and paranoia.

PCP reduces and distorts sensory input, especially proprioception—the sensation of body position and movement—and creates a state of sensory deprivation. PCP was initially used as an anesthetic but was unsatisfactory because it caused agitation, confusion, and delirium. The effects of ketamine are similar to those of PCP—confusion, agitation, aggression, and lack of coordination—but they tend to be less predictable. Tolerance to either drug can develop rapidly.

Mescaline, derived from the peyote cactus, is the ceremonial drug of the Native American Church. It causes effects similar to LSD, including altered perception and feeling; increased body temperature, heart rate, and blood pressure; weakness and trembling; and sleeplessness. Mescaline is expensive, so most street mescaline is diluted LSD or a mixture of other drugs. Hallucinogenic effects can be obtained from certain mushrooms (*Psilocybe mexicana,* or "magic mushrooms"), certain morning glory seeds, nutmeg, jimsonweed, and other botanical products, but unpleasant side effects, such as dizziness, have limited the popularity of these products.

Inhalants

Inhaling certain chemicals can produce effects ranging from heightened pleasure to delirium and death. Inhalants fall into several major groups; (1) volatile solvents, which are found in products such as paint thinner, glue, and gasoline); (2) aerosols, which are sprays that contain propellants and solvents; (3) nitrites, such as butyl nitrite and amyl nitrite); and (4) anesthetics, which include nitrous oxide (laughing gas).

Ask Yourself

QUESTIONS FOR CRITICAL THINKING AND REFLECTION

Do you know any young teens who may be at risk for using inhalants? If so, would you try to intervene in some way? What would you tell a youngster to convince him or her to stop inhaling chemicals?

TERMS

synesthesia A condition in which a stimulus evokes not only the sensation appropriate to it but also another sensation of a different character, such as when a color evokes a specific smell.

altered states of consciousness Profound changes in mood, thinking, and perception.

flashback A perceptual distortion or bizarre thought that recurs after the chemical effects of a drug have worn off.

Inhalant use tends to be highest among younger adolescents and declines with age. Inhalant use is difficult to control because inhalants are easy to obtain. They are present in a variety of seemingly harmless products, from dessert-topping sprays to underarm deodorants, that are both inexpensive and legal. Using the drugs also requires no illegal or suspicious paraphernalia. Inhalant users get high by sniffing, snorting, "bagging" (inhaling fumes from a plastic bag), or "huffing" (placing an inhalant-soaked rag in the mouth).

Although different in makeup, nearly all inhalants produce effects similar to those of anesthetics, which slow down body functions. Low doses may cause users to feel slightly stimulated; at higher doses, users may feel less inhibited and less in control. Sniffing high concentrations of the chemicals in solvents or aerosol sprays can cause a loss of consciousness, heart failure, and death. High concentrations of any inhalant can also cause death from suffocation by displacing oxygen in the lungs and central nervous system. Deliberately inhaling from a bag or in a closed area greatly increases the chances of suffocation. Other possible effects of the excessive or long-term use of inhalants include damage to the nervous system; hearing loss; increased risk of cancer; and damage to the liver, kidneys, and bone marrow.

Synthetic Recreational Drugs

In recent years herbal or synthetic recreational drugs have become increasingly available. These "designer drugs" are intended to have pharmacological effects similar to those of illicit drugs but to be chemically distinct from them and therefore either legal or impossible to detect in drug screening. The drugs fall into two main groups. One group is marketed as synthetic marijuana and sold as "herbal incense," or "herbal highs" with names such as Spice, K2, Genie, and Nice Guy. The other group is marketed as stimulants with properties like those of cocaine or amphetamine and is sold as "bath salts" with names such as Zoom, Ivory Wave, and White Rush.

Spice and other synthetic mimics of THC are distributed in the form of dried leaves or powder. They are typically smoked, using a pipe or by rolling in a cigarette paper, but can also be ingested as an infusion such as tea or inhaled. The active ingredients in Spice and similar products are synthetic cannabinoids that act on brain cells to produce effects similar to those of THC, such as physical relaxation, changes in perception, elevated mood, and mild euphoria.

More than 1 in 10 American high school seniors (11.4%) report using synthetic marijuana in the prior year, according to the "Monitoring the Future" survey conducted by the University of Michigan. This level of use is four times the rate reported for inhalants or cocaine and eight times the rate for methamphetamine.

Spice and similar products have not been included in any wide-scale animal or human studies, and little information is available in international medical databases. The blends of ingredients vary widely, but these products typically contain more than a dozen different plant-derived compounds, which give rise to a wide variety of drug combinations. Calls to poison control centers for exposure to synthetic marijuana doubled between 2010 and 2011, with patients describing symptoms that include rapid heart rate, vomiting, agitation, confusion, and hallucinations. In March 2011 the U.S. Drug Enforcement Administration (DEA) banned five synthetic cannabinoids used in Spice and similar products.

"Bath salts," marketed as cocaine or methamphetamine substitutes, are widely available on the Internet. They contain the synthetic stimulants mephedrone, methylone, or methylenedioxypyrovalerone (MDPV). Similar in effect to MDMA, MDPV is a synthetic version of the active ingredient found in the stimulant khat, which is widely used in countries of the Middle East. The products are sold in small packets of salt-like crystals with warnings like "novelty only" and "not for human consumption." Bath salts can be ingested by smoking, eating, or injecting or by crushing them and snorting the powder. The speed of onset is up to 15 minutes depending on how the drug is ingested, and the effects may last as long as six hours.

The effects of bath salts can be severe and include combative violent behavior, extreme agitation, confusion, hallucinations, hypertension, chest pain, and suicidal thoughts. In 2010 poison centers in the United States received 304 calls about reactions to bath salts; the number rose to 6,138 calls in 2011. In September 2011 the DEA banned three of the drugs found in bath salts. Possession or sale of the chemicals or products that contain them is now illegal in the United States.

DRUG USE: THE DECADES AHEAD

Although the use of some drugs, both legal and illegal, has declined dramatically since the 1970s, the use of others has held steady or increased. Mounting public concern has led to debate about what should be done about drug abuse. Efforts to combat the problem include workplace drug testing, tougher law enforcement and prosecution, and treatment and education. With drugs being produced domestically and entering the country on a massive scale from South America, Southeast Asia, and elsewhere, and being distributed through tightly controlled drug-smuggling organizations and street gangs, the success of any program is uncertain.

Drugs, Society, and Families

According to the Department of Justice, National Drug Intelligence Center, and Institute on Drug Abuse, the cost to society of illicit drug abuse alone is $193 billion annually. That figure is higher than the cost of many major health problems, including diabetes, obesity, and smoking. But the costs are more than just financial—they are also paid in human pain and suffering.

The criminal justice system is inundated with people accused of crimes related to drug possession, sale, or use. The FBI reports that more than 1.7 million arrests are made annually for drug violations. In 2009, the most recent year for which data are available, 18% of state prison inmates (252,000) were serving time for drug offenses. In 2010 about half of federal inmates (107,000) were in prison because of drug offenses. The Bureau of Justice Statistics reports that about half of all state and federal prisoners—roughly 850,000 men and women—meet diagnostic criteria for drug abuse or addiction. Many assaults and murders are committed when people try to acquire or protect drug territories, settle disputes about drugs, or steal from dealers. Violence and gun use are common in neighborhoods where drug trafficking is prevalent. Addicts commit more robberies and burglaries than criminals not on drugs. People under the influence of drugs, especially alcohol, are more likely to commit violent crimes like rape and murder than people who do not use drugs (see the box "Drug Use and Ethnicity").

Drug abuse is also a health care issue for society. In the United States, illegal drug use leads to more than 800,000 emergency department admissions and nearly 20,000 deaths annually. Although it is in the best interest of society to treat addicts who want help, there is not nearly enough space in treatment facilities to help the millions of Americans who need immediate treatment.

Drug abuse also takes a toll on individuals and families. Children born to women who use drugs such as alcohol, tobacco, or cocaine may have long-term health problems. Drug abuse in families can become a vicious cycle. Children who observe the adults around them using drugs assume it is acceptable. Abuse, neglect, lack of opportunity, and unemployment become contributing factors to drug use and perpetuate the cycle.

Legalizing Drugs

Pointing out that many of the social problems associated with drugs are related to prohibition rather than to the effects of the drugs themselves, some people have argued for various forms of drug legalization or decriminalization. Proposals range from making drugs such as marijuana and heroin available by prescription to allowing licensed dealers to sell some of these drugs to adults. Proponents argue that legalizing some currently illicit drugs—but putting controls on them similar to those used for alcohol, tobacco, and prescription drugs—could eliminate many problems. Some jurisdictions have adopted policies that make personal use and possession of small amounts of marijuana misdemeanor crimes without significant penalties. In 2010 California removed even the misdemeanor status of possession of less than an ounce of marijuana, making it an infraction comparable to a traffic ticket.

Many American businesses **require workers to take drug tests;** a substantial number of employers offer counseling and treatment support for workers who test positive.

QUICK STATS

In 2010, **4.1 million** people aged 12 or older received treatment for a problem related to the use of alcohol or illicit drugs.

—NSDUH, 2011

Opponents of drug legalization argue that allowing easier access to drugs would expose many more people to possible abuse and dependence. Drugs would be cheaper and easier to obtain, and drug use would be more socially acceptable. Legalizing drugs could cause an increase in drug use among children and teenagers. Opponents point out that alcohol and tobacco—drugs that already are legal—are major causes of disease and death in our society.

Drug Testing

According to data from recent surveys, the majority of substance users hold full-time jobs. Drug use in the workplace not only creates health problems for individual users, but also has a negative effect on productivity and on safety of coworkers.

Statistics from the federal government show that 8.4% of full-time workers were illicit drug users in 2007, the most recent year for which data are available. In absolute numbers, approximately 13.1 million current illicit drug users and 13 million heavy alcohol users were full-time workers in 2007. Illicit drug use is highest among workers in the food industry and construction sectors, while heavy alcohol use is greatest among construction, mining, and repair workers. The economic burden of lost productivity resulting from premature death, illness, and disability is estimated to run as high as $114 billion for drug abuse and $179 billion for heavy alcohol use.

The extent of the problem has given rise to the development of workplace policies to help workers regain their health and well-being. Workplace policies developed to address the problem often include drug testing and referral services. Despite controversial aspects of drug testing in the workplace, a growing number of U.S. workers recognize the need for such screening. Most drug testing involves a urine test. A test for alcohol involves a blood test or a breath test. If a person tests positive for drugs, the employer may provide drug counseling or treatment, suspend the employee until he or she tests negative, or fire the individual.

Treatment for Drug Addiction

Regardless of the therapeutic approach used, many individuals undergoing treatment will often slide back into their drug habits.

Preventing relapse and maintaining long-term cessation of drug use are complex medical goals. Relapse prevention research is instead increasingly focusing on expanding the repertoire of behavioral skills individuals need to overcome drug dependence. Medications are also used in treating addiction.

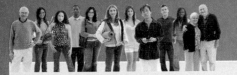

DIVERSITY MATTERS
Drug Use And Ethnicity

Surveys of the U.S. population find a variety of trends in drug use and abuse among ethnic groups (see the accompanying table). In addition to these general trends, there are also trends relating to the use of specific drugs among different groups. However, as is true for many areas of health, ethnic trends are influenced by a complex interplay of other factors:

- *Educational status:* Adults with four or more years of college are more likely to have *tried* illicit drugs than are people of the same age who never finished high school. *Current* drug use, however, is lower among college graduates than among people with less education. Among teens, poor school performance is associated with a higher risk of drug use.

- *Employment status:* Most adult drug users are employed, but rates of current drug use are much higher among people who are unemployed or who work part-time compared with those who are employed full-time.

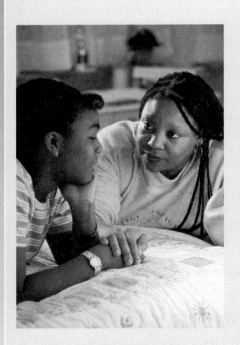

LIFETIME AND PAST MONTH ILLICIT DRUG USE AMONG PEOPLE AGED 12 OR OLDER

	NATIONAL SURVEY RESULTS, 2010	
	LIFETIME DRUG USE (PERCENT)	PAST MONTH DRUG USE (PERCENT)
White	50.7	9.1
Black or African American	46.1	10.7
Hispanic or Latino	36.4	8.1
Asian American	21.2	3.5
American Indian and Alaska Native	57.6	N/A
Native Hawaiian and Pacific Islander American	N/A	N/A
Two or more races	56.1	22.2

NOTE: Results shown in percentages of each population group.

N/A = Data not available.

- *Parental education and socioeconomic status:* Students from poor families have higher rates of *early* drug use compared with students from wealthier families. By the 12th grade the differences disappear. Socioeconomic status and parental education are closely linked.

- *Geographic area:* Current drug use in the United States is highest in the West and Midwest; drug use is also higher in metropolitan and urban areas compared with more rural areas. People living in communities with high rates of poverty, crime, and unemployment have higher-than-average rates of drug use and abuse. Specific drugs may also be more available—and their abuse more prevalent—in certain regions or communities.

Strong cultural identity is associated with reduced risk of drug use and abuse among all groups. The following factors may contribute to lower rates of drug use among such groups:

- *Parental and community disapproval of drug and alcohol use:* Parents of Asian American children tend to have more restrictive drug and alcohol use norms than African American and white parents. Black parents tend to monitor their children's

activities and friendships more closely than white parents. Parental disapproval of drug use is often tied to greater perceived risk of drug use—and lower rates of drug use—among teens.

- *Close family ties:* Asian American teens are the likeliest to come from intact homes. Respect for authority and family loyalty are strongly valued among many Asian American populations. Black teens, although least likely to come from intact homes, often come from single-parent households with close extended family ties. Teens from cohesive and stable families are less likely to use drugs.

- *Focus on schooling and education:* Teens from families who value education and where parents help with homework and limit weeknight time with friends have lower rates of drug use.

SOURCES: Johnston, L. D., et al. 2012. *Monitoring the Future: Overview of Key Findings, 2011.* Ann Arbor, MI: Institute for Social Research, The University of Michigan; Substance Abuse and Mental Health Services Administration. 2011. *Results from the 2010 National Survey on Drug Use and Health: National Findings.* Rockville, MD: Office of Applied Studies, NSDUH Series H-36, HHS Publication No. SMA 11-4434.

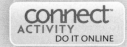
ACTIVITY
DO IT ONLINE

Medication-Assisted Treatment Medications can reduce the craving for the abused drug or to block or oppose its effects. Perhaps the best-known medication for drug abuse is methadone, a synthetic drug used as a substitute for heroin. Methadone prevents withdrawal reactions and reduces the craving for heroin. Its use enables heroin-addicted people to function normally in social and vocational activities, although they remain dependent on methadone. The drug buprenorphine, approved for treatment of opioid addiction, also reduces cravings.

Medication therapy is relatively simple and inexpensive and is therefore popular among patients, health care providers, and insurance companies. However, the relapse rate is high. Combining drug therapy with psychological and social services improves success rates, underscoring the importance of psychological factors in drug dependence.

Treatment Centers Treatment centers offer a variety of short-term and long-term services, including hospitalization, detoxification, counseling, and other mental health services. The therapeutic community is a specific type of center, a residential program run in a completely drug-free atmosphere. Administered by ex-addicts, these programs use confrontation, strict discipline, and unrelenting peer pressure to attempt to resocialize the addict with a different set of values. Halfway houses, which are transitional settings between a 24-hour-a-day program and independent living, are an important phase of treatment for some people."

Groups and Peer Counseling Groups such as Alcoholics Anonymous (AA) and Narcotics Anonymous (NA) have helped many people. People treated in drug substitution programs or substance abuse treatment centers are often urged or required to join a self-help group as part of their recovery. These groups follow a 12-step program. Group members' first step is to acknowledge that they have a problem over which they have no control. Peer support is a critical ingredient of these programs, and members usually meet at least once a week. Each member is paired with a sponsor to call on for advice and support if the temptation to relapse becomes overwhelming. Chapters of AA and NA meet on some college campuses; community-based chapters are listed in local newspapers and on the Internet.

Many colleges also have peer counseling programs, in which students are trained to help other students who have drug problems. A peer counselor's role may be as limited as referring a student to a professional or as involved as helping arrange a leave of absence from school for participation in a drug treatment program (see the box "If Someone You Know Has a Drug Problem . . .").

Harm Reduction Strategies Because many attempts at treatment are at first unsuccessful, some experts advocate the use of harm reduction strategies. The goal of harm reduction is to minimize the negative effects of drug use and abuse: a common example is the use of designated drivers to reduce alcohol-related motor vehicle crashes. Drug substitution programs such as methadone maintenance are a form of harm reduction—although participants remain drug dependent, the negative individual and social consequences of their drug use are reduced. Syringe exchange programs, designed to reduce transmission of HIV and hepatitis C, are another harm reduction approach. Some experts have also suggested free testing of street drugs for purity and potency to help users avoid unintentional toxicity or overdose.

Codependency Drug abuse takes a toll on friends and family members, and counseling can help people work through painful feelings of guilt and powerlessness. **Codependency,** in which a person close to the drug abuser is controlled by the abuser's behavior, sometimes develops. Codependent people may come to believe that love, approval, and security are contingent on their taking care of the abuser. People can become codependent because they want to help when someone they love becomes dependent on a drug. They may assume that their good intentions will persuade the drug user to stop.

Codependent people often engage in behaviors that remove or soften the effects of drug use on the user—so-called *enabling* behaviors. The habit of enabling can inhibit a drug abuser's recovery because the person never has to experience the consequences of his or her behavior. For this reason, many treatment programs involve the whole family.

Have you ever been an enabler in a relationship? You may have if you've ever done any of the following:

- Given someone one more chance to stop abusing drugs, then another, and another
- Made excuses or lied for someone to his or her friends, teachers, or employer
- Joined someone in drug use and blamed others for your behavior
- Lent money to someone to continue drug use
- Stayed up late waiting for or gone out searching for someone who uses drugs
- Felt embarrassed or angry about the actions of someone who uses drugs
- Ignored the drug use because the person got defensive when you brought it up
- Avoided confronting a friend or relative who was obviously intoxicated or high on a drug

If you come from a codependent family or see yourself developing codependency relationships or engaging in enabling behaviors, consider acting now to make changes in your patterns of interaction.

> **TERMS**
>
> **codependency** A relationship in which a non–substance-abusing partner or family member is controlled by the abuser's behavior; codependent people frequently engage in enabling behaviors.

Changes in behavior and mood in someone you know may signal a growing dependence on drugs. Signs that a person's life is beginning to focus on drugs include the following:

- Sudden withdrawal or emotional distance
- Rebellious or unusually irritable behavior
- A loss of interest in usual activities or hobbies
- A decline in school performance
- A sudden change in the chosen group of friends
- Changes in sleeping or eating habits
- Frequent borrowing of money or stealing
- Secretive behavior about personal possessions, such as a backpack or the contents of a drawer
- Deterioration of physical appearance

If you believe a family member or friend has a drug problem, locate information about drug treatment resources available on campus or in your community. Communicate your concern, provide him or her with information about treatment options, and offer your support during treatment. If the person continues to deny having a problem, talk with an experienced counselor about setting up an intervention—a formal, structured confrontation designed to end denial by having family, friends, and other caring people present their concerns to the drug user. Participants in an intervention would indicate the ways in which the individual is hurting others as well as himself or herself. If your friend or family member agrees to treatment, encourage him or her to attend a support group such as Narcotics Anonymous or Alcoholics Anonymous.

And finally, examine your relationship with the abuser for signs of codependency. If necessary, get help for yourself; friends and family of drug users can often benefit from counseling.

Preventing Drug Abuse

The best solution to drug abuse is prevention. Government attempts at controlling the drug problem have historically focused on stopping the production, importation, and distribution of illegal drugs. A new national drug policy announced in 2010, however, redirects federal funding and efforts into stopping the demand for drugs. Developing persuasive antidrug educational programs may offer the best hope for solving the drug problem in the future.

Indirect approaches to prevention involve building young people's self-esteem, improving their academic skills, and increasing their recreational opportunities. Direct approaches involve providing information about the adverse effects of drugs and teaching tactics that help students resist peer pressure to use drugs in various situations. Developing strategies for resisting peer pressure is one of the more effective techniques.

Prevention efforts need to focus on the different motivations individuals have for using and abusing specific drugs at different ages. For example, adolescents are often responsive to peer counselors. Many young adults tend to be influenced by efforts that focus on health education. For all ages, it is important to provide nondrug alternatives—such as recreational facilities, counseling, greater opportunities for leisure activities, and places to socialize—that speak to the individual's or group's specific reasons for using drugs. Reminding young people that most people, no matter what age, do not use drugs is a critical part of preventing substance abuse.

Ask Yourself

Do you know someone who may have a drug problem? What steps, if any, have you taken to help that person? If you were using drugs and felt that things had gone out of control, what would you want your friends to do for you?

connect

Connect to Your Choices

Have you ever thought about why you make the choices you do about drugs? Many factors can influence the drug-related choices we make, some not as obvious as others. If you use drugs—or if you don't—have you been influenced by attitudes toward drug use in your family or peer group? Do you take drugs when they're offered at parties because it's easier than saying no? Are you influenced by the lyrics of songs that make drug use sound glamorous?

What are the external factors that influence your drug-related choices? What are your inner motivations and core values, and how do they affect your choices? Based on what you learned in this chapter, will you make some different choices in the future? If so, what will they be?

Go online to Connect to complete this activity: www.mcgraw-hillconnect.com

SUMMARY

- Addictive behaviors are self-reinforcing. Addicts experience a strong compulsion for the behavior and a loss of control over it; an escalating pattern of abuse with serious negative consequences may result.

- The sources or causes of addiction include heredity, personality, lifestyle, and environmental factors. People may use an addictive behavior as a means of alleviating stress or painful emotions.

- Some common behaviors are potentially addictive, including gambling, shopping, sexual activity, Internet use, eating, and working.

- Drug abuse is a maladaptive pattern of drug use that persists despite adverse social, psychological, or medical consequences.

- Drug addiction involves taking a drug compulsively, which includes neglecting constructive activities because of it and continuing to use it despite experiencing adverse effects resulting from its use. Tolerance and withdrawal symptoms are often present.

- Reasons for using drugs include the lure of the illicit; curiosity; rebellion; peer pressure; and the desire to alter one's mood or escape boredom, anxiety, depression, or other psychological problems.

- Psychoactive drugs affect the mind and body by altering brain chemistry. The effect of a drug depends on its properties and on how it's used (drug factors), the physical and psychological characteristics of the user (user factors), and the physical and social environment surrounding the drug use (social factors).

- Opioids relieve pain, cause drowsiness, and induce euphoria; they reduce anxiety and produce lethargy, apathy, and an inability to concentrate.

- CNS depressants slow down the overall activity of the central nervous system; they reduce anxiety and cause mood changes, impaired muscular coordination, slurring of speech, and drowsiness or sleep.

- CNS stimulants speed up the activity of the central nervous system, causing acceleration of the heart rate, a rise in blood pressure, dilation of the pupils and bronchial tubes, and an increase in gastric and adrenal secretions.

- Marijuana usually causes euphoria and a relaxed attitude at low doses; very high doses produce feelings of depersonalization and sensory distortion.

- Hallucinogens alter perception, feelings, and thoughts and may cause an altered sense of time, visual disturbances, and mood changes.

- Inhalants are present in a variety of everyday products; they can cause delirium. Their use can lead to loss of consciousness, heart failure, suffocation, and death.

- Economic and social costs of drug abuse include the financial costs of law enforcement, treatment, and health care and the social costs of crime, violence, and family problems. Drug testing and drug legalization have been proposed to address some of the problems related to drug abuse.

- Approaches to treatment include medication, treatment centers, self-help groups, and peer counseling; many programs also offer counseling to family members.

FOR MORE INFORMATION

BOOKS

Hanson, G. R., et al. 2011. *Drugs and Society*, 11th ed. Boston: Jones & Bartlett. *Discusses the impact of drug abuse on individuals' lives and on the broader society.*

Kegan, K. 2008. *Chasing the High: A Firsthand Account of One Young Person's Experience with Substance Abuse.* New York: Oxford University Press. *The personal story of the author's descent into heroin addiction, homelessness, and crime and his redemption and recovery; both a memoir and a resource for young people struggling with substance dependence.*

Ksir, C., C. L. Hart, and O. S. Ray. 2010. *Drugs, Society, and Human Behavior*, 14th ed. New York: McGraw-Hill. *Examines drugs and behavior from the behavioral, pharmacological, historical, social, legal, and clinical perspectives.*

Mohammed, A. R., and E. Fritsvold. 2009. *Dorm Room Dealers: Drugs and the Privileges of Race and Class.* Boulder, CO: Lynn Rienner Publishers. *An exploration of drug dealing among middle-class students at a private four-year university, touching on issues of class, race, and deviance.*

Reding, N. 2010. *Methland: The Death and Life of an American Small Town.* New York: Bloomsbury USA. *The author chronicles the epidemic of meth production and addiction that overtook rural America—and one tiny Iowa town—as small farms and businesses declined in the wake of globalization.*

Rosen Publishing. 2009. *Drug Abuse and Society Series.* New York: Rosen Publishing. *A series of short books, each exploring a different type of drugs—from prescription medicine to club drugs—and their use and abuse.*

ORGANIZATIONS, HOTLINES, AND WEBSITES

Club Drugs. Provides information about drugs commonly classified as "club drugs."
http://www.drugabuse.gov/drugs-abuse/club-drugs

Drug Enforcement Administration: Drug Information. Provides basic facts about major drugs of abuse, including penalties for drug trafficking.

http://www.justice.gov/dea/concern/concern.htm

Gamblers Anonymous. Includes questions to help diagnose gambling problems and resources for getting help.

http://www.gamblersanonymous.org/ga/

Higher Education Center for Alcohol and Other Drug Abuse and Violence Prevention. Gives information about alcohol and drug abuse on campus and links to related sites.

http://www.higheredcenter.org

Narcotics Anonymous (NA). Similar to Alcoholics Anonymous, NA sponsors 12-step meetings and provides other support services for drug abusers.

http://www.na.org

There are also 12-step programs that focus on specific drugs:

Cocaine Anonymous

http://www.ca.org

Marijuana Anonymous

http://www.marijuana-anonymous.org

National Center on Addiction and Substance Abuse (CASA) at Columbia University. Provides information about the costs of substance abuse to individuals and society.

http://www.casacolumbia.org

National Council on Problem Gambling. Provides information and help for people with gambling problems and their families, including a searchable directory of counselors.

http://www.ncpgambling.org

National Drug Information, Treatment, and Referral Hotlines. Sponsored by the SAMHSA Center for Substance Abuse Treatment, these hotlines provide information on drug abuse and on HIV infection as it relates to substance abuse; referrals to support groups and treatment programs are available.

800-662-HELP

800-729-6686 (Spanish)

800-487-4889 (TDD for hearing impaired)

National Institute on Drug Abuse. Develops and supports research on drug abuse prevention programs.

http://www.drugabuse.gov

Substance Abuse and Mental Health Services Administration (SAMHSA). Provides statistics, information, and other resources related to substance abuse prevention and treatment.

http://www.samhsa.gov

SELECTED BIBLIOGRAPHY

American Psychiatric Association. 2000. *Diagnostic and Statistical Manual of Mental Disorders,* 4th ed., text revision. *(DSM-IV-TR).* Washington, DC: American Psychiatric Association.

Centers for Disease Control and Prevention. 2012. *HIV Surveillance Report, 2010; vol. 22* (http://www.cdc.gov/hiv/surveillance/resources/reports/2010report/index.htm).

Daniello, A., E. Flevisohn, and T. S. Gregory. Modeling the effects of caffeine on the sleep/wake cycle. *Biomedical Sciences Instrumentation* 48: 73-80.

Dever, B. V., et al. 2012. Predicting risk-taking with and without substance use: The effects of parental monitoring, school bonding, and sports participation. *Prevention Science,* Sept. 8 (Epub ahead of print).

Drug Enforcement Administration, U.S. Department of Justice. 2011. *Drugs of Abuse: A DEA Resource Guide, 2011 Edition* (http://www.justice.gov/dea/pubs/drugs_of_abuse.pdf).

Elliot, J. C., and K. B. Carey. Pros and cons: Prospective predictors of marijuana use on a college campus. *Psychology of Addictive Behaviors,* Sept. 17 (Epub ahead of print).

Giles, G. E. , et al. 2012. Differential cognitive effects of energy drink ingredients: Caffeine, taurine, and glucose. *Pharmacology, Biochemistry, and Behavior* 102(4): 569–577.

Johnston, L. D., et al. 2012. *Monitoring the Future: Overview of Key Findings, 2011.* Ann Arbor, MI: Institute for Social Research, The University of Michigan.

King, D. L., et al. 2012. Cognitive-behavioral approaches to outpatient treatment of Internet addiction in children and adolescents. *Journal of Clinical Psychology,* Sept. 13 (Epub ahead of print).

Koester, P., et al. 2012. Cortical thinning in amphetamine-type stimulant users. *Neuroscience* 221: 182–192.

Kurtz, S., et al. 2012. Interview as intervention: The case of young adult multidrug users in the club scene. *Journal of Substance Abuse Treatment,* Sept. 10 (Epub ahead of print).

Lucas, P. Cannabis as an adjunct to or substitute for opiates in the treatment of chronic pain. *Journal of Psychoactive Drugs* 44(2): 125–133.

Lyons, T., et al. 2010. Breaking the bond between stimulant use and risky sex: A qualitative study. *Substance Abuse* 31(4), 224–230.

National Council on Problem Gambling. 2010. *What Is Problem Gambling?* (http://www.ncpgambling.org/i4a/pages/index.cfm?pageid=1).

National Institute on Drug Abuse. 2008, rev. 2010. *Comorbidity: Addiction and Other Mental Illnesses.* Bethesda, MD: National Institute on Drug Abuse, NIH Publication No. 10-5771.

Office of National Drug Control Policy. 2012. *2010 National Strategy* (http://www.http://www.whitehouse.gov/ondcp/2012-national-drug-control-strategy/).

Patrick, M. E., et al. 2012. HIV/AIDS risk behaviors and substance use by young adults in the United States. *Prevention Science* 13(5): 532–538.

Pensers, T. M., R. E. Gestring, and D. A. Vilensky. 2012. Excited delirium following use of synthetic cathinones (bath salts). *General Hospital Psychiatry,* Aug. 13 (Epub ahead of print).

Porter, R. S., et. al. 2011. *The Merck Manual of Diagnosis and Therapy,* 19th ed. New York: Wiley.

Reith, G. 2012. Beyond addiction and compulsion: The continuing role of environment in the case of pathological gambling. *Addiction* 107(10): 1736–1737.

Rugani, F., et al. 2012. Symptomatological features of patients with and without Ecstasy use during their first psychotic episode. *International Journal of Environmental Research and Public Health* 9(7): 2283–2292.

Savoca, M. R., et al. 2005. Association of ambulatory blood pressure and dietary caffeine in adolescents. *American Journal of Hypertension* 18(1): 116–120.

Singer, L. T., et al. 2012. One-year outcomes of prenatal exposure to MDMA and other recreational drugs. *Pediatrics* 130(3): 407–413.

Substance Abuse and Mental Health Services Administration. 2011. *Results from the 2010 National Survey on Drug Use and Health: National Findings.* Rockville, MD: Office of Applied Studies, NSDUH Series H-36, HHS Publication No. SMA 11-4434.

Substance Abuse and Mental Health Services Administration, Center for Behavioral Health Statistics and Quality. 2011. *Drug Abuse Warning Network, 2008: National Estimates of Drug-Related Emergency Department Visits.* HHS Publication No. SMA 11-4618. Rockville, MD.

Tashkin, D. P., M. S. Simmons, and C. H. Tseng. 2012. Impact of changes in regular use of marijuana and/or tobacco on chronic bronchitis. *COPD* 9(4): 367–374.

U.S. Department of Justice, Federal Bureau of Investigation. 2009. *Crime in the United States: 2009* (http://www2.fbi.gov/ucr/cius2009/index.htm).

Van Ryzin, M. J., G. M. Fosco, and T. J. Dishion. 2012. Family and peer predictors of substance use from early adolescence to early adulthood: An 11-year prospective analysis. *Addictive Behaviors* 37(12): 1314–1324.

This behavior change strategy focuses on one of the most commonly used drugs—caffeine. If you are concerned about your use of a different drug or another type of addictive behavior, you can devise your own plan based on this one and on the steps outlined in Chapter 1.

Like many Americans, you may find yourself relying on coffee (or tea, chocolate, or cola) to get through a busy schedule. When you are studying for exams, for example, the forced physical inactivity and the need to concentrate even when fatigued may lead you to overuse caffeine. But caffeine doesn't help unless you are already sleepy. And it does not relieve any underlying condition (you are just more tired when it wears off). How can you change this pattern?

Self-Monitoring

Keep a log of how much caffeine you eat or drink. Be sure to include all forms, such as chocolate and OTC medications, as well as colas, tea, and coffee. Using Table 7.3, convert the amounts you drink into an estimate expressed in milligrams of caffeine.

Self-Assessment

At the end of the week, add up your daily totals and divide by 7 to get your daily average in milligrams. At more than 250 mg per day, you may be experiencing some adverse symptoms. If you are experiencing at least five of the following symptoms, you may want to cut down: restlessness, nervousness, excitement, insomnia, flushed face, excessive sweating, gastrointestinal problems, muscle twitching, rambling thoughts and speech, irregular heartbeat, periods of inexhaustibility, and excessive pacing or movement.

Set Limits

Can you restrict your caffeine intake to a daily total, and stick to this contract? If so, set a cutoff point, such as the amount of caffeine in one cup of coffee. If you cannot stick to your limit, you may want to cut out caffeine altogether: abstinence can be easier than moderation for some people. If you experience caffeine withdrawal symptoms (headache, fatigue), you may want to cut your intake more gradually.

Find Other Ways to Keep Up Your Energy

Get enough sleep or exercise more, rather than drowning the problem in coffee or tea. Remember that exercise raises your metabolic rate for hours afterward—a handy fact to exploit when you need to feel more awake and want to avoid an irritable caffeine jag. And if you've been compounding your fatigue by not eating properly, try filling up on complex carbo-

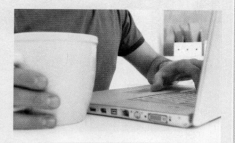

hydrates such as whole-grain bread or crackers instead of candy bars.

Tips for Cutting Out Caffeine

Here are some more ways to decrease your consumption of caffeine:

- Keep some noncaffeinated drinks on hand.
- Alternate between hot and very cold liquids.
- Fill your coffee cup only halfway.
- Avoid the office or school lunchroom or cafeteria and the chocolate sections of the grocery store. (Often people drink coffee or tea and eat chocolate simply because they're available.)
- Read labels of over-the-counter medications to check for hidden sources of caffeine.

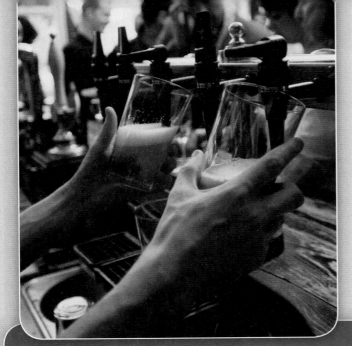

LOOKING AHEAD...

After reading this chapter, you should be able to

- Explain how alcohol is absorbed and metabolized by the body
- Describe the immediate and long-term effects of drinking alcohol
- Describe the different forms of alcohol abuse and their consequences
- List the reasons why people start using tobacco and why they continue to use it
- Explain the short- and long-term health risks associated with tobacco use
- Describe strategies for using alcohol responsibly, and develop plans for quitting tobacco use and avoiding environmental tobacco smoke

8

Alcohol and Tobacco

Alcohol and tobacco are the most common and widely used drugs in the United States. They are also the ones responsible for the most illnesses, injuries, and deaths.

Alcohol has a mixed role in human life. Used in moderation, it can enhance social occasions by loosening inhibitions and creating a pleasant feeling of relaxation. But like other drugs, alcohol has physiological effects that can impair functioning in the short term and cause devastating damage in the long term. For some people, alcohol use becomes an addiction, leading to a lifetime of recovery or, for a few, to debilitation and death.

Smoking is the leading preventable cause of death in the United States, taking 13 years of life from the average male smoker and 15 years from the average female smoker. Smoking affects those who don't smoke too. Exposure to environmental tobacco smoke (secondhand smoke) kills thousands of nonsmokers every year. Yet one in five Americans continues to smoke. This chapter examines the complex realities of alcohol and tobacco use in the United States today.

THE NATURE OF ALCOHOL

If you have ever been around people who are drinking, you probably noticed that alcohol seems to affect different people in different ways. One person may seem to get drunk after just a drink or two, while another appears to tolerate a great deal of alcohol without becoming intoxicated. These differences make alcohol's effects on the body seem mysterious and help explain why many misconceptions have evolved about alcohol use. The following sections explain how alcohol works in the body.

Alcoholic Beverages

Technically speaking, there are many kinds of **alcohol,** but in this book, the term *alcohol* refers only to ethyl alcohol (or ethanol, often abbreviated as ETOH). Other kinds of alcohol, such as methanol (wood alcohol) and isopropyl alcohol (rubbing alcohol), highly toxic; and can cause death if consumed.

Common Alcoholic Beverages   There are several basic types of alcoholic beverages. Ethanol is the psychoactive ingredient in each of them:

- Beer is a mild intoxicant brewed from a mixture of grains. By volume, beer usually contains 3–6% alcohol.

- Ales and malt liquors, which are similar to beer, typically contain 6–8% alcohol by volume.

- Wines are made by fermenting the juices of grapes or other fruits. In table wines, the concentration of alcohol is

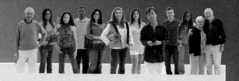

Metabolizing Alcohol: Our Bodies Work Differently

Do you and your friends react differently to alcohol? If so, your reactions may be affected by genetic differences in alcohol metabolism associated with ethnicity. Alcohol is metabolized mainly in the liver, where it is converted by an enzyme, alcohol dehydrogenase, into a toxic substance called acetaldehyde. Acetaldehyde causes many of alcohol's noxious effects. Ideally it is quickly broken down to a less active by-product, acetate, by another enzyme, acetaldehyde dehydrogenase (ALDH). Acetate can then separate into water and carbon dioxide and easily be eliminated.

Some people, primarily those of Asian descent, inherit ineffective or inactive variations of acetaldehyde dehydrogenase. Others, including some of African and Jewish descent, have forms of alcohol dehydrogenase that metabolize alcohol to acetaldehyde very quickly. Either way, toxic acetaldehyde builds up when these people drink alcohol. They experience a reaction called *flushing syndrome*. Their skin feels hot, their heart and respiration rates increase, and they may get a headache, vomit, or break out in hives. Drinking makes some people so uncomfortable that they are unlikely to develop alcohol addiction.

The body's response to acetaldehyde is the basis for treating alcohol abuse with the drug disulfiram (Antabuse), which inhibits the action of acetaldehyde dehydrogenase. When a person taking disulfiram ingests alcohol, acetaldehyde levels increase rapidly, and he or she develops an intense flushing reaction along with weakness, nausea, vomiting, and other disagreeable symptoms.

How people behave in relation to alcohol is influenced in complex ways by a wide range of factors, including liver size, body mass, and social and cultural influences. But individual choices and behavior are strongly influenced by specific genetic characteristics.

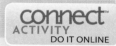

about 9–14%. Fortified wines—such as sherry, port, and Madeira—contain about 20% alcohol.

- Hard liquor—such as gin, whiskey, rum, tequila, vodka, and liqueur—is made by *distilling* brewed or fermented grains or other plant products. Hard liquors usually contain 35–50% alcohol.

The concentration of alcohol in a beverage is indicated by its **proof value,** which is two times the percentage concentration. For example, if a beverage is 100 proof, it contains 50% alcohol by volume. Two ounces of 100-proof whiskey contain one ounce of pure alcohol. The proof value of hard liquor can usually be found on the bottle's label.

"Standard Drinks" versus Actual Servings When discussing alcohol consumption, the term **one drink** (or *a standard drink*) means the amount of a beverage that typically contains about 0.6 ounce of alcohol. A 12-ounce bottle of beer, a 5-ounce glass of wine, and a 1.5-ounce shot of hard liquor are all considered one drink.

In practice, a typical serving of most alcoholic beverages is larger (sometimes significantly larger) than a single standard drink. This is particularly true of mixed drinks, which often include more than one type of hard liquor.

Caloric Content Alcohol provides 7 calories per gram, and the alcohol in one drink (14–17 grams) supplies about 100–120 calories. Most alcoholic beverages also contain some carbohydrate; for example, one beer provides about 150 total calories. The "light" in light beer refers to calories; a light beer typically has close to the same alcohol content as a regular beer and about 100 calories. A 5-ounce glass of red wine has 100 calories; white wine has 96. A 3-ounce margarita supplies 157 calories, a 6-ounce cosmopolitan has 143 calories, and a 6-ounce rum and Coke contains about 180 calories.

Absorption

When a person ingests alcohol, about 20% is rapidly absorbed from the stomach into the bloodstream. About 75% is absorbed through the upper part of the small intestine. Any remaining alcohol enters the bloodstream farther along the gastrointestinal tract. Once in the bloodstream, alcohol produces sensations of intoxication.

The rate of absorption is affected by a variety of factors. For example, the carbonation in a beverage like champagne increases the rate of alcohol absorption. Artificial sweeteners (commonly used in drink mixers) have the same effect. Food in the stomach slows the rate of absorption, as does the drinking of highly concentrated alcoholic beverages such as hard liquor.

Metabolism and Excretion

Because alcohol easily moves through most biological membranes, it is rapidly distributed throughout most body tissues. Alcohol **metabolizes** mainly in the liver, though a small amount of alcohol is metabolized in the stomach (see the box "Metabolizing Alcohol: Our Bodies Work Differently").

TERMS

alcohol The intoxicating ingredient in fermented or distilled beverages; a colorless, pungent liquid.

tobacco The leaves of cultivated tobacco plants prepared for smoking, chewing, or use as snuff.

proof value Two times the percentage of alcohol, by volume, in an alcoholic beverage; a "100-proof" beverage is 50% alcohol by volume.

one drink The amount of a beverage that typically contains about 0.6 ounce of alcohol; also called a *standard drink*.

metabolism The chemical transformation of food and other substances in the body into energy and wastes.

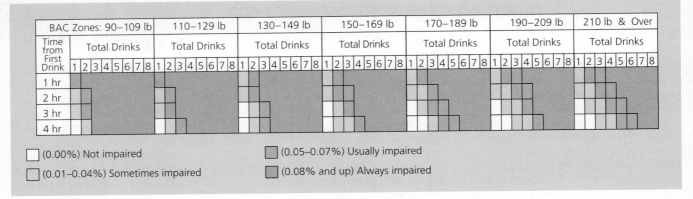

FIGURE 8.1 Approximate blood alcohol concentration and body weight. This chart illustrates the BAC an average person of a given weight would reach after drinking the specified number of drinks in the time shown. The legal limit for BAC is 0.08%; for drivers under 21 years of age, many states have zero-tolerance laws that set BAC limits of 0.01% or 0.02%.

About 2–10% of ingested alcohol is not metabolized in the liver or other tissues but is excreted unchanged by the lungs, kidneys, and sweat glands. Excreted alcohol causes the telltale smell on a drinker's breath and is the basis of breath and urine analyses for alcohol levels.

Alcohol readily enters the human brain, affecting neurotransmitters, the chemicals that carry messages between brain cells. These changes are temporary, creating many of the immediate effects of drinking alcohol. With chronic heavy usage, however, alcohol's effects become permanent, resulting in permanent disruption of brain function and changes in brain structure.

Alcohol Intake and Blood Alcohol Concentration

Blood alcohol concentration (BAC) is the amount of alcohol in a person's blood by volume, expressed as the percentage of alcohol measured in a deciliter of blood. BAC is

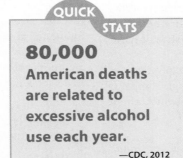

QUICK STATS

80,000
American deaths are related to excessive alcohol use each year.
—CDC, 2012

TERMS

blood alcohol concentration (BAC) The amount of alcohol in the blood, expressed as the percentage of alcohol in a deciliter of blood; used as a measure of intoxication.

affected by the amount of alcohol consumed in a given amount of time and by individual factors:

- *Body weight:* In most cases, a smaller person develops a higher BAC than a larger person after drinking the same amount of alcohol (Figure 8.1). A smaller person has less overall body tissue into which alcohol can be distributed.

- *Percentage body fat:* A person with a higher percentage of body fat will usually develop a higher BAC than a more muscular person of the same weight. Alcohol does not concentrate as much in fatty tissue as in muscle and most other tissues, in part because fat has fewer blood vessels.

- *Sex:* Women metabolize less alcohol in the stomach than men do because the stomach enzyme that breaks down alcohol before it enters the bloodstream is four times more active in men than in women. This means that more unmetabolized alcohol is released into the bloodstream in women. Because women are also generally smaller than men and have a higher percentage of body fat, women will have a higher BAC than men after consuming the same amount of alcohol. Hormonal fluctuations may also affect the rate of alcohol metabolism, making a woman more susceptible to high BACs at certain times during her menstrual cycle, usually just prior to the onset of menstruation.

BAC also depends on the balance between the rate of alcohol absorption and the rate of alcohol metabolism. A man who weighs 150 pounds and has normal liver function metabolizes about 0.3 ounce of alcohol per hour, the equivalent of about half a 12-ounce bottle of beer or half a 5-ounce glass of wine.

The rate of alcohol metabolism varies among individuals and is largely determined by genetic factors and drinking behavior. Although the rate of alcohol absorption can be slowed by factors like food, the metabolic rate *cannot* be influenced by exercise, breathing deeply, eating, drinking coffee, or taking other drugs. The rate of alcohol metabolism is the same whether a person is asleep or awake.

If a person absorbs slightly less alcohol each hour than he or she can metabolize in an hour, the BAC remains low. People can drink large amounts of alcohol this way over a long period of time without becoming noticeably intoxicated. Regardless, they run the risk of long-term health problems (described later in the chapter). If a person drinks alcohol more quickly than it can be metabolized, the BAC will steadily increase, and he or she will become more and more drunk.

ALCOHOL AND HEALTH

The effects of alcohol consumption on health depend on the individual, the circumstances, and the amount of alcohol consumed.

The Immediate Effects of Alcohol

Alcohol depresses the central nervous system (CNS), and its effects vary with the BAC. The effects of alcohol are more pronounced when the BAC is rapidly increasing than when it is slowly increasing, steady, or decreasing. The effects of alcohol are more pronounced if a person drinks on an empty stomach because alcohol is absorbed more quickly and the BAC rises more quickly.

Low Concentrations of Alcohol   The effects of alcohol can first be felt at a BAC of about 0.03–0.05%. These effects may include lightheadedness, relaxation, and a release of inhibitions. Most drinkers experience mild euphoria and become more sociable. When people drink in social settings, alcohol often seems to act as a stimulant, enhancing conviviality or assertiveness. This apparent stimulation occurs because alcohol depresses inhibitory centers in the brain.

Higher Concentrations of Alcohol   At higher concentrations, the pleasant effects tend to be replaced by more negative ones: interference with motor coordination, verbal performance, and intellectual functions. When the BAC reaches 0.1%, most sensory and motor functioning is reduced, and many people become sleepy. At 0.2% most drinkers are completely unable to function, either physically or psychologically, because of the pronounced depression of the central nervous system, muscles, and other body systems. Coma usually occurs at a BAC of 0.35%, and any higher level can be fatal.

Alcohol Hangover   The symptoms of a hangover include headache, shakiness, nausea, diarrhea, fatigue, and impaired mental functioning. During a hangover, heart rate and blood pressure increase, making some individuals more vulnerable to heart attacks. Electroencephalography (brain wave measurement) shows diffuse slowing of brain waves for up to 16 hours after BAC drops to 0.0%. Studies of pilots, drivers, and skiers all indicate that coordination and cognition are impaired in a person with a hangover, increasing the risk of injury. A hangover is probably caused by a combination of the toxic products of alcohol breakdown, dehydration, and hormonal effects.

Alcohol Poisoning   Drinking large amounts of alcohol in a short time can rapidly raise the BAC into the lethal range. Death from alcohol poisoning may be caused either by central nervous system and respiratory depression or by inhaling fluid or vomit into the lungs. The amount of alcohol that renders a person unconscious is dangerously close to a fatal dose. Although passing out may prevent someone from drinking more, BAC can keep rising during unconsciousness because the body continues to absorb ingested alcohol into the bloodstream. Special care should be taken to ensure the safety of anyone who has been drinking heavily, especially if he or she passes out (see the box "Dealing with an Alcohol Emergency").

Using Alcohol with Other Drugs   Alcohol–drug combinations are a leading cause of drug-related deaths. Using alcohol while taking a medication that causes CNS depression increases the effects of both drugs, potentially leading to coma, respiratory depression, and death. Such drugs include barbiturates, Valium-like drugs, narcotics such as codeine, and OTC antihistamines such as Benadryl. For people who consume three or more drinks per day, use of OTC pain relievers like aspirin, ibuprofen, or acetaminophen increases the risk of stomach bleeding or liver damage. Some antibiotics and diabetes medications can also interact dangerously with alcohol.

Many illegal drugs are especially dangerous when combined with alcohol. Life-threatening overdoses occur at much lower doses when heroin and other narcotics are combined with alcohol. When cocaine and alcohol are used together, they form a toxic substance called cocaethylene, which is responsible for more than half of all cocaine-related deaths. A recent trend among young drinkers is mixing alcoholic beverages with caffeinated ones, especially highly caffeinated energy drinks. (see the box "Alcoholic Energy Drinks: The Dangers of Being 'Drunk and Wide Awake'").

Alcohol-Related Injuries and Violence   The combination of impaired judgment, weakened sensory perception, reduced inhibitions, impaired motor coordination, and increased aggressiveness and hostility that characterizes alcohol intoxication can be dangerous. Through homicide, suicide, automobile crashes, and other traumatic incidents, alcohol use is linked to more than 80,000 American deaths each year. The majority of people who attempt suicide have

TAKE CHARGE
Dealing with an Alcohol Emergency

Being very drunk is potentially life-threatening. Helping a drunken friend could save a life.

- Get the person out of harm's way. Don't let her drive, wander outside, or drink any more alcohol.

- If the person is unconscious, don't assume she is just "sleeping it off." Place her on her side with her knees up. This position helps prevent choking if she vomits.

- Monitor airway, breathing, and circulation (check pulse).

- Stay with the person. You need to be ready to help if she vomits or stops breathing.

- Don't try to give the person anything to eat or drink, including coffee or other drugs. Don't give cold showers or try to make her walk around. None of these things help anyone to sober up, and they can be dangerous.

Call 911 immediately in any of the following instances:

- You can't wake the person even with shouting or shaking.

- The person is taking fewer than eight breaths per minute, or her breathing seems shallow or irregular.

- You think the person took other drugs with alcohol.

- The person has had an injury, especially a blow to the head.

- The person drank a large amount of alcohol in a short period of time and then became unconscious. Death caused by alcohol poisoning most often occurs when the blood alcohol level rises very quickly due to rapid ingestion of alcohol.

If you aren't sure what to do, call 911. Alcohol poisoning is a medical emergency.

---

been drinking. Alcohol use more than triples the risk of fatal injuries during leisure activities such as swimming and boating. More than 50% of fatal falls and serious burns happen to people who have been drinking.

Alcohol and Aggression In 2008 more than 2,720,000 arrests were made for alcohol-related offenses (driving under the influence of alcohol, public drunkenness, and liquor law violations). Alcohol use contributes to over 50% of all murders, assaults, and rapes. Alcohol is frequently found in the bloodstream of victims as well as perpetrators. Some people become violent under alcohol's influence; these people may be predisposed to aggressive, impulsive behavior, tendencies are exacerbated by alcohol.

Alcohol abuse can wreak havoc on home life. Marital discord and domestic violence often occur in the presence of excessive alcohol consumption. Heavy drinking by parents is associated with child abuse.

Alcohol and Sexual Decision Making Alcohol seriously impairs a person's ability to make wise decisions about sex. Heavy drinkers are also more likely to have multiple sex partners and to engage in other forms of high-risk sexual behavior. Rates of sexually transmitted diseases (including HIV) and unwanted pregnancy are higher among people who drink heavily than among people who drink moderately or not at all.

> **QUICK STATS**
>
> **15.1%** of American males and **7.9%** of females aged 16 and older drove under the influence of alcohol in 2010.
> —SAMHSA, 2011

Women who binge-drink are at increased risk of rape and other forms of nonconsensual sex. Having sex with a person who is drunk or unconscious is sexual assault.

Drinking and Driving

In 2009, 10,839 Americans were killed in accidents involving drivers with a BAC of 0.08% or higher—about 32% of all traffic fatalities for the year. Each year more than 275,000 people are injured in alcohol-related car crashes—an average of one person injured every two minutes. In the 2010 National Survey on Drug Use and Health, 15.1% of Americans aged 18–20 admitted driving under the influence of alcohol at least once.

People who drink are unable to drive safely because their judgment is impaired, their reaction time is slower, and their coordination is reduced. Some driving skills are affected at BACs of 0.02% and lower.

The *dose-response function* is the relationship between the amount of alcohol or drug consumed and the type and intensity of the resulting effect. Higher doses of alcohol are associated with a much greater probability of automobile crashes (Figure 8.2). A person driving with a BAC of 0.14% is over 40 times more likely to be involved in a crash than someone with no alcohol in his or her blood.

In addition to an increased risk of injury and death, driving while intoxicated can have serious legal consequences. Drunk driving is against the law. The legal limit for BAC is

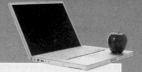

Over the past decade, the practice of blending alcoholic beverages with highly caffeinated energy drinks has grown increasingly popular, particularly among young adults and underage drinkers. According to the CDC, 31% of 12- to 17-year-olds and 34% of 18- to 24-year-olds regularly drink caffeinated alcoholic beverages (CABs), also known as alcoholic energy drinks (AEDs). The caffeine in a CAB masks the depressant effects of the alcohol, producing a "drunk and wide awake" state of alert intoxication, potentially leading the drinker to consume more alcohol than he or she would otherwise. Caffeine does nothing to speed the metabolism of the alcohol by the liver.

More than 13,000 ER visits related to the highly caffeinated drinks were reported in 2009, according to researchers from the U.S. Substance Abuse and Mental Health Services Administration (SAMHSA). Nearly half the emergencies occurred after the beverages were mixed with alcohol or other drugs, and young adults aged 18 to 25 accounted for more than half of those cases, the researchers found.

Commercial CABs are typically malt- or distilled-spirits-based and have higher alcohol content than beer (5–12% alcohol by volume compared to 6–8% for beer). The amount of caffeine and other stimulants in a CAB is usually not reported by the manufacturer. Health officials are concerned that many CABs contain much higher levels of caffeine than are found in soft drinks, which are limited by the FDA to 200 parts per million—the amount that meets the criteria for being "generally regarded as safe (GRAS)" for human consumption. However, SAMHSA researchers found some energy drinks that contained as much as 500 mg of caffeine—four to five times the amount in a cup of coffee.

A growing body of evidence highlights the risks associated with the use of caffeinated alcoholic beverages. For example, studies cited by the CDC have reported the following:

- Being in a "drunk/awake" state can lead to risky behaviors such as drunk driving, unplanned sex or sexual assault, and aggression.

- CAB drinkers are three times as likely as non-CAB drinkers to binge-drink.

- CAB drinkers are about twice as likely as non-CAB drinkers to report being taken advantage of sexually, taking advantage of someone sexually, or riding with a driver who was under the influence of alcohol.

- Emerging evidence indicates that CAB use, especially by adolescents, may lead to an increased risk of alcohol or drug dependence later in life.

These concerns and others led the FDA to launch an investigation into the safety, and even the legality, of commercial CABs. Prior to this investigation, two manufacturers of CABs voluntarily removed their products from the market and committed to discontinuing production of such beverages permanently. In light of this development, and skepticism among scientists that CABs can be proven safe, the CAB market may start to shrink—if not disappear altogether—in the near future.

SOURCES: Arria, A. M., et al. 2009. *Letter to the FDA Regarding the Use of Caffeine in Alcoholic Beverages* (http://www.fda.gov/downloads/food/foodingredientspackaging/ucm190372.pdf); Centers for Disease Control and Prevention. 2010. *Alcohol and Public Health: Caffeinated Alcoholic Beverages* (http://www.cdc.gov/alcohol/fact-sheets/cab.htm); U.S. Food and Drug Administration. 2010. Caffeinated Alcoholic Beverages (http://www.fda.gov/food/foodingredientspackaging/ucm190366.htm); U.S. Substance Abuse and Mental Health Services Administration, *Emergency Department Visits Involving Energy Drinks,* (http://www.nlm.nih.gov/medlineplus/news/fullstory_118979.html).

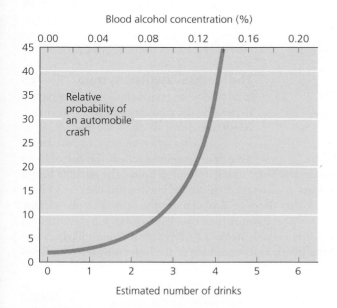

FIGURE 8.2 The dose-response relationship between BAC and automobile crashes.

0.08% in all states, the District of Columbia, and Puerto Rico. There are stiff penalties for drunk driving, including fines, loss of license, confiscation of vehicle, and jail time. Under current zero-tolerance laws in many states, drivers under age 21 who have consumed *any* alcohol may have their licenses suspended. If you are out of your home and drinking, find alternative transportation or appoint a *designated driver* who doesn't drink and can provide safe transportation home.

It's more difficult to protect yourself against someone else who drinks and drives. Learn to be alert to the erratic driving that signals an impaired driver. Warning signs include wide, abrupt, and illegal turns; straddling the center line or lane marker; driving against traffic; driving on the shoulder; weaving, swerving, or nearly striking objects or other vehicles; following too closely; erratic speed; driving with headlights off at night; and driving with the windows down in very cold weather. If you see any of these signs in another driver, avoid that vehicle by pulling off the road or turning at the nearest intersection. Report the driver to the police.

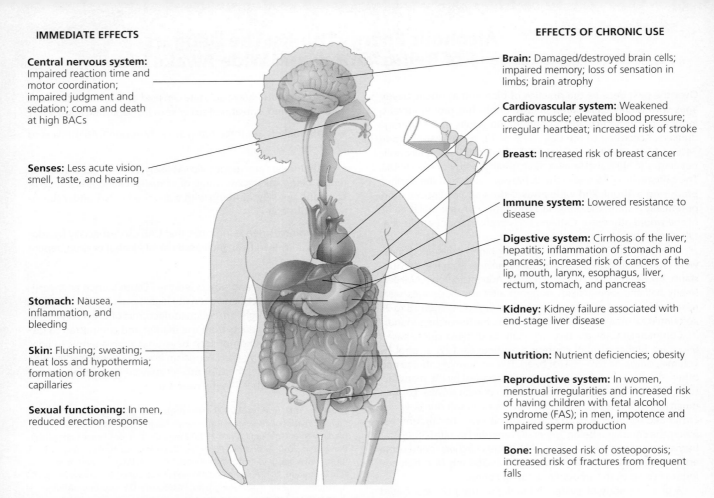

Central nervous system: Impaired reaction time and motor coordination; impaired judgment and sedation; coma and death at high BACs

Senses: Less acute vision, smell, taste, and hearing

Stomach: Nausea, inflammation, and bleeding

Skin: Flushing; sweating; heat loss and hypothermia; formation of broken capillaries

Sexual functioning: In men, reduced erection response

Brain: Damaged/destroyed brain cells; impaired memory; loss of sensation in limbs; brain atrophy

Cardiovascular system: Weakened cardiac muscle; elevated blood pressure; irregular heartbeat; increased risk of stroke

Breast: Increased risk of breast cancer

Immune system: Lowered resistance to disease

Digestive system: Cirrhosis of the liver; hepatitis; inflammation of stomach and pancreas; increased risk of cancers of the lip, mouth, larynx, esophagus, liver, rectum, stomach, and pancreas

Kidney: Kidney failure associated with end-stage liver disease

Nutrition: Nutrient deficiencies; obesity

Reproductive system: In women, menstrual irregularities and increased risk of having children with fetal alcohol syndrome (FAS); in men, impotence and impaired sperm production

Bone: Increased risk of osteoporosis; increased risk of fractures from frequent falls

FIGURE 8.3 The immediate and long-term effects of alcohol abuse.

The Effects of Chronic Abuse

Because alcohol is distributed throughout most of the body, it can affect many different organs and tissues (Figure 8.3).

The Digestive System   Even in the short term, alcohol can alter the functioning of the liver. Within just a few days of heavy alcohol consumption, fat begins to accumulate in liver cells, resulting in the development of "fatty liver." If drinking continues, inflammation of the liver can occur, resulting in alcoholic hepatitis, a frequent cause of hospitalization and death in alcoholics. Both fatty liver and alcoholic hepatitis are potentially reversible if the person stops drinking. With continued alcohol use, however, liver cells are progressively damaged and then destroyed. The destroyed cells are replaced by fibrous scar tissue, a condition known as **cirrhosis.** People with cirrhosis who continue to drink have only a 50% chance of surviving five or more years.

Alcohol can inflame the pancreas, causing nausea, vomiting, abnormal digestion, and severe pain. Unlike cirrhosis,

The U.S. Department of Health and Human Services has listed **alcohol as a known human carcinogen**.

which usually occurs after years of fairly heavy alcohol use, pancreatitis can occur after one or two severe binge-drinking episodes. Acute pancreatitis is often fatal; in survivors it can become a chronic condition.

The Cardiovascular System   The effects of alcohol on the cardiovascular system depend on the amount of alcohol consumed. Moderate doses of alcohol—one drink or less a day for women and one to two drinks a day for men—may reduce the risk of heart disease and heart attack in some people. (The possible health benefits of alcohol are discussed later in this chapter.) However, higher doses of alcohol harm the cardiovascular system. In some people, more than two drinks a day will elevate blood pressure, making stroke and heart attack more likely. Some alcoholics show a weakening of the heart muscle, a condition

cirrhosis   A disease in which the liver is severely damaged by alcohol, other toxins, or infection.

TERMS

known as **cardiac myopathy.** Binge drinking can cause "holiday heart," a syndrome characterized by serious abnormal heart rhythms, which usually appear within 24 hours of a binge episode.

Cancer In 2000 the U.S. Department of Health and Human Services added alcoholic beverages to its list of known human carcinogens. Chronic alcohol consumption is a clear risk factor for cancers of the mouth, throat, larynx, and esophagus. Five or six daily drinks, especially combined with smoking, increase the risk of these cancers by a factor of 50 or more. Alcohol also is largely responsible for the most common form of liver cancer.

Alcohol increases the risk of breast cancer, but quantifying the risk is complicated. A study published in 2011 shows that regularly drinking even a small quantity of alcohol—three to six drinks a week—could significantly increase the risk of breast cancer. Research conducted in 2009 indicates that even moderate drinking may encourage the recurrence of breast cancer in women who have survived the disease before.

Brain Damage Imaging studies document that many alcoholics experience brain shrinkage with loss of both gray and white matter, reduced blood flow, and slowed metabolic rates in some brain regions. About half of the alcoholics in the United States have cognitive impairments, ranging from mild to severe. These include memory loss, dementia, and compromised problem-solving and reasoning abilities. Malnutrition, particularly thiamine deficiency, contributes to severe brain damage.

Mortality Excessive alcohol consumption is a factor in several leading causes of death for Americans. Average life expectancy among alcoholics is about 15 years less than among nonalcoholics. About half the deaths caused by alcohol are due to chronic conditions such as cirrhosis and cancer; the

Experts warn that there is no safe level of alcohol consumption during pregnancy.

other half are due to acute conditions or events such as car crashes, falls, and suicide.

QUICK STATS

12.2% (about one in eight) of pregnant women drink alcohol, and almost **2%** (about 1 in 50) are binge drinkers.

—CDC, 2012

Alcohol Use during Pregnancy

During pregnancy, alcohol and its metabolic product acetaldehyde readily cross the placenta, harming the developing fetus. Damage to the fetus depends on the amount of alcohol consumed and the stage of the pregnancy. Early in pregnancy, heavy drinking can cause spontaneous abortion or miscarriage. Alcohol in early pregnancy, during critical fetal development periods, can also cause a collection of birth defects known as *fetal alcohol syndrome (FAS)*.

FAS is a permanent, incurable condition that causes lifelong disability; it is among the most common preventable causes of mental retardation in the Western world. Full-blown FAS occurs in up to 15 out of every 10,000 live births in the United States. About three times as many

TERMS

cardiac myopathy Weakening of the heart muscle through disease.

babies are born with **alcohol-related neurodevelopmental disorder (ARND).** Children with ARND appear physically normal but often have significant learning and behavioral disorders. The whole range of FAS and ARND is commonly called *fetal alcohol spectrum disorder (FASD).*

No one is sure exactly how much alcohol causes FASD or ARND. A 2002 study found that children born to mothers who drank as little as one and a half alcoholic drinks per week during their pregnancy weighed less and were shorter at age 14 than children of mothers who drank nothing during pregnancy. Such findings have led experts to assert that no amount of alcohol during pregnancy is safe.

Women who are trying to conceive, or who are sexually active without using effective contraception, should abstain from alcohol to avoid inadvertently harming their fetus in the first few days or weeks of pregnancy, before they know they're expecting. And because any alcohol consumed by a nursing mother quickly enters breast milk, many physicians advise nursing mothers to abstain from drinking.

Possible Health Benefits of Alcohol

Numerous studies have shown that, on average, light to moderate drinkers (no more than one drink per day for women, no more than two drinks per day for men) live longer than either abstainers or heavy drinkers. Alcohol consumption appears to confer health benefits primarily to older individuals.

The benefits of alcohol relate to heart health. The lowest rates of death from coronary heart disease (CHD) occur with moderate alcohol use, which in studies had a positive effect on both healthy people and individuals at risk for CHD. In a 2006 study of men age 50 and over, those who drank moderately each day reduced their risk of CHD by about 40% compared to men who never drank. The difference was not as great in women. Moderate drinking may improve heart health by raising blood levels of HDL (the beneficial form of cholesterol), by thinning the blood, or by reducing inflammation and the risk of dangerous blood clots, all of which can contribute to the risk of a heart attack. Some evidence also suggests that moderate drinkers may be less likely to develop or better able to manage a variety of other conditions, including diabetes, high blood pressure, strokes, arterial blockages in the legs, cognitive decline (including Alzheimer's disease), and benign prostate enlargement.

ALCOHOL ABUSE AND DEPENDENCE

The CDC estimates that about 60% of Americans age 18 and older drink alcohol routinely or infrequently. Approximately 15% of Americans are former drinkers, and 25% are lifetime abstainers. According to the National Survey on Drug Abuse and Health for 2010, almost 7% of Americans were classified as heavy alcohol users. Excessive alcohol use is responsible for

80,000 deaths per year among Americans and is the third leading lifestyle-related cause of death.

Abuse versus Dependence

Alcohol abuse is recurrent alcohol use that has negative consequences, such as drinking in dangerous situations (before driving, for instance) or drinking patterns that result in academic, professional, interpersonal, or legal difficulties. One does not have to be an alcoholic to have problems with alcohol. **Alcohol dependence,** or **alcoholism,** involves more extensive problems with alcohol use, usually involving physical tolerance and withdrawal.

How can you tell if you or someone you know is becoming alcohol-dependent? Look for the following warning signs:

- Drinking alone or secretively
- Using alcohol deliberately and repeatedly to perform or get through difficult situations
- Using alcohol as a way to "self-medicate" in order to dull strong emotions or negative feelings
- Feeling uncomfortable on certain occasions when alcohol is not available
- Escalating alcohol consumption beyond an already established drinking pattern
- Consuming alcohol heavily in risky situations, such as before driving
- Getting drunk regularly or more frequently than in the past
- Drinking in the morning or at other unusual times

Binge Drinking

Binge drinking is a pattern of rapid, periodic drinking that brings a person's blood alcohol concentration up to 0.08% or higher. This typically happens for men if they drink five or more drinks in about two hours, and for women if they drink four or more drinks in about two hours.

TERMS

alcohol-related neurodevelopmental disorder (ARND) Cognitive and behavioral problems seen in people whose mothers drank alcohol during pregnancy.

alcohol abuse The use of alcohol to a degree that causes physical damage, impairs functioning, or results in behavior harmful to others.

alcohol dependence or **alcoholism** A pathological use of alcohol or impairment in functioning due to alcohol; characterized by tolerance and withdrawal symptoms.

binge drinking Periodically drinking alcohol to the point of severe intoxication, usually from consuming five or more drinks in about two hours (men) or four or more drinks in about two hours (women).

Table 8.1 — The Effects of Binge Drinking on College Students

ALCOHOL-RELATED PROBLEM	PERCENTAGE OF STUDENTS EXPERIENCING PROBLEMS	
	NON–BINGE DRINKERS	FREQUENT BINGE DRINKERS
Drove after drinking alcohol	18	58
Did something they regretted	17	62
Argued with friends	10	43
Engaged in unplanned sex	9	41
Missed a class	9	60
Got behind in schoolwork	9	42
Had unprotected sex	4	21
Got hurt or injured	4	28
Got into trouble with police	2	14
Had five or more of these problems since school year began	4	48

SOURCE: Wechsler, H., and B. Wuethrich. 2003. *Dying to Drink: Confronting Binge Drinking on College Campuses,* reprint ed. Emmaus, PA: Rodale.

More than 38 million adults in the United States binge-drink about four times a month. Binge-drinking is the most common drinking pattern among men aged 18–34. Among Americans under 21 years old, most drinking occurs in the form of bingeing, and over 90% of the alcohol they drink is consumed while binge drinking. Over half the alcohol consumed by all adults in the United States is downed during binge drinking.

Binge drinking profoundly affects students' lives (see the box "College Binge Drinking"). Frequent binge drinkers are three to seven times more likely than non–binge drinkers to engage in unplanned or unprotected sex, to drive after drinking, and to get hurt or injured (Table 8.1). Binge drinkers are also more likely to miss classes, fall behind in schoolwork, and argue with friends. The more frequent the binges, the more problems these students encounter.

Alcoholism

Alcoholism (or alcohol dependence) is usually characterized by tolerance to alcohol and withdrawal symptoms when consumption stops.

Patterns and Prevalence   Alcoholism occurs among people of all ethnic groups and at all socioeconomic levels. There are different patterns of alcohol dependence, including these four common ones:

- Regular daily intake of large amounts
- Regular heavy drinking limited to weekends
- Long periods of sobriety interspersed with binges of daily heavy drinking lasting for weeks or months
- Heavy drinking limited to periods of stress

Once established, alcoholism often exhibits a pattern of exacerbations and remissions. Alcoholism is not hopeless, however; many alcoholics achieve permanent abstinence.

Health Effects   *Tolerance* means that a drinker needs more alcohol to achieve intoxication or the desired effect, that the effects of continued use of the same amount of alcohol are diminished, or that the drinker can function adequately at doses or a BAC that would produce significant impairment in a casual user. Heavy users of alcohol may need to consume about 50% more than they originally needed in order to experience the same degree of intoxication.

Withdrawal symptoms include trembling hands (shakes or jitters), a rapid pulse and accelerated breathing rate, insomnia, nightmares, anxiety, and gastrointestinal upset.

More severe withdrawal symptoms occur in about 5% of alcoholics. These include seizures, confusion, and **hallucinations.** Still less common is **delirium tremens (the DTs),** a medical emergency characterized by severe disorientation, confusion, epileptic-like seizures, and vivid hallucinations. The mortality rate from DTs can be as high as 15%.

Alcoholics face all the physical health risks associated with intoxication and chronic drinking described earlier in the chapter. Some damage is compounded by nutritional deficiencies that often accompany alcoholism. A mental problem associated with alcohol use is profound memory gaps (commonly known as blackouts).

Social and Psychological Effects   Alcohol use causes more serious social and psychological problems than all other forms of drug abuse combined. For every person who is an alcoholic, another three or four people are directly affected.

Alcoholics frequently suffer from mental disorders in addition to their substance dependence. Alcoholics are much more likely than nonalcoholics to suffer from clinical depression, panic disorder, schizophrenia, borderline personality disorder, and antisocial personality disorders. People with anxiety or panic attacks may try to use alcohol to lessen their anxiety, even though alcohol often makes these disorders worse.

QUICK STATS

Nearly **17** million Americans are heavy drinkers.

—SAMHSA, 2011

TERMS

hallucination   A false perception that does not correspond to external reality, such as seeing visions or hearing voices that are not there.

delirium tremens (the DTs)   A state of confusion brought on by the reduction of alcohol intake in an alcohol-dependent person; other symptoms are sweating, trembling, anxiety, hallucinations, and seizures.

Although college binge drinking has been a serious problem for decades, it has recently come under a harsh spotlight due largely to highly publicized alcohol-related tragedies on campus. Deaths from alcohol overdose, alcohol-related injuries (including motor vehicle crashes), violent crimes, student riots, and serious vandalism have all drawn attention to the epidemic of heavy drinking on college campuses.

Drinking on campus is pervasive. Approximately 61% of college students report having drunk alcohol at least once in the past month. According to the 2008 National Survey on Drug Use and Health, nearly 41% of college students reported binge drinking at least once in the past month, and 16% reported being heavy drinkers.

Every year, more than 1800 college students aged 18–24 die from alcohol-related injuries. Another 600,000 sustain unintentional alcohol-related injuries, 700,000 are assaulted by other students who have been drinking, and 100,000 are victims of alcohol-related date rape or sexual assault.

These statistics have shocked many students, administrators, and parents into demanding changes in college attitudes and policies regarding alcohol. In response, the Task Force of the National Advisory Council on Alcohol Abuse and Alcoholism was formed. Its report documents the extent of the alcohol problem and is a call to action for colleges and their surrounding communities to reexamine their alcohol policies and overhaul the campus drinking culture. These efforts, according to the Task Force, must focus on three levels:

1. Ultimately *each student* is accountable and must take responsibility for his or her own behavior. Needed are programs that encourage and support development of healthy attitudes toward alcohol. These programs should target students at increased risk of developing alcohol problems: first-year students, Greek organization members, and athletes.

2. The *student body as a whole* must work to discourage alcohol abuse. These efforts include promoting alcohol-free activities, reducing availability of alcohol, and avoiding social and commercial promotion of alcohol on campus. There should be an environment of acceptance of students who choose to abstain, and disapproval of students who drink to excess.

3. *Colleges and surrounding communities* must cooperate to discourage excessive drinking. Those who enable students to drink irresponsibly must be held accountable.

In 2007 the U.S. Surgeon General's Call to Action to Prevent and Reduce Underage Drinking suggested eliminating alcohol sponsorship of athletic events and other social activities. Working together, students, faculty, administrators, parents, and the community have begun to change the culture of heavy drinking on college campuses. Some schools have attempted to shift classes to Fridays and even Saturdays after it was found that binge drinking increases when students don't have Friday classes. Increasingly, incoming students are required to take a three-hour online class about alcohol. And there is stricter punishment for underage drinking and public drunkenness on some campuses, with the likelihood of suspension for repeat offenders.

Causes of Alcoholism   The precise causes of alcoholism are unknown, but many factors are probably involved. Some studies suggest that as much as 50–60% of a person's risk for alcoholism is determined by genetic factors. Not all children of alcoholics become alcoholics, however, and it is clear that other factors are involved. A person's risk of developing alcoholism may be increased by certain personality disorders, having grown up in a violent or otherwise troubled household, and imitating the alcohol abuse of peers and other role models. People who begin drinking excessively in their teens are especially prone to binge drinking and alcoholism later in life. Certain social factors have also been linked with alcoholism, including urbanization, disappearance of the extended family, a general loosening of kinship ties, increased mobility, and changing values.

Treatment   Some alcoholics recover without professional help. How often this occurs is unknown, but possibly as many as one-third stop drinking on their own or reduce their drinking enough to eliminate problems. Often these spontaneous recoveries are linked to an alcohol-related crisis, such as a blackout or alcohol-related automobile crash, a health problem (especially one that can be made worse by alcohol use), or the threat of losing one's job.

Most alcoholics, however, require a treatment program of some kind in order to stop drinking. Many different kinds of programs exist. No single treatment works for everyone, so a person may have to try different programs before finding the right one.

One of the oldest and best-known recovery programs is Alcoholics Anonymous (AA). AA consists of self-help groups that meet several times each week in many communities and follow a 12-step program. Important steps for people in these programs include recognizing that they are "powerless over alcohol" and must seek help from a "higher power" to regain control of their lives. By verbalizing these steps, the alcoholic

Alcohol treatment programs **achieve extended sobriety for about 50% of alcoholics** who participate.

directly addresses the denial that is often prominent in alcoholism and other addictions. Many AA members have a sponsor of their choosing who is available by phone 24 hours a day for individual support and crisis intervention.

Other recovery approaches are available. Some, like Rational Recovery and Women for Sobriety, deliberately avoid any emphasis on higher spiritual powers. A more controversial approach to problem drinking is offered by the group Moderation Management, which encourages people to manage their drinking behavior by limiting intake or abstaining.

Al-Anon is a companion program to AA for families and friends of alcoholics. In Al-Anon, spouses and others explore how they enable the alcoholic to drink by denying, rationalizing, or covering up his or her drinking and how they can change this codependent behavior.

Inpatient hospital rehabilitation is useful for some alcoholics, especially if they have serious medical or mental problems or if life stressors threaten to overwhelm them. There are also several medical treatments for alcoholism.

- *Disulfiram* (Antabuse) inhibits the metabolic breakdown of acetaldehyde and causes patients to flush and feel ill when they drink, thus theoretically inhibiting impulse drinking.

- *Naltrexone* (ReVia, Depade) binds to a brain pleasure center that reduces the craving for alcohol and decreases its pleasant, reinforcing effects.

- *Injectable naltrexone* (Vivtrol) is a single monthly shot administered by a health professional.

- *Acamprosate* (Campral) helps people maintain abstinence after they have stopped drinking.

Alcohol treatment programs are successful in achieving an extended period of sobriety for about half of those who participate. Success rates of conventional treatment programs are about the same for men and women and for people from different ethnic groups. AA remains the mainstay of treatment for most people and is often a component of even the most expensive treatment programs.

Gender and Ethnic Differences

Alcohol abusers come from all socioeconomic levels and cultural groups, but notable differences appear in drinking patterns between men and women and among different ethnic groups (Table 8.2).

Men   Among white American men, excessive drinking often begins in the teens or 20s and progresses gradually through the 30s until the man is clearly identifiable as an alcoholic by the time he is in his late 30s or early 40s. Other men may remain controlled drinkers until later in life, sometimes becoming alcoholic in association with retirement, the loss of friends and loved ones, boredom, illness, or psychological disorders.

Women   Women tend to become alcoholic at later ages and with fewer years of heavy drinking. It is not unusual for

Table 8.2   Users and Abusers of Alcohol in the United States by Demographic Characteristics: 2010

	PAST YEAR PREVALENCE (PERCENTAGE)	
	ALCOHOL USE	ALCOHOL ABUSE OR DEPENDENCE
Gender		
Male	69.4	9.5
Female	63.5	4.7
Ethnicity		
White	70.8	7.4
Black or African American	57.8	5.7
American Indian and Alaska Native	51.2	14.0
Native Hawaiian/Pacific Islander	N/A	5.0
Asian American	55.6	3.2
Hispanic or Latino	58.8	7.6
Two or more races	62.8	7.4
Total population	**66.4**	**7.0**

N/A = Not available.

SOURCE: Substance Abuse and Mental Health Services Administration. 2011. *Results from the 2010 National Survey on Drug Use and Health: Summary of National Findings*. Rockville, MD: Substance Abuse and Mental Health Services Administration, NSDUH Series H-41, HHS Publication No. (SMA) 11-4658.

women in their 40s or 50s to succumb to alcoholism after years of controlled drinking.

Women alcoholics develop cirrhosis and other medical complications more often and after a shorter period of heavier drinking than men, and have higher death rates—including deaths from cirrhosis—than male alcoholics. Female alcoholics are less likely to seek early treatment for drinking problems, possibly because of the social stigma attached to problem drinking. In addition, women may have an inherently greater biological risk for drinking alcohol.

African Americans   As a group, African Americans use less alcohol than most other groups (including whites), but they face disproportionately high levels of alcohol-related birth defects, cirrhosis, cancer, hypertension, and other medical problems. African American women are more likely to abstain from alcohol use than white women, but among black women who drink there is a higher percentage of heavy drinkers.

AA groups of predominantly African Americans are effective, perhaps because essential elements of AA—sharing common experiences, mutual acceptance of one another as human beings, and trusting a higher power—are already a part of African American culture.

Latinos Drinking patterns among Latinos vary significantly, depending on their specific cultural background and how long they and their families have lived in the United States. Drunk driving and cirrhosis are the most common causes of alcohol-related death and injury among Hispanic men. Hispanic women are more likely to abstain from alcohol than white or black women, but those who drink are at special risk for problems. Treating the entire family as a unit is an important part of treatment because family pride, solidarity, and support are important aspects of Latino culture.

Asian Americans As a group, Asian Americans have lower-than-average rates of alcohol abuse. However, acculturation may somewhat weaken the generally strong Asian taboos and community sanctions against alcohol misuse. For many Asian Americans, though, the genetically based physiological aversion to alcohol remains a deterrent to abuse. Ethnic agencies, health care professionals, and ministers seem to be the most effective sources of treatment for members of this group, when needed.

American Indians and Alaska Natives Alcohol abuse is one of the most widespread and severe health problems among American Indians and Alaska Natives, especially for adolescents and young adults. Excessive drinking varies from tribe to tribe but is generally high in both men and women. The rate of alcoholism among American Indians is twice that of the general population, and the death rate from alcohol-related causes is about eight times higher. Treatment may be more effective if it reflects tribal values.

Helping Someone with an Alcohol Problem

Helping a friend or relative with an alcohol problem requires skill and tact. Start by making sure you are not enabling someone to continue excessively using alcohol. Enabling takes many forms, such as making excuses for the alcohol abuser—for example, saying "he has the flu" when it is really a hangover. Another important step is open, honest labeling—"I think you have a problem with alcohol." Such explicit

statements usually elicit emotional rebuttals and may endanger a relationship. However, you are not helping your friends by allowing them to deny their problems with alcohol or other drugs. Taking action shows that you care. Even when problems are acknowledged, there is usually reluctance to get help. Your best role might be to obtain information about the available resources and persistently encourage their use.

WHO USES TOBACCO?

Despite the known health hazards, an estimated 69.6 million Americans aged 12 or older currently use tobacco. According to the 2011 National Health Interview Survey, nearly 20% of Americans aged 18 and older are current smokers, meaning they smoke cigarettes every day or most days. Young adults aged 18–25 have the highest rates of tobacco use, at more than 40%.

According to the survey, about 21.5% of men and 17.3% of women currently smoke cigarettes. Rates of smoking vary based on gender, age, ethnicity, and education level (Table 8.3). Adults with less than a 12th-grade education are much more likely to smoke cigarettes than those with a college degree.

As of June 2010, federal regulations made it a federal crime to sell tobacco products to anyone under 18 years of age. Even so, minors smoke an estimated 800 million packs of cigarettes each year; more than half of these cigarettes are purchased at retail stores. Each day roughly 1000 teenagers

> **QUICK STATS**
>
> ## 2.0 million
> **Americans aged 12–17 are current tobacco users.**
> —SAMHSA, 2011

Ask Yourself

QUESTIONS FOR CRITICAL THINKING AND REFLECTION

Do you know anyone with a serious alcohol problem? From what you have read in this chapter, would you say that person abuses alcohol or is dependent on it? What effects, if any, has this person's problem had on your life? Have you thought about getting support or help?

Table 8.3	Who Smokes?		
	PERCENTAGE OF SMOKERS		
	MEN	**WOMEN**	**TOTAL**
Ethnic Group (Age ≥ 18)			
White	22.6	19.6	21.0
Black	24.8	17.1	20.6
Asian	14.7	4.3	9.2
American Indian/ Alaskan Native	N/A	36	31.4
Latino	15.8	9.0	12.5
Education (Age ≥ 25)			
≤ 8 years	20.3	11.2	16.2
9–11 years	38.3	29.8	33.8
12 years (no diploma)	22.4	21.2	21.7
GED	46.4	44.1	45.2
High school graduate	27.4	20.6	23.8
Associate degree	21.8	16.4	18.8
Undergraduate degree	10.2	9.5	9.9
Graduate degree	7.1	5.4	6.3
Total	**21.5**	**17.3**	**19.3**

SOURCE: Centers for Disease Control and Prevention. 2011. Vital signs: current cigarette smoking among adults aged ≥18 years—United States, 2005–2010. *Morbidity and Mortality Weekly Report* 60(35): 1189–1232.

become regular smokers; at least one-third of them will die prematurely because of tobacco. According to the 2011 Monitoring the Future survey, nearly one-fifth of American teens become current smokers by the time they leave high school.

Men and women with other drug abuse problems frequently use tobacco. Smoking also is more prevalent among people with mental disorders than among the rest of the population: 40% of people with major depression, social phobias, and generalized anxiety disorder are smokers, as are 80% of people with schizophrenia. Such findings suggest that underlying psychological or physiological traits may predispose people to drug use, including tobacco.

WHY PEOPLE USE TOBACCO

Although people start smoking for a variety of reasons, they usually become long-term smokers after becoming addicted to nicotine—the key psychoactive ingredient in tobacco smoke.

Nicotine Addiction

The primary reason people continue to use tobacco is that they have become addicted to a powerful psychoactive drug: **nicotine.** Many researchers consider nicotine to be the most physically addictive of all the psychoactive drugs, including cocaine and heroin.

Some neurological studies indicate that nicotine acts on the brain in much the same way as cocaine and heroin. Nicotine reaches the brain via the bloodstream seconds after it is inhaled or, in the case of spit tobacco, absorbed through membranes of the mouth or nose. It triggers the release of powerful chemical messengers in the brain, including epinephrine, norepinephrine, and dopamine. But unlike street drugs, most of which are used to achieve a high, nicotine's primary attraction seems to lie in its ability to modulate everyday emotions.

At low doses, nicotine acts as a stimulant. It increases heart rate and blood pressure. In adults, nicotine can enhance

Spit tobacco users maintain blood nicotine levels as high as those of cigarette smokers.

> **nicotine** A poisonous, addictive substance found in tobacco and responsible for many of the effects of tobacco.
>
> **TERMS**

Ask Yourself

QUESTIONS FOR CRITICAL THINKING AND REFLECTION

Do any of your friends or family members smoke or use smokeless tobacco? What effect has it had on their health and relationships? Have you ever discussed their tobacco use with them? Why or why not?

alertness, concentration, information processing, memory, and learning. In some circumstances, nicotine acts as a mild sedative. Most commonly, nicotine relieves symptoms such as anxiety, irritability, and mild depression in tobacco users who are experiencing withdrawal. Nicotine addiction fulfills the criteria for substance dependence, including loss of control, tolerance, and withdrawal.

Loss of Control   About 69% of smokers say they want to quit completely, and about 52.4% of smokers try to quit each year. Regular tobacco users live according to a rigid cycle of need and gratification. On average, they can go no more than 40 minutes between doses of nicotine; otherwise they begin feeling edgy and irritable and have trouble concentrating. Tobacco users may plan their daily schedule around opportunities to satisfy their nicotine cravings; this loss of control and personal freedom can affect all the dimensions of wellness.

Tolerance and Withdrawal   Tobacco users build up tolerance to nicotine. Whereas one cigarette may make a beginning smoker nauseated and dizzy, a long-term smoker may have to chain-smoke a pack or more to experience the same effects. For most regular tobacco users, sudden abstinence from nicotine produces predictable withdrawal symptoms. These symptoms, which come on several hours after the last dose of nicotine, can include severe cravings, insomnia, confusion, tremors, difficulty concentrating, fatigue, muscle pains, headache, nausea, irritability, anger, and depression. Although most of these symptoms of physical dependence pass in two or three days, the craving associated with addiction can persist for weeks or months before gradually subsiding.

Social and Psychological Factors

Social and psychological forces combine with physiological addiction to maintain the tobacco habit. Many people, for example, have established habits of smoking while doing something else—while talking, working, drinking, and so on. The spit tobacco habit is also associated with certain situations—studying, drinking coffee, or playing sports. These associations can make it more difficult for users to break their habits because the activities they associate with tobacco use continue to trigger their urge.

Why Start in the First Place?

In the United States, nearly 90% of all adult smokers started smoking before age 18. The average age for starting smokers and smokeless tobacco users is around 15. The earlier people begin smoking, the more likely they are to become heavy smokers—and to die of tobacco-related disease.

Young people start using tobacco for a variety of reasons. Many young, white, male athletes, for example, begin using

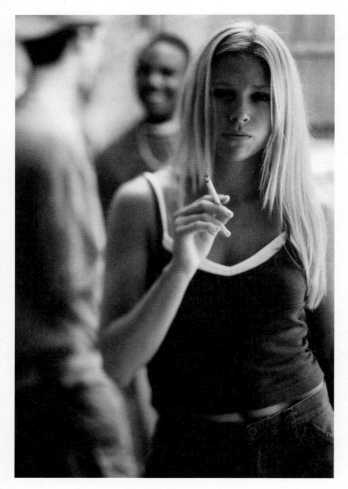

Most adult smokers began as teenagers.

stop smoking when they want. In fact, adolescents are more vulnerable to nicotine than are older tobacco users. Compared with older smokers, adolescents are more likely to become heavy smokers and develop dependence after fewer cigarettes. Nicotine addiction can start within a few days of smoking and after just a few cigarettes. In polls, about 75% of smoking teens state they wish they had never started.

Emulating Smoking in the Media   Both the Institute of Medicine and the National Cancer Institute have identified media portrayals of smoking as a key influence on young people who start smoking. In fact, studies by the National Cancer Institute have concluded that a direct causal relationship exists between media portrayals of smoking and actual smoking initiation by young moviegoers.

In general, the portrayal of smoking in films does not reflect U.S. patterns of tobacco use. The prevalence of smoking among lead characters is three to four times that among comparable Americans. Films typically show smokers as white, male, well educated, successful, and attractive. In reality, smokers tend to be poor and to have less education. Public campaigns to reduce images of smoking in movies have succeeded to an extent; smoking is shown less often in film and television shows now than even just a few years ago. Still, anti-smoking advocates say that films are still a critical and highly successful form of advertising for the tobacco industry.

HEALTH HAZARDS

Tobacco adversely affects nearly every part of the body, including the brain, stomach, mouth, and reproductive organs.

spit tobacco to emulate professional athletes. Young women commonly take up smoking because they think it will help them lose weight or stay thin. Most often, however, young people start smoking simply because their peers are already doing it.

Rationalizing the Dangers   Making the decision to smoke requires minimizing or denying the health risks of tobacco use. A sense of invincibility, characteristic of many adolescents and young adults, also contributes to the decision to use tobacco. Many teenagers believe they can

> **Nicotine addiction can start within a few days of smoking** and after just a few cigarettes.

Tobacco Smoke: A Toxic Mix

Tobacco smoke contains thousands of chemical substances, including acetone (nail polish remover), ammonia, hexamine (lighter fluid), and toluene (industrial solvent). Smoke from a typical unfiltered cigarette contains about 5 billion particles per cubic millimeter—50,000 times as many as are found in an equal volume of smoggy urban air. These particles, when condensed, form a brown, sticky mass called **cigarette tar.**

Carcinogens and Poisons   At least 69 chemicals in tobacco smoke are linked to the development of cancer. Some, such as benzo(a)pyrene and urethane, are **carcinogens**—that is, they directly cause cancer. Other chemicals, such as formaldehyde,

cigarette tar   A brown, sticky mass created when the chemical particles in tobacco smoke condense.

carcinogen   Any substance that causes cancer.

TERMS

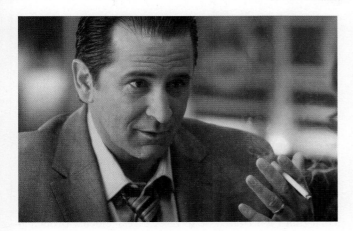

Anti-smoking advocates commonly criticize movies for their inclusion of characters who use tobacco.

are **cocarcinogens;** they do not themselves cause cancer but combine with other chemicals to stimulate the growth of certain cancers, at least in laboratory animals. Tobacco also contains poisonous substances, including arsenic and hydrogen cyanide. In addition to being an addictive psychoactive drug, nicotine is a poison that can be fatal in high doses.

Cigarette smoke contains carbon monoxide, the deadly gas in automobile exhaust, in concentrations 400 times greater than is considered safe in industrial workplaces. Carbon monoxide displaces oxygen in red blood cells, depleting the body's supply of oxygen needed for extra work. Carbon monoxide also impairs visual acuity, especially at night.

Additives Tobacco manufacturers use additives to manipulate the taste and effect of cigarettes and other tobacco products. Additives include sugars and other flavoring agents to mask the harsh, bitter taste of tobacco, so smokers can inhale more smoke and absorb more nicotine. Other flavor components act as bronchodilators, opening the lungs' airways and making it easier for nicotine to get into the bloodstream.

Some additives are intended to make **sidestream smoke** (the uninhaled smoke from a burning cigarette) less obvious and objectionable. Nearly 600 chemicals used in manufacturing cigarettes are approved as safe when used as food additives but may form carcinogens when heated or burned.

"Reduced Harm" Cigarettes Some smokers choose low-tar, low-nicotine, or filtered cigarettes because they believe them to be less dangerous alternatives. The tobacco industry has long promoted such products as "reduced harm" cigarettes, but there is no such thing as a safe cigarette. Smokers who switch to a low-nicotine brand often compensate by smoking more cigarettes, inhaling more deeply, taking larger or more frequent puffs, or blocking ventilation holes with lips or fingers to offset the effects of filters. In 2010, the use of terms like "light," "mild," and "low" on cigarette labels was banned by federal law.

Federal laws prohibit the use of terms such as "light" and "mild" on cigarette packaging.

Menthol Cigarettes About 70% of African American smokers smoke menthol cigarettes, as compared to 30% of whites. Studies have found that blacks absorb more nicotine than other groups and metabolize it more slowly; they also have lower rates of successful quitting. The anesthetizing effect of menthol, which may allow smokers to inhale more deeply and hold smoke in their lungs for a longer period, may be partly responsible for these differences.

The Immediate Effects of Smoking

The beginning smoker often has symptoms of mild nicotine poisoning: dizziness; faintness; rapid pulse; cold, clammy skin; nausea; vomiting; and diarrhea.

The effects of nicotine on smokers vary, depending greatly on the size of the nicotine dose and how much tolerance one has built up through previous smoking. Nicotine can either excite or tranquilize the nervous system, depending on dosage.

Nicotine has many other immediate effects. It stimulates the part of the brain called the **cerebral cortex.** It also stimulates the adrenal glands to discharge adrenaline. Nicotine inhibits the formation of urine; constricts the blood vessels, especially in the skin; accelerates the heart rate; and elevates blood pressure. Smoking depresses hunger sensations and dulls the taste buds.

The Long-Term Effects of Smoking

Smoking is linked to many deadly and disabling diseases. Research indicates that the total amount of tobacco smoke inhaled is a key factor contributing to disease. People who smoke more cigarettes per day, inhale deeply, puff frequently, smoke cigarettes down to the butts, or begin smoking at early ages run a greater risk of disease than do those who smoke more moderately or who do not smoke at all.

Cardiovascular Disease Although lung cancer tends to receive the most publicity, one form of cardiovascular disease, **coronary heart disease (CHD),** is actually the most widespread single cause of death for cigarette smokers. CHD

TERMS

cocarcinogen   A substance that works with a carcinogen to cause cancer.

sidestream smoke   The uninhaled smoke from a burning cigarette.

cerebral cortex   The outer layer of the brain, which controls complex behavior and mental activity.

coronary heart disease (CHD)   Cardiovascular disease caused by hardening of the arteries that supply oxygen to the heart muscle; also called *coronary artery disease.*

often results when the arteries that supply the heart muscle with blood develop **atherosclerosis.** In atherosclerosis, fatty deposits called **plaques** form on the inner walls of arteries, causing them to narrow and stiffen. Smoking and exposure to environmental tobacco smoke (ETS) permanently accelerate the rate of plaque accumulation in the coronary arteries—50% for smokers, 25% for ex-smokers, and 20% for people regularly exposed to ETS. The plaque completely blocks the flow of blood to a portion of the heart, a heart attack (**myocardial infarction**) occurs. CHD can also interfere with the heart's electrical activity, resulting in disturbances of the normal heartbeat rhythm.

Smokers have a death rate from CHD that is 70% higher than that of nonsmokers. The risks of CHD decrease rapidly when a person stops smoking. This is particularly true for younger smokers, whose coronary arteries have not yet been extensively damaged. Cigarette smoking has been linked to other cardiovascular diseases, including the following:

- *Stroke:* a sudden interference with the circulation of blood in a part of the brain, resulting in the destruction of brain cells.

- *Aortic aneurysm:* a bulge in the aorta caused by a weakening in its walls.

- *Pulmonary heart disease:* a disorder of the right side of the heart, caused by changes in the blood vessels of the lungs.

Lung Cancer and Other Cancers   Cigarette smoking is the primary cause of lung cancer. Those who smoke two or more packs of cigarettes a day have lung cancer death rates 12–25 times greater than those of nonsmokers. The dramatic rise in lung cancer rates among women in the past 40 years parallels the increase of smoking in this group; lung cancer now exceeds breast cancer as the leading cause of cancer deaths among women. The risk of developing lung cancer increases with the number of cigarettes smoked each day and the number of years of smoking. Greater your risk of developing a smoking-related cancer. Evidence suggests that after 1 year without smoking, the risk of lung cancer decreases substantially. After 10 years, the risk of lung cancer among ex-smokers is 50% lower than that of continuing smokers.

Research has also linked smoking to cancers of the trachea, mouth, pharynx, esophagus, larynx, pancreas, bladder, kidney, breast, cervix, stomach, liver, colon, and skin.

Chronic Obstructive Pulmonary Disease A smoker's lungs are constantly exposed to dangerous chemicals and irritants, so they must work harder to function adequately. The stresses placed on the lungs by smoking can permanently damage lung function and lead to *chronic obstructive pulmonary disease (COPD)*, also known as chronic obstructive lung disease (COLD), or chronic lower respiratory disease. COPD was the third leading cause of death in the United States in 2008 (the most recent year for which complete data

are available). This progressive and disabling disorder consists of several different but related diseases; emphysema and chronic bronchitis are two of the most common.

Emphysema is a disabling condition in which the air sacs in the walls of the lungs lose their elasticity and are gradually destroyed. The lungs' ability to take in oxygen and expel carbon dioxide is impaired. A person with emphysema is often breathless, gasps for air, and has the feeling of drowning. The heart must pump harder and may become enlarged. People with emphysema often die from a damaged heart. There is no known way to reverse this disease.

Chronic bronchitis is a persistent, recurrent inflammation of the bronchial tubes. When the cell lining of the bronchial tubes is irritated, it secretes excess mucus. Bronchial congestion is followed by a chronic cough, which makes breathing more and more difficult. If smokers have chronic bronchitis, they face a greater risk of lung cancer, no matter how old they are or how many cigarettes they smoke. Chronic bronchitis seems to be a shortcut to lung cancer.

Even when a smoker shows no signs of lung impairment or disease, cigarette smoking damages the respiratory system. Normally the cells lining the bronchial tubes secrete *mucus*, a sticky fluid that collects particles of soot, dust, and other substances in inhaled air. Mucus is carried up to the mouth by the continuous motion of *cilia*, which are hairlike structures that protrude from the inner surface of the bronchial tubes. If the cilia are destroyed or impaired, or if inhaled air contains more pollutants than the system can remove, the protection provided by cilia is lost.

Cigarette smoke first slows and then stops the action of the cilia. Eventually it destroys them, leaving delicate membranes exposed to injury from substances inhaled in cigarette smoke or from the polluted air. This interference with the functioning of the respiratory system often leads rapidly to the conditions known as *smoker's throat* and *smoker's cough*, as well as to shortness of breath. Other respiratory effects of smoking include a worsening of allergy and

> **QUICK STATS**
>
> **Smoking accounts for at least 30% of cancer deaths and 80% of all lung cancer deaths.**
> —American Cancer Society, 2012

TERMS

atherosclerosis   Cardiovascular disease caused by the deposit of fatty substances (called *plaque*) in the walls of the arteries.

plaque   A deposit on the inner wall of blood vessels; blood can coagulate around plaque and form a clot.

angina pectoris   Chest pain due to coronary heart disease.

myocardial infarction   A heart attack caused by the complete blockage of a main coronary artery.

emphysema   A disease characterized by a loss of lung tissue elasticity and destruction of the air sacs, impairing the lungs' ability to take in oxygen and expel carbon dioxide.

chronic bronchitis   Recurrent, persistent inflammation of the bronchial tubes.

asthma symptoms and an increase in the smoker's susceptibility to colds.

Additional Health, Cosmetic, and Economic Concerns

People who smoke are more likely to develop peptic ulcers because smoking impairs the body's healing ability. Smoking also increases the risk of gastroesophageal reflux, which causes heartburn. Smoking affects blood flow in the veins and arteries of the penis and is an independent risk factor for erectile dysfunction. Smoking is also linked to reduced fertility in both men and women. Smokers are at increased risk for tooth decay and gum and periodontal diseases, with symptoms appearing by the mid-20s. Smoking dulls the senses of taste and smell. Over time it increases the risk of hearing loss and of blindness. Smokers have higher rates of motor vehicle crashes, fire-related injuries, and back pain. Smoking can cause premature skin wrinkling, premature baldness, stained teeth, discolored fingers, and a persistent tobacco odor in clothes and hair. In September 2011 the average per-pack price of cigarettes was $5.29. A pack-a-day habit cost more than $1900 per year for cigarettes alone. In addition, smoking contributes to osteoporosis, increases the risk of complications from diabetes, and accelerates the course of multiple sclerosis.

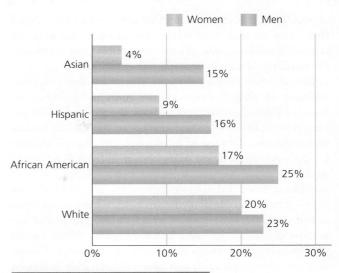

FIGURE 8.4 Differences in smoking prevalence between American men and women: United States, 2010.

SOURCE: American Cancer Society. 2012. *Cancer Facts and Figures, 2012*. Atlanta: American Cancer Society.

Cumulative Effects

The cumulative effects of tobacco use fall into two general categories. The first category is reduced life expectancy. A male who takes up smoking before age 15 and continues to smoke is only half as likely to live to age 75 as a male who never smokes. Females who have similar smoking habits also have a reduced life expectancy.

The second category involves quality of life. A national health survey begun in 1964 shows that smokers spend one-third more time away from their jobs because of illness than nonsmokers. Both male and female smokers show a greater rate of acute and chronic disease than people who have never smoked. Smokers become disabled at younger ages than nonsmokers and have more years of unhealthy life as well as shorter life spans.

Gender Differences in Health Hazards

As the rate of smoking among women approaches that of men (Figure 8.4), so do rates of tobacco-related illness and death. Although overall risks of tobacco-related illness are similar for women and men, sex appears to make a difference in some diseases. Women, for example, are more at risk for smoking-related blood clots and strokes than are men, and the risk is even greater for women using oral contraceptives. Among men and women with the same smoking history, the odds for developing three major types of cancer, including lung cancer, is 1.2–1.7 times higher in women than in men. Women who smoke have higher rates of osteoporosis (a bone-thinning disease that can lead to fractures), thyroid-related diseases, and depression than women who don't smoke.

QUICK STATS

In 2007 the total health care and productivity costs of smoking amounted to **$227 billion**.
—American Cancer Society, 2012

Women who smoke also have risks associated with reproduction and the reproductive organs. Smoking is associated with greater menstrual bleeding, greater duration of painful menstrual cramps, and more variability in menstrual cycle length. Smokers have a more difficult time becoming pregnant, and when they do become pregnant, they face increased chances of miscarriage or placental disorders that lead to bleeding and premature delivery. Rates of ectopic pregnancy, preeclampsia, and stillbirth are also higher among women who smoke. In addition, smoking is a risk factor for cervical cancer.

Other Forms of Tobacco Use

Many smokers have switched from cigarettes to other forms of tobacco, such as spit (smokeless) tobacco, cigars, pipes, clove cigarettes, bidis, and e-cigarettes. These alternatives, however, are far from safe.

Spit (Smokeless) Tobacco

More than 8.1 million adults and about 9% of all high school students are current spit tobacco users. Spit tobacco comes in two major forms: snuff and chewing tobacco (chew). In snuff, the tobacco leaf is processed into a coarse, moist powder and mixed with flavorings. Snuff is usually sold in small tins. Users place a "pinch," "dip," or "quid" between the lower lip or cheek and gum and suck on it. In chewing tobacco, the tobacco leaf may be shredded ("leaf"), pressed into bricks or cakes ("plugs"), or dried and twisted into ropelike strands ("twists"). Chew is usually sold in pouches. Users place a wad of tobacco in their mouth and then chew or suck it to release the nicotine. All types of smokeless tobacco cause an increase in saliva production, and the resulting tobacco juice is spit out or swallowed.

The nicotine in spit tobacco—along with flavorings and additives—is absorbed through the gums and lining of the mouth. Holding an average-size dip in the mouth for 30 minutes delivers about the same amount of nicotine as two or three cigarettes. Because of its nicotine content, spit tobacco is highly addictive. Some users keep it in their mouth even while sleeping.

Although not as dangerous as smoking cigarettes, the use of spit tobacco carries many health risks. Changes can occur in the mouth after only a few weeks of use. Gums and lips become dried and irritated and may bleed. White or red patches may appear inside the mouth; this condition, known as *leukoplakia*, can lead to oral cancer. About 25% of regular spit tobacco users have *gingivitis* (inflammation) and recession of the gums and bone loss around the teeth, especially where the tobacco is usually placed. The senses of taste and smell are usually dulled.

One of the most serious effects of spit tobacco is an increased risk of oral cancer—cancers of the lip, tongue, cheek, throat, gums, roof and floor of the mouth, and larynx. Spit tobacco contains at least 28 chemicals known to cause cancer, and long-term snuff use may increase the risk of oral cancer by as much as 50 times. Surgery to treat oral cancer is often disfiguring and may involve removing parts of the face, tongue, cheek, or lip.

Cigars and Pipes

Cigars are most popular among white males aged 18–44 with higher-than-average income and education, but women are also smoking cigars in record numbers. Cigar use is also growing among young people: in government surveys, 14% of American high school students reported having smoked at least one cigar in the previous month. Fewer than 1% of Americans, mostly males who also smoke cigarettes, are pipe smokers.

Cigars are made from rolled whole tobacco leaves; pipe tobacco is made from shredded leaves and is often flavored. Users absorb nicotine through the gums and lining of the mouth. Cigars contain more tobacco than cigarettes and so contain more nicotine and produce more tar when smoked. Large cigars may contain as much tobacco as a whole pack of cigarettes and take one or two hours to smoke.

The smoke from cigars contains many of the same toxins and carcinogens as the smoke from cigarettes, some in much higher quantities. The health risks of cigars depend on the number of cigars smoked and whether the smoker inhales. Because most cigar and pipe users do not inhale, they have a lower risk of cancer and cardiovascular and respiratory diseases than cigarette smokers. However, their risks are substantially higher than those of nonsmokers.

Nicotine addiction is another concern. Most adults who smoke cigars do so only occasionally, and there is little evidence

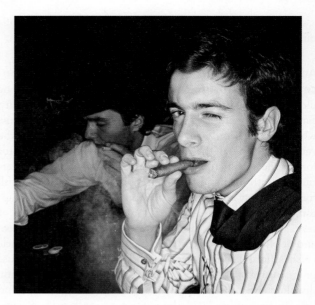

Occasional cigar smoking may be more likely to lead to nicotine addiction in teens than in adults.

that use of cigars by adults leads to addiction. The recent rise in cigar use among teens has raised concerns, however, because nicotine addiction almost always develops in the teen or young adult years.

> A large cigar may contain **as much tobacco as a whole pack of cigarettes**.

Clove Cigarettes and Bidis

Clove cigarettes, also called "kreteks" or "chicartas," are made of tobacco mixed with chopped cloves; they are imported primarily from Indonesia and Pakistan. Clove cigarettes contain almost twice as much tar, nicotine, and carbon monoxide as conventional cigarettes and so present all the same health hazards. Some chemical constituents of cloves may also be dangerous. There have been a number of serious respiratory injuries and deaths from the use of clove cigarettes.

Bidis, or "beadies," are small cigarettes imported from India that contain species of tobacco different from those used by U.S. cigarette manufacturers. The tobacco in bidis is hand-rolled in Indian ebony leaves and often flavored; clove, mint, chocolate, and fruit varieties are available. Bidis contain up to four times more nicotine than U.S. cigarettes and twice as much tar.

E-Cigarettes

The electronic cigarette, also known as an *e-cig*, is a battery-powered device that resembles a real cigarette. Instead of containing tobacco, the device uses a changeable filter that contains one or more chemicals, such as nicotine, flavorings, and other compounds. The user "smokes" an e-cig by sucking the filtered end; the device's battery heats the chemicals to create an inhalable vapor. During use, the device's tip even glows like the burning end of a real cigarette.

Marketers of e-cigs have claimed that the devices deliver only nicotine, making them a safe cigarette that does not cause cancer and that can serve as an alternative to other nicotine replacement products such as gum and patches. However, the

FDA has warned consumers not to purchase or use e-cigs because analysis of nearly 20 e-cig cartridges revealed that they contained carcinogens, including at least one of the same carcinogens found in real cigarettes.

THE EFFECTS OF SMOKING ON THE NONSMOKER

Tens of thousands of nonsmokers die each year because of exposure to secondhand smoke. Further, the medical and societal costs of tobacco use are enormous.

Environmental Tobacco Smoke

The U.S. Environmental Protection Agency (EPA) has designated **environmental tobacco smoke (ETS)**—more commonly called *secondhand smoke*—a Class A carcinogen. The Surgeon General has concluded that there is no safe level of exposure to ETS; even brief exposure can cause serious harm.

Environmental tobacco smoke consists of mainstream smoke and sidestream smoke. Smoke exhaled by smokers is referred to as **mainstream smoke.** Sidestream smoke enters the atmosphere from the burning end of a cigarette, cigar, or pipe. Nearly 85% of the smoke in a room where someone is smoking comes from sidestream smoke. Undiluted sidestream smoke, because it is not filtered through either a cigarette filter or a smoker's lungs, has twice as much tar and nicotine, three times as much benzo(a)pyrene, almost three times as much carbon monoxide, and three times as much ammonia.

In rooms where people are smoking, levels of carbon monoxide can exceed those permitted by Federal Air Quality Standards for outside air. The carcinogens in the secondhand smoke from a single cigar exceed those of three cigarettes, and cigar smoke contains up to 30 times more carbon monoxide. The CDC estimates that 88 million nonsmoking Americans (including 54% of children aged 3–11 years) are exposed to some level of ETS every year.

ETS Effects Nonsmokers subjected to ETS frequently develop coughs, headaches, nasal discomfort, and eye irritation. Other symptoms range from breathlessness to sinus problems. People with allergies tend to suffer the most.

> According to the U.S. Surgeon General, **there is no safe level of exposure to secondhand smoke.**

ETS causes 3400 lung cancer deaths and about 46,000 deaths from heart disease each year in people who do not smoke. ETS aggravates asthma and increases the risk for breast and cervical cancers.

Scientists have been able to measure changes that contribute to lung tissue damage and potential tumor promotion in the bloodstreams of healthy young test subjects who spend just three hours in a smoke-filled room. After just 30 minutes of exposure to ETS, the function in the coronary arteries of healthy nonsmokers is reduced to the same level as that of smokers.

Infants, Children, and ETS Infants exposed to smoke are more likely to die of sudden infant death syndrome (SIDS) than are babies not exposed to ETS. Children under age 5 whose primary caregiver smokes 10 or more cigarettes per day have measurable blood levels of nicotine and tobacco carcinogens. Chemicals in tobacco smoke also show up in breast milk, and breastfeeding may pass more chemicals to the infant of a smoking mother than direct exposure to ETS.

ETS triggers bronchitis, pneumonia, and other respiratory infections in infants and toddlers, resulting in as many as 15,000 hospitalizations each year. ETS is a risk factor for asthma and aggravates the symptoms of children who already have asthma. ETS is also linked to reduced lung function and fluid buildup in the middle ear, a contributing factor in middle-ear infections, a leading reason for childhood surgery. Later in life, people exposed to ETS as children are at increased risk for lung cancer, emphysema, and chronic bronchitis.

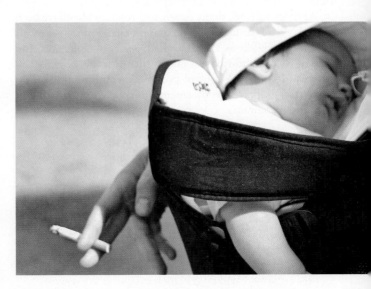

Millions of American infants and children are regularly exposed to environmental tobacco smoke.

TERMS

environmental tobacco smoke (ETS) Smoke that enters the atmosphere from the burning end of a cigarette, cigar, or pipe, as well as smoke that is exhaled by smokers; also called *secondhand smoke*.

mainstream smoke Smoke that is inhaled by a smoker and then exhaled into the atmosphere.

Smoking and Pregnancy

Smoking almost doubles a pregnant woman's chance of having a miscarriage, and it significantly increases her risk of ectopic pregnancy. Maternal smoking causes hundreds of infant deaths in the United States each year, primarily due to premature delivery and smoking-related problems with the placenta. Maternal smoking is a major factor in low birth weight, which puts newborns at high risk for infections and other serious problems. If a nonsmoking mother is regularly exposed to ETS, her infant is also at greater risk for low birth weight.

Babies born to mothers who smoke more than two packs a day perform poorly on developmental tests in the first hours after birth, compared to babies of nonsmoking mothers. Later in life, obesity, hyperactivity, short attention span, and lower scores on spelling and reading tests all occur more frequently in children whose mothers smoked during pregnancy than in those born to nonsmoking mothers. Prenatal tobacco exposure has also been associated with behavioral problems in children.

WHAT CAN BE DONE?

There are many ways to act against this public health threat.

Action at Many Levels

There are now thousands of local ordinances across the nation designed to discourage smoking in public places. An assessment made in 2010 found that nearly 80% of Americans live in municipalities that restrict or ban smoking in public buildings, workplaces, restaurants, and bars. Hundreds of colleges and universities now have totally smoke-free campuses or prohibit smoking in residential buildings. As local nonsmoking laws proliferate, evidence mounts that environmental restrictions are effective in encouraging smokers to quit.

At the state level, many tough anti-tobacco laws have been passed. As of January 2012, comprehensive smoke-free air laws were in effect in 35 states, the District of Columbia, and Puerto Rico. California has one of the most aggressive—and successful—tobacco control programs, combining taxes on cigarettes, graphic advertisements, and bans on smoking in bars and restaurants.

Ask Yourself

QUESTIONS FOR CRITICAL THINKING AND REFLECTION

What are your views on the government's role in regulating tobacco products? Is there currently enough regulation, or should the government go further in controlling the production and marketing of these products? What events or experiences have shaped your views on this issue?

Until 2009, the U.S. FDA did not have the power to regulate tobacco products. That changed when Congress passed.

The Family Smoking Prevention and Tobacco Control Act, giving the FDA broad regulatory powers over the production, marketing, and sale of tobacco products. The law gives the FDA the power to eliminate or control levels of the thousands of chemical additives used to make tobacco more appealing and addictive. In addition, the legislation strengthens health warnings and places even greater limits on tobacco advertising.

The World Health Organization has taken the lead in international anti-tobacco efforts by sponsoring the Framework Convention on Tobacco Control. Another international activity is the annual commemoration of World No Tobacco Day (May 31), on which smokers are encouraged to stop smoking for one day. Such local, state, national, and international efforts represent progress, but health activists warn that tobacco industry influence remains strong. The tobacco industry contributes heavily to sympathetic legislative officeholders and candidates, spending millions of federal lobbying activities. The tobacco industry has also focused increasing attention on the developing world, exporting its products to countries where there are few or no consumer protection laws in place.

Individual Action

Nonsmokers have the right not only to breathe clean air but also to take action to help solve one of society's most serious public health threats. Here are a few actions you can take. When a smoker violates a no-smoking designation, complain. If your favorite restaurant or shop doesn't have a nonsmoking policy, ask the manager to adopt one. If you see children buying tobacco, report this illegal activity to the facility manager or the police. Learn more about addiction and tobacco cessation so you can better support the tobacco users you know. Vote for candidates who support anti-tobacco measures; contact local, state, and national representatives to express your views.

You can also cancel your subscriptions to magazines that carry tobacco advertising; send a letter to the publisher explaining your decision. Voice your opinion about other positive representations of tobacco use. (A recent study found that more than two-thirds of children's animated feature films have featured tobacco or alcohol use with no clear message that such practices were unhealthy.) Volunteer with the American Lung Association, the American Cancer Society, or the American Heart Association.

HOW A TOBACCO USER CAN QUIT

Giving up tobacco is a long-term process. Research shows that tobacco users move through predictable stages—from being uninterested in stopping, to thinking about change, to making a serious effort to stop, to finally maintaining abstinence. But most smokers attempt to quit several times before they finally succeed. Relapse is a normal part of the process.

Table 8.4   Benefits of Quitting Smoking

Within 20 minutes of your last cigarette:
- You stop polluting the air.
- Blood pressure drops to normal.
- Pulse rate drops to normal.
- Temperature of hands and feet increases to normal.

8 hours:
- Carbon monoxide level in blood drops to normal.
- Oxygen level in blood increases to normal.

24 hours:
- Chance of heart attack decreases.

48 hours:
- Nerve endings start regrowing.
- Ability to smell and taste is enhanced.

2–3 months:
- Circulation improves.
- Walking becomes easier.
- Lung function increases up to 30%.

1–9 months:
- Coughing, sinus congestion, fatigue, and shortness of breath all decrease.

1 year:
- Heart disease death rate is half that of a smoker.

5 years:
- Stroke risk drops nearly to the risk for nonsmokers.

10 years:
- Lung cancer death rate drops to 50% of that of continuing smokers.
- Incidence of other cancers (mouth, throat, larynx, esophagus, bladder, kidney, and pancreas) decreases.
- Risk of ulcer decreases.

15 years:
- Risk of lung cancer is about 25% of that of continuing smokers.
- Risks of heart disease and death are close to those of nonsmokers.

The Benefits of Quitting

Giving up tobacco provides immediate health benefits to men and women of all ages (Table 8.4). The younger people are when they stop smoking, the more pronounced the health improvements. And these improvements gradually increase as the period of nonsmoking lengthens. It's never too late to quit. According to a U.S. Surgeon General's report, people who quit smoking, regardless of age, live longer than people who continue to smoke.

Options for Quitting

Most tobacco users—76% in a recent survey—want to quit, and half of those who want to quit will make an attempt this year. What are their options? No single method works

> **It's never too late to stop smoking,** and smokers have a variety of options for quitting.

for everyone, but each does work for some people some of the time.

Behavioral Strategies Choosing to quit requires developing a strategy for success. Some people quit cold turkey, whereas others taper off slowly. There are over-the-counter and prescription products that help many people. Behavioral factors that have been shown to increase the chances of success are support from others and regular exercise. Support can come from friends and family and/or formal group programs sponsored by organizations such as the American Cancer Society and the American Lung Association, or by your college health center or community hospital.

Most smokers in the process of quitting experience both physical and psychological effects of nicotine withdrawal, and exercise can help with both. For many smokers, tobacco use is associated with certain times and places—following a meal, for example. Resolving to walk after dinner instead of lighting up provides a distraction from cravings and eliminates the cues that trigger a desire to smoke. In addition, many people worry about weight gain associated with quitting. Although most ex-smokers do gain a few pounds, at least temporarily, incorporating exercise into a new tobacco-free routine lays the foundation for healthy weight management. The health risks of adding a few pounds are minimal compared to the risks of continued smoking.

Free telephone quitlines are a popular and effective strategy to help stop smoking. Quitlines are staffed by trained counselors who help each caller plan a personal quitting strategy, usually including a combination of nicotine replacement therapy, changes in daily habits, and emotional support. The Department of Health and Human Services has a national toll-free number, 1-800-QUITNOW (1-800-784-8669), to serve as a single access point for smokers seeking information and assistance in quitting.

As with any significant change in health-related behavior, giving up tobacco requires planning, sustained effort, and support. It is an ongoing process, not a one-time event. The "Behavior Change Strategy" section describes the steps that successful quitters follow.

Smoking Cessation Products People who want to stop smoking can also try smoking cessation aids. Although pharmacological options are limited, the few available drugs have proved successful.

CHANTIX (VARINICLINE) The newest smoking cessation drug, marketed under the name Chantix, works in two ways: it reduces nicotine cravings, easing the withdrawal process, and it blocks the pleasant effects of nicotine. The drug acts on neurotransmitter receptors in the brain.

Unlike most smoking cessation products currently on the market, Chantix is not a nicotine replacement. For this reason, smokers may be advised to continue smoking for the first few days of treatment to avoid withdrawal and to allow the drug to build up in their bodies. The approved course of treatment is 12 weeks, but the duration and recommended dosage depend on several factors, including the smoker's general health and the length and severity of his or her nicotine addiction.

Side effects reported with Chantix include nausea, headaches, vomiting, sleep disruptions, and changes in taste perception. People with kidney problems or who take certain medications should not take Chantix, and it is not recommended for women who are pregnant or nursing. In 2008 the FDA issued a public health advisory warning that some Chantix users suffered adverse reactions, such as behavioral changes, agitation, depression, suicidal thoughts, and attempted suicide. Anyone taking Chantix should immediately notify his or her doctor of any sudden change in mood or behavior.

ZYBAN (BUPROPION) Bupropion is an antidepressant (prescribed under the name Wellbutrin) as well as a smoking cessation aid (prescribed under the name Zyban). As a smoking cessation aid, bupropion eases the symptoms of nicotine withdrawal and reduces the urge to smoke. Like Chantix, it acts on neurotransmitter receptors in the brain.

Bupropion users have reported an array of side effects, but they are rare. Side effects may be reduced by changing the dosage, taking the medicine at a different time of day, or taking it with or without food. Zyban and Wellbutrin should not be taken together.

NICOTINE REPLACEMENT PRODUCTS The most widely used smoking cessation products replace the nicotine that the user would normally get from tobacco. The user continues to get nicotine, so withdrawal symptoms and cravings are reduced. Although still harmful, nicotine replacement products provide a cleaner form of nicotine without the thousands of poisons and tars produced by burning tobacco. Less of the product is used over time as the need for nicotine decreases.

Nicotine replacement products come in several forms, including patches, gum, lozenges, nasal sprays, and inhalers. They are available in a variety of strengths and can be worked into many different smoking cessation strategies. Most are available without a prescription.

The nicotine patch is popular because it can be applied and forgotten until it needs to be removed or changed, usually every 16 or 24 hours. Placed on the upper arm or torso, it releases a steady stream of nicotine, which is absorbed through the skin. The main side effects are skin irritation and redness. Nicotine gum and nicotine lozenges have the advantage of allowing the smoker to use them whenever he or she craves nicotine. Side effects of nicotine gum include mouth sores and headaches; nicotine lozenges can cause nausea and heartburn. Nicotine nasal sprays and inhalers are available only by prescription.

Although all these products have proved to be effective in helping users stop smoking, experts recommend them only as one part of a complete smoking cessation program. Such a program should include regular professional counseling and physician monitoring.

Connect to Your Choices

Have you ever thought about why you make the drinking and smoking decisions you do? Many factors can influence our choices, some not as obvious as others. Did your parents drink or smoke, and did their choices influence your decisions? Is your desire to drink or smoke affected when either behavior is glamourized in the movies? Is drinking normalized on your campus by sponsorship of athletic events by alcoholic beverage companies? Do you live in a state where the tobacco industry is strong and smoking is socially accepted, or do you live where there are strict regulations on smoking?

What are the external factors that influence your choices about tobacco use? What are your inner motivations and core values, and how do they affect your choices? Based on what you learned in this chapter, will you make some different choices in the future? If so, what will they be?

Go online to Connect to complete this activity: www.mcgraw-hillconnect.com

TIPS FOR TODAY AND THE FUTURE

The responsible use of alcohol means drinking in moderation or not at all. The best approach to tobacco use is never to start.

RIGHT NOW YOU CAN:
- Consider whether there is a history of alcohol abuse or dependence in your family.
- Take stock of the number of alcoholic beverages in your home. Does there always seem to be a lot on hand? Do you find yourself purchasing alcohol frequently? What do your purchasing habits say about your drinking?
- If you smoke, think about the next time you'll want a cigarette. Visualize yourself enjoying this activity without smoking.

IN THE FUTURE YOU CAN:
- Think about the next party you plan to attend. Decide how much you will drink at the party, and how you will get home afterward.
- If you have a family member who smokes, resolve to talk to that person, offering support and assistance if he or she is interested in quitting.
- If you smoke, resolve to quit. Research your options for quitting and choose the one you think will work best for you.

SUMMARY

• After being absorbed into the bloodstream in the stomach and small intestine, alcohol is transported throughout the body. The liver metabolizes alcohol as blood circulates through it.

• Alcohol is a CNS depressant. At low doses, it tends to make people feel relaxed. At higher doses, it interferes with motor and mental functioning; at very high doses, alcohol poisoning, coma, and death can occur.

• Alcohol use increases the risk of injury and violence; drinking before driving is particularly dangerous, even at low doses.

• Chronic alcohol use has negative effects on the digestive and cardiovascular systems and increases cancer risk and overall mortality.

• Pregnant women who drink risk giving birth to children with a cluster of birth defects known as fetal alcohol syndrome (FAS). Even occasional drinking during pregnancy can cause brain injury in the fetus.

• Alcohol abuse involves drinking in dangerous situations or drinking to a degree that causes academic, professional, interpersonal, or legal difficulties.

• Alcohol dependence, or alcoholism, is characterized by more extensive problems with alcohol, usually involving tolerance and withdrawal.

• Binge drinking is a common form of alcohol abuse on college campuses that has negative effects on both drinking and nondrinking students.

• Physical consequences of alcoholism include the direct effects of tolerance and withdrawal, as well as all the problems associated with chronic drinking. Psychological problems include memory loss and additional mental disorders such as depression.

• Alcoholism treatment approaches include mutual support groups like AA, job- and school-based programs, inpatient hospital programs, and pharmacological treatments.

• Smoking is the largest preventable cause of ill health and death in the United States. Nevertheless, millions of Americans use tobacco.

• People who begin smoking are usually imitating others or responding to seductive advertising. Smoking is associated with low education level and the use of other drugs.

• Tobacco smoke is made up of hundreds of different chemicals, including some that are carcinogenic or poisonous or that damage the respiratory system.

• Nicotine acts on the nervous system as a stimulant or a depressant. It can cause blood pressure and heart rate to increase, straining the heart.

• Cardiovascular disease is the most widespread cause of death for cigarette smokers. Cigarette smoking is the primary cause of lung cancer and is linked to many other cancers and respiratory diseases.

• The use of spit tobacco leads to nicotine addiction and is linked to a variety of cancers of the head and neck.

• Cigars, pipes, clove cigarettes, and bidis are not safe alternatives to cigarettes.

• Environmental tobacco smoke (ETS) contains high concentrations of toxic chemicals and can cause headaches, eye and nasal irritation, and sinus problems. Long-term exposure to ETS causes cancer and heart disease.

• Smoking during pregnancy increases the risk of miscarriage, stillbirth, congenital abnormalities, premature birth, and low birth weight. SIDS, behavior problems, and long-term impairments in development are also risks.

• Giving up smoking is a difficult and long-term process. Although most ex-smokers quit on their own, some smokers benefit from stop-smoking programs, OTC and prescription medications, and support groups.

FOR MORE INFORMATION

BOOKS

American Lung Association. 2004. *How to Quit Smoking without Gaining Weight.* New York: American Lung Association. *Provides methods for smokers who want to quit but are afraid they'll gain weight as a result.*

Carr, A. 2010. *The Easy Way to Stop Smoking.* New York: Sterling. *A best-selling self-help book for smokers who want to stop.*

Committee on Secondhand Smoke Exposure and Acute Coronary Events, Institute of Medicine. 2010. *Secondhand Smoke Exposure and Cardiovascular Effects: Making Sense of the Evidence.* Washington, D.C.: National Academies Press. *A review of the available research and literature on the relationship between secondhand smoke and heart disease; includes an evaluation of smoking bans in several locales around the world.*

Dean, M. 2007. *Empty Cribs: The Impact of Smoking on Child Health.* New York: Arts & Sciences Publishing. *Examines the effects of smoking on children, before and after birth.*

Kinney, J. 2011. *Loosening the Grip: A Handbook of Alcohol Information,* 10th ed. New York: McGraw-Hill. *An authoritative source of information on alcohol use and its impact on families and society.*

Marlatt, G. A., M. E. Larimer, and K. Wittiewitz (eds.). 2011. *Harm Reduction: Pragmatic Strategies for Managing High-Risk Behaviors,* 2nd ed. New York: Guilford. *An introductory guide to the complexities of harm reduction approaches, whether applied to alcohol or drug abuse, tobacco use, or risky sexual behavior.*

Sheff, N. 2012. *We All Fall Down: Living with Addiction.* New York: Little, Brown. *A compelling memoir about one man's struggle with alcohol and drugs, detox, rehab, relapse, and recovery.*

Vander Ven, T. 2011. *Getting Wasted: Why College Students Drink Too Much and Party So Hard.* New York: NYU Press. *A sociologist looks with both personal and scientific interest at the drinking culture on American college campuses; he focuses on the social process of alcohol use—the way students drink together—and comes to some surprising conclusions.*

Vaknin, J. 2007. *Smoke Signals: 100 Years of Tobacco Advertising.* London: Middlesex University Press. *An exploration of the many ways tobacco products have been marketed to consumers.*

ORGANIZATIONS, HOTLINES, AND WEBSITES

Action on Smoking and Health (ASH). An advocacy group that provides statistics, news briefs, and other information.

> http://ash.org

Al-Anon Family Group Headquarters. Provides information and referrals to local Al-Anon and Alateen groups. The website includes a self-quiz to determine if you are affected by someone's drinking.

> http://www.al-anon.alateen.org

Alcoholics Anonymous (AA) World Services. Provides general information about AA, literature about alcoholism, and information about AA meetings and related 12-step organizations.

> http://www.aa.org

Alcohol Treatment Referral Hotline. Provides referrals to local intervention and treatment providers.

> 800-ALCOHOL

American Cancer Society (ACS). Sponsor of the annual Great American Smokeout; provides information about the dangers of tobacco, as well as tools for prevention and cessation for both smokers and users of spit tobacco.

> http://www.cancer.org

American Lung Association. Provides information about lung diseases, tobacco control, and environmental health.

> http://www.lungusa.org

Bacchus and Gamma Peer Education Network. An association of college- and university-based peer education programs that focus on prevention of alcohol abuse.

> http://www.bacchusgamma.org

CDC's Tobacco Information and Prevention Source (TIPS). Provides research results, educational materials, and tips on how to quit smoking; website includes special sections for kids and teens.

> http://www.cdc.gov/tobacco

The College Alcohol Study. Harvard School of Public Health. Provides information about and results from the recent studies of binge drinking on college campuses.

> http://www.hsph.harvard.edu/cas

Mothers Against Drunk Driving (MADD). Supports efforts to develop solutions to the problems of drunk driving and underage drinking; provides news, information, and brochures about many topics, including a guide for giving a safe party.

> http://www.madd.org

National Association for Children of Alcoholics (NACoA). Provides information and support for children of alcoholics.

> http://www.nacoa.net

National Council on Alcoholism and Drug Dependence (NCADD). Provides information and counseling referrals.

> 212-269-7797; 800-NCA-CALL (24-hour Hope Line)

> http://www.ncadd.org

National Institute on Alcohol Abuse and Alcoholism (NIAAA). Provides booklets and other publications on a variety of alcohol-related topics, including fetal alcohol syndrome, alcoholism treatment, and alcohol use and minorities.

> http://www.niaaa.nih.gov

Environmental Protection Agency Indoor Air Quality/ETS. Provides information and links about secondhand smoke.

> http://www.epa.gov/smokefree

Nicotine Anonymous. A 12-step program for tobacco users.

> http://www.nicotine-anonymous.org

Rational Recovery. A free self-help program that offers an alternative to 12-step programs; the emphasis is on learning the skill of abstinence.

> http://www.rational.org

Smokefree.Gov. Provides step-by-step strategies for quitting as well as expert support via telephone or instant messaging.

> http://www.smokefree.gov

Substance Abuse and Mental Health Services Administration. Provides statistics and information about alcohol abuse, including resources for people who want to help friends and family members overcome alcohol abuse problems.

> http://store.samhsa.gov/home

World Health Organization Tobacco Free Initiative. Promotes the goal of a tobacco-free world.

> http://www.who.int/tobacco/en

World No Tobacco Day (WNTD). Provides information about the annual worldwide event to encourage people to quit smoking; includes general information about tobacco use and testimonials of ex-smokers.

> http://www.who.int/tobacco/wntd/2012/announcement/en/index.html

SELECTED BIBLIOGRAPHY

American Cancer Society. 2012. *Cancer Facts and Figures, 2012.* Atlanta: American Cancer Society.

American Lung Association. 2011. *Trends in Tobacco Use* (http://www.lungusa.org/finding-cures/our-research/trend-reports/Tobacco-Trend-Report.pdf).

American Lung Association. 2012. *State of Tobacco Control 2012* (http://www.stateoftobaccocontrol.org/SOTC_2012.pdf).

Campaign for Tobacco-Free Kids. 2011. *State Cigarette Excise Tax Rates and Rankings.* Washington, DC: Campaign for Tobacco-Free Kids.

Centers for Disease Control and Prevention. 2009. Alcohol use among pregnant and nonpregnant women of childbearing age: United States, 1991–2005. *Morbidity and Mortality Weekly Report* 58(19): 529–532.

Centers for Disease Control and Prevention. 2009. Cigarette smoking among adults and trends in smoking cessation—United States, 2008. *Morbidity and Mortality Weekly Report* 58(44): 1227–1232.

Centers for Disease Control and Prevention. 2010. *Smoking and Tobacco Use Fact Sheet: Tobacco-Related Mortality* (http://www.cdc.gov/tobacco/data_statistics/fact_sheets/health_effects/tobacco_related_mortality).

Centers for Disease Control and Prevention. 2010. Vital signs: nonsmokers' exposure to secondhand smoke—United States, 1999–2009. *Morbidity and Mortality Weekly Report* 59(35): 1141–1146.

Centers for Disease Control and Prevention. 2010. Youth risk behavior surveillance—United States, 2009. *Morbidity and Mortality Weekly Report* 59(SS-05): 1–148.

Centers for Disease Control and Prevention. 2011. Quitting smoking among adults—United States, 2001–2010. *Morbidity and Mortality Weekly Report* 60(44).

Centers for Disease Control and Prevention. 2011. Vital signs: current cigarette smoking among adults aged ≥18 years—United States, 2005–2010. *Morbidity and Mortality Weekly Report* 60(35): 1189–1232.

Centers for Disease Control and Prevention. 2012. *Alcohol and Public Health* (http://www.cdc.gov/alcohol/index.htm).

Chen, W. Y., et al. 2011. Moderate alcohol consumption during adult life, drinking patterns, and breast cancer risk. *Journal of the American Medical Association* 306(17): 1884–1890.

College Drinking Prevention. 2012. *A Snapshot of Annual High-Risk College Drinking Consequences* (http://www.collegedrinkingprevention.gov/StatsSummaries/snapshot.aspx).

Collins, G. B., et al. 2006. Drug adjuncts for treating alcohol dependence. *Cleveland Clinic Journal of Medicine* 73(7): 641–644.

Costello, R. M. 2006. Long-term mortality from alcoholism: A descriptive analysis. *Journal of Studies on Alcohol* 67(5): 694–699.

Federal Trade Commission. 2011. *Federal Trade Commission Cigarette Report for 2007 and 2008.* Washington, DC: Federal Trade Commission.

Fucito, L. M., et al. 2012. Cigarette smoking predicts differential benefit from naltrexone for alcohol dependence. *Biological Psychiatry*, April 25 (Epub ahead of print).

Gorsane, M. A., et al. 2012. Is baclofen a revolutionary medication in alcohol addiction management? Review and recent updates. *Substance Abuse* 33(4):336–349.

Johnston, L. D., P. M. O'Malley, J. G. Bachman, & J. E. Schulenberg. 2011. *Monitoring the Future National Survey Results on Drug Use, 1975–2010: Volume I, Secondary School Students.* Ann Arbor: Institute for Social Research, The University of Michigan.

National Center for Health Statistics. 2010. National Hospital Ambulatory Medical Care Survey: 2007 Emergency Department Summary. *National Health Statistics Reports* 26. Hyattsville, MD: National Center for Health Statistics.

National Center for Health Statistics. 2011. Deaths: final data for 2008. *National Vital Statistics Reports* 59(10).

National Highway Traffic Safety Administration. 2009. *Traffic Safety Facts 2008: Alcohol-Impaired Driving.* Washington, DC: National Highway Traffic Safety Administration, DOT Pub. 811 155.

Parker-Pope, Tara. 2012. *America's Drinking Binge* (http://well.blogs.nytimes.com/2012/01/11/americas-drinking-binge).

Science Daily. 2012. *Early Intervention May Curb Dangerous College Drinking.* (http://www.sciencedaily.com/releases/2012/01/120130131204.htm).

Substance Abuse and Mental Health Services Administration. 2011. *Results from the 2010 National Survey on Drug Use and Health: Summary of National Findings.* Rockville, MD: Office of Applied Studies, NSDUH Series H-41, HHS Publication No. SMA 11-4658.

Substance Abuse and Mental Health Services Administration. 2012. *Nearly Half of College Student Treatment Admissions Were for Primary Alcohol Abuse* (http://www.samhsa.gov/data/spotlight/Spotlight054College2012.pdf).

Titus-Ernstoff, L., et al. 2008. Longitudinal study of viewing smoking in movies and initiation of smoking by children. *Pediatrics* 121(1): 15–21.

U.S. Food and Drug Administration Center for Tobacco Products. 2010. *2009–2010: Inaugural Year in Review.* Washington, DC: U.S. Food and Drug Administration.

U.S. Surgeon General. 2006. *The Health Consequences of Involuntary Exposure to Tobacco Smoke* (http://www.surgeongeneral.gov/library/secondhandsmoke/report/).

BEHAVIOR CHANGE STRATEGY
Kicking the Tobacco Habit

You can look forward to a longer and healthier life if you join the 48 million Americans who have quit using tobacco. The steps for quitting described here are discussed in terms of the most popular tobacco product in the United States—cigarettes—but they can be adapted for all forms of tobacco.

Gather Information

Collect personal smoking information in a detailed journal about your smoking behavior. Write down the time you smoke each cigarette of the day, the situation you are in, how you feel, where you smoke, and how strong your craving for the cigarette is, plus any other information that seems relevant. Part of the job is to identify patterns of smoking that are connected with routine situations (for example, the after-dinner cigarette, the coffee break smoke, the tension reduction cigarette). Use this information to discover the behavior patterns involved in your smoking habit.

Make the Decision to Quit

Choose a date in the near future when you expect to be relatively stress-free and can give quitting the energy and attention it will require. Don't choose a date right before or during finals week, for instance. Consider making quitting a gift: choose your birthday as your quit date, for example, or make quitting a Father's Day or Mother's Day present. You might also want to coordinate your quit date with a buddy—a fellow tobacco user who wants to quit or a nonsmoker who wants to give up another bad habit or begin an exercise program. Tell your friends and family when you plan to quit. Ask them to offer encouragement and help hold you to your goal.

Decide what approach to quitting will work best for you. Will you go cold turkey, or will you taper off? Will you use nicotine patches or gum? Will you join a support group or enlist the help of a buddy? Prepare a contract for quitting, as discussed in Chapter 1. Set firm dates and rewards, and sign the contract. Post it in a prominent place.

Prepare to Quit

One of the most important things you can do to prepare to quit is to develop and practice nonsmoking relaxation techniques. Many smokers find that they use cigarettes to help them unwind in tense situations or to relax at other times. If this is true for you, you'll need to find and develop effective substitutes. It takes time to become proficient at relaxation techniques, so begin practicing before your quit date. Refer to the detailed discussion of relaxation techniques in Chapter 2.

Other things you can do to help prepare for quitting include the following:

- Make an appointment to see your physician. Ask about OTC and prescription aids for tobacco cessation and whether one or more might be appropriate for you.
- Make a dentist's appointment to have your teeth cleaned the day after your target quit date.
- Start an easy exercise program if you're not exercising regularly already.
- Buy some sugarless gum. Stock your kitchen with low-calorie snacks.
- Clean and air out your car, and air out your house.
- Throw away all your cigarette-related paraphernalia (ashtrays, lighters, and so on).
- The night before your quit day, get rid of all your cigarettes. Have fun with this—get your friends or family to help you tear them up.

- Make your last few days of smoking inconvenient: smoke only outdoors and when alone. Don't do anything else while you smoke.

Quitting

Your first few days without cigarettes will probably be the most difficult. It's hard to give up such a strongly ingrained habit, but remember that millions of Americans have done it—and you can, too. Plan and rehearse the steps you will take when you experience a powerful craving. Avoid or control situations that you know from your journal are powerfully associated with your smoking (see the accompanying table). If your hands feel empty without a cigarette, try holding or fiddling with a small object such as a paper clip, pencil, or small toy.

Social support can also be a big help. Arrange with a buddy to help you with your weak moments, and call him or her whenever you feel overwhelmed by an urge to smoke. Tell people you've just quit. You may discover many inspiring former smokers who can encourage you and reassure you that it's possible to quit and lead a happier, healthier life. Find a formal support group to join if you think it will help.

Maintaining Nonsmoking

The lingering smoking urges that remain once you've quit should be carefully tracked and controlled because they can cause relapses if left unattended. Keep track of these urges in your journal to help you deal with them. If certain situations still trigger the urge for a cigarette, change something about those situations to break past associations. If stress or boredom causes strong smoking urges, use a relaxation technique, take a brisk walk, have a stick of gum, or substitute some other activity for smoking.

Don't set yourself up for a relapse. If you allow yourself to get overwhelmed at school or work or to gain weight, it will be easier to convince yourself that now isn't the right time to quit. This *is* the right time. Continue to practice time management and relaxation techniques. Exercise regularly, eat sensibly, and get enough sleep. These habits not only will ensure your success at remaining tobacco-free but also will serve you well in stressful times throughout your life. In fact, former smokers who have quit for at least three months report reduced stress levels, probably because quitting smoking lowers overall arousal.

Watch out for patterns of thinking that can make not smoking more difficult. Focus on the positive aspects of not smoking, and give yourself lots of praise—you deserve it. Stick with the schedule of rewards you developed for your contract.

Keep track of the emerging benefits that come from having quit. Items that might appear on your list include improved stamina, an increased sense of pride at having kicked a strong addiction, a sharper sense of taste and smell, no more smoker's cough, and so on. Keep track of the money you're saving by not smoking, and spend it on things you really enjoy. And if you do lapse, be gentle with yourself. Lapses are a normal part of quitting. Forgive yourself, and pick up where you left off.

SOURCES: Adapted from *Postgraduate Medicine* 90(1), Kramer, S. E., and K. E. Graham. Helping your patients who smoke quit for good: A quick and easy approach, pp. 238–248. Copyright 1991, with permission from JTE Multimedia..

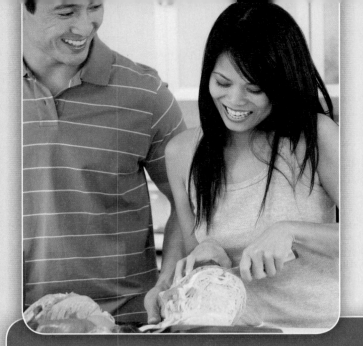

LOOKING AHEAD...

After reading this chapter, you should be able to

- List the essential nutrients, and describe the functions they perform in the body
- Describe the guidelines that have been developed to help people choose a healthy diet, avoid nutritional deficiencies, and reduce their risk of diet-related chronic diseases
- Discuss nutritional guidelines for vegetarians and for special population groups
- Explain how to use food labels and other consumer tools to make informed choices about foods
- Put together a personal nutrition plan based on affordable foods that you enjoy and that promote wellness, today as well as in the future

Nutrition Basics

9

n your lifetime, you'll spend about six years eating—about 70,000 meals and 60 tons of food. What you eat can have profound effects on your health and well-being. Your nutritional habits help determine your risk of major chronic diseases, including heart disease, cancer, stroke, and diabetes. Choosing foods that provide the nutrients you need while limiting the substances linked to disease should be an important part of your daily life.

Choosing a healthy diet is a two-part process. First, you have to know which nutrients you need and in what amounts. Second, you have to translate those requirements into a diet consisting of foods you like that are both available and affordable and that fit into your lifestyle. Once you know what constitutes a healthy diet for you, you can adjust your current diet to bring it into line with your goals.

This chapter explains the basic principles of **nutrition.** It introduces the six classes of essential nutrients and explains their roles in the functioning of the body. It also provides guidelines that you can use to design a healthy diet plan.

NUTRITIONAL REQUIREMENTS: COMPONENTS OF A HEALTHY DIET

You probably think about your diet in terms of the foods you like to eat. More important for your health, though, are the nutrients contained in those foods. Your body requires proteins, fats, carbohydrates, vitamins, minerals, and water—about 45 **essential nutrients.** In this context, the word *essential* means that you must get these substances from food because your body is unable to manufacture them, or at least do so fast enough, to meet your physiological needs.

The body needs some essential nutrients in relatively large amounts; these **macronutrients** include protein, fat, carbohydrate, and water. **Micronutrients,** such as vitamins and minerals, are required in much smaller amounts. Your body obtains nutrients through the process of **digestion,** in which the foods you eat are broken down into compounds your gastrointestinal tract can absorb and your body can use (Figure 9.1).

The energy in foods is expressed as **kilocalories.** One kilocalorie represents the amount of heat required to raise the temperature of 1 liter of water 1°C. A person needs about 2000 kilocalories per day to meet his or her energy needs. In common usage, people usually refer to kilocalories as *calories,* which is technically a much smaller energy unit (1 kilocalorie contains 1000 calories). This text uses the familiar word *calorie* to stand for the larger energy unit; you'll also find the word *calorie* used on food labels.

Of the six classes of essential nutrients, three supply energy:

- Fat = 9 calories per gram
- Protein = 4 calories per gram
- Carbohydrate = 4 calories per gram

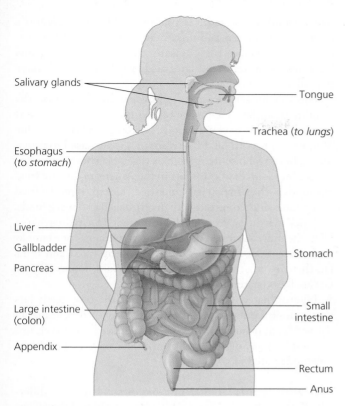

Salivary glands

Tongue

Trachea (*to lungs*)

Esophagus (*to stomach*)

Liver

Gallbladder

Pancreas

Stomach

Large intestine (colon)

Small intestine

Appendix

Rectum

Anus

FIGURE 9.1 **The digestive system.** Food is partially broken down by being chewed and mixed with saliva in the mouth. After traveling to the stomach via the esophagus, food is broken down further by stomach acids and other secretions. As food moves through the digestive tract, it is mixed by muscular contractions and broken down by chemicals. Most absorption of nutrients occurs in the small intestine, aided by secretions from the pancreas, gallbladder, and intestinal lining. The large intestine reabsorbs excess water; the remaining solid wastes are collected in the rectum and excreted through the anus.

Alcohol, though not an essential nutrient, also supplies energy, providing 7 calories per gram. The high caloric content of fat is one reason why experts often advise against high fat consumption. Most people do not need the extra calories to meet energy needs. Regardless of their source, calories consumed in excess of energy needs are converted to fat and stored in the body. Just meeting energy needs is not enough, however. Your body needs enough of the essential nutrients to function properly.

Proteins—The Basis of Body Structure

Proteins form important parts of the body's main structural components: muscles and bones. Proteins also form important parts of blood, enzymes, some hormones, and cell membranes. When consumed, proteins also provide energy (4 calories per gram) for the body.

Amino Acids The building blocks of proteins are called **amino acids.** Twenty common amino acids are found in

food. Nine of these are essential (or indispensable). The other eleven amino acids can be produced by the body, given the presence of the needed components supplied by foods.

Complete and Incomplete Proteins Individual protein sources are considered *complete* if they supply all the essential amino acids in adequate amounts and *incomplete* if they do not. Meat, fish, poultry, eggs, milk, cheese, and soy provide complete proteins. Incomplete proteins, which come from other plant sources such as legumes and nuts, are good sources of most essential amino acids but are usually low in one or more.

Certain combinations of vegetable proteins, such as wheat and peanuts in a peanut butter sandwich, allow each vegetable protein to make up for the amino acids missing in the other protein. The combination yields a complete protein. Many traditional food pairings, such as beans and rice or corn and beans, may have emerged as dietary staples because they are complementary proteins. Vegetarians should include a variety of vegetable protein sources in their diets to make sure they get all the essential amino acids in adequate amounts. About two-thirds of the protein in the typical American diet comes from animal sources (meat and dairy products); therefore, the American diet is rich in essential amino acids.

Recommended Protein Intake Adequate daily intake of protein for adults is 0.8 gram per kilogram (0.36 gram per pound) of body weight, corresponding to 50 grams of protein per day for someone who weighs 140 pounds and 65 grams of protein for someone who weighs 180 pounds.

Most Americans meet or exceed the protein intake needed for adequate nutrition. If you consume more protein than

TERMS

nutrition The science of food and how the body uses it in health and disease.

essential nutrients Substances the body must get from foods because it cannot manufacture them at all or fast enough to meet its needs. These nutrients include proteins, fats, carbohydrates, vitamins, minerals, and water.

macronutrient An essential nutrient required by the body in relatively large amounts.

micronutrient An essential nutrient required by the body in minute amounts.

digestion The process of breaking down foods into compounds the gastrointestinal tract can absorb and the body can use.

kilocalorie A measure of energy content in food; 1 kilocalorie represents the amount of heat needed to raise the temperature of 1 liter of water 1°C; commonly referred to as a *calorie.*

protein An essential nutrient that forms important parts of the body's main structures (muscles and bones) as well as blood, enzymes, hormones, and cell membranes; also provides energy.

amino acid One of the building blocks of proteins; 20 common amino acids are found in foods.

your body needs, the extra energy from protein is synthesized into fat for storage or burned for energy requirements. A little extra protein is not harmful, but it can contribute excess calories and fat to the diet because protein-rich foods can be high in fat (especially saturated fat), as well.

Recommendations for protein intake (and intake of other nutrients) as a percentage of total daily calorie intake have been published by the Food and Nutrition Board of the Institute of Medicine. These recommendations, called Acceptable Macronutrient Distribution Ranges (AMDRs), are based on ensuring adequate intake of essential nutrients while also reducing the risk of chronic diseases. A fairly broad range of protein intakes is associated with good health; the AMDR for protein is 10–35% of total daily calorie intake, depending on the individual's age. Because most people in the United States meet the recommendations for protein, the 2010 Dietary Guidelines for Americans emphasize a variety of low-fat protein choices to encourage people to avoid consuming too many calories.

Fats—Essential in Small Amounts

Fats, also known as *lipids*, are the most concentrated source of energy, at 9 calories per gram. The fats stored in your body represent usable energy, they help insulate your body, and they support and cushion your organs. Fats in the diet help your body to absorb fat-soluble vitamins, and they add important flavor and texture to foods. Fats are the major fuel for the body during rest and light activity. Two fats, linoleic acid and alpha-linolenic acid, are essential components of the diet.

Types and Sources of Fats   Most of the fats in foods are fairly similar in composition, generally including a molecule of glycerol (an alcohol) with three fatty acid chains attached to it. The resulting structure is called a *triglyceride*.

Within a triglyceride, differences in the fatty acid structure result in different types of fats. Depending on this structure, a fat may be unsaturated, monounsaturated, polyunsaturated, or saturated. (The essential fatty acids—linoleic and alpha-linolenic acids—are both polyunsaturated.) The different types of fatty acids have different characteristics and different effects on your health.

Food fats are usually composed of both saturated and unsaturated fatty acids; the dominant type of fatty acid determines the fat's characteristics. Food fats containing large amounts of saturated fatty acids are usually solid at room temperature; they are generally found naturally in animal products. The leading sources of saturated fat in the American diet are red meats (hamburger, steak, roasts), whole milk, cheese, hot dogs, and lunch meats. Food fats containing large amounts of monounsaturated and polyunsaturated fatty acids usually come from plant sources and are liquid at room temperature. Olive, canola, safflower, and peanut oils contain mostly monounsaturated fatty acids. Soybean, corn, and cottonseed oils contain mostly polyunsaturated fatty acids.

Hydrogenation and Trans Fats   When unsaturated vegetable oils undergo the chemical process known as

hydrogenation, the result is a more solid fat that contains a mixture of saturated and unsaturated fatty acids. Hydrogenation also changes some unsaturated fatty acids to **trans fatty acids**—unsaturated fatty acids with an atypical shape that affects their behavior in the body.

Food manufacturers use hydrogenation to increase the stability of an oil so it can be reused for deep frying, to improve the texture of certain foods, and to extend the shelf life of foods made with oil. Hydrogenation is also used to transform a liquid oil into margarine or vegetable shortening.

Leading sources of trans fats in the American diet are fried fast foods such as french fries and fried chicken (typically fried in vegetable shortening rather than oil), baked and snack foods, and stick margarine. In general, the more solid a hydrogenated oil is, the more saturated or trans fats it contains; for example, stick margarines typically contain more saturated and trans fats than do tub or squeeze margarines. Small amounts of trans fats are found naturally in meat and milk.

Hydrogenated vegetable oils are not the only plant fats that contain saturated fats. Palm and coconut oils, although derived from plants, are also highly saturated. However, fish oils, unlike many oils derived from animal sources, are rich in polyunsaturated fats.

Fats and Health   Different types of fats have very different effects on health. Many studies have examined the effects of dietary fat intake on blood **cholesterol** levels and the risk of heart disease. Saturated and trans fatty acids raise blood levels of **low-density lipoprotein (LDL),** or "bad" cholesterol. Unsaturated fatty acids lower LDL. Monounsaturated fatty acids, such as those found in olive and canola oils, may also increase levels of **high-density lipoproteins (HDL),** or "good" cholesterol, providing even greater benefits for heart health. In large amounts, trans fatty acids may lower HDL. Thus it is important to choose unsaturated fats instead of saturated and trans fats to reduce the risk of heart disease.

Most Americans consume 4–5 times as much saturated fat as trans fat (8–10% versus 2% of total daily calories).

TERMS

hydrogenation   A chemical process by which hydrogen atoms are added to molecules of unsaturated fats, increasing the degree of saturation and turning liquid oils into solid fats. Hydrogenation produces a mixture of saturated fatty acids and standard and trans forms of unsaturated fatty acids.

trans fatty acid   A type of unsaturated fatty acid produced during the process of hydrogenation; trans fats have an atypical shape that affects their chemical activity.

cholesterol   A waxy substance in the blood and cells, needed for synthesis of cell membranes, vitamin D, and hormones.

low-density lipoprotein (LDL)   Blood fat that transports cholesterol to organs and tissues; excess amounts result in the accumulation of deposits on artery walls.

high-density lipoprotein (HDL)   Blood fat that helps transport cholesterol out of the arteries, thereby protecting against heart disease.

Touring Lifestyle Behaviors

Alcohol Use: Stages of Intoxication

Tobacco Use: Immediate Effects and Long-Term Health Risks

Exercise: Immediate Effects and Long-Term Health Benefits

The Greenhouse Effect, Climate Change, and You

GOALS OF THE TOUR

1. **Alcohol Use.** Describe the stages of intoxication and the effects experienced in each stage.

2. **Tobacco Use.** Identify and describe the immediate effects and long-term health risks of tobacco use.

3. **Exercise.** Identify and describe the immediate effects and long-term health benefits of exercise.

4. **The Greenhouse Effect.** Explain the greenhouse effect and describe actions individuals can take to reduce their carbon footprint.

Alcohol Use: Stages of Intoxication

1 Describe the stages of intoxication and the effects experienced at each stage.

Blood alcohol concentration (BAC) rises quickly with alcohol consumption, but alcohol is metabolized at a relatively slow rate—about 1 drink per hour. Note that rate of alcohol metabolism varies widely depending on sex, body weight, ethnicity, age, food in the stomach, genetics, and other factors—so the effects at different BACs also vary.

One drink =

a 12-ounce beer

or

a 1.5-ounce shot

or

a 5-ounce glass of wine

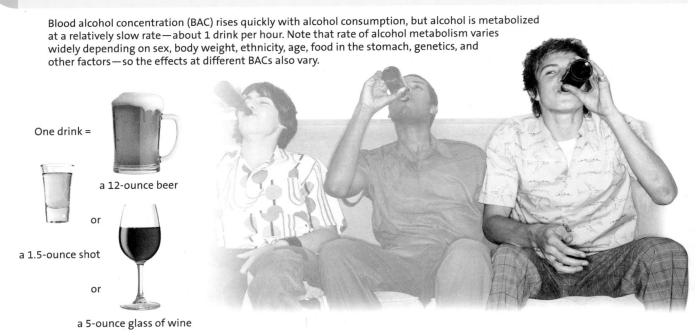

Number of drinks in 1 hour before the legal BAC limit of 0.08 is reached

Weight in pounds	Drinks in 1 hour
90–109	1
110–129	1
130–149	2
150–169	2
170–189	2
190–200+	3

150 lbs   130 lbs   180 lbs   170 lbs   102 lbs   200 lbs

BAC
0.00   0.10
0.02   0.05   0.08   0.15

effects

BAC: 0.01–0.05
Relaxation; mild euphoria; reduced inhibition; decreased alertness; impaired motor coordination and judgment.
Approximate time to metabolize: 2–3 hours

BAC: 0.10–0.15
Mood swings; aggression; staggering gait; impaired balance; slurred speech.
Approximate time to metabolize: 7–10 hours

BAC: 0.05–0.10
Emotional instability; exaggerated feelings and behaviors; impaired reasoning, judgment, and visual tracking; slowed information processing, reflexes, and reaction time; sleepiness; nausea. Legally intoxicated at 0.08% in all 50 states.
Approximate time to metabolize: 3–6 hours

Tobacco Use: Immediate Effects and Long-Term Health Risks

Identify and describe the immediate effects and long-term health risks of tobacco use.

2

Immediate Effects

Brain
• Nicotine triggers release of sedating and stimulating chemicals in brain

Skin
• Nicotine constricts blood vessels, reducing blood flow to skin

Heart
• Nicotine increases heart rate, elevates blood pressure
• Heart must work harder to deliver oxygen to cells

Lungs, bronchi
• Smoke is absorbed into bloodstream and carried throughout the body
• Oxygen delivery to cells is impaired

Liver
• Nicotine causes liver to convert glycogen to glucose and release it into bloodstream, raising blood sugar levels

Adrenal glands
• Nicotine triggers release of adrenaline, causing stimulating effects throughout the body and reduced body temperature in extremities

Kidneys
• Nicotine inhibits production of urine

Digestive system
• Nicotine depresses appetite and hunger contractions

Reproductive system
• In pregnant women, nicotine and chemicals are passed to fetus

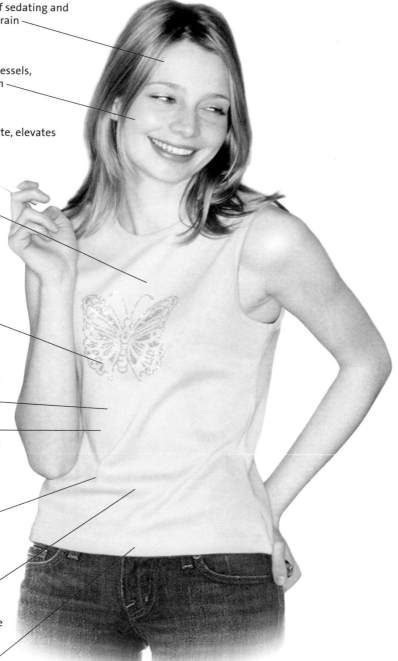

Exercise: Immediate Effects and Long-Term Health Benefits

3 Identify and describe the immediate effects and long-term health benefits of exercise.

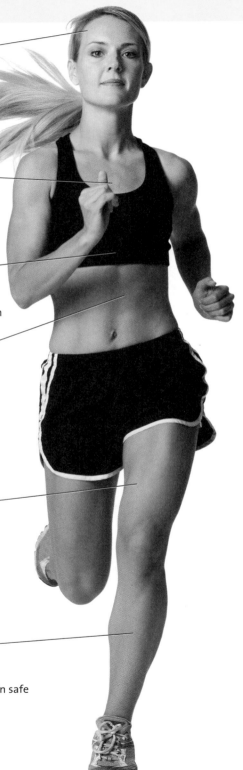

Immediate Effects

Brain
- Increased oxygen and nutrients to brain
- Increased levels of neurotransmitters

Heart
- Increased heart rate
- Greater volume of blood pumped to body

Lungs
- Increased breathing rate
- Increased oxygen consumption

Stomach
- Reduced blood flow to digestive system

Muscles
- Increased blood flow to muscles
- Increased energy production in muscles

Skin
- Increased blood flow to skin
- Increased sweating to maintain safe body temperature

The Greenhouse Effect, Climate Change, and You

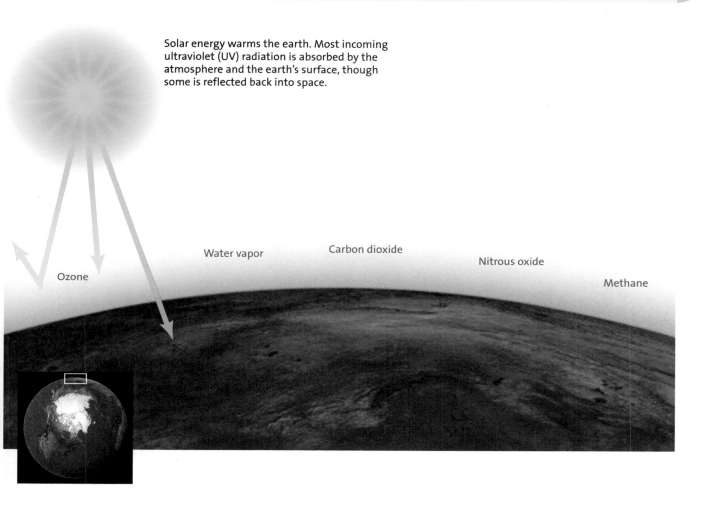

Solar energy warms the earth. Most incoming ultraviolet (UV) radiation is absorbed by the atmosphere and the earth's surface, though some is reflected back into space.

Water vapor

Carbon dioxide

Nitrous oxide

Ozone

Methane

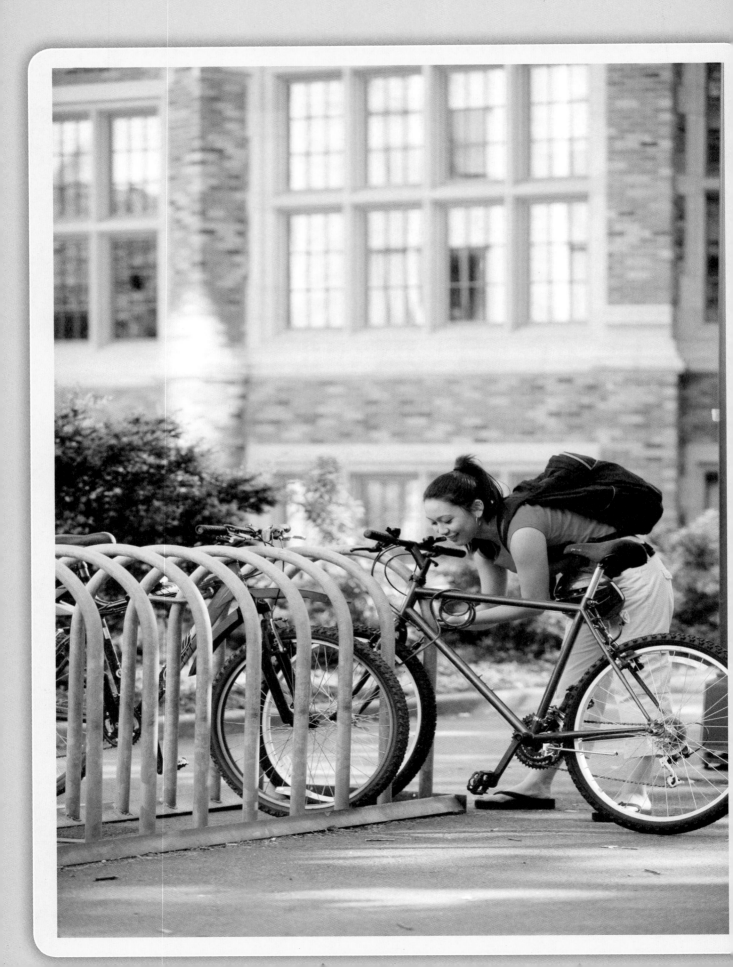

Table 9.1 Types of Fatty Acids and Their Possible Effects on Health

TYPE OF FATTY ACID	FOUND IN[a]	POSSIBLE EFFECTS ON HEALTH
Keep Intake Low — Saturated	• Animal fats (especially fatty meats and poultry fat and skin) • Butter, cheese, and other high-fat dairy products • Palm and coconut oils	• Raises total cholesterol and LDL cholesterol • May increase risk of heart disease • May increase risk of certain types of cancers
Trans	• Deep-fried fast foods • Stick margarines, shortening • Packaged cookies and crackers • Processed snacks and sweets	• Raises total cholesterol and LDL cholesterol • Lowers HDL cholesterol • May increase risk of heart disease and some cancers
Monounsaturated	• Olive, canola, and safflower oils • Avocados, olives • Peanut butter (without added fat) • Many nuts, including almonds, cashews, pecans, and pistachios	• Lowers total cholesterol and LDL cholesterol • May reduce blood pressure and lower triglycerides (a risk factor for heart disease) • May reduce risk of heart disease, stroke, and some cancers
POLYUNSATURATED (two groups)[b]		
Choose Moderate Amounts — Omega-3	• Fatty fish, including salmon, white albacore tuna, mackerel, anchovies, and sardines • Lesser amounts in walnut, flaxseed, canola, and soybean oils; tofu, walnuts; flaxseeds; and dark green leafy vegetables	• Reduces blood clotting and inflammation and inhibits abnormal heart rhythms • Lowers triglycerides • May lower blood pressure in some people • May reduce risk of fatal heart attack, stroke, and some cancers
Omega-6	• Corn, soybean, and cottonseed oils (often used in margarine, mayonnaise, and salad dressings)	• Lowers total cholesterol and LDL cholesterol • May lower HDL cholesterol • May reduce risk of heart disease • May slightly increase risk of cancer if omega-6 intake is high and omega-3 intake is low

[a]Food fats contain a combination of types of fatty acids in various proportions. For example, canola oil is composed mainly of monounsaturated fatty acids (62%) but also contains polyunsaturated (32%) and saturated (6%) fatty acids. Food fats are categorized here according to their predominant fatty acid.

[b]The essential fatty acids are polyunsaturated: linoleic acid is an omega-6 fatty acid and alpha-linolenic acid is an omega-3 fatty acid.

However, health experts are particularly concerned about trans fats because of their double-negative effect on heart health—they both raise LDL and lower HDL. Consuming trans fats increases the risk of both cardiovascular disease and type 2 diabetes. By federal regulation, the trans fat content of packaged food items is listed on their labels. Consumers can also check for the presence of trans fats by examining the ingredient list of a food for partially hydrogenated oil or vegetable shortening.

Although saturated and trans fats pose health hazards, other fats can be beneficial. When used in place of saturated fats, monounsaturated fatty acids—found in avocados, most nuts, and olive, canola, peanut, and safflower oils—improve cholesterol levels and may help protect against some cancers. **Omega-3 fatty acids,** a form of polyunsaturated fat found primarily in fish, may be even more healthful. Foods rich in omega-3s are important because they contain the essential nutrient alpha-linolenic acid. Omega-3s and the compounds the body makes from them have a number of heart-healthy effects. Nutritionists recommend that Americans increase the proportion of omega-3s in their diet by eating fish two or more times a week. Salmon, tuna, trout, mackerel, herring, sardines, and anchovies are all good sources of omega-3s. Lesser amounts are found in plant foods, including dark-green leafy vegetables; walnuts; flaxseeds; and canola, walnut, and flaxseed oils.

Most of the polyunsaturated fats currently consumed by Americans are **omega-6 fatty acids,** primarily from corn oil and soybean oil. Foods rich in omega-6s are important because they contain the essential nutrient linoleic acid. The American Heart Association (AHA) recommends consuming at least 5–10% of energy from omega-6 fatty acids as part of a low-saturated-fat and low-cholesterol diet, to reduce the risk of coronary heart disease.

In addition to its effects on heart disease risk, dietary fat can affect health in other ways. Diets high in fatty red meat are associated with an increased risk of certain forms of cancer, especially colon cancer. A high-fat diet can also make weight management more difficult. The types of fatty acids and their effects on health are summarized in Table 9.1.

omega-3 fatty acids Polyunsaturated fatty acids commonly found in fish oils; beneficial to cardiovascular health.

omega-6 fatty acids Polyunsaturated fatty acids found commonly in soybean and corn oil; beneficial for cardiovascular health.

TERMS

TAKE CHARGE
Setting Intake Goals for Protein, Fat, and Carbohydrate

The Food and Nutrition Board has established goals to help ensure adequate intake of the essential amino acids, fatty acids, and carbohydrate. The daily goals for adults follow:

	MEN	WOMEN
Protein	56 grams	46 grams
Fat: linoleic acid	17 grams	12 grams
Alpha-linolenic acid	1.6 grams	1.1 grams
Carbohydrate	130 grams	130 grams

Protein intake goals can be calculated more specifically by multiplying your body weight in kilograms by 0.8 or your body weight in pounds by 0.36. (Refer to the "Nutrition Resources" section at the end of the chapter for information for specific age groups and life stages.)

To meet your daily energy needs, you need to consume more than the minimally adequate amounts of the energy-providing nutrients listed here, which alone supply only about 800–900 calories.

The Food and Nutrition Board provides additional guidance in the form of Acceptable Macronutrient Distribution Ranges (AMDRs), as noted in the text. The ranges can help you balance your intake of the energy-providing nutrients in ways that ensure adequate intake while reducing the risk of chronic disease. The AMDRs for protein, total fat, and carbohydrate follow:

Protein	10–35% of total daily calories
Total fat	20–35% of total daily calories
Carbohydrate	45–65% of total daily calories

To set individual goals, begin by estimating your total daily energy (calorie) needs. If your weight is stable, your current energy intake is the number of calories needed to maintain your weight at your current activity level. Next select percentage goals for protein, fat, and carbohydrate. You can allocate your total daily calories among the three classes of macronutrients to suit your preferences, but make sure that the three percentages you select total 100% and that you meet the minimum intake goals listed.

To translate your own percentage goals into daily intake goals expressed in calories and grams, multiply the appropriate percentages by total calorie intake and then divide the results by the corresponding calories per gram. For example, a fat limit of 35% applied to a 2200-calorie diet would be calculated as follows: 0.35 × 2200 = 770 calories of total fat; 770 ÷ 9 calories per gram = 86 grams of total fat. (Remember that fat has 9 calories per gram and that protein and carbohydrate have 4 calories per gram.)

SOURCE: From Food and Nutrition Board, Institute of Medicine. 2010. *Dietary Reference Intakes: The Essential Guide to Nutrient Requirements*. Washington, DC: National Academies Press. Available online at http://www.nap.edu/openbook.php?record_id=11537&page1. Reprinted with permission from the National Academies Press, Copyright 2010, National Academy of Sciences.

Recommended Fat Intake To meet the body's demand for essential fats, adult men need about 17 grams per day of linoleic acid and 1.6 grams per day of alpha-linolenic acid; adult women need 12 grams of linoleic acid and 1.1 grams of alpha-linolenic acid. It takes only 3–4 teaspoons (15–20 grams) of vegetable oil per day incorporated into your diet to supply the essential fats. Most Americans consume sufficient amounts of the essential fats; limiting unhealthy fats is a much greater health concern.

Limits for total fat, saturated fat, and trans fat intake have been set by a number of government and research organizations. As with protein, a range of levels of fat consumption is associated with good health; the AMDR for total fat is 20–35% of total calories. Although more difficult for consumers to monitor, AMDRs have also been set for omega-6 fatty acids (5–10%) and omega-3 fatty acids (0.6–1.2%) as part of total fat intake. Because any amount of saturated and trans fats increases the risk of heart disease, the Food and Nutrition Board recommends that saturated fat and trans fat intake be kept as low as possible; most fat in a healthy diet should be unsaturated.

For advice on setting individual intake goals, see the box "Setting Intake Goals for Protein, Fat, and Carbohydrate." To determine how close you are to meeting your personal intake goals for fat, keep a running total over the course of the day.

For prepared foods, food labels list the numbers of grams of fat, protein, and carbohydrate. Nutrition information is also available in many grocery stores, in inexpensive published nutrition guides, and online. By checking these resources, you can keep track of the total grams of fat, protein, and carbohydrate you eat and assess your current diet. You can still eat high-fat foods, as long as you limit the size of your portions and balance your intake with low-fat foods.

Carbohydrates—An Ideal Source of Energy

Carbohydrates are needed in the diet primarily to supply energy for body cells. Some cells, such as those found in the brain and other parts of the nervous system and in blood, use only the carbohydrate glucose for fuel. During high-intensity exercise, muscles also use energy from carbohydrates as their primary fuel source.

carbohydrate An essential nutrient, required for energy for cells; sugars, starches, and dietary fiber are all carbohydrates.

TERMS

Simple and Complex Carbohydrates Carbohydrates are classified into two groups: simple and complex. *Simple carbohydrates* include single sugar molecules (monosaccharides) and double sugar molecules (disaccharides). The monosaccharides are glucose, fructose, and galactose. The disaccharides are pairs of single sugars; they include sucrose, maltose, and lactose. Simple carbohydrates add sweetness to foods; they are found naturally in fruits and milk and are added to soft drinks, fruit drinks, candy, and sweet desserts. There is no evidence that any type of simple carbohydrate is more nutritious than any others.

Complex carbohydrates include starches and most types of dietary fiber. Starches are found in a variety of plants, especially grains (wheat, rye, rice, oats, barley, millet), legumes (dry beans, peas, and lentils), and tubers (potatoes and yams). Most other vegetables contain a mixture of complex and simple carbohydrates.

During digestion, your body breaks down carbohydrates into simple sugar molecules, such as **glucose,** for absorption. Once glucose is in the bloodstream, the pancreas releases the hormone insulin, which allows cells to take up glucose and use it for energy. The liver and muscles take up glucose to provide carbohydrate storage in the form of a starch called **glycogen.** Some people have problems controlling blood glucose levels, a disorder called *diabetes mellitus*.

Refined Carbohydrates versus Whole Grains Complex carbohydrates can be further divided into refined, or processed, carbohydrates and unrefined carbohydrates, or whole grains. Before they are processed, all grains are **whole grains,** consisting of an inner layer, the germ; a middle layer, the endosperm; and an outer layer, the bran. During processing, the germ and bran are often removed, leaving just the starchy endosperm. The refinement of whole grains transforms whole-wheat flour into white flour, brown rice into white rice, and so on.

Refined carbohydrates usually retain all the calories of their unrefined counterparts, but they tend to be much lower in fiber, vitamins, minerals, and other beneficial compounds. Unrefined carbohydrates tend to take longer to chew and digest than refined ones; they also enter the bloodstream more slowly. This slower digestive pace tends to make people feel full sooner and for a longer period. Also, a slower rise in blood glucose levels following the consumption of complex carbohydrates may help in the management of diabetes. Whole grains are also high in dietary fiber and so have all the benefits of fiber (discussed later).

Consumption of whole grains has been linked to a reduced risk of heart disease, diabetes, and cancer and plays an important role in gastrointestinal health and body weight management. For all these reasons, whole grains are recommended over those that have been refined (see the box "Choosing More Whole-Grain Foods".)

Glycemic Index Insulin and glucose levels rise and fall following a meal or snack containing any type of carbohydrate. Some foods cause a quick and dramatic rise in glucose and insulin levels, while others have a slower, more moderate effect. A food that has a rapid effect on blood glucose levels is said to have a high **glycemic index.** The glycemic index of a food indicates the type of carbohydrate in that food.

Attempting to base food choices on glycemic index is a difficult task. For people with particular health concerns, such as diabetes, glycemic index may be an important consideration in choosing foods. But for most people, the best bet is to choose a variety of vegetables daily and to limit foods that are high in added sugars and low in other nutrients.

Recommended Carbohydrate Intake On average, Americans consume 200–300 grams of carbohydrate per day—well above the 130 grams needed to meet the body's requirement for essential carbohydrate. A range of intakes is associated with good health; the AMDR for carbohydrates is 45–65% of total daily calories. That's about 225–325 grams of carbohydrate for someone who consumes 2000 calories per day. The focus should be on consuming a variety of foods rich in complex carbohydrates, especially whole grains. Athletes in training can benefit from high-carbohydrate diets (60–70% of total daily calories), which enhance the amount of carbohydrates stored in their muscles and therefore provide more fuel for use during endurance events or long workouts.

Added sugars—sugars that are added to foods—should not be a major contributor to the diet. Added sugars include the white and brown sugar and high-fructose corn syrup that are added to foods like candy, baked goods, and sodas and other sugar-sweetened beverages. Currently, added sugars contribute 16% of the total calories in the typical American diet. Foods high in added sugars are generally high in calories and low in nutrients and fiber, thus providing "empty calories." The USDA Food Patterns recommendations (based on the Dietary Guidelines for Americans) are designed so that people can meet nutrient needs and have no more than 5–15% of calories from solid fats AND added sugars together. To reduce your intake of added sugars, limit soft drinks, candy, desserts, and sweetened fruit drinks. The sugars in your diet should come mainly from fruits, which are excellent sources of vitamins and minerals, and from low-fat or fat-free milk and other dairy products, which are high in protein and calcium.

Fiber—A Closer Look

Fiber is the term given to nondigestible carbohydrates provided by plants. Instead of being digested, like starch, fiber moves through the intestinal tract and provides bulk for feces

---

TERMS

glucose A simple sugar that is the body's basic fuel.

glycogen A starch stored in the liver and muscles.

whole grain The entire edible portion of a grain (such as wheat, rice, or oats), consisting of the germ, endosperm, and bran; processing removes parts of the grain, often leaving just the endosperm.

glycemic index A measure of how a particular food affects blood glucose levels.

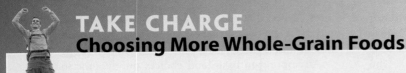

TAKE CHARGE
Choosing More Whole-Grain Foods

Because whole-grain foods offer so many health benefits, federal dietary guidelines recommend six or more servings of grain products every day, with at least half of those servings from whole grains.

What Are Whole Grains?

The first step in increasing your intake of whole grains is to correctly identify them. The following are whole grains:

Whole wheat   Whole-grain corn
Whole rye   Popcorn
Whole oats   Brown rice
Oatmeal   Whole-grain barley

More unusual choices include bulgur (cracked wheat), millet, kasha (roasted buckwheat kernels), quinoa, wheat and rye berries, amaranth, wild rice, graham flour, whole-grain kamut, whole-grain spelt, and whole-grain triticale.

Wheat flour, unbleached flour, enriched flour, and degerminated corn meal are not whole grains. Wheat germ and wheat bran are also not whole grains, but they are the constituents of wheat typically left out when wheat is processed and so are healthier choices than regular wheat flour, which typically contains just the grain's endosperm.

Checking Packages for Whole Grains

To find packaged foods that are rich in whole grains, read the list of ingredients and check for special health claims related to whole grains. The *first* item on the list of ingredients should be one of the whole grains in the preceding list. The FDA allows manufacturers to include special health claims for foods that contain 51% or more whole-grain ingredients. Such products may display a statement such as the following on their packaging: "Rich in whole grain.", "Made with 100% whole grain.", or "Diets rich in whole-grain foods may help reduce the risk of heart disease and certain cancers." However, many whole-grain products do not carry such claims. This is one more reason to check the ingredient list for whole grains.

---

in the large intestine, which in turn facilitates elimination. In the large intestine, bacteria break down some types of fiber into acids and gases, which explains why consuming too much fiber can lead to intestinal gas. Even though humans don't digest fiber, it is necessary for good health.

Types of Fiber   The Food and Nutrition Board has defined two types of fiber:

- **Dietary fiber** refers to the nondigestible carbohydrates (and the noncarbohydrate substance *lignin*) that are naturally present in plants such as grains, legumes, and vegetables.

- **Functional fiber** refers to nondigestible carbohydrates that have been either isolated from natural sources or synthesized in a lab and then added to a food product or dietary supplement.

Total fiber is the sum of dietary and functional fiber in one's diet. Fibers have different properties that lead to different physiological effects in the body. For example, **soluble (viscous) fiber** such as that found in oat bran or legumes can delay stomach emptying, slow the movement of glucose into the blood after eating, and reduce absorption of cholesterol. **Insoluble fiber,** such as that found in wheat bran or psyllium seed, increases fecal bulk and helps prevent constipation, hemorrhoids, and other digestive disorders.

A high-fiber diet can help reduce the risk of type 2 diabetes, heart disease, and pulmonary disease, as well as improve gastrointestinal health and aid in the management of metabolic syndrome and body weight. Some studies have linked high-fiber diets with a reduced risk of colon and rectal cancer. Other studies have suggested that other characteristics of diets rich in fruits, vegetables, and whole grains may be responsible for this reduction in risk.

Sources of Fiber   All plant foods contain some dietary fiber. Fruits, legumes, oats (especially oat bran), and barley all contain the viscous types of fiber that help lower blood glucose and cholesterol levels. Wheat (especially wheat bran), other grains and cereals, and vegetables are good sources of cellulose and other fibers that help prevent constipation.

> **TERMS**
>
> **dietary fiber**   Nondigestible carbohydrates and lignin that are intact in plants.
>
> **functional fiber**   Nondigestible carbohydrates either isolated from natural sources or synthesized; these may be added to foods and dietary supplements.
>
> **total fiber**   The total amount of dietary fiber and functional fiber in the diet.
>
> **soluble (viscous) fiber**   Fiber that dissolves in water or is broken down by bacteria in the large intestine.
>
> **insoluble fiber**   Fiber that does not dissolve in water and is not broken down by bacteria in the large intestine.

Psyllium, which is often added to cereals or used in fiber supplements and laxatives, improves intestinal health and also helps control glucose and cholesterol levels. The processing of packaged foods can remove fiber, so it is important to rely on fresh fruits and vegetables and foods made from whole grains as your main sources of fiber.

Recommended Fiber Intake   To reduce the risk of chronic disease and maintain intestinal health, the Food and Nutrition Board recommends a daily fiber intake of 38 grams for adult men and 25 grams for adult women. Americans currently consume about half this amount. Fiber should come from foods, not supplements, which should be used only under medical supervision.

Vitamins—Organic Micronutrients

Vitamins are organic (carbon-containing) substances required in small amounts to regulate various processes within living cells (Table 9.2). Humans need 13 vitamins; of these, 4 are fat-soluble (A, D, E, and K), and 9 are water-soluble (C, and the B-complex vitamins thiamin, riboflavin, niacin, vitamin B-6, folate, vitamin B-12, biotin, and pantothenic acid).

Functions of Vitamins   Many vitamins help chemical reactions take place. They provide no energy to the body directly but help unleash the energy stored in carbohydrates, proteins, and fats. Other vitamins are critical in the production of red blood cells and the maintenance of the nervous, skeletal, and immune systems. Some vitamins act as **antioxidants,** which help preserve the health of cells. Key vitamin antioxidants include vitamin E, vitamin C, and the vitamin A precursor beta-carotene.

Sources of Vitamins   The human body does not manufacture most of the vitamins it requires and must obtain them from foods. Vitamins are abundant in fruits, vegetables, and grains. In addition, many processed foods, such as flour and breakfast cereals, contain added vitamins. A few vitamins are made in certain parts of the body: the skin makes vitamin D when it is exposed to sunlight, and intestinal bacteria make vitamin K.

Vitamin Deficiencies   If your diet lacks a particular vitamin, characteristic symptoms of deficiency can develop. (Table 9.2 lists the signs of certain vitamin deficiencies.) For example, *scurvy* is a potentially fatal illness caused by a long-term lack of vitamin C. Children who do not get enough vitamin D can develop *rickets*, which leads to potentially disabling bone deformations. Vitamin A deficiency may cause

blindness, and anemia can develop in people whose diet lacks vitamin B-12. Low intake of folate and vitamins B-6 and B-12 has been linked to an increased risk of heart disease.

New research is tying vitamin deficiencies with other health risks, as well. For example, experts once thought that vitamin D was the only vitamin that played a role in bone health. Now scientists know that vitamins C and K, as well as several B vitamins, are also important in the prevention of osteoporosis. A great deal of recent research has focused on vitamin D, with surprising results. A systematic review of 17 studies suggests that vitamin D supplementation can reduce the risk of cardiovascular disease. Other studies also link low vitamin D levels to an increased risk of several cancers.

Vitamin deficiency diseases are most often seen in developing countries; they are relatively rare in the United States because vitamins are readily available from our food supply. Still, many Americans consume lower-than-recommended amounts of several vitamins. Even in the face of new findings, however, experts warn that there is not yet enough evidence to suggest that everyone should begin taking vitamin supplements. Supplementation is discussed in detail later in this chapter.

Extra vitamins in the diet can also be harmful, especially when taken as supplements. Megadoses of fat-soluble vitamins are particularly dangerous because the excess is stored in the body rather than excreted, increasing the risk of toxicity. Even when vitamins are not taken in excess, relying on supplements for an adequate intake of vitamins can be a problem. There are many substances in foods other than vitamins and minerals, and some of these compounds may have important health effects.

Minerals—Inorganic Micronutrients

Minerals are inorganic (non-carbon-containing) elements you need in relatively small amounts to help regulate body functions, aid in the growth and maintenance of body tissues,

> Even though we don't digest fiber, **it is necessary for good health**.

> **QUICK STATS**
>
> An estimated 10 million Americans have osteoporosis, and **34 million** more are at risk due to low bone mass.
> —National Osteoporosis Foundation, 2012

TERMS

vitamins   Carbon-containing substances needed in small amounts to help promote and regulate chemical reactions and processes in the body.

antioxidant   A substance that can reduce the breakdown of food or body constituents by free radicals; the actions of antioxidants include binding oxygen, donating electrons to free radicals, and repairing damage to molecules.

minerals   Inorganic compounds needed in relatively small amounts for regulation, growth, and maintenance of body tissues and functions.

Table 9.2	Facts about Vitamins			
VITAMIN	IMPORTANT DIETARY SOURCES	MAJOR FUNCTIONS	SIGNS OF PROLONGED DEFICIENCY	TOXIC EFFECTS OF MEGADOSES
Fat-soluble				
Vitamin A	Liver, milk, butter, cheese, fortified margarine, carrots, spinach, orange and deep-green vegetables and fruits	Immune function and maintenance of vision, skin, linings of the nose, mouth, digestive and urinary tracts	Night blindness, scaling skin, increased susceptibility to infection, loss of appetite, anemia, kidney stones	Liver damage, miscarriage, birth defects, headache, vomiting, diarrhea, vertigo, double vision, bone abnormalities
Vitamin D	Fortified milk and margarine, fish oils, butter, egg yolks (sunlight on skin also produces vitamin D)	Development and maintenance of bones and teeth, promotion of calcium absorption	Rickets (bone deformities) in children; bone softening, loss, and fractures in adults	Kidney damage, calcium deposits in soft tissues, depression, death
Vitamin E	Vegetable oils, whole grains, nuts and seeds, green leafy vegetables, asparagus, peaches	Protection and maintenance of cellular membranes	Red blood cell breakage and anemia, weakness, neurological problems, muscle cramps	Relatively nontoxic, but may cause excess bleeding or formation of blood clots
Vitamin K	Green leafy vegetables; smaller amounts widespread in other foods	Production of factors essential for blood clotting and bone metabolism	Hemorrhaging	None reported
Water-soluble				
Biotin	Cereals, yeast, egg yolks, soy flour, liver; widespread in foods	Synthesis of fat, glycogen, and amino acids	Rash, nausea, vomiting, weight loss, depression, fatigue, hair loss	None reported
Folate	Green leafy vegetables, yeast, oranges, whole grains, legumes, liver	Amino acid metabolism, synthesis of RNA and DNA, new cell synthesis	Anemia, weakness, fatigue, irritability, shortness of breath, swollen tongue	Masking of vitamin B-12 deficiency
Niacin	Eggs, poultry, fish, milk, whole grains, nuts, enriched breads and cereals, meats, legumes	Conversion of carbohydrates, fats, and protein into usable forms of energy	Pellagra (symptoms include diarrhea, dermatitis, inflammation of mucous membranes, dementia)	Flushing of the skin, nausea, vomiting, diarrhea, liver dysfunction, glucose intolerance
Pantothenic acid	Animal foods, whole grains, broccoli, potatoes; widespread in foods	Metabolism of fats, carbohydrates, and proteins	Fatigue, numbness and tingling of hands and feet, gastrointestinal disturbances	None reported
Riboflavin	Dairy products, enriched breads and cereals, lean meats, poultry, fish, green vegetables	Energy metabolism, maintenance of skin, mucous membranes, and nervous system structures	Cracks at corners of mouth, sore throat, skin rash, hypersensitivity to light, purple tongue	None reported
Thiamin	Whole-grain and enriched breads and cereals, organ meats, lean pork, nuts, legumes	Conversion of carbohydrates into usable forms of energy, maintenance of appetite and nervous system function	Beriberi (symptoms include muscle wasting, mental confusion, anorexia, enlarged heart, nerve changes)	None reported
Vitamin B-6	Eggs, poultry, fish, whole grains, nuts, soybeans, liver, kidney, pork	Metabolism of amino acids and glycogen	Anemia, convulsions, cracks at corners of mouth, dermatitis, nausea, confusion	Neurological abnormalities and damage
Vitamin B-12	Meat, fish, poultry, fortified cereals	Synthesis of blood cells, other metabolic reactions	Anemia, fatigue, nervous system damage, sore tongue	None reported
Vitamin C	Peppers, broccoli, spinach, brussels sprouts, citrus fruits, strawberries, tomatoes, potatoes, cabbage, other fruits and vegetables	Maintenance and repair of connective tissue, bones, teeth, and cartilage; promotion of healing; absorption of iron	Scurvy, anemia, reduced resistance to infection, loosened teeth, joint pain, poor wound healing, hair loss, poor iron absorption	Urinary stones in some people, acid stomach from ingesting supplements in pill form, nausea, diarrhea, headache, fatigue

SOURCES: Food and Nutrition Board, Institute of Medicine. 2006. *Dietary Reference Intakes: The Essential Guide to Nutrient Requirements.* Washington, DC: The National Academies Press. Available online at http://www.nap.edu/openbook.php?record_id=11537&page1; Shils, M. E., et al., eds. 2005. *Modern Nutrition in Health and Disease,* 10th ed. Baltimore: Lippincott Williams & Wilkins.

Table 9.3	Facts about Selected Minerals			
MINERAL	IMPORTANT DIETARY SOURCES	MAJOR FUNCTIONS	SIGNS OF PROLONGED DEFICIENCY	TOXIC EFFECTS OF MEGADOSES
Calcium	Milk and milk products, tofu, fortified orange juice and bread, green leafy vegetables, bones in fish	Formation of bones and teeth, control of nerve impulses, muscle contraction, blood clotting	Stunted growth in children, bone mineral loss in adults, urinary stones	Kidney stones, calcium deposits in soft tissues, inhibition of mineral absorption, constipation
Fluoride	Fluoridated water, tea, marine fish eaten with bones	Maintenance of tooth and bone structure	Higher frequency of tooth decay	Increased bone density, mottling of teeth, impaired kidney function
Iodine	Iodized salt, seafood, processed foods	Essential part of thyroid hormones, regulation of body metabolism	Goiter (enlarged thyroid), cretinism (birth defect)	Depression of thyroid activity, hyperthyroidism in susceptible people
Iron	Meat and poultry, fortified grain products, dark green vegetables, dried fruit	Component of hemoglobin, myoglobin, and enzymes	Iron-deficiency anemia, weakness, impaired immune function, gastrointestinal distress	Nausea, diarrhea, liver and kidney damage, joint pains, sterility, disruption of cardiac function, death
Magnesium	Widespread in foods and water (except soft water); especially found in grains, legumes, nuts, seeds, green vegetables, milk	Transmission of nerve impulses, energy transfer, activation of many enzymes	Neurological disturbances, cardiovascular problems, kidney disorders, nausea, growth failure in children	Nausea, vomiting, diarrhea, central nervous system depression, coma; death in people with impaired kidney function
Phosphorus	Present in nearly all foods, especially milk, cereal, peas, eggs, meat	Bone growth and maintenance, energy transfer in cells	Impaired growth, weakness, kidney disorders, cardiorespiratory and nervous system dysfunction	Drop in blood calcium levels, calcium deposits in soft tissues, bone loss
Potassium	Meats, milk, fruits, vegetables, grains, legumes	Nerve function and body water balance	Muscular weakness, nausea, drowsiness, paralysis, confusion, disruption of cardiac rhythm	Cardiac arrest
Selenium	Seafood, meat, eggs, whole grains	Defense against oxidative stress, regulation of thyroid hormone action	Muscle pain and weakness, heart disorders	Hair and nail loss, nausea and vomiting, weakness, irritability
Sodium	Salt, soy sauce, salted foods, tomato juice	Body water balance, acid–base balance, nerve function	Muscle weakness, loss of appetite, nausea, vomiting; deficiency is rarely seen	Edema (excess fluid buildup), hypertension in sensitive people
Zinc	Whole grains, meat, eggs, liver, seafood (especially oysters)	Synthesis of proteins, RNA, and DNA; wound healing; immune response; ability to taste	Growth failure, loss of appetite, impaired taste acuity, skin rash, impaired immune function, poor wound healing	Vomiting, impaired immune function, decline in blood HDL levels, impaired copper absorption

SOURCES: Food and Nutrition Board, Institute of Medicine. 2006. *Dietary Reference Intakes: The Essential Guide to Nutrient Requirements.* Washington, DC: The National Academies Press. Available online at http://www.nap.edu/openbook.php?record_id=11537&page1; Shils, M. E., et al., eds. 2005. *Modern Nutrition in Health and Disease,* 10th ed. Baltimore: Lippincott Williams & Wilkins.

and help release energy (Table 9.3). There are about 17 essential minerals. The major minerals, which the body needs in amounts exceeding 100 milligrams per day, include calcium, phosphorus, magnesium, sodium, potassium, and chloride. The essential trace minerals, which you need in minute amounts, include copper, fluoride, iodide, iron, selenium, and zinc.

Characteristic symptoms develop if an essential mineral is consumed in a quantity too small or too large for good health. The minerals commonly lacking in the American diet are iron, calcium, potassium, and magnesium. Iron-deficiency **anemia** is a problem in many age groups, and researchers fear that poor calcium intakes in childhood are sowing the seeds for future **osteoporosis,** especially in women (see the box "Eating for Healthy Bones").

TERMS

anemia   A deficiency in the oxygen-carrying material in the red blood cells.

osteoporosis   A condition in which the bones become thin and brittle over time and break easily; due largely to insufficient calcium intake.

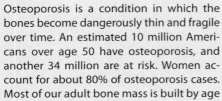

Osteoporosis is a condition in which the bones become dangerously thin and fragile over time. An estimated 10 million Americans over age 50 have osteoporosis, and another 34 million are at risk. Women account for about 80% of osteoporosis cases. Most of our adult bone mass is built by age 18 in girls and age 20 in boys. After bone density peaks between ages 25 and 35, bone mass is lost over time. To prevent osteoporosis, the best strategy is to build as much bone as possible during your youth and do everything you can to maintain it as you age. Up to 50% of bone loss is determined by controllable lifestyle factors. Key nutrients for bone health include the following:

- **Calcium.** Getting enough calcium is important throughout life to build and maintain bone mass. Milk, yogurt, and calcium-fortified orange juice, bread, and cereals are all good sources.

- **Vitamin D.** Vitamin D is necessary for bones to absorb calcium; a daily intake of 600 IU is recommended for individuals aged 1–70. Vitamin D can be obtained from foods and is manufactured by the skin when exposed to sunlight. Candidates for vitamin D supplements include people who don't eat many foods rich in vitamin D; those who don't expose their faces, arms, and hands to the sun (without sunscreen) for 5–15 minutes a few times each week; and people who live north of an imaginary line

roughly between Boston and the Oregon–California border (where the sun is weaker).

- **Vitamin K.** Vitamin K promotes the synthesis of proteins that help keep bones strong. Broccoli and leafy green vegetables are rich in vitamin K.

- **Other nutrients.** Other nutrients that may play an important role in bone health include vitamin C, magnesium, potassium, phosphorus, fluoride, manganese, zinc, copper, and boron.

Several dietary substances may have a *negative* effect on bone health, especially if consumed in excess. These include alcohol, sodium, caffeine, and retinol (a form of vitamin A). Drinking lots of soda, which often replaces milk in the diet, has been shown to increase the risk of bone fractures in teenage girls.

The effect of protein intake on bone mass depends on other nutrients. Protein helps build bone as long as calcium and vitamin D intake are adequate. But if intake of calcium and vitamin D is low, high protein intake can lead to bone loss.

Weight-bearing aerobic exercise helps maintain bone mass throughout life, and strength training improves bone density, muscle mass, strength, and balance. Drinking alcohol only in moderation, refraining from smoking, and managing depression and stress are also important for maintaining strong bones. For people who develop osteoporosis, a variety of medications are available to treat the condition.

Water—Vital but Often Ignored

Water is the major component in both foods and the human body: we are composed of about 50–60% water. Our need for other nutrients, in terms of weight, is much less than our need for water. We can live up to 50 days without food but only a few days without water.

Water is distributed all over the body, among lean and other tissues and in blood and other body fluids. Water is used in the digestion and absorption of food and is the medium in which most of the chemical reactions take place within the body. Some water-based fluids, like blood, transport substances around the body, whereas other fluids serve as lubricants or cushions. Water also helps regulate body temperature.

Water is contained in almost all foods, particularly in liquids, fruits, and vegetables. The foods and beverages you consume provide 80–90% of your daily water intake; the remainder is generated through metabolism. You lose water each day in urine, feces, and sweat and through evaporation from your lungs.

Most people can maintain a healthy water balance by consuming beverages at meals and drinking fluids in response to thirst. The Food and Nutrition Board has set levels of adequate water intake to maintain hydration. All fluids, including those containing caffeine, can count toward your total daily fluid intake. Under these guidelines, men need about 3.7 total liters of

water daily, with 3.0 liters (about 13 cups) coming from beverages; women need 2.7 total liters, with 2.2 liters (about 9 cups) coming from beverages. (See Table 1 in the Nutrition Resources section at the end of the chapter for information about specific age groups.) If you exercise vigorously or live in a hot climate, you need to consume additional fluids to maintain a balance between water consumed and water lost.

Other Substances in Food

Many substances in food are not essential nutrients but may influence health.

Antioxidants   When the body uses oxygen or breaks down certain fats or proteins as a normal part of metabolism, it gives rise to substances called **free radicals.** Environmental factors such as cigarette smoke, exhaust fumes, radiation, excessive

---

free radical   An electron-seeking compound that can react with fats, proteins, and DNA, damaging cell membranes and mutating genes in its search for electrons; produced through chemical reactions in the body and by exposure to environmental factors such as sunlight and tobacco smoke.   **TERMS**

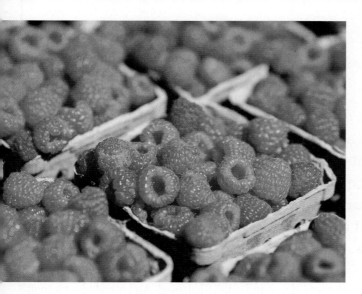

Berries are rich in antioxidants, vitamins, and dietary fiber.

30 years, researchers have identified and studied hundreds of different compounds found in foods, and many findings are promising. For example, certain substances found in soy foods may help lower cholesterol levels. Sulforaphane, a compound isolated from broccoli and other **cruciferous vegetables,** may render some carcinogenic compounds harmless. Allyl sulfides, a group of chemicals found in garlic and onions, appear to boost the activity of immune cells. Carotenoids found in green vegetables may help preserve eyesight with age.

If you want to increase your intake of phytochemicals, it is best to eat a variety of fruits, vegetables, and grains rather than relying on supplements. Like many vitamins and minerals, isolated phytochemicals may be harmful if taken in high doses. In many cases, their health benefits could be the result of many chemical substances working in combination.

NUTRITIONAL GUIDELINES: PLANNING YOUR DIET

Scientific and government groups have created a variety of tools to help people design healthy diets. The **Dietary Reference Intakes (DRIs)** are standards for nutrient intake designed to prevent nutritional deficiencies and reduce the risk of chronic diseases. The **Dietary Guidelines for Americans** were established to promote health and reduce the risk of major chronic diseases through diet and physical activity. **MyPlate (formerly MyPyramid)** provides a food guidance system to help people apply the Dietary Guidelines for Americans to their own diets.

Dietary Reference Intakes (DRIs)

The Food and Nutrition Board establishes dietary standards, or recommended intake levels, for Americans of all ages. The current set of standards, called Dietary Reference Intakes

sunlight, certain drugs, and stress can increase free radical production. A free radical is a chemically unstable molecule that reacts with fats, proteins, and DNA, damaging cell membranes and mutating genes. Free radicals have been implicated in aging, cancer, cardiovascular disease, and other degenerative diseases like arthritis.

Antioxidants found in foods can help protect the body from damage by free radicals in several ways. Some prevent or reduce the formation of free radicals; others remove free radicals from the body; still others repair some types of free radical damage after it occurs. Some antioxidants, such as vitamin C, vitamin E, and selenium, are also essential nutrients. Others—such as the carotenoids found in yellow, orange, and deep-green vegetables—are not. Some of the top antioxidant-containing foods and beverages include blackberries, walnuts, strawberries, artichokes, cranberries, brewed coffee, raspberries, pecans, blueberries, cloves, grape juice, unsweetened baking chocolate, sour cherries, and red wine. Also high in antioxidants are brussels sprouts, kale, cauliflower, and pomegranates.

Phytochemicals   Antioxidants fall into the broader category of **phytochemicals,** which are substances found in plant foods that may help prevent chronic disease. In just the past

TERMS

phytochemical   A naturally occurring substance found in plant foods that may help prevent and treat chronic diseases like cancer and heart disease; *phyto* means plant.

cruciferous vegetables   Vegetables of the cabbage family, including cabbage, broccoli, brussels sprouts, kale, and cauliflower; the flower petals of these plants form the shape of a cross, hence the name.

Dietary Reference Intakes (DRIs)   An umbrella term for four types of nutrient standards designed to prevent nutritional deficiencies and reduce the risk of chronic diseases. Estimated Average Requirement (EAR), Adequate Intake (AI), Recommended Dietary Allowance (RDA), and Tolerable Upper Intake Level (UL).

Dietary Guidelines for Americans   National nutritional recommendations issued jointly by the U.S. Department of Agriculture and the U.S. Department of Health and Human Services every five years; designed to promote health and reduce the risk of chronic diseases.

MyPlate   The USDA food guidance system designed to help Americans make healthy food choices.

(DRIs), was introduced in 1997. The DRIs are frequently reviewed and are updated as substantial new nutrition-related information becomes available. The DRIs present different categories of nutrients in easy-to-read table format. The DRIs have a broad focus, being based on research that looks not just at the prevention of nutrient deficiencies but also at the role of nutrients in promoting health and preventing chronic diseases such as cancer, osteoporosis, and heart disease.

The DRIs include standards for both recommended intakes and maximum safe intakes. The recommended intake of each nutrient is expressed as either *Recommended Dietary Allowance (RDA)* or *Adequate Intake (AI)*. An AI is set when there is not enough information available to set an RDA value; regardless of the type of standard used, however, the DRI represents the best available estimate of intake for optimal health. The *Tolerable Upper Intake Level (UL)* is the maximum daily intake that is unlikely to cause health problems in a healthy person.

Because of lack of data, ULs have not been set for all nutrients. This does not mean that people can tolerate chronic intakes of these vitamins and minerals above recommended levels. Like all chemical agents, nutrients can produce adverse effects if intakes are excessive. There is no established benefit from consuming nutrients at levels above the RDA or AI. The DRIs can be found in the "Nutrition Resources" section at the end of the chapter.

Because the DRIs are too cumbersome to use as a basis for food labels, the U.S. Food and Drug Administration (FDA) uses another set of dietary standards, the **Daily Values.** The Daily Values are based on several different sets of guidelines and include standards for fat, cholesterol, carbohydrate, dietary fiber, and selected vitamins and minerals. The Daily Values represent appropriate intake levels for a 2000-calorie diet. The percentage Daily Value shown on a food label shows how well that food contributes to your recommended daily intake.

Dietary Guidelines for Americans

To provide general guidance for choosing a healthy diet, the U.S. Department of Agriculture (USDA) and the U.S. Department of Health and Human Services (DHHS) issue the Dietary Guidelines for Americans,

> Two-thirds of Americans are overweight or obese, yet many are **undernourished in several key nutrients**.

revising them every five years. These guidelines are intended for all healthy Americans, including children aged 2 and older. Following these guidelines promotes health and reduces risk of chronic disease, including heart disease, cancer, diabetes, stroke, osteoporosis, and obesity. Each of the guidelines is supported by an extensive review of scientific and medical evidence.

The 2010 Dietary Guidelines are designed to help Americans make healthy and informed food choices. The main objective of the 2010 report is to encourage improved nutrition and physical activity in the American population, two-thirds of whom are overweight or obese and yet undernourished in several key nutrients. It focuses on the total diet and how to integrate the recommendations into a practical eating pattern that is nutrient-dense and calorie-balanced. And it includes findings on the broad environmental and societal aspects of the American diet—that is, the "food environment."

The 2010 Dietary Guidelines point out the large discrepancy between the recommendations and the actual American diet, which includes too few vegetables, fruits, high-fiber whole grains, low-fat milk and milk products, and seafood and too much added sugar, solid fat, refined grains, and sodium. A variety of dietary patterns can help Americans meet the recommendations.

General Guidelines   The Dietary Guidelines present two overarching recommendations:

- *Maintain calorie balance over time to achieve and sustain a healthy weight.*

- *Focus on consuming nutrient-dense foods and beverages.*

The guidelines highlight several key areas—balancing calories to manage weight, reducing certain dietary components, increasing other dietary components, building healthy eating patterns, and making healthy choices in the context of the current food and physical activity environment.

> The environment affects both sides of the calorie balance equation— **promoting overconsumption of calories and discouraging calorie expenditure** in the form of physical activity.

Balancing Calories to Manage Weight Calorie balance—the balance between calories consumed and calories expended—is the key to weight management. Current high rates of overweight and obesity can be attributed at least in part to people consuming more calories in foods and beverages than they expend in physical activity. In other words, many Americans are overweight because they are in calorie imbalance.

The guidelines recognize that many aspects of American life promote obesity, leading to an "obesogenic food environment." The environment affects both sides of the calorie balance equation—promoting overconsumption of calories and

---

Daily Values   A simplified version of the RDAs used on food labels; also included are values for nutrients with no RDA per se.

TERMS

discouraging calorie expenditure in the form of physical activity. Factors contributing to this environment include an increase in the number of fast-food restaurants in communities, an increase in meals eaten outside the home, increased portion sizes, sedentary work and home environments, limited availability of safe outdoor walking and recreational spaces, and increased dependence on transportation and technological advances that lead to lower calorie expenditure on everyday tasks.

Still, managing body weight means that individuals need to carefully consider their total calorie intake, and for people who are overweight or obese, this means consuming fewer calories from foods and beverages. The guidelines encourage people to become more conscious of what, when, why, and how much they eat; to deliberately make better choices; to seek ways to be more physically active, striving to meet the recommendations in the 2008 Physical Activity Guidelines for Americans; and to maintain a healthy weight at all stages of life. The guidelines also urge people to cook at home more and eat out less, to eat smaller portions, to limit screen time, and not to eat while watching TV.

Foods and Food Components to Reduce   In addition to overall calories, Americans tend to eat certain foods and food components in excess—in particular, sodium, solid fats, added sugars, and refined grains. Foods high in these items often replace foods with needed nutrients in the diet. Key recommendations include the following:

• Reduce daily sodium intake to less than 2,300 milligrams (mg) and further reduce intake to 1,500 mg if you are 51 or older, are African American, or have hypertension, diabetes, or chronic kidney disease. High sodium intake is associated with high blood pressure.

• Limit intake of saturated fats, trans fats, and dietary cholesterol. Consume less than 10% of calories from saturated fatty acids by replacing them with monounsaturated and polyunsaturated fatty acids. Keep trans fatty acid consumption as low as possible. Consume less than 300 mg per day of dietary cholesterol.

• Reduce the intake of calories from solid fats and added sugars. Most people should consume no more than 5–15% of daily calories from foods in these categories.

• Limit the consumption of foods that contain refined grains, especially refined grain foods that contain solid fats, added sugars, and sodium.

• If alcohol is consumed, it should be consumed in moderation—up to one drink per day for women and two drinks per day for men.

Foods and Nutrients to Increase   In general, Americans don't eat a wide enough variety of nutrient-dense foods to obtain all the nutrients they need in the amounts for optimal health. Recommendations include these:

• Eat more fruits and vegetables, and eat a variety of vegetables, especially dark-green, red, and orange vegetables and beans and peas.

• Consume at least half of all grains as whole grains, which are a source of iron, B vitamins, and dietary fiber.

• Increase intake of fat-free or low-fat milk and milk products, such as milk, yogurt, cheese, or fortified soy beverages. They are important sources of calcium, potassium, magnesium, vitamin D, and vitamin A.

• Choose a variety of protein foods, including seafood, lean meat and poultry, eggs, beans and peas, soy products, and unsalted nuts and seeds. Increase the amount and variety of seafood, and reduce protein foods that are high in solid fats and calories. In addition to protein, these foods provide B vitamins, vitamin E, zinc, and magnesium.

• Use oils to replace solid fats where possible.

• Choose foods that provide more potassium, dietary fiber, calcium, and vitamin D, which are nutrients of concern in American diets. These foods include vegetables, fruits, whole grains, and milk and milk products.

• Other nutrients are a concern for certain specific population groups, such as folic acid and iron for women who are pregnant or may become pregnant and vitamin B12 for adults aged 50 or older.

Building Healthy Eating Patterns   There are many different ways to incorporate the individual recommendations of the 2010 Dietary Guidelines into healthy eating patterns that (1) meet nutrient needs; (2) stay within calorie limits; (3) accommodate cultural, ethnic, traditional, and personal preferences; and (4) take into account food cost and availability. In other words, people can eat healthfully in many different ways.

Three eating plans that show how to put the Dietary Guidelines recommendations into action are the USDA Food Patterns, vegetarian adaptations of the USDA Food Patterns, and the DASH Eating Plan. A general principle in all these diets is that people should eat nutrient-dense foods—foods with little or no solid fats and added sugars—so they get all the needed nutrients without exceeding calorie limits. Another principle is that people should get their nutrients from foods rather than from dietary supplements, although supplements or fortification may be helpful for certain populations.

The USDA Food Patterns set recommended amounts of food to eat from each of five food groups and subgroups at different calorie levels. They also allow a certain amount of oils, and they limit the number of calories that should be consumed from solid fats and added sugars (SoFAS). You can use the chart shown in Figure 9.2 to find out the recommended intake of foods in each food group at your calorie level. For help determining your calorie level, refer to Table 9.4.

The vegetarian adaptations of the USDA Food Patterns include changes in the protein group and, for vegans, in the dairy group. The vegetarian variations, especially the vegan variation, rely on some fortified foods to ensure that the diet provides all required nutrients, such as calcium and vitamin B12.

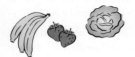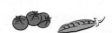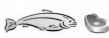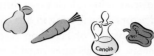

Daily Amount of Food from Each Group
Food group amounts shown in cups (c) or ounce-equivalents (oz-eq)

Calorie level of pattern	1600	1800	2000	2200	2400	2600	2800	3000
Fruits	1.5 c	1.5 c	2 c	2 c	2 c	2 c	2.5 c	2.5 c
Vegetables	2 c	2.5 c	2.5 c	3 c	3 c	3.5 c	3.5 c	4 c
Dark-green	1.5 c/wk	1.5 c/wk	1.5 c/wk	2 c/wk	2 c/wk	2.5 c/wk	2.5 c/wk	2.5 c/wk
Red and orange	4 c/wk	5.5 c/wk	5.5 c/wk	6 c/wk	6 c/wk	7 c/wk	7 c/wk	7.5 c/wk
Beans and peas (legumes)	1 c/wk	1.5 c/wk	1.5 c/wk	2 c/wk	2 c/wk	2.5 c/wk	2.5 c/wk	3 c/wk
Starchy	4 c/wk	5 c/wk	5 c/wk	6 c/wk	6 c/wk	7 c/wk	7 c/wk	8 c/wk
Other	3.5 c/wk	4 c/wk	4 c/wk	5 c/wk	5 c/wk	5.5 c/wk	5.5 c/wk	7 c/wk
Grains	5 oz-eq	6 oz-eq	6 oz-eq	7 oz-eq	8 oz-eq	9 oz-eq	10 oz-eq	10 oz-eq
Whole grains	3 oz-eq	3 oz-eq	3 oz-eq	3.5 oz-eq	4 oz-eq	4.5 oz-eq	5 oz-eq	5 oz-eq
Enriched grains	2 oz-eq	3 oz-eq	3 oz-eq	3.5 oz-eq	4 oz-eq	4.5 oz-eq	5 oz-eq	5 oz-eq
Protein foods	5 oz-eq	5 oz-eq	5.5 oz-eq	6 oz-eq	6.5 oz-eq	6.5 oz-eq	7 oz-eq	7 oz-eq
Seafood	8 oz/wk	8 oz/wk	8 oz/wk	9 oz/wk	10 oz/wk	10 oz/wk	11 oz/wk	11 oz/wk
Meat poultry, eggs	24 oz/wk	24 oz/wk	26 oz/wk	29 oz/wk	31 oz/wk	31 oz/wk	34 oz/wk	34 oz/wk
Nuts, seeds, soy products	4 oz/wk	4 oz/wk	4 oz/wk	4 oz/wk	5 oz/wk	5 oz/wk	5 oz/wk	5 oz/wk
Dairy	3 c	3 c	3 c	3 c	3 c	3 c	3 c	3 c
Oils	22 g	24 g	27 g	29 g	31 g	34 g	36 g	44 g
Maximum SoFAS limit, calories (% of calories)	121 (8%)	161 (9%)	258 (13%)	266 (12%)	330 (14%)	362 (14%)	395 (14%)	459 (15%)

FIGURE 9.2 USDA Food Patterns. To determine an appropriate amount of food from each food group, find the column for your estimated daily calorie level. That column shows the recommended daily intake from each group. For a personalized intake plan, visit ChooseMyPlate.gov.

SOURCE: U.S. Department of Agriculture and U.S. Department of Health and Human Services. 2010. *Dietary Guidelines for Americans, 2010*. 7th edition. Washington, DC: U.S. Government Printing Office.

The DASH Eating Plan emphasizes fruits, vegetables, fat-free and low-fat milk and milk products, whole grains, fish, poultry, seeds, and nuts. The DASH Eating Plan has been shown to help people lower their blood pressure and cholesterol levels, and it is associated with a lower risk of cardiovascular disease.

The eating pattern associated with many cultures bordering the Mediterranean Sea and referred to as the Mediterranean diet or the Mediterranean-style eating pattern has many features in common with the USDA Food Patterns and the DASH Eating Plan. It emphasizes fruits and

vegetables, nuts, olive oil, and grains, often whole grains, and includes only small amounts of meat and full-fat milk and milk products. The Mediterranean diet has been associated with lower rates of heart disease and lower rate of total mortality.

Helping Americans Make Healthy Choices A final area covered by the 2010 Dietary Guidelines for Americans is the environment in which people make their food choices. To make healthy choices, individuals need opportunities to obtain healthy foods and engage in physical activity. Significant

Table 9.4	Estimated Daily Calorie Needs		
AGE (YEARS)	SEDENTARY[a]	MODERATELY ACTIVE[b]	ACTIVE[c]
Female			
2–3	1000	1000–1400	1000–1400
4–8	1200–1400	1400–1600	1400–1800
9–13	1400–1600	1600–2000	1800–2200
14–18	1800	2000	2400
19–30	1800–2000	2000–2200	2400
31–50	1800	2000	2200
51+	1600	1800	2000–2200
Male			
2–3	1000–1200	1000–1400	1000–1400
4–8	1400–1600	1400–1600	1600–2000
9–13	1600–2000	1800–2200	2000–2600
14–18	2000–2400	2400–2800	2800–3200
19–30	2400–2600	2600–2800	3000
31–50	2200–2400	2400–2600	2800–3000
51+	2000–2200	2200–2400	2400–2800

[a]A lifestyle that includes only the light physical activity associated with typical day-to-day life

[b]A lifestyle that includes physical activity equivalent to walking about 1.5 to 3 miles per day at 3 to 4 miles per hour (30–60 minutes a day of moderate physical activity), in addition to the light physical activity associated with typical day-to-day life

[c]A lifestyle that includes physical activity equivalent to walking more than 3 miles per day at 3 to 4 miles per hour (60 or more minutes a day of moderate physical activity), in addition to the light physical activity associated with typical day-to-day life

SOURCE: U.S. Department of Health and Human Services and U.S. Department of Agriculture. 2011. *Dietary Guidelines for Americans, 2010* (http://www.cnpp.usda.gov/publications/dietaryguidelines/2010/policydoc/policydoc.pdf).

numbers of Americans—notably members of racial and ethnic minorities, people with disabilities, and people with lower incomes—lack access to affordable, nutritious foods and/or opportunities for safe physical activity in their neighborhoods.

The guidelines also recognize the need for *food security* in the United States—defined as the ability to acquire adequate food to meet nutritional needs in a socially acceptable manner. Nearly 15% of the population is not able to obtain sufficient food to meet basic nutritional needs. The guidelines call on all elements of society, ranging from educators to communities to government policymakers, to implement strategies aimed at improving the food and activity environment in the United States.

USDA's MyPlate

To further help consumers put the Dietary Guidelines for Americans into practice, the USDA also issues the food guidance system known as MyPlate (formerly MyPyramid).

MyPlate provides a simple graphic showing how to use the five good groups to build a healthy plate at each meal (Figure 9.3). Key messages include the following:

- Balancing calories:
  - Enjoy your food, but eat less.
  - Avoid oversized portions.
- Foods to increase:
  - Make half your plate fruits and vegetables.
  - Make at least half your grains whole grains.
  - Switch to fat-free or low-fat (1%) milk.
- Foods to reduce:
  - Compare sodium in foods like soup, bread, and frozen meals and choose the foods with lower numbers.
  - Drink water instead of sugary drinks.

You can get a personalized version of MyPlate recommendations by visiting www.ChooseMyPlate.gov. Using the daily food plan feature, you can determine the amount of each food group you need daily based on your calorie allowance. Your plan is personalized based on your age, gender, weight, height, and level of physical activity. Another feature available at ChooseMyPlate.gov is the SuperTracker, which helps consumers create a personalized food and activity plan.

Each food group is described briefly in the following sections. Many Americans have trouble identifying serving sizes, so recommended daily intakes from each group are given in terms of cups and ounces; see the box "Judging Portion Sizes" for additional advice.

Whole and Refined Grains A 2000-calorie diet should include 6 ounce-equivalents of grains each day, with half of those servings from whole grains. The key message

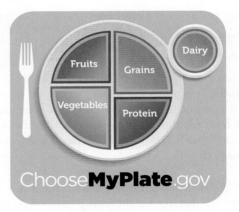

FIGURE 9.3 How to eat for health. Released in 2011, the USDA's MyPlate is designed as a simple graphic to help Americans apply the Dietary Guidelines for Americans to their own diets.

SOURCE: U.S. Department of Agriculture. 2010. *Choose MyPlate* (http://www.choosemyplate.gov).

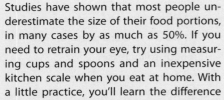

Studies have shown that most people underestimate the size of their food portions, in many cases by as much as 50%. If you need to retrain your eye, try using measuring cups and spoons and an inexpensive kitchen scale when you eat at home. With a little practice, you'll learn the difference between 3 and 8 ounces of chicken or meat and what a half-cup of rice really looks like. For quick estimates, use the following equivalents:

- 1 teaspoon of margarine = the tip of your thumb

- 1 ounce of cheese = your thumb, four dice stacked together, or an ice cube

- 3 ounces of chicken or meat = a deck of cards

- 1 cup of pasta = a small fist or a tennis ball

- ½ cup of rice or cooked vegetables = an ice cream scoop or one-third of a can of soda

- 2 tablespoons of peanut butter = a ping-pong ball or a large marshmallow

- 1 medium potato = a computer mouse

- 2-ounce muffin or roll = a plum or a large egg

- 2-ounce bagel = a hockey puck or a yo-yo

- 1 medium fruit (apple or orange) = a baseball

- ¼ cup nuts = a golf ball

- small cookie or cracker = a poker chip

---

for consumers is this: *Make at least half of your grains whole grains.* The following items count as a 1 ounce-equivalent:

- 1 slice of bread
- 1 small (2½-inch diameter) muffin
- 1 cup ready-to-eat cereal flakes
- ½ cup cooked cereal, rice, grains, or pasta
- 1 6-inch tortilla

Vegetables   A 2000-calorie diet should include 2½ cups of vegetables daily. The key message for the vegetable group is this: *Make half your plate fruits and vegetables.* Each of the following counts as 1 cup from the vegetable group:

- 1 cup raw or cooked vegetables
- 2 cups raw leafy salad greens
- 1 cup vegetable juice

Because vegetables vary in the nutrients they provide, it is important to eat a variety of vegetables to obtain maximum nutrition. MyPlate recommends weekly servings from five different subgroups within the vegetables group (see Figure 9.2). Try to eat vegetables from several subgroups each day.

Fruits   A 2000-calorie diet should include 2 cups of fruits daily. The key message for the fruit group is this: *Make half your plate fruits and vegetables.* Each of the following counts as 1 cup from the fruit group:

- 1 cup fresh, canned, or frozen fruit.
- 1 cup fruit juice (100% juice).

- 1 small whole fruit.
- ½ cup dried fruit.

Choose whole fruits often; they are higher in fiber and often lower in calories than fruit juices. Fruit *juices* typically contain more nutrients and less added sugar than fruit *drinks*.

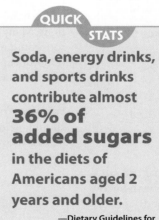

QUICK STATS

Soda, energy drinks, and sports drinks contribute almost **36% of added sugars** in the diets of Americans aged 2 years and older.

—Dietary Guidelines for Americans, 2010

Dairy   Dairy choices should be fat-free or low-fat as much as possible to reduce calories and limit saturated fats. The key message for the dairy group is this: *Switch to fat-free or low-fat (1%) milk.* A 2000-calorie diet should include 3 cups of milk or the equivalent daily. Each of the following counts as the equivalent of 1 cup:

- 1 cup milk
- 1 cup yogurt
- ½ cup ricotta cheese
- 1½ ounces natural cheese
- 2 ounces processed cheese

Cottage cheese is lower in calcium than most other cheeses; ½ cup is equivalent to ¼ cup milk.

Protein Foods   A 2000-calorie diet should include 5½ ounce-equivalents daily. Each of the following counts as equivalent to 1 ounce:

- 1 ounce cooked lean meat, poultry, or fish
- ¼ cup cooked dried beans (legumes) or tofu
- 1 egg
- 1 tablespoon peanut butter
- ½ ounce nuts or seeds

Choose lean meats and skinless poultry, select a variety of protein foods, and watch serving sizes carefully. Choose at least one serving of plant proteins, such as black beans, lentils, or tofu, every day, and include at least 8 ounces of cooked seafood per week.

Oils Oils are major sources of vitamin E and unsaturated fatty acids, including essential fatty acids, but they are not a food group. A 2000-calorie diet should include 6 teaspoons (27g) of oils per day. One teaspoon is the equivalent of the following:

- 1 teaspoon vegetable oil or soft margarine
- 1 tablespoon mayonnaise-type salad dressing

Foods that are mostly oils include nuts, olives, avocados, and some fish. The following portions include about 1 teaspoon of oil: 8 large olives, 1/6 medium avocado, 1/2 tablespoon peanut butter, and 1/3 ounce roasted nuts.

Solid Fats and Added Sugars (SoFAs) If you consistently choose nutrient-dense foods that are fat-free or low-fat and that contain no added sugars, you can also have a small amount of additional calories in the form of solid fats and added sugars (SoFAS). Figure 9.2 shows the maximum number of SoFAS calories allowed at each calorie level in MyPlate.

The current American diet includes higher levels of sugar intake and more calories per day from sugar than recommended. In particular, experts advise consumers to be wary of products containing high-fructose corn syrup. Although this sweetener is not harmful in itself, it is high in calories and very low in nutritional value. High-fructose corn syrup is found in many products, especially soft drinks and processed foods. Research has linked high consumption of high-fructose corn syrup with obesity, diabetes, and other health problems.

Physical Activity The Dietary Guidelines for Americans and MyPlate strongly encourage all Americans to be physically active as much as possible. Daily physical activity improves health, reduces the risk of chronic diseases, and helps people manage body weight. The MyPlate recommendation for adults is 2 1/2 hours of moderate physical activity or 1 1/4 hours of vigorous physical activity per week, equivalent to the 150 minutes of moderate activity or 75 minutes of vigorous activity recommended in the 2008 Physical Activity Guidelines for Americans.

The Vegetarian Alternative

Vegetarians choose a diet that restricts or excludes foods of animal origin (meat, poultry, fish, eggs, and milk). Vegetarian diets tend to be lower in total calories and calories from fat,

saturated fat, cholesterol, and animal protein while being higher in complex carbohydrates, dietary fiber, potassium, folate, vitamins C and E, carotenoids, and phytochemicals. Individuals who follow a vegetarian diet generally have a lower body mass index than nonvegetarians. Many people adopt a vegetarian diet for health reasons, while others do so out of concern for the environment, for financial reasons, or for reasons related to ethics or religion.

Types of Vegetarian Diets There are various vegetarian styles. The wider the variety of the diet eaten, the easier it is to meet nutritional needs. *Vegans* eat only plant foods. *Lacto-vegetarians* eat plant foods and dairy products. *Lacto-ovo-vegetarians* eat plant foods, dairy products, and eggs. Others can be categorized as partial vegetarians, semivegetarians, or pescovegetarians. These people eat plant foods, dairy products, eggs, and usually a small selection of poultry, fish, and other seafood.

A Food Plan for Vegetarians Adapting the USDA Food Patterns and MyPlate for vegetarians requires only a few key modifications. For the meat and beans group, vegetarians can focus on the nonmeat choices of dry beans, nuts, seeds, eggs, and soy foods like tofu. Vegans and other vegetarians who do not consume any dairy products must find other rich sources of calcium. Fruits, vegetables, and whole grains are healthy choices for people following all types of vegetarian diets.

A healthy vegetarian diet emphasizes a wide variety of plant foods. Although plant proteins are generally of lower quality than animal proteins, choosing a variety of plant foods will supply all of the essential amino acids. Choosing minimally processed and unrefined foods will maximize nutrient value and provide ample dietary fiber. Daily consumption of a variety of plant foods in amounts that meet total energy needs can provide all needed nutrients, except vitamin B-12 and possibly calcium, iron, zinc, and vitamin D.

Dietary Challenges for Various Population Groups

The Dietary Guidelines for Americans and MyPlate can help nearly anyone create a healthy diet. However, some population groups face special dietary challenges.

College Students Convenient foods are not always the healthiest choices. Students who eat in buffet-style dining halls can easily overeat, and the foods offered are not necessarily high in nutrients or low in fat. The same is true of meals at fast-food restaurants. See the box "Eating Strategies for College Students" for tips on healthy, inexpensive choices.

TERMS

vegetarian Someone who follows a diet that restricts or eliminates foods of animal origin.

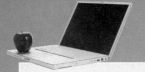
All the Time

- Eat a colorful, varied diet. The more colorful your diet is, the more varied and rich in fruits and vegetables it will be. Fruits and vegetables are typically inexpensive, delicious, nutritious, and low in fat and calories.

- Eat breakfast. You'll have more energy in the morning and be less likely to grab an unhealthy snack later on.

- Choose healthy snacks—fruits, vegetables, whole grains, and cereals.

- Drink nonfat milk, water, mineral water, or 100% fruit juice more often than soft drinks or sweetened beverages.

- Pay attention to portion sizes.

- Combine physical activity with healthy eating.

Eating in the Dining Hall

- Choose a meal plan that includes breakfast.

- Decide what you want to eat before you get in line, and stick to your choices.

- Build your meals around whole grains and vegetables.

- Choose leaner poultry, fish, or bean dishes rather than high-fat meats and fried entrees.

- Ask that gravies and sauces be served on the side.

- Choose broth-based or vegetable soups, not cream soups.

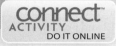

connect
ACTIVITY
DO IT ONLINE

- At the salad bar, load up on leafy greens, beans, and fresh vegetables. Avoid mayonnaise-coated salads, bacon, croutons, and high-fat dressings. Put dressing on the side, and dip your fork into it rather than pouring it over the salad.

- Choose fruit for dessert rather than baked goods.

Eating in Fast-Food Restaurants

- Order small single burgers with no cheese instead of double burgers with many toppings.

- Ask for items to be prepared without mayonnaise, tartar sauce, sour cream, or other high-fat sauces. Ketchup, mustard, and fat-free mayonnaise or sour cream are better choices and are available at many fast-food restaurants.

- Choose whole-grain bread for burgers and sandwiches.

- Choose chicken items made from chicken breast, not processed chicken.

- Order vegetable pizzas without extra cheese.

- Try a salad or fruit as a side item. If you can't resist french fries or onion rings, get the smallest size.

Eating on the Run

- Carry healthy snacks in your backpack or a small insulated lunch sack (with a frozen gel pack).

- Include fresh fruits or vegetables, snack-size cereal boxes, whole-grain crackers, pretzels, nuts or seeds, baked chips, low-fat popcorn, low-fat granola bars, or water.

Older Adults   Nutrient needs do not change much as people age, but because older adults tend to become less active, they don't need as many calories to maintain body weight. At the same time, older adults absorb some nutrients less efficiently because of age-related changes in the digestive tract. For these reasons, older adults should focus on eating nutrient-dense foods. Foods fortified with vitamin B-12 and/or B-12 supplements are recommended for people over age 50, and calcium and vitamin D supplements may be recommended for older adults to reduce bone loss and lower the risk of osteoporosis.

Athletes   Key dietary concerns for athletes are meeting their increased energy requirements and drinking enough fluids during practice and throughout the day to remain fully hydrated. Endurance athletes and athletes in heavy training may also benefit from increasing the amount of carbohydrate in the diet to 60–70% of total daily calories; this increase should take the form of complex, rather than simple, carbohydrates. Athletes who need to maintain a low body weight—such as skaters, gymnasts, and wrestlers—must avoid unhealthy eating patterns, which can lead to eating disorders.

People with Special Health Concerns   Many Americans have special health concerns that affect their dietary needs. For example, women who are pregnant or breastfeeding require extra calories, vitamins, and minerals. People with diabetes benefit from a well-balanced diet that is low in simple sugars, high in complex carbohydrates, and rich in monounsaturated fats. People with high blood pressure need to control their weight and limit their sodium consumption. If you have a health concern that requires a special diet, discuss your situation with a physician or registered dietitian.

A PERSONAL PLAN: MAKING INFORMED CHOICES ABOUT FOOD

Understanding the basics of good nutrition should get you started on creating a healthy diet that works for you. But eating for health involves other skills too, including knowing how to read food labels and dietary supplement labels, knowing how to handled and prepare food safely, and understanding food industry practices so you can make informed choices about what you eat.

Reading Food Labels

All processed foods regulated by either the FDA or the USDA include standardized nutrition information on their labels. Every food label shows serving sizes and the amounts of fat, saturated fat, trans fat, cholesterol, sodium, total carbohydrate, dietary fiber, sugars, and protein in each serving. To make intelligent choices about food, learn to read and *understand* food labels (see the box "Using Food Labels").

Dietary Supplements

All government food guidance systems encourage people to meet their nutritional needs with food rather than with vitamin and mineral supplements. Supplements lack the fiber and potentially beneficial phytochemicals that are found only in whole foods. Most Americans can get the vitamins and minerals they need by eating a nutritionally balanced diet of various foods. The use of supplements to reduce heart disease or cancer risk remains controversial, so experts suggest that you avoid taking any nutrient at a level exceeding the Tolerable Upper Intake Level (UL).

Although dietary supplements are sold over the counter, that doesn't necessarily mean they are safe. Some vitamins and minerals are dangerous when taken in excess. Large doses of particular nutrients can also cause health problems by affecting the absorption of certain vitamins or minerals. For this reason, ask your doctor or a dietician before taking any high-dosage supplement.

People Who Benefit from Supplements   In setting the DRIs, the Food and Nutrition Board recommended supplements of particular nutrients for specific groups:

• Women who are capable of getting pregnant should get 400 μg per day of folic acid (the synthetic form of the vitamin folate) from fortified foods and/or supplements in addition to folate from a varied diet. This level of folate can reduce the risk of neural tube defects in a developing fetus. Enriched breads, flours, cornmeal, rice, noodles, and other grain products are fortified with folic acid. Folate is found naturally in leafy green vegetables, legumes, oranges, and strawberries.

• As noted earlier, people over age 50 should eat foods fortified with vitamin B-12, take a B-12 supplement, or com-

bine the two to meet the RDA of 2.4 μg daily. Up to 30% of people over 50 may have trouble absorbing protein-bound B-12 in foods.

• Because of the oxidative stress caused by smoking, smokers should get 35 mg more vitamin C per day than the RDA set for their age and sex. Supplements aren't usually necessary, however, because this extra vitamin C can easily be found in foods. For example, an 8-ounce glass of orange juice has about 100 mg of vitamin C.

Supplements may be recommended in other cases. Women with heavy menstrual flows, for example, may need extra iron. Older adults, people with dark skin, and people exposed to little sunlight may need extra vitamin D. Other people may benefit from supplementation based on their physical condition, the medicines they take, or their dietary habits.

Before deciding whether to take a vitamin or mineral supplement, consider whether you already eat a fortified breakfast cereal every day. Many breakfast cereals contain almost as many nutrients as a multivitamin pill. If you elect to take a supplement, choose one that contains 50–100% of the Daily Values for vitamins and minerals. Avoid supplements containing large doses of particular nutrients.

Reading Supplement Labels   Dietary supplements include vitamins, minerals, amino acids, herbs, glandular extracts, enzymes, and other compounds. Although dietary supplements are often thought to be safe and "natural," they can contain powerful bioactive chemicals that have the potential for harm.

In the United States, dietary supplements are not legally considered drugs and are not regulated the same way drugs are. The FDA does not authorize or test dietary supplements, and supplement manufacturers are not required to demonstrate either safety or effectiveness prior to marketing.

Dietary supplement manufacture is not as closely regulated as the manufacture of drugs, and there is no guarantee that a product even contains a given ingredient, let alone in the appropriate amount. In addition, herbs can be contaminated or misidentified at any stage from harvest to packaging. To provide consumers with more reliable and consistent information about supplements, the FDA requires supplements to have labels similar to those found on foods (see the box "Using Dietary Supplement Labels" for more information).

Protecting Yourself against Foodborne Illness

Many people worry about additives or pesticide residues in their food, but a greater threat comes from microorganisms that cause foodborne illnesses. Raw or undercooked animal products, such as chicken, hamburger, and oysters, pose the greatest threat, although in recent years contaminated fruits and vegetables have been catching up.

Symptoms of foodborne illness include diarrhea, vomiting, fever, pain, headache, and weakness. Although the effects of foodborne illnesses are usually not serious, some groups,

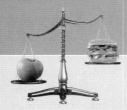

CRITICAL CONSUMER
Using Food Labels

The Nutrition Facts panel on a food label is designed to help consumers make food choices based on the nutrients that are most important to good health. In addition to listing nutrient content by weight, the label puts the information in the context of a daily diet of 2000 calories that includes no more than 65 grams of fat (approximately 30% of total calories). For example, if a serving of a particular product has 13 grams of fat, the label will show that the serving represents 20% of the daily fat allowance. If your daily diet contains fewer or more than 2000 calories, you need to adjust these calculations accordingly.

Food labels contain uniform serving sizes. This means that if you look at different brands of salad dressing, for example, you can compare calories and fat content based on the serving amount. It is important to keep in mind, however that food label serving sizes may be larger or smaller than MyPlate serving size equivalents. Regulations also require that foods meet strict definitions if their packaging includes the terms *light, low-fat,* or *high-fiber*. Health claims such as "good source of dietary fiber" or "low in saturated fat" on packages are signals that those products can wisely be included in your diet. Overall, the food label is an important tool to help you choose a diet that conforms to MyPlate and the Dietary Guidelines.

Selected Nutrient Claims and What They Mean

Healthy A food that is low in fat, is low in saturated fat, has no more than 360–480 mg of sodium and 60 mg of cholesterol, *and* provides 10% or more of the Daily Value for vitamin A, vitamin C, protein, calcium, iron, or dietary fiber.

Light or lite 33% fewer calories or 50% less fat than a similar product.

Reduced or fewer At least 25% less of a nutrient than a similar product; can be applied to fat ("reduced fat"), saturated fat, cholesterol, sodium, and calories.

Extra or added 10% or more of the Daily Value per serving when compared to what a similar product has.

Good source 10–19% of the Daily Value for a particular nutrient per serving.

High, rich in, or excellent source of 20% or more of the Daily Value for a particular nutrient per serving.

Low calorie 40 or fewer calories per serving.

High fiber 5 g or more of fiber per serving.

Good source of fiber 2.5–4.9 g of fiber per serving.

Fat-free Less than 0.5 g of fat per serving.

Low-fat 3 g of fat or less per serving.

Saturated fat-free Less than 0.5 g of saturated fat and 0.5 g of trans fatty acids per serving.

Low saturated fat 1 g or less of saturated fat per serving and no more than 15% of total calories.

Cholesterol-free Less than 2 mg of cholesterol and 2 g or less of saturated fat per serving.

Low cholesterol 20 mg or less of cholesterol and 2 g or less of saturated fat per serving.

Low sodium 140 mg or less of sodium per serving.

Very low sodium 35 mg or less of sodium per serving.

Lean Cooked seafood, meat, or poultry with less than 10 g of fat, 4.5 g or less of saturated fat, and less than 95 mg of cholesterol per serving.

Extra lean Cooked seafood, meat, or poultry with less than 5 g of fat, 2 g of saturated fat, and 95 mg of cholesterol per serving.

NOTE: The FDA has not yet defined nutrient claims relating to carbohydrates, so foods labeled low- or reduced-carbohydrate do not conform to any approved standard.

SOURCE: FDA, Food. Appendix C: Health Claims (http://www.fda.gov/Food/GuidanceComplianceRegulatoryInformation/GuidanceDocuments/FoodLabelingNutrition/FoodLabelingGuide/ucm064919.htm).

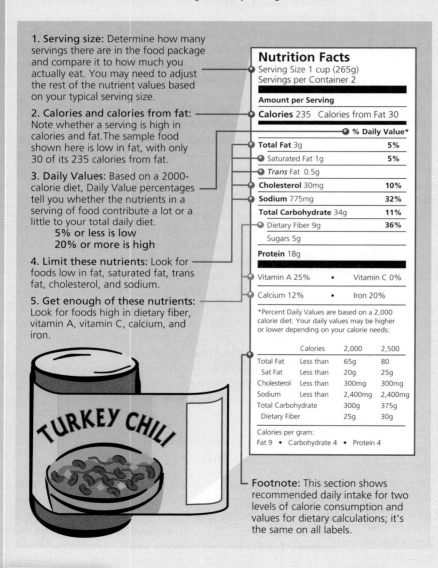

1. Serving size: Determine how many servings there are in the food package and compare it to how much you actually eat. You may need to adjust the rest of the nutrient values based on your typical serving size.

2. Calories and calories from fat: Note whether a serving is high in calories and fat. The sample food shown here is low in fat, with only 30 of its 235 calories from fat.

3. Daily Values: Based on a 2000-calorie diet, Daily Value percentages tell you whether the nutrients in a serving of food contribute a lot or a little to your total daily diet.
 5% or less is low
 20% or more is high

4. Limit these nutrients: Look for foods low in fat, saturated fat, trans fat, cholesterol, and sodium.

5. Get enough of these nutrients: Look for foods high in dietary fiber, vitamin A, vitamin C, calcium, and iron.

Footnote: This section shows recommended daily intake for two levels of calorie consumption and values for dietary calculations; it's the same on all labels.

Nutrition Facts

Serving Size 1 cup (265g)
Servings per Container 2

Amount per Serving

Calories 235   Calories from Fat 30

	% Daily Value*
Total Fat 3g	**5%**
Saturated Fat 1g	**5%**
Trans Fat 0.5g	
Cholesterol 30mg	**10%**
Sodium 775mg	**32%**
Total Carbohydrate 34g	**11%**
Dietary Fiber 9g	**36%**
Sugars 5g	
Protein 18g	

Vitamin A 25%	•	Vitamin C 0%
Calcium 12%	•	Iron 20%

*Percent Daily Values are based on a 2,000 calorie diet. Your daily values may be higher or lower depending on your calorie needs:

	Calories	2,000	2,500
Total Fat	Less than	65g	80
Sat Fat	Less than	20g	25g
Cholesterol	Less than	300mg	300mg
Sodium	Less than	2,400mg	2,400mg
Total Carbohydrate		300g	375g
Dietary Fiber		25g	30g

Calories per gram:
Fat 9 • Carbohydrate 4 • Protein 4

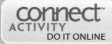
ACTIVITY DO IT ONLINE

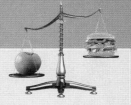

Since 1999 specific types of information have been required on the labels of dietary supplements. In addition to basic information about the product, labels include a "Supplement Facts" panel, modeled after the "Nutrition Facts" panel used on food labels (see the label illustrated here). Under the Dietary Supplement Health and Education Act (DSHEA) and food labeling laws, supplement labels can make three types of health-related claims:

- *Nutrient content claims,* such as "high in calcium," "excellent source of vitamin C," or "high potency." The claims "high in" and "excellent source of" mean the same as they do on food labels. A "high-potency" single-ingredient supplement must contain 100% of that nutrient's Daily Value; a "high-potency" multi-ingredient product must contain 100% or more of the Daily Value of at least two-thirds of the nutrients present for which Daily Values have been established.

- *Health claims,* if they have been authorized by the FDA or another authoritative scientific body. The association between adequate calcium intake and lower risk of osteoporosis is an example of an approved health claim. Since 2003 the FDA has also allowed so-called *qualified* health claims for situations in which there is emerging but as yet inconclusive evidence for a particular claim. Such claims must include qualifying language such as "scientific evidence suggests but does not prove" the claim.

- *Structure–function claims,* such as "antioxidants maintain cellular integrity" or "this product enhances energy levels." Because these claims are not reviewed by the FDA, they must carry a disclaimer (see the sample label).

Tips for Choosing and Using Dietary Supplements

- Check with your physician before taking a supplement. Many are not meant for children, older adults, women who are pregnant or breast-feeding, people with chronic illnesses or upcoming surgery, or people taking prescription or OTC medications.

- Choose brands made by nationally known food and drug manufacturers or house brands from large retail chains. Due to their size and visibility, such sources are likely to have high manufacturing standards.

- Look for the USP verification mark on the label, indicating that the product meets minimum safety and purity standards developed under the Dietary Supplement Verification Program by the United States Pharmacopeia (USP). The USP mark means that the product (1) contains the listed ingredients, (2) has the declared amount and strength of ingredients, (3) will dissolve effectively, (4) has been screened for harmful contaminants, and (5) has been manufactured using safe, sanitary, and well-controlled procedures. The National Nutritional Foods Association (NNFA) has a self-regulatory testing program for its members; other associations and labs, including ConsumerLab.Com, also test and rate dietary supplements.

- Follow the label's cautions, directions for use, and dosage.

- If you experience side effects, stop using the product and contact your physician. Report any serious reactions to the FDA's MedWatch monitoring program (800-FDA-1088 or online at http://www.fda.gov/Safety/MedWatch/default.htm).

For More Information about Dietary Supplements

ConsumerLab.Com: http://www.consumerlab.com

Food and Drug Administration: http://www.fda.gov/food/DietarySupplements/default.htm

National Institutes of Health, Office of Dietary Supplements: http://ods.od.nih.gov

U.S. Department of Agriculture: http://fnic.nal.usda.gov/dietary-supplements

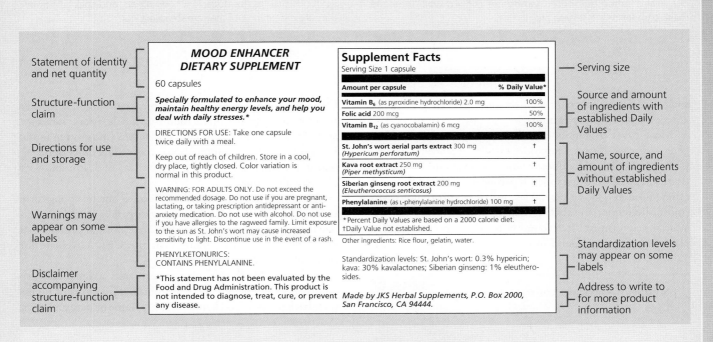

Statement of identity and net quantity

MOOD ENHANCER DIETARY SUPPLEMENT

60 capsules

Specially formulated to enhance your mood, maintain healthy energy levels, and help you deal with daily stresses.*

Structure-function claim

DIRECTIONS FOR USE: Take one capsule twice daily with a meal.

Keep out of reach of children. Store in a cool, dry place, tightly closed. Color variation is normal in this product.

Directions for use and storage

WARNING: FOR ADULTS ONLY. Do not exceed the recommended dosage. Do not use if you are pregnant, lactating, or taking prescription antidepressant or anti-anxiety medication. Do not use with alcohol. Do not use if you have allergies to the ragweed family. Limit exposure to the sun as St. John's wort may cause increased sensitivity to light. Discontinue use in the event of a rash.

Warnings may appear on some labels

PHENYLKETONURICS: CONTAINS PHENYLALANINE.

Disclaimer accompanying structure-function claim

*This statement has not been evaluated by the Food and Drug Administration. This product is not intended to diagnose, treat, cure, or prevent any disease.

Supplement Facts
Serving Size 1 capsule

Amount per capsule	% Daily Value*
Vitamin B$_6$ (as pyroxidine hydrochloride) 2.0 mg	100%
Folic acid 200 mcg	50%
Vitamin B$_{12}$ (as cyanocobalamin) 6 mcg	100%
St. John's wort aerial parts extract 300 mg (*Hypericum perforatum*)	†
Kava root extract 250 mg (*Piper methysticum*)	†
Siberian ginseng root extract 200 mg (*Eleutherococcus senticosus*)	†
Phenylalanine (as L-phenylalanine hydrochloride) 100 mg	†

* Percent Daily Values are based on a 2000 calorie diet.
† Daily Value not established.

Other ingredients: Rice flour, gelatin, water.

Standardization levels: St. John's wort: 0.3% hypericin; kava: 30% kavalactones; Siberian ginseng: 1% eleutherosides.

Made by JKS Herbal Supplements, P.O. Box 2000, San Francisco, CA 94444.

Serving size

Source and amount of ingredients with established Daily Values

Name, source, and amount of ingredients without established Daily Values

Standardization levels may appear on some labels

Address to write to for more product information

- Don't buy food in containers that leak, bulge, or are severely dented. Refrigerated foods should be cold and frozen foods should be solid when you buy them.

- Refrigerate perishable items as soon as possible after purchase. Use or freeze fresh meats within 3–5 days and fresh poultry, fish, and ground meat within 1–2 days.

- Store raw meat, poultry, fish, and shellfish in containers in the refrigerator so that the juices don't drip onto other foods. Keep these items away from other foods, surfaces, utensils, or serving dishes to prevent cross-contamination.

- Thaw frozen food in the refrigerator or in the microwave oven, not on the kitchen counter. Cook foods immediately after thawing.

- Thoroughly wash your hands with warm soapy water for 20 seconds before and after handling food, especially raw meat, fish, shellfish, poultry, or eggs.

- Make sure counters, cutting boards, dishes, utensils, and other equipment are thoroughly cleaned before and after use using hot soapy water. Wash dishcloths frequently.

- If possible, use separate cutting boards for meat, poultry, and seafood and for foods that will be eaten raw. Replace cutting boards once they become worn or develop hard-to-clean grooves.

- Thoroughly rinse and scrub fruits and vegetables with a brush, if possible, or peel off the skin.

- Cook foods thoroughly, especially beef, poultry, fish, pork, wild game, and eggs; cooking kills most microorganisms. Use a food thermometer to ensure that foods are cooked to a safe temperature. Hamburgers should be cooked to at least 160°F. Turn or stir microwaved food to make sure it is heated evenly throughout. When eating out, order hamburger cooked well-done and make sure foods are served piping hot.

- Keep hot foods hot (140°F or above) and cold foods cold (40°F or below). Harmful bacteria can grow rapidly between these two temperatures. Refrigerate foods within two hours of purchase or preparation, and within one hour if the air temperature is above 90°F. Refrigerate foods at or below 40°F and freeze at or below 0°F. Use refrigerated leftovers within 3–4 days.

- Don't eat raw animal products, including raw eggs in homemade hollandaise sauce or eggnog. Use only pasteurized milk and juice, and look for pasteurized eggs, which are now available in some states.

- Cook eggs until they're firm, and fully cook foods containing eggs. Store eggs in the coldest part of the refrigerator, not in the door, and use them within 3–5 weeks.

- Avoid raw sprouts. Even sprouts grown under clean conditions in the home can be risky because bacteria may be present in the seeds. Cook sprouts before eating them.

- Read the food label and package information, and follow safety instructions such as "Keep Refrigerated" and the "Safe Handling Instructions."

- According to the USDA, "When in doubt, throw it out." Even if a food looks and smells fine, it may not be safe. If you aren't sure that a food has been prepared, served, and stored safely, don't eat it.

Additional precautions are recommended for people at particularly high risk for foodborne illness—pregnant women, young children, older people, and people with weakened immune systems or certain chronic illnesses. If you are a member of one of these groups, don't eat or drink any of the following products: unpasteurized juices; raw sprouts; unpasteurized (raw) milk and products made from unpasteurized milk; raw or undercooked meat, poultry, eggs, fish, and shellfish; and soft cheeses such as feta, Brie, Camembert, or blue-veined cheeses. To protect against *Listeria,* avoid ready-to-eat foods such as hot dogs, luncheon meats, and cold cuts unless they are reheated until they are steaming hot.

---

such as children, pregnant women, and the elderly, are more at risk for severe complications.

Most cases of foodborne illness are caused by **pathogens**—disease-causing microorganisms. According to the CDC, about 90% of foodborne illnesses, hospitalizations, and deaths in 2010 were due to seven pathogens: *Salmonella* (most often found in eggs, on vegetables, and on poultry); norovirus (most often found in salad ingredients and shellfish); *Campylobacter jejuni* (most often found in meat and poultry); *Toxoplasma* (most often found in meat); *Escherichia coli* (*E. coli*)

O157:H7 (most often found in meat and water); *Listeria monocytogenes* (most often found in lunch meats, sausages, and hot dogs); and *Clostridium perfringens* (most often found in meat and gravy). Salmonella was the leading cause of hospitalizations and deaths, accounting for 28% of deaths and 35% of hospitalizations.

Another potential threat from food is bovine spongiform encephalopathy (BSE), or "mad cow disease", a fatal degenerative neurological disease caused by an abnormal protein that forms deposits in the brain. Visit the USDA website for more information (www.usda.gov).

Although foodborne illness outbreaks associated with food-processing plants make headlines, most cases of illness trace back to poor food handling in the home or in restaurants.

| **pathogen** A microorganism that causes disease. | **TERMS** |

The Dietary Guidelines for Americans encourage people to follow four basic food safety principles:

- **Clean** hands, food contact surfaces, and vegetables and fruits.
- **Separate** raw, cooked, and ready-to-eat foods while shopping, storing, and preparing foods.
- **Cook** foods to a safe temperature.
- **Chill** (refrigerate) perishable foods promptly.

If you think you may be having a bout of foodborne illness, drink plenty of fluids to prevent dehydration and consult a physician. For more details on handling food safely, see the box "Safe Food Handling."

Although pathogens are usually destroyed during cooking, the U.S. government has taken steps to bring down levels of contamination by improving national surveillance and testing. Raw meat and poultry products are now sold with safe handling and safe cooking instructions, and all packaged, unpasteurized fresh fruit and vegetable juices carry warnings about potential contamination. In 2011 the Food Safety Modernization Act (FSMA) was signed into law to reform the food safety system in the United States and further ensure the safety of the U.S. food supply. The FSMA allows the FDA to focus more on preventing food safety problems than on reacting to problems after they occur.

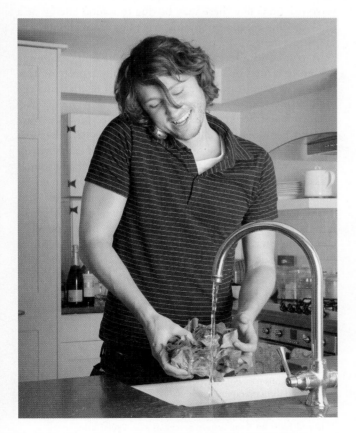

Careful food handing greatly reduces the risk of foodborne illness.

Organic Foods

Some people who are concerned about pesticides and other environmental contaminants choose to buy foods that are **organic.** To be certified as organic by the USDA, foods must meet strict production, processing, handling, and labeling criteria. Organic crops must meet limits on pesticide residues. For meat, milk, eggs, and other animal products to be certified organic, animals must be given organic feed and access to the outdoors and may not be given antibiotics or growth hormones. The use of genetic engineering, ionizing radiation, and sewage sludge is prohibited. Products can be labeled "100% organic" if they contain all organic ingredients and "organic" if they contain at least 95% organic ingredients; all such products may carry the USDA organic seal. A product with at least 70% organic ingredients can be labeled "made with organic ingredients" but cannot use the USDA seal.

Some experts recommend that consumers who want to buy organic produce spend their money on those fruits and vegetables that have the highest levels of pesticide residue when grown conventionally (the "dirty dozen"): apples, bell peppers, celery, cherries, imported grapes, nectarines, peaches, pears, potatoes, red raspberries, spinach, and strawberries. Experts also recommend buying organic beef, poultry, eggs, dairy products, and baby food. Fruits and vegetables that carry little pesticide residue whether grown conventionally or organically include asparagus, avocadoes, bananas, broccoli, cauliflower, corn, kiwi, mangoes, onions, papaya, pineapples, and peas. All foods are subject to strict pesticide limits; the debate about the health effects of small amounts of residue is ongoing.

Whether organic foods are better for your health or not, organic farming is better for the environment. Benefits include sustainable farming practices, preservation of biodiversity, healthier soil, protection of water supplies, reduced use of fossil fuels, improved animal welfare, protection of ecosystems, and safer conditions for farmworkers. Buying organic food, buying locally grown foods, and participating in a community garden are ways to support food production that benefits and sustains the environment.

Guidelines for Fish Consumption

A specific area of concern has been mercury contamination in fish. Overall, fish and shellfish are healthy sources of protein, omega-3 fats, and other nutrients. Prudent choices can minimize the risk of any possible negative health effects.

However, according to FDA and Environmental Protection Agency (EPA) guidelines, as well as the Dietary Guidelines for

organic A designation applied to foods grown and produced according to strict guidelines limiting the use of pesticides, nonorganic ingredients, hormones, antibiotics, irradiation, genetic engineering, and other practices.

TERMS

Americans, women who are or who may become pregnant and nursing mothers should follow these guidelines to minimize their exposure to mercury:

- Do not eat shark, swordfish, king mackerel, or tilefish.
- Eat 8–12 ounces a week of a variety of fish and shellfish that is lower in mercury, such as shrimp, canned light tuna, salmon, pollock, and catfish. Limit consumption of albacore tuna to 6 ounces per week.
- Check advisories about the safety of recreationally caught fish from local lakes, rivers, and coastal areas; if no information is available, limit consumption to 6 ounces per week.

The same FDA/EPA guidelines apply to children, although they should consume smaller servings.

Additives in Food

Approximately 3000 substances are intentionally added to foods to maintain or improve nutritional quality, to maintain freshness, to help in processing or preparation, or to alter taste or appearance. The most widely used food additives are sugar, salt, and corn syrup; these three plus citric acid, baking soda, vegetable colors, mustard, and pepper account for 98% by weight of all food additives used in the United States.

Additives having potential health concerns include nitrates and nitrites, used in processed meats and associated with the synthesis of cancer-causing agents in the stomach; BHA and BHT, used to maintain freshness and possibly associated with an increased risk of some cancers; sulfites, used to keep vegetables from turning brown and associated with severe reactions in sensitive people; and monosodium glutamate (MSG), used as a flavor enhancer and associated with episodes of increased blood pressure and sweating in sensitive people. If you are sensitive to an additive, check food labels when you shop, and ask questions when you eat out.

Food Biotechnology

Modern biotechnology tools, such as genetic engineering and cloning, allow for more precise, productive, and efficient development of crops and livestock. The USDA, FDA, and EPA are the three federal agencies in charge of the regulatory oversight of biotechnology.

Food irradiation is the treatment of foods with gamma rays, X-rays, or high-voltage electrons to kill potentially harmful pathogens, including bacteria, parasites, insects, and fungi that cause foodborne illness. Irradiation also reduces spoilage and extends a product's shelf life. Even though irradiation has been generally endorsed by agencies such as the WHO, the CDC, and the American Medical Association (AMA), few irradiated foods are currently on the market due to consumer resistance and skepticism. All primary irradiated foods (meat, vegetables, and so on) are labeled with the flowerlike radura symbol and a brief information label;

spices and foods that are merely ingredients do not have to be so labeled.

Genetic engineering involves altering the characteristics of a plant, animal, or microorganism by adding, rearranging, or replacing genes in its DNA; the result is a **genetically modified (GM) organism.** Many GM crops are already grown in the United States. Products made with GM organisms include juice, soda, nuts, tuna, frozen pizza, spaghetti sauce, canola oil, chips, salad dressings, and soup.

The potential benefits of GM foods cited by supporters include improved yields overall and in difficult growing conditions, increased disease resistance, improved nutritional content, lower prices, and less pesticide use. Critics argue that unexpected effects may occur. Gene manipulation could elevate levels of naturally occurring toxins or allergens, permanently change the gene pool, reduce biodiversity, and produce pesticide-resistant insects through the transfer of genes. Experience has shown that GM products are difficult to keep separate from non-GM products. Animal escapes, cross-pollination, and contamination during processing are just a few ways in which GM organisms could potentially appear unexpectedly in the food supply or the environment.

Food Allergies and Food Intolerances

For some people, consuming a particular food causes symptoms such as itchiness, swollen lips, or abdominal pain. Adverse reactions like these may be due to a food allergy or a food intolerance, and symptoms may range from annoying to life-threatening.

A true **food allergy** is a reaction of the body's immune system to a food or food ingredient, usually a protein. This immune reaction can occur within minutes of ingesting the food, resulting in symptoms that affect the skin (hives), gastrointestinal tract (cramps or diarrhea), respiratory tract (asthma), or mouth (swelling of the lips or tongue). The most severe response is a systemic reaction called *anaphylaxis*, which involves a potentially life-threatening drop in blood pressure. People at risk are usually advised to carry medications to treat anaphylaxis, such as injectable epinephrine.

Although numerous food allergens have been identified, just eight foods account for more than 90% of the food allergies in the United States: cow's milk, eggs, peanuts, tree nuts (walnuts, cashews, and so on), soy, wheat, fish, and shellfish.

TERMS

food irradiation The treatment of foods with gamma rays, X-rays, or high-voltage electrons to kill potentially harmful pathogens and increase shelf life.

genetically modified (GM) organism A plant, animal, or microorganism in which genes have been added, rearranged, or replaced through genetic engineering.

food allergy An adverse reaction to a food or food ingredient in which the immune system perceives a particular substance (allergen) as foreign and acts to destroy it.

Food labels are now required to state the presence of the eight most common allergens in plain language in the ingredient list.

Many people who believe they have food allergies may actually suffer from a **food intolerance.** In this case, the body may not be able to adequately digest a food or food component, often because of some type of chemical deficiency, or it may react to a particular compound in a food. Lactose intolerance is a fairly common food intolerance. A more serious condition is intolerance of gluten, a protein component of some grains; in affected individuals, consumption of gluten damages the lining of the small intestine. Sulfite, a common food additive, can produce severe asthmatic reactions in sensitive individuals.

Food intolerance reactions often produce symptoms similar to those of food allergies, such as diarrhea or cramps, but reactions are typically localized and not life-threatening. Exceptions are gluten and sulfite, which must be avoided by sensitive individuals. Through trial and error, most people with food intolerances can adjust their intake of the trigger food to an appropriate level.

> **TERMS**
>
> **food intolerance** An adverse reaction to a food or food ingredient that doesn't involve an immune reaction.

SUMMARY

- To function at its best, the human body requires about 45 essential nutrients in specific proportions. People get these nutrients from foods; the body cannot synthesize most of them.

- Proteins, made up of amino acids, form muscles and bones and help make up blood, enzymes, hormones, and cell membranes. Foods from animal sources provide complete proteins; plants provide incomplete proteins. Protein intake should be 10–35% of total daily calories.

- Fats, a concentrated source of energy, also help insulate the body and cushion the organs; 1 tablespoon of vegetable oil per day supplies the essential fats. Dietary fat intake should be 20–35% of total daily calories. Unsaturated fats should be favored over saturated and trans fats.

- Carbohydrates supply energy to the brain and other parts of the nervous system as well as to red blood cells. The body needs about 130 grams of carbohydrates a day, but more is recommended. Carbohydrates should make up 45–65% of total daily calories.

- Fiber includes nondigestible carbohydrates provided mainly by plants. Adequate intake of fiber (38 grams per day for men and 25 grams per day for women) can help people manage diabetes and high cholesterol levels and improve intestinal health.

- The 13 vitamins needed in the diet are organic substances that promote specific chemical and cell processes within living tissue. Deficiencies or excesses can cause serious illnesses and even death.

- The approximately 17 minerals needed in the diet are inorganic substances that regulate body functions, aid in the growth and maintenance of body tissues, and help in the release of energy from foods.

• Water is used to digest and absorb food, transport substances around the body, and regulate body temperature.

• Foods contain other substances such as phytochemicals, which may not be essential nutrients but may help reduce chronic disease risk.

• Dietary Reference Intakes (DRIs) are recommended intakes for essential nutrients that meet the needs of healthy people.

• The Dietary Guidelines for Americans are designed to help people make healthy and informed food choices. Following the guidelines promotes health and reduces the risk of chronic disease. The 2010 Dietary Guidelines for Americans present recommendations in several areas: balancing calories to manage weight, reducing certain food components, increasing other food components, building healthy eating patterns, and making healthy choices in the context of the current food and physical activity environment.

• Choosing the right amount of foods from each food group in MyPlate every day ensures that you get enough necessary nutrients without overconsuming calories.

• A vegetarian diet can meet human nutritional needs.

• Almost all foods have labels that show how much fat, cholesterol, protein, fiber, and sodium they contain. Serving sizes are standardized, and health claims are carefully regulated. Dietary supplements also have uniform labels.

• Foodborne illnesses are a greater threat to health than additives and environmental contaminants. Other dietary issues of concern to some people include organic foods, food irradiation, genetic modification of foods, and food allergies and intolerances.

FOR MORE INFORMATION

BOOKS

Byrd-Bredbenner, C., et al. 2012. *Wardlaw's Perspectives in Nutrition*, 9th ed. New York: McGraw-Hill. *An easy-to-understand review of major concepts in nutrition.*

Duyff, R. L. 2012. *ADA Complete Food and Nutrition Guide*, 4th ed. Hoboken, NJ: Wiley. *An excellent review of current nutrition information.*

Insel, P., D. Ross, K. McMahon, and M. Bernstein. 2011. *Nutrition*, 4th ed. Sudbury, MA: Jones & Bartlett. *An introductory nutrition textbook covering a variety of key topics.*

Nestle, M. 2007. *What to Eat*. New York: North Point Press. *A nutritionist examines the marketing of food and explains how to interpret food-related information while shopping.*

Selkowitz, A. 2005. *The College Student's Guide to Eating Well on Campus*, revised ed. Bethesda, MD: Tulip Hill Press. *Provides practical advice for students, including how to make healthy choices when eating in a dorm or restaurant and how to stock a first pantry.*

Warshaw, H. 2008. *Eat Out Eat Right: The Guide to Healthier Restaurant Eating*. 3rd ed. Agate Surrey. *A registered dietitian provides realistic, informative guidelines for restaurant eating to enable diners to make healthy menu choices from a wide variety of foods and cuisines.*

NEWSLETTERS

Environmental Nutrition (http://www.environmentalnutrition.com)

Nutrition Action Health Letter (http://cspinet.org/nah)

Tufts University Health & Nutrition Letter (http://www.tuftshealthletter.com)

ORGANIZATIONS, HOTLINES, AND WEBSITES

American Diabetes Association. An organization with the aim of leading the fight against the deadly consequences of diabetes and fighting for those affected by diabetes.

http://www.diabetes.org

Academy of Nutrition and Dietetics (formerly the American Dietetic Association). Provides a wide variety of nutrition-related educational materials.

http://www.eatright.org

The *Dietary Guidelines*. The official site for the Dietary Guidelines for Americans, 2010.

http://www.dietaryguidelines.gov

FDA Center for Food Safety and Applied Nutrition. Offers information about topics such as food labeling, food additives, dietary supplements, and foodborne illness.

http://www.fda.gov/food

Food Safety Hotlines. Provide information on safe purchase, handling, cooking, and storage of food.

888-SAFEFOOD (FDA)

800-535-4555 (USDA)

Fruit and Veggies: More Matters. A nonprofit organization designed to increase consumption of fruits and vegetables to five or more servings a day to improve the health of Americans.

http://www.fruitsandveggiesmorematters.org

Gateways to Government Nutrition Information. Provide access to government resources relating to food safety and nutrition.

http://www.foodsafety.gov

http://www.nutrition.gov

Harvard School of Public Health: The Nutrition Source. Provides recent key research findings, an overview of the Healthy Eating Plate, and suggestions for building a healthful diet.

http://www.hsph.harvard.edu/nutritionsource

Mayo Clinic: Nutrition Basics. Medical, nutrition, and health information and tools for healthy living.

http://www.mayoclinic.com/health/nutrition-and-healthy-eating/MY00431

MyPlate. Provides personalized dietary plans and interactive food and activity tracking tools.

http://www.ChooseMyPlate.gov

National Academies' Food and Nutrition Board. Provides information about the Dietary Reference Intakes and related guidelines.

http://iom.edu/About-IOM/Leadership-Staff/Boards/Food-and-Nutrition-Board.aspx

USDA Center for Nutrition Policy and Promotion. Includes information about the Dietary Guidelines and MyPlate.

http://www.cnpp.usda.gov/

USDA Food and Nutrition Information Center. Provides a variety of materials and extensive links relating to the Dietary Guidelines, food labels, MyPlate, and many other topics.

http://www.nal.usda.gov/fnic

SELECTED BIBLIOGRAPHY

A guide to the best and worst drinks. 2006. *Consumer Reports on Health*, July: 8–9.

American Heart Association. 2012. *Diet and Lifestyle Recommendations* (http://www.heart.org/HEARTORG/GettingHealthy/Diet-and-Life-style-Recommendations_UCM_305855_Article.jsp).

American Heart Association. 2012. *Fish and Omega-3 Fatty Acids* (http://www.heart.org/HEARTORG/GettingHealthy/NutritionCenter/HealthyDietGoals/Fish-and-Omega-3-Fatty-Acids_UCM_303248_Article.jsp).

American Heart Association. 2012. Frequently Asked Questions about "Bad" Fats (http://www.heart.org/HEARTORG/General/Frequently-Asked-Questions-About-Bad-Fats_UCM_306349_Article.jsp).

Centers for Disease Control and Prevention. 2011. Vital signs: Incidence and trends of infection with pathogens transmitted commonly through food—Foodborne Diseases Active Surveillance Network, 10 U.S. sites, 1996–2010. *Morbidity and Mortality Weekly Report*, 60(2): 749–755.

Centers for Disease Control and Prevention. 2012. *CDC and the Food Safety Modernization Act* http://www.cdc.gov/foodsafety/fsma.html).

Centers for Disease Control and Prevention. 2012. Vital signs: Food categories contributing the most to sodium consumption—United States, 2007–2008. *Morbidity and Mortality Weekly Report* 61(5): 92–98.

Council for Responsible Nutrition. 2009. *Dietary Supplements: Safe, Regulated and Beneficial* (http://www.crnusa.org/pdfs/CRN_FACT_DSSafeRegulatedBeneficial_09.pdf).

Fink, S. W. 2012. Key articles of dietary interventions that influence cardiovascular mortality. *Pharmacotherapy*, 32(4): e54-87.

Finkelstein, E. A., et al. 2012. Obesity and severe obesity forecasts through 2030. *American Journal of Preventive Medicine Online* (http://www.ajpmonline.org/webfiles/images/journals/amepre/AMEPRE_33853-stamped2.pdf).

Food and Nutrition Board, Institute of Medicine. 2005. *Dietary Reference Intakes for Energy, Carbohydrate, Fiber, Fat, Fatty Acids, Cholesterol, Protein, and Amino Acids*. Washington, DC: National Academy Press.

Food and Nutrition Board, Institute of Medicine. 2005. *Dietary Reference Intakes for Water, Potassium, Sodium, Chloride, and Sulfate*. Washington, DC: National Academy Press.

Food and Nutrition Board, Institute of Medicine. 2011. *Dietary Reference Intakes for Calcium and Vitamin D*. Washington, DC: National Academy Press.

Harris, W. S., et al. 2009. Omega-6 fatty acids and risk for cardiovascular disease: A science advisory from the American Heart Association Nutrition Subcommittee of the Council on Nutrition, Physical Activity, and Metabolism; Council on Cardiovascular Nursing; and Council on Epidemiology and Prevention. *Circulation* 119(6): 902–907.

Harvard School of Public Health, Department of Nutrition. 2010. *The Nutrition Source: Knowledge for Healthy Eating* (http://www.hsph.harvard.edu/nutritionsource).

Johnson, R. K., et al. 2009. Dietary sugars intake and cardiovascular health: A scientific statement from the American Heart Association. *Circulation* 120(11): 1011–1020.

Jonnalagadda, S. S., et al. 2011. Putting the whole grain puzzle together: Health benefits associated with whole grains—Summary of American Society for Nutrition 2010 Satellite Symposium. *Journal of Nutrition*, 14(5): 1011S-1022S.

Lasater, G., C. Piernas, and B. M. Popkin. 2011. Beverage patterns and trends among school-age children in the U.S., 1989–2008. *Nutrition Journal* 10:103.

Mosaffarian, D., et al. 2006. Trans fatty acids and cardiovascular disease. *New England Journal of Medicine* 354(15): 1601–1613.

Nicholls, S. J., et al. 2006. Consumption of saturated fat impairs the anti-inflammatory properties of high-density lipoproteins and endothelial function. *Journal of the American College of Cardiology* 48(4): 715–720.

Siri-Tarino, P. W., et al. 2010. Meta-analysis of prospective cohort studies evaluating the association of saturated fat with cardiovascular disease. *American Journal of Clinical Nutrition* 91(3): 535–546.

Trump, D. L., et al. 2010. Vitamin D: Considerations in the continued development as an agent for cancer prevention and therapy. *Cancer Journal* 16(1): 1–9.

Tucker, K. L. 2009. Osteoporosis prevention and nutrition. *Current Osteoporosis Reports* 7(4): 111–117.

U.S. Department of Agriculture. 2011. Choose MyPlate (http://www.choose-myplate.gov).

U.S. Department of Agriculture and Centers for Disease Control and Prevention. 2010. *What We Eat in America* (http://www.ars.usda.gov/Services/docs.htm?docid=15044).

U.S. Department of Health and Human Services and U.S. Department of Agriculture. 2010. *Dietary Guidelines for Americans, 2010.* 7th edition. Washington, DC: U.S. Government Printing Office.

U.S. Environmental Protection Agency. 2012. *Fish Consumption Advisories* (http://www.epa.gov/hg/advisories.htm).

U.S. Food and Drug Administration. 2012. *Food Allergies: What You Need to Know* (http://www.fda.gov/food/resourcesforyou/consumers/ucm079311.htm).

BEHAVIOR CHANGE STRATEGY
Improving Your Diet by Choosing Healthy Beverages

This Behavior Change Strategy focuses on choosing healthy beverages to increase intake of nutrients and decrease intake of empty calories from added sugars and fat. This model can be applied to any change you want to make to your diet.

Gather Data and Establish a Baseline

Begin by tracking your beverage consumption in a journal. Write down the types and amounts of beverages you drink, including water. Also note where you were at the time and whether you got the beverage there or brought it with you. At the same time, investigate your options. Find out what other beverages you can easily find during your daily routine. This information will help you put together a successful plan for change.

Analyze Your Data and Set Goals

Evaluate your beverage consumption by dividing your typical daily consumption between healthy and less healthy choices. Use the following guide as a basis, and add other beverages to the lists as needed:

Choose More Often	Servings Daily	Choose Less Often	Servings Daily
Water: plain, mineral, sparkling		Regular soda	
Low-fat or fat-free milk		Whole milk	
Fruit juice (100%)		Fruit beverages made with little fruit juice	
Unsweetened herbal tea		Sugar-sweetened beverages such as iced tea and sports drinks	
Others		Others	

How many beverages do you consume daily from each category? What would be a healthy and realistic goal for change? For example, if your beverage consumption is currently evenly divided between the "choose more often" and "choose less often" categories (four from each list), you might set a final goal for your behavior change program of increasing your healthy choices by two (to six from the "more often" list and two from the "less often" list).

Develop a Plan for Change

Once you've set your goal, you need to develop strategies that will help you choose healthy beverages more often. Consider the following possibilities:

* Keep healthy beverages on hand. If you live in a dorm, rent a small refrigerator or keep water in a reusable bottle and other healthy choices in the dorm kitchen's refrigerator.

* Plan ahead, and carry a reusable bottle with water or 100% juice in your backpack every day.

* Check food labels on beverages for serving sizes, calories, and nutrients; comparison shop to find the healthiest choices, and watch your serving sizes. Use this information to make your "choose more often" list longer and more specific.

* If you eat out frequently, examine all the beverages available at the places you typically eat your meals. You'll probably find that plain water or other healthy choices are available.

You may also need to make changes in your routine to decrease the likelihood that you'll make unhealthy choices. For example, your journal might reveal that you always buy a soda after class when you pass a particular vending machine. If this is the case, try another route that bypasses the machine. Guard against impulse buying by carrying water or a healthy snack with you every day.

To complete your plan, try some of the other behavior change strategies described in Chapter 1: develop and sign a contract, set up a system of rewards, involve other people in your program, and develop strategies for challenging situations. Once your plan is complete, take action. Keep track of your progress by continuing to monitor and evaluate your beverage consumption.

Table 1 — Dietary Reference Intakes (DRIs): Recommended Levels for Individual Intake

LIFE STAGE	GROUP	BIOTIN (μG/DAY)	CHOLINE (MG/DAY)[a]	FOLATE (MG/DAY)[b]	NIACIN (MG/DAY)[c]	PANTOTHENIC ACID (MG/DAY)	RIBOFLAVIN (MG/DAY)
Infants	0–6 months	5	125	65	2	1.7	0.3
	7–12 months	6	150	80	4	1.8	0.4
Children	1–3 years	8	200	**150**	**6**	2	**0.5**
	4–8 years	12	250	**200**	**8**	3	**0.6**
Males	9–13 years	20	375	**300**	**12**	4	**0.9**
	14–18 years	25	550	**400**	**16**	5	**1.3**
	19–30 years	30	550	**400**	**16**	5	**1.3**
	31–50 years	30	550	**400**	**16**	5	**1.3**
	51–70 years	30	550	**400**	**16**	5	**1.3**
	>70 years	30	550	**400**	**16**	5	**1.3**
Females	9–13 years	20	375	**300**	**12**	4	**0.9**
	14–18 years	25	400	**400**[i]	**14**	5	**1.0**
	19–30 years	30	425	**400**[i]	**14**	5	**1.1**
	31–50 years	30	425	**400**[i]	**14**	5	**1.1**
	51–70 years	30	425	**400**[i]	**14**	5	**1.1**
	>70 years	30	425	**400**	**14**	5	**1.1**
Pregnancy	≤18 years	30	450	**600**[i]	**18**	6	**1.4**
	19–30 years	30	450	**600**[j]	**18**	6	**1.4**
	31–50 years	30	450	**600**[j]	**18**	6	**1.4**
Lactation	≤18 years	35	550	**500**	**17**	7	**1.6**
	19–30 years	35	550	**500**	**17**	7	**1.6**
	31–50 years	35	550	**500**	**17**	7	**1.6**
Tolerable Upper Intake Levels for Adults (19–70)			3500	1000[k]	35[k]		

LIFE STAGE	GROUP	THIAMIN (MG/DAY)	VITAMIN A (μG/DAY)[d]	VITAMIN B-6 (MG/DAY)	VITAMIN B-12 (μG/DAY)	VITAMIN C (MG/DAY)[e]	VITAMIN D (IU/DAY)[f]	VITAMIN E (MG/DAY)[g]
Infants	0–6 months	0.2	400	0.1	0.4	40	400*	4
	7–12 months	0.3	500	0.3	0.5	50	400*	5
Children	1–3 years	**0.5**	**300**	**0.5**	**0.9**	**15**	600	6
	4–8 years	**0.6**	**400**	**0.6**	**1.2**	**25**	600	7
Males	9–13 years	**0.9**	**600**	**1.0**	**1.8**	**45**	600	11
	14–18 years	**1.2**	**900**	**1.3**	**2.4**	**75**	600	15
	19–30 years	**1.2**	**900**	**1.3**	**2.4**	**90**	600	15
	31–50 years	**1.2**	**900**	**1.3**	**2.4**	**90**	600	15
	51–70 years	**1.2**	**900**	**1.7**	**2.4**[h]	**90**	600	15
	>70 years	**1.2**	**900**	**1.7**	**2.4**[h]	**90**	800	15
Females	9–13 years	**0.9**	**600**	**1.0**	**1.8**	**45**	600	11
	14–18 years	**1.0**	**700**	**1.2**	**2.4**	**65**	600	15
	19–30 years	**1.1**	**700**	**1.3**	**2.4**	**75**	600	15
	31–50 years	**1.1**	**700**	**1.3**	**2.4**	**75**	600	15
	51–70 years	**1.1**	**700**	**1.5**	**2.4**[h]	**75**	600	15
	>70 years	**1.1**	**700**	**1.5**	**2.4**[h]	**75**	800	15
Pregnancy	≤18 years	**1.4**	**750**	**1.9**	**2.6**	**80**	600	15
	19–30 years	**1.4**	**770**	**1.9**	**2.6**	**85**	600	15
	31–50 years	**1.4**	**770**	**1.9**	**2.6**	**85**	600	15
Lactation	≤18 years	**1.4**	**1200**	**2.0**	**2.8**	**115**	600	19
	19–30 years	**1.4**	**1300**	**2.0**	**2.8**	**120**	600	19
	31–50 years	**1.4**	**1300**	**2.0**	**2.8**	**120**	600	19
Tolerable Upper Intake Levels for Adults (19–70)			3000	100		2000	4000	1000[k]

NOTE: The table includes values for the type of DRI standard—Adequate Intake (AI) or Recommended Dietary Allowance (RDA)—that has been established for that particular nutrient and life stage; RDAs are shown in **bold type**. The final row of the table shows the Tolerable Upper Intake Levels (ULs) for adults; refer to the full DRI report for information on other ages and life stages. A UL is the maximum level of daily nutrient intake that is likely to pose no risk of adverse effects. There are insufficient data to set ULs for all nutrients, but this does not mean that there is no potential for adverse effects; source of intake should be from food only to prevent high levels of intake of nutrients without established ULs. In healthy individuals, there is no established benefit from nutrient intakes above the RDA or AI.

[a]Although AIs have been set for choline, there are few data to assess whether a dietary supply of choline is needed at all stages of the life cycle, and it may be that the choline requirement can be met by endogenous synthesis at some of these stages.

[b]As dietary folate equivalents (DFE): 1 DFE = 1 μg food folate = 0.6 μg folate from fortified food or as a supplement consumed with food = 0.5 μg of a supplement taken on an empty stomach.

[c]As niacin equivalents (NE): 1 mg niacin = 60 mg tryptophan.

[d]As retinol activity equivalents (RAEs): 1 RAE = 1 μg retinol, 12 μg β-carotene, or 24 μg α-carotene or β-cryptoxanthin. Preformed vitamin A (retinol) is abundant in animal-derived foods; provitamin A carotenoids are abundant in some dark yellow, orange, red, and deep-green fruits and vegetables. For preformed vitamin A and for provitamin A carotenoids in supplements, 1RE = 1 RAE; for provitamin A carotenoids in foods, divide the REs by 2 to obtain RAEs. The UL applies only to preformed vitamin A.

LIFE STAGE	GROUP	VITAMIN K (μG/DAY)	CALCIUM (MG/DAY)	CHROMIUM (μG/DAY)	COPPER (μG/DAY)	FLUORIDE (MG/DAY)	IODINE (μG/DAY)
Infants	0–6 months	2.0	200*	0.2	200	0.01	110
	7–12 months	2.5	260*	5.5	220	0.5	130
Children	1–3 years	30	700	11	340	0.7	90
	4–8 years	55	1000	15	440	1	90
Males	9–13 years	60	1300	25	700	2	120
	14–18 years	75	1300	35	890	3	150
	19–30 years	120	1000	35	900	4	150
	31–50 years	120	1000	35	900	4	150
	51–70 years	120	1000	30	900	4	150
	>70 years	120	1200	30	900	4	150
Females	9–13 years	60	1300	21	700	2	120
	14–18 years	75	1300	24	890	3	150
	19–30 years	90	1000	25	900	3	150
	31–50 years	90	1000	25	900	3	150
	51–70 years	90	1200	20	900	3	150
	>70 years	90	1200	20	900	3	150
Pregnancy	≤8 years	75	1300	29	1000	3	220
	19–30 years	90	1000	30	1000	3	220
	31–50 years	90	1000	30	1000	3	220
Lactation	≤18 years	75	1300	44	1300	3	290
	19–30 years	90	1000	45	1300	3	290
	31–50 years	90	1000	45	1300	3	290
Tolerable Upper Intake Levels for Adults (19–70)			2500		10,000	10	1100

LIFE STAGE	GROUP	IRON (MG/DAY)[l]	MAGNESIUM (MG/DAY)	MANGANESE (MG/DAY)	MOLYBDENUM (μG/DAY)	PHOSPHORUS (MG/DAY)	SELENIUM (MG/DAY)	ZINC (MG/DAY)[m]
Infants	0–6 months	0.27	30	0.003	2	100	15	2
	7–12 months	11	75	0.6	3	275	20	3
Children	1–3 years	7	80	1.2	17	460	20	3
	4–8 years	10	130	1.5	22	500	30	5
Males	9–13 years	8	240	1.9	34	1250	40	8
	14–18 years	11	410	2.2	43	1250	55	11
	19–30 years	8	400	2.3	45	700	55	11
	31–50 years	8	420	2.3	45	700	55	11
	51–70 years	8	420	2.3	45	700	55	11
	>70 years	8	420	2.3	45	700	55	11
Females	9–13 years	8	240	1.6	34	1250	40	8
	14–18 years	15	360	1.6	43	1250	55	9
	19–30 years	18	310	1.8	45	700	55	8
	31–50 years	18	320	1.8	45	700	55	8
	51–70 years	8	320	1.8	45	700	55	8
	>70 years	8	320	1.8	45	700	55	8
Pregnancy	≤8 years	27	400	2.0	50	1250	60	13
	19–30 years	27	350	2.0	50	700	60	11
	31–50 years	27	360	2.0	50	700	60	11
Lactation	≤18 years	10	360	2.6	50	1250	70	14
	19–30 years	9	310	2.6	50	700	70	12
	31–50 years	9	320	2.6	50	700	70	12
Tolerable Upper Intake Levels for Adults (19–70)		45	350[k]	11	2000	4000	400	40

[e]Individuals who smoke require an additional 35 mg/day of vitamin C over that needed by nonsmokers; nonsmokers regularly exposed to tobacco smoke should ensure they meet the RDA for vitamin C.

[f]As cholecalciferol: 1 μg cholecalciferol = 40 IU vitamin D. DRI values are based on the absence of adequate exposure to sunlight.

[g]As α-tocopherol. Includes naturally occurring RRR-α-tocopherol and the 2R-stereoisomeric forms from supplements; does not include the 2S-stereoisomeric forms from supplements.

[h]Because 10–30% of older people may malabsorb foodbound B-12, those over age 50 should meet their RDA mainly with supplements or foods fortified with B-12.

[i]In view of evidence linking folate intake with neural tube defects in the fetus, it is recommended that all women capable of becoming pregnant consume 400 μg from supplements or fortified foods in addition to consuming folate from a varied diet.

[j]It is assumed that women will continue consuming 400 μg from supplements or fortified food until their pregnancy is confirmed and they enter prenatal care, which ordinarily occurs after the end of the periconceptional period—the critical time for formation of the neural tube.

[k]The UL applies only to intake from supplements, fortified foods, and/or pharmacological agents and not to intake from foods.

[l]Because the absorption of iron from plant foods is low compared to that from animal foods, the RDA for strict vegetarians is approximately 1.8 times higher than the values established for omnivores (14 mg/day for adult male vegetarians; 33 mg/day for premenopausal female vegetarians). Oral contraceptives (OCs) reduce menstrual blood losses, so women taking them need less daily iron; the RDA for premenopausal women taking OCs is 10.9 mg/day. For more on iron requirements for other special situations, refer to *Dietary Reference Intakes for Vitamin A, Vitamin K, Arsenic, Boron, Chromium, Copper, Iodine, Iron, Manganese, Molybdenum, Nickel, Silicon, Vanadium, and Zinc* (visit http://www.nap.edu for the complete report).

[m]Zinc absorption is lower for those consuming vegetarian diets, so the zinc requirement for vegetarians is approximately twofold greater than for those consuming a nonvegetarian diet.

LIFE STAGE	GROUP	POTASSIUM (G/DAY)	SODIUM (G/DAY)	CHLORIDE (G/DAY)	CARBOHYDRATE RDA/AI (G/DAY)	CARBOHYDRATE AMDR[o] (%)	TOTAL FIBER RDA/AI (G/DAY)	TOTAL FAT AMDR[o] (%)
Infants	0–6 months	0.4	0.12	0.18	**60**	ND[q]	ND	[r]
	7–12 months	0.7	0.37	0.57	**95**	ND[q]	ND	[r]
Children	1–3 years	3.0	1.0	1.5	**130**	45–65	19	30–40
	4–8 years	3.8	1.2	1.9	**130**	45–65	25	25–35
Males	9–13 years	4.5	1.5	2.3	**130**	45–65	31	25–35
	14–18 years	4.7	1.5	2.3	**130**	45–65	38	25–35
	19–30 years	4.7	1.5	2.3	**130**	45–65	38	20–35
	31–50 years	4.7	1.5	2.3	**130**	45–65	38	20–35
	51–70 years	4.7	1.3	2.0	**130**	45–65	30	20–35
	>70 years	4.7	1.2	1.8	**130**	45–65	30	20–35
Females	9–13 years	4.5	1.5	2.3	**130**	45–65	26	25–35
	14–18 years	4.7	1.5	2.3	**130**	45–65	26	25–35
	19–30 years	4.7	1.5	2.3	**130**	45–65	25	20–35
	31–50 years	4.7	1.5	2.3	**130**	45–65	25	20–35
	51–70 years	4.7	1.3	2.0	**130**	45–65	21	20–35
	>70 years	4.7	1.2	1.8	**130**	45–65	21	20–35
Pregnancy	≤18 years	4.7	1.5	2.3	**175**	45–65	28	20–35
	19–30 years	4.7	1.5	2.3	**175**	45–65	28	20–35
	31–50 years	4.7	1.5	2.3	**175**	45–65	28	20–35
Lactation	≤18 years	5.1	1.5	2.3	**210**	45–65	29	20–35
	19–30 years	5.1	1.5	2.3	**210**	45–65	29	20–35
	31–50 years	5.1	1.5	2.3	**210**	45–65	29	20–35
Tolerable Upper Intake Levels for Adults (19–70)			2.3	3.6				

LIFE STAGE	GROUP	LINOLEIC ACID RDA/AI (G/DAY)	LINOLEIC ACID AMDR[o] (%)	ALPHA-LINOLENIC ACID RDA/AI (G/DAY)	ALPHA-LINOLENIC ACID AMDR[o] (%)	PROTEIN[n] RDA/AI (G/DAY)	PROTEIN[n] AMDR[o] (%)	WATER[p] (L/DAY)
Infants	0–6 months	4.4	ND[q]	0.5	ND[q]	9.1	ND[q]	0.7
	7–12 months	4.6	ND[q]	0.5	ND[q]	**13.5**	ND[q]	0.8
Children	1–3 years	7	5–10	0.7	0.6–1.2	**13**	5–20	1.3
	4–8 years	10	5–10	0.9	0.6–1.2	**19**	10–30	1.7
Males	9–13 years	12	5–10	1.2	0.6–1.2	**34**	10–30	2.4
	14–18 years	16	5–10	1.6	0.6–1.2	**52**	10–30	3.3
	19–30 years	17	5–10	1.6	0.6–1.2	**56**	10–35	3.7
	31–50 years	17	5–10	1.6	0.6–1.2	**56**	10–35	3.7
	51–70 years	14	5–10	1.6	0.6–1.2	**56**	10–35	3.7
	>70 years	14	5–10	1.6	0.6–1.2	**56**	10–35	3.7
Females	9–13 years	10	5–10	1.0	0.6–1.2	**34**	10–30	2.1
	14–18 years	11	5–10	1.1	0.6–1.2	**46**	10–30	2.3
	19–30 years	12	5–10	1.1	0.6–1.2	**46**	10–35	2.7
	31–50 years	12	5–10	1.1	0.6–1.2	**46**	10–35	2.7
	51–70 years	11	5–10	1.1	0.6–1.2	**46**	10–35	2.7
	>70 years	11	5–10	1.1	0.6–1.2	**46**	10–35	2.7
Pregnancy	≤18 years	13	5–10	1.4	0.6–1.2	**71**	10–35	3.0
	19–30 years	13	5–10	1.4	0.6–1.2	**71**	10–35	3.0
	31–50 years	13	5–10	1.4	0.6–1.2	**71**	10–35	3.0
Lactation	≤18 years	13	5–10	1.3	0.6–1.2	**71**	10–35	3.8
	19–30 years	13	5–10	1.3	0.6–1.2	**71**	10–35	3.8
	31–50 years	13	5–10	1.3	0.6–1.2	**71**	10–35	3.8

[n]Daily protein recommendations are based on body weight for reference body weights. To calculate for a specific body weight, use the following values: 1.5 g/kg for infants, 1.1 g/kg for 1–3 years, 0.95 g/kg for 4–13 years, 0.85 g/kg for 14–18 years, 0.8 g/kg for adults, and 1.1 g/kg for pregnant (using prepregnancy weight) and lactating women.

[o]Acceptable Macronutrient Distribution Range (AMDR), expressed as a percentage of total daily calories, is the range of intake for a particular energy source that is associated with reduced risk of chronic disease while providing intakes of essential nutrients. If an individual consumes in excess of the AMDR, there is a potential for increasing the risk of chronic diseases and/or insufficient intakes of essential nutrients.

[p]Total water intake from fluids and food.

[q]Not determinable due to lack of data of adverse effects in this age group and concern with regard to lack of ability to handle excess amounts. Source of intake should be from food only to prevent high levels of intake.

[r]For infants, adequate intake of total fat is 31 grams/day (0–6 months) and 30 grams per day (7–12 months) from breast milk and, for infants 7–12 months, complementary food and beverages.

SOURCE: From Food and Nutrition Board, Institute of Medicine, National Academies, 2010, Dietary Reference Intakes: The Essential Guide to Nutrient Requirements. Washington, D. C.: National Academies Press (http://www.iom.edu/Activities/Nutrition/SummaryDRIs/DRI-Tables.aspx. Reprinted with permission from the National Academies Press, Copyright 2010, National Academy of Sciences.

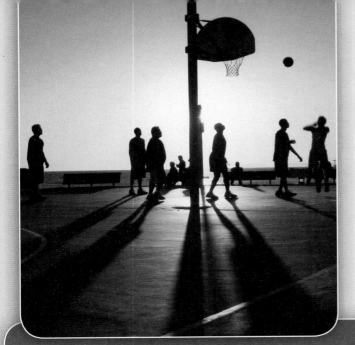

LOOKING AHEAD...

After reading this chapter, you should be able to

- Define physical fitness, and list the health-related components of fitness
- Explain the wellness benefits of physical activity and exercise
- Describe how to develop each of the health-related components of fitness
- Describe how to choose appropriate exercise equipment, how to eat and drink for exercise, and how to prevent and manage injuries
- Put together a personalized exercise program that you enjoy and that will enable you to achieve your fitness goals

Exercise for Health and Fitness

10

Your body is a wonderful moving machine, made to work best when it is physically active. It readily adapts to practically any level of activity and exercise: the more you ask of your body, the stronger and more fit it becomes. The opposite is also true. Left unchallenged, bones lose their density, joints stiffen, muscles become weak, and the body's energy systems degenerate. To be truly healthy, human beings must be active. If approached correctly, physical activity and exercise can contribute immeasurably to overall wellness, add fun and joy to life, and provide the foundation for a lifetime of fitness.

WHAT IS PHYSICAL FITNESS?

Physical fitness is a set of physical attributes that allow the body to respond or adapt to the demands and stress of physical effort—to perform moderate to vigorous levels of physical activity without becoming overly tired.

Some components of fitness are related to specific activities or sports, while others relate to general health. **Health-related fitness** includes cardiorespiratory endurance, muscular strength, muscular endurance, flexibility, and body composition. Health-related fitness helps you withstand physical challenges and protects you from diseases.

Cardiorespiratory Endurance

Cardiorespiratory endurance is the ability to perform prolonged, large-muscle, dynamic exercise at moderate to high intensity. When cardiorespiratory fitness is low, the heart has to work hard during normal daily activities and may not be able to work hard enough to sustain high-intensity physical activity in an emergency. Poor cardiorespiratory fitness is linked with heart disease, diabetes, colon cancer, stroke, depression, anxiety, and premature death from all causes.

Regular **cardiorespiratory endurance training,** however, conditions the heart. Endurance training makes the heart stronger and improves the function of the entire cardiorespiratory system. As cardiorespiratory fitness improves, related physical functions also improve. The heart pumps more blood per heartbeat, resting heart rate slows and resting blood pressure decreases, blood volume increases, blood supply to tissues improves, the body can cool itself better, and metabolic health improves, which helps the body process fuels and regulate cell function.

A healthy heart can better withstand the strains of daily life, the stress of occasional emergencies, and the wear and tear of time. You can develop cardiorespiratory endurance through activities that involve continuous, rhythmic movements of large muscle groups, such as the legs. Such activities include walking, jogging, cycling, and aerobic dancing.

Muscular Strength

Muscular strength is the amount of force a muscle can produce with a single maximum effort. It depends on such factors as the size of muscle cells and the ability of nerves to activate muscle cells. Strong muscles are important for everyday activities, such as climbing stairs, as well as for emergencies. They help keep the skeleton in proper alignment, preventing back and leg pain and providing the support necessary for good posture. Muscular strength has obvious importance in recreational activities. Strong people can hit a tennis ball harder, kick a soccer ball farther, and ride a bicycle uphill more easily.

Muscle tissue is an important element of overall body composition. Greater muscle mass makes possible a higher rate of metabolism and faster energy use, which help maintain a healthy body weight. Strength training helps maintain muscle mass, function, and balance in older people, which greatly enhances their quality of life and

prevents injuries. Strength training promotes cardiovascular health, reduces the risk of osteoporosis (bone loss), and prevents premature death from all causes. Muscular strength can be developed by training with weights or by using the weight of the body for resistance during calisthenic exercises such as push-ups and curl-ups.

Muscular Endurance

Muscular endurance is the ability to resist fatigue and sustain a given level of muscle tension—that is, to hold a muscle contraction for a long time or to contract a muscle over and over again. It depends on factors such as the size of muscle cells, the ability of muscles to store fuel, the content of mitochondria (cell energy centers), and the blood supply to muscles.

Muscular endurance is important for good posture and for injury prevention. Muscular endurance helps people cope with the physical demands of everyday life and enhances performance in sports and work. Stressing the muscles with a greater load (weight) than they are used to develops muscle endurance as well as muscular strength. The degree to which strength or endurance develops depends on the type and amount of stress that is applied.

Flexibility

Flexibility is the ability of joints to move through their full range of motion. Flexible, pain-free joints are important for good health and well-being. Inactivity causes the joints to become stiffer with age. Stiffness, in turn, often causes older people to assume unnatural body postures that can stress

Cardiorespiratory endurance is a critical component of fitness.

TERMS

physical fitness   The body's ability to respond or adapt to the demands and stress of physical effort.

health-related fitness   Physical capabilities that contribute to health, including cardiorespiratory endurance, muscular strength, muscular endurance, flexibility, and body composition.

cardiorespiratory endurance   The ability of the body to perform prolonged, large-muscle, dynamic exercise at moderate to high levels of intensity.

cardiorespiratory endurance training   Exercise intended to improve cardiorespiratory endurance.

muscular strength   The amount of force a muscle can produce with a single maximum effort.

muscular endurance   The ability of a muscle or group of muscles to remain contracted or to contract repeatedly for a long period of time.

flexibility   The joints' ability to move through their full range of motion.

joints and muscles. Stretching exercises can help ensure a healthy range of motion for all major joints.

Body Composition

Body composition refers to the proportion of fat and **fat-free mass** (muscle, bone, and water) in the body. Healthy body composition involves a high proportion of fat-free mass and an acceptably low level of body fat, adjusted for age and sex. A person with excessive body fat—especially in the abdomen—is more likely to experience health problems, including heart disease, high blood pressure, stroke, joint problems, diabetes, gallbladder disease, cancer, and back pain. The best way to lose fat is through a lifestyle that includes a sensible diet and exercise. The best way to add muscle mass is through resistance training such as weight training.

> **The best way to lose fat** is through a lifestyle that includes a sensible diet and exercise.

Skill-Related Components of Fitness

In addition to the five health-related components of physical fitness, the ability to perform a particular sport or activity may depend on **skill-related fitness** components such as speed, power, agility, balance, coordination, and reaction time.

Skill-related fitness tends to be sport-specific and is best developed through practice. Playing a sport can be fun, can help build fitness, and may contribute to other areas of wellness.

PHYSICAL ACTIVITY AND EXERCISE FOR HEALTH AND FITNESS

Physical activity is any body movement carried out by the skeletal muscles that requires energy. Quick, easy movements such as standing up or walking down a hallway require little energy or effort. More intense, sustained activities such as cycling five miles or running in a race require considerably more.

Exercise refers to a subset of physical activity—planned, structured, repetitive movement of the body intended specifically to improve or maintain physical fitness. To develop fitness, a person must perform enough physical activity to stress the body and cause long-term physiological changes. Moderate-intensity physical activity is essential to health and confers wide-ranging health benefits, but more intense exercise is necessary to improve physical fitness.

In 2011 the American College of Sports Medicine (ACSM) released the newest version of its exercise guidelines for healthy adults. This followed the 2010 U.S. Surgeon General report overweight and obesity in American children and adults, *The Surgeon General's Vision for a Healthy and Fit Nation*, and the landmark 2008 report from the U.S. Department of Health and Human Services, *Physical Activity Guidelines for Americans*. Although each of these reports has a somewhat different focus, they all stress the importance of regular physical activity for health, wellness, and the prevention of chronic diseases and premature death.

The 2008 guidelines include the following key guidelines for adults:

• For substantial health benefits, adults should do at least 150 minutes (2½ hours) a week of moderate-intensity aerobic physical activity, or 75 minutes (1 hour and 15 minutes) a week of vigorous-intensity aerobic physical activity, or an equivalent combination of moderate- and vigorous-intensity aerobic activity. Activity should preferably be spread throughout the week.

• For additional and more extensive health benefits, adults should increase their aerobic physical activity to 300 minutes (5 hours) a week of moderate-intensity activity, or 150 minutes (2½ hours) a week of vigorous-intensity activity, or an equivalent combination of moderate- and vigorous-intensity activity.

• Adults should also do muscle-strengthening activities that are moderate or high intensity and involve all major muscle groups on two or more days a week.

• Everyone should avoid inactivity.

These levels of physical activity promote health and wellness by lowering the risk of high blood pressure, stroke, heart disease, type 2 diabetes, colon cancer, and osteoporosis and

---

TERMS

body composition The proportion of fat and fat-free mass (muscle, bone, and water) in the body.

fat-free mass The nonfat components of the human body, consisting of skeletal muscle, bone, and water.

skill-related fitness Physical abilities that contribute to performance in a sport or activity, including speed, power, agility, balance, coordination, and reaction time.

physical activity Any body movement carried out by the skeletal muscles that requires energy.

exercise Planned, structured, repetitive movement of the body intended to improve or maintain physical fitness.

Ask Yourself

QUESTIONS FOR CRITICAL THINKING AND REFLECTION

When you think about exercise, do you think of only one or two of the five components of health-related fitness, such as muscular strength or body composition? If so, where do you think your ideas come from? What role do the media play in shaping your ideas about fitness?

"Too little time" is a common excuse for not being physically active. Learning to manage your time successfully is crucial if you are to maintain a wellness lifestyle. Begin by keeping a record of how you currently spend your time. List each type of activity and the total time you engaged in it on a given day—for example, sleeping, 7 hours; eating, 1.5 hours; studying, 3 hours; and so on. Prioritize your activities according to how important they are to you, from essential to somewhat important to not important at all.

Make changes in your daily schedule by subtracting time from some activities in order to make time for physical activity. Look carefully at your leisure-time activities and your methods of transportation—these are areas where it is easy to build in physical activity. For example, you may choose to reduce the total amount of time you spend playing computer games to make time for an after-dinner bike ride or a walk with a friend. You may decide to watch 10 fewer minutes of television in the morning to change your 5-minute drive to class into a 15-minute walk.

Here are a few ways to incorporate more physical activity into your daily routine:

• Take the stairs instead of the elevator or escalator.

• Walk to the mailbox, post office, store, bank, or library whenever possible.

• Do at least one chore every day that requires physical activity: wash the windows or your car, clean your room or house, mow the lawn, or rake the leaves.

• Take study or work breaks to avoid sitting for more than 30 minutes at a time. Get up and walk around the library, your office, or your home or dorm; go up and down a flight of stairs.

• When you take public transportation, get off one stop early and walk to your destination.

• Take the dog for a walk every day.

• If weather or neighborhood safety rule out walking outside, look for alternative locations—an indoor track, an enclosed shopping mall, or even a long hallway.

• Seize every opportunity to get up and walk around. Move more and sit less.

---

by reducing feelings of mild to moderate depression and anxiety. For people who need to prevent weight gain, lose weight, or maintain weight loss, 150 minutes per week of physical activity may not be enough. They may need to increase physical activity to 300 minutes or more per week, up to 90 minutes per day.

What's the difference between moderate- and vigorous-intensity physical activity? *Physical Activity Guidelines for Americans* defines moderate-intensity physical activity as activity that causes a noticeable increase in heart rate, such as brisk walking. Vigorous-intensity physical activity is activity that causes rapid breathing and a substantial increase in heart rate, such as jogging. Brisk walking, dancing, swimming, cycling, and yardwork can all help you meet the physical activity recommendations. You can burn the same number of calories by doing a moderate-intensity activity for a longer time or higher-intensity activity for a shorter time.

Ask Yourself

QUESTIONS FOR CRITICAL THINKING AND REFLECTION

Does your current lifestyle include enough physical activity—150 minutes of moderate-intensity activity a week—to support health and wellness? Do you go beyond this level to include enough vigorous activity and exercise to build physical fitness? What changes could you make in your lifestyle to start developing physical fitness?

The daily total of physical activity can be accumulated in multiple bouts of 10 or more minutes—for example, two 10-minute bike rides to and from class and a brisk 10-minute walk to the store. In this lifestyle approach to physical activity, people can choose activities that they find enjoyable and that fit into their daily routine. Everyday tasks at school, work, and home can be structured to contribute to the daily activity total (see the box "Making Time for Physical Activity").

THE BENEFITS OF EXERCISE

The greater the demands made on the human body, the more it adjusts to meet the demands—it becomes fit. Over time, immediate, short-term adjustments translate into long-term changes and improvements. (See page T1-4 of the color transparency insert "Touring Lifestyle Behaviors" in Chapter 8) The goal of regular physical activity is to bring about these kinds of long-term changes and improvements in the body's functioning.

Reduced Risk of Premature Death

Physically active people have a reduced risk of dying prematurely from all causes, with the greatest benefits found in the most active people (Figure 13.3). Physical inactivity increases the risk of premature death and is as important a risk factor as smoking, high blood pressure, obesity, and diabetes. Poor muscle strength also increases the risk of premature death.

Improved Cardiorespiratory Functioning

During exercise, the cardiorespiratory system (heart, lungs, and circulatory system) must work harder to meet the body's increased demand for oxygen. Regular cardiorespiratory endurance exercise improves the functioning of the heart and the ability of the cardiorespiratory system to carry oxygen to body tissues. Exercise directly affects the health of your arteries, keeping them from stiffening or clogging with plaque and reducing the risk of cardiovascular disease. Exercise also improves sexual function and general vitality.

More Efficient Metabolism and Improved Cell Health

Endurance exercise improves metabolism—the process that converts food to energy and builds tissue. This process involves oxygen, nutrients, hormones, and enzymes. A physically fit person's body can more efficiently use energy from carbohydrates and fats and better regulate hormones. Exercise may also protect cells from damage from free radicals, which are destructive chemicals produced normally during metabolism, and from inflammation caused by obesity, high blood pressure or cholesterol, nicotine, and overeating. Training activates antioxidants that prevent free radical damage and maintain cell health. Regular physical activity prevents the deterioration of telomeres, which form the protective ends of chromosomes that are vital for cell health and repair.

Improved Body Composition

Exercise can improve body composition in several ways. Endurance exercise significantly increases daily calorie expenditure. It can also slightly raise *metabolic rate*, the rate at which the body burns calories, for several hours after an exercise session. Strength training increases muscle mass, thereby tipping the body composition ratio toward fat-free mass and away from fat. It can also help with losing fat because metabolic rate is directly proportional to fat-free mass: the more muscle mass, the higher the metabolic rate.

Disease Prevention and Management

Regular physical activity lowers your risk of many chronic, disabling diseases.

Cardiovascular Disease   A sedentary lifestyle is one of the six major risk factors for cardiovascular disease (CVD),

including heart attack and stroke. Sedentary people have CVD death rates significantly higher than those of fit individuals. Physical inactivity increases the risk of CVD by as much as 240%. The benefits of physical activity begin at moderate levels of exercise and increase as the amount and intensity of activity rises. Exercise positively affects the risk factors for CVD, including cholesterol levels, insulin resistance, and blood pressure. Exercise also directly interferes with the disease process itself, lowering the risk of heart disease and stroke.

> Any increase in physical activity will **contribute to your health and well-being**.

Cancer   Studies have shown a relationship between increased physical activity and a reduced risk of cancer, but these findings are not conclusive. There is evidence that exercise reduces the risk of colon cancer and promising data that it reduces the risk of cancer of the breast and reproductive organs in women and prostate cancer in men.

Osteoporosis   A special benefit of exercise, especially for women, is protection against osteoporosis, a disease that results in loss of bone density and poor bone strength. Weight-bearing exercise, which includes almost everything except swimming, helps build bone during childhood and the teens and twenties. Strength training and impact exercises such as jumping rope can increase bone density throughout life. With stronger bones and muscles and better balance, fit people are less likely to experience debilitating falls and bone fractures.

QUICK STATS

70,551 Americans died of diabetes in 2008, making it the 7th leading cause of death that year.
—CDC, 2011

Type 2 Diabetes   People with diabetes are prone to heart disease, blindness, and severe problems of the nervous and circulatory systems. Exercise prevents the development of type 2 diabetes, the most common form of the disease. Exercise burns excess sugar and makes cells more sensitive to insulin. Exercise also helps keep body fat at healthy levels, which is important because obesity is a key risk factor for type 2 diabetes. For people who have diabetes, physical activity is an important part of treatment.

Improved Psychological and Emotional Wellness

Physically active people enjoy many social, psychological, and emotional benefits, including the following:

* *Reduced anxiety and depression.* Exercise reduces symptoms of anxiety, such as worry and self-doubt, and is associated with a lower risk for panic attacks. Exercise also relieves feelings of sadness and hopelessness and can be as effective as psychotherapy in treating mild to moderate cases of depression.

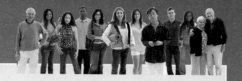

If you have a special health concern and hesitate to become more active, one helpful strategy is to take a class or join an exercise group specifically designed for your condition. Many health centers and support groups sponsor specially tailored programs. A class or group activity can provide you with expert advice and exercise partners who share your concerns and goals. If you prefer to exercise at home, exercise videos are available for people with a variety of conditions.

The fitness recommendations for the general population presented in this chapter can serve as general guidelines for any exercise program. However, for people with special health concerns, certain precautions and monitoring may be required. *Anyone with special health concerns should consult a physician before beginning an exercise program.*

Asthma

• Carry medication during workouts and avoid exercising alone. Use your inhaler before exercise, if recommended by your physician.

• Exercise regularly, and warm up and cool down slowly to reduce the risk of acute attacks.

• When starting a fitness program, choose self-paced endurance activities, especially those involving interval training (short bouts of exercise followed by rest periods).

• When possible, avoid circumstances that may trigger an asthma attack, including dust, pollen, or cold dry air. Drink water to keep your airways moist, and in cold weather, cover your mouth with a mask or scarf to warm and humidify the air you breathe. Swimming is a good activity for people with asthma.

Diabetes

• Don't exercise alone. Wear a bracelet or necklace that identifies you as a diabetic.

• If you take insulin or another medication, you may need to adjust the timing and amount of each dose as you learn to balance your energy intake and output and your medication dosage.

• To prevent abnormally rapid absorption of injected insulin, inject it over a muscle that won't be exercised and wait at least an hour after injection before exercising.

• Check blood sugar levels before, during, and after exercise, and adjust your diet or insulin dosage if needed.

• Avoid exercise if your blood sugar level is above 250 mg/dl, and ingest carbohydrates prior to exercise if your blood sugar level is below 100 mg/dl. Keep high-carbohydrate foods available during a workout.

• Check your skin regularly for blisters and abrasions, especially on your feet.

Obesity

• For maximum benefit and minimum risk, start with low- to moderate-intensity activities and increase intensity slowly as fitness improves.

• To lose weight or maintain lost weight, exercise moderately for 30–60 minutes or more daily and reduce food intake.

• Start your program with non- or low-weight-bearing activities like swimming, water exercises, cycling, or walking.

• Stay alert for symptoms of heat-related problems during exercise.

• Include as much lifestyle physical activity in your daily routine as possible.

• Add strength training to your program to build or maintain muscle mass.

Heart Disease and Hypertension

• Warm-ups and cool-downs should be gradual and last at least 10 minutes.

• Exercise at a moderate rather than high intensity. Monitor your heart rate during exercise, and stop if you experience dizziness or chest pain.

• Increase exercise frequency, intensity, and time very gradually.

• Don't hold your breath and strain when exercising. This can cause a sudden, steep increase in blood pressure.

• Discuss the effects of your medication with your physician. If your physician has prescribed nitroglycerine, keep it with you during exercise.

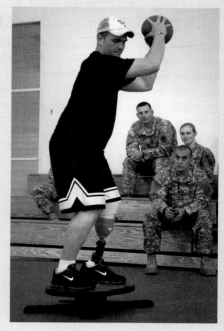

Arthritis

• Begin an exercise program as early as possible in the course of the disease.

• Warm up thoroughly before each workout to loosen stiff muscles and lower the risk of injury.

• Avoid high-impact activities that may damage arthritic joints. Swimming or water aerobics may be good choices for someone with arthritis.

• In strength training, pay special attention to muscles that support and protect affected joints. Add weight very gradually.

• Do flexibility exercises regularly.

Osteoporosis

• If possible, choose low-impact, weight-bearing activities to help safely maintain bone density.

• To prevent fractures, avoid any activity or movement that stresses the back or carries a risk of falling.

• Weight-train to improve strength and balance and to reduce the risk of falls and fractures, but avoid lifting heavy weights.

- *Improved sleep.* Regular physical activity helps people fall asleep more easily; it also improves sleep quality.

- *Reduced stress.* Exercise reduces the body's overall response to all forms of stressors and helps people deal more effectively with stress.

- *Enhanced self-esteem, self-confidence, and self-efficacy.* Exercise can boost self-esteem and self-confidence by providing opportunities for people to succeed and excel. Exercise also improves body image. Sticking with an exercise program increases people's belief in their ability to be active, thereby boosting self-efficacy.

- *Enhanced creativity and intellectual functioning.* Exercise improves alertness and memory in the short term and helps maintain reaction time, short-term memory, and nonverbal reasoning skills over time.

- *Improved work productivity.* Studies show that workers' quality of work, time management abilities, and mental and interpersonal performance are better on days they exercise.

- *Increased opportunities for social interaction.* Exercise provides many chances for people to have positive interactions with other people.

Improved Immune Function

Exercise can have either positive or negative effects on the immune system—the physiological processes that protect us from disease. Moderate endurance exercise boosts immune function, whereas excessive training depresses it. Physically fit people get fewer colds and upper respiratory tract infections than people who are not fit.

Prevention of Injuries and Low-Back Pain

Increased muscle strength provides protection against injury because it helps people maintain spinal stability, good posture, and appropriate body mechanics when performing everyday activities such as walking, lifting, and carrying. Good muscle endurance in the abdomen, hips, lower back, and legs supports the back in proper alignment and helps prevent low-back pain, which afflicts more than 85% of Americans at some time in their lives.

Improved Wellness for Life

Although people differ in the maximum levels of fitness they can achieve through exercise, the wellness benefits of exercise are available to everyone (see the box "Exercise for People with Special Health Concerns"). Exercising regularly may be the single most important thing you can do now to improve the quality of your life in the future.

DESIGNING YOUR EXERCISE PROGRAM

The best exercise program has two primary characteristics: it promotes your health, and it's fun for you to do. Exercise can provide some of the most pleasurable moments of your day, once you make it a habit.

Figure 10.1 shows a physical activity pyramid to guide you in meeting goals for physical activity. If you are sedentary, start at the bottom of the pyramid and gradually increase the moderate-intensity physical activity in your daily life. You don't have to

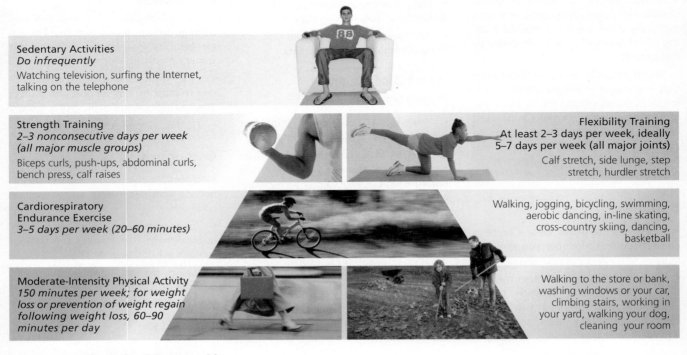

Sedentary Activities
Do infrequently
Watching television, surfing the Internet, talking on the telephone

Strength Training
2–3 nonconsecutive days per week (all major muscle groups)
Biceps curls, push-ups, abdominal curls, bench press, calf raises

Flexibility Training
At least 2–3 days per week, ideally 5–7 days per week (all major joints)
Calf stretch, side lunge, step stretch, hurdler stretch

Cardiorespiratory Endurance Exercise
3–5 days per week (20–60 minutes)

Walking, jogging, bicycling, swimming, aerobic dancing, in-line skating, cross-country skiing, dancing, basketball

Moderate-Intensity Physical Activity
150 minutes per week; for weight loss or prevention of weight regain following weight loss, 60–90 minutes per day

Walking to the store or bank, washing windows or your car, climbing stairs, working in your yard, walking your dog, cleaning your room

FIGURE 10.1 Physical activity pyramid.

exercise vigorously, but you should experience a moderate increase in your heart and breathing rates. If weight management is a concern for you, begin by achieving the goal of 150 minutes per week and then gradually increase your activity level to 300 minutes per week or more while reducing caloric intake.

For even greater benefits, move up to the next two levels of the pyramid, which illustrate parts of a formal exercise program. These recommendations are from the ACSM's exercise guidelines, which include cardiorespiratory endurance (aerobic) exercise, strength training, flexibility training, and balance training (for older adults). Such a program will develop all the health-related components of physical fitness. For a summary of the health and fitness benefits of different levels of physical activity, see Figure 10.2.

First Steps

Are you thinking about starting a formal exercise program? A little planning can help make it a success.

Medical Clearance   Previously inactive men over 40 and women over 50 should get a medical examination before

Ask Yourself

QUESTIONS FOR CRITICAL THINKING AND REFLECTION

Which benefits of exercise are most important to you, and why? For example, is there a history of heart disease or diabetes in your family? Have you thought about how regular exercise could reduce your risks for specific diseases?

beginning an exercise program. Diabetes, asthma, heart disease, and extreme obesity are conditions that may call for a modified program. If you have an increased risk of heart disease because of smoking, high blood pressure, or obesity, get a physical checkup, including an **electrocardiogram (ECG or EKG),** before beginning an exercise program.

electrocardiogram (ECG or EKG)   A recording of the changes in electrical activity of the heart.   **TERMS**

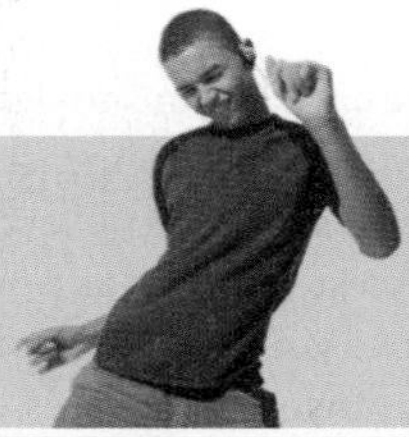

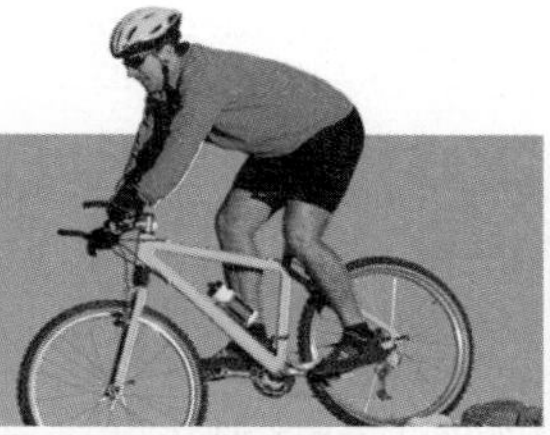

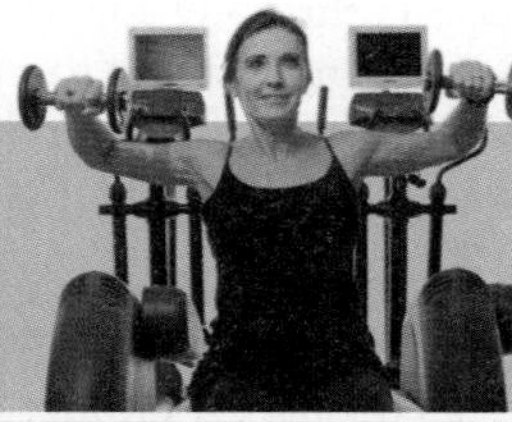

	Lifestyle physical activity	Moderate exercise program	Vigorous exercise program
Description	Moderate physical activity (150 minutes per week; muscle-strengthening exercises 2 or more days per week)	Cardiorespiratory endurance exercise (20–60 minutes, 3–5 days per week); strength training (2–3 nonconsecutive days per week); and stretching exercises (2 or more days per week)	Cardiorespiratory endurance exercise (20–60 minutes, 3–5 days per week); interval training; strength training (3–4 nonconsecutive days per week); and stretching exercises (5–7 days per week)
Sample activities or program	*One of the following:* • Walking to and from work, 15 minutes each way • Cycling to and from class, 10 minutes each way • Yard work for 30 minutes • Dancing (fast) for 30 minutes • Playing basketball for 20 minutes	• Jogging for 30 minutes, 3 days per week • Weight training, 1 set of 8 exercises, 2 days per week • Stretching exercises, 3 days per week	• Running for 45 minutes, 3 days per week • Intervals: running 400 m at high effort, 4 sets, 2 days per week • Weight training, 3 sets of 10 exercises, 3 days per week • Stretching exercises, 6 days per week
Health and fitness benefits	Better blood cholesterol levels, reduced body fat, better control of blood pressure, improved metabolic health, and enhanced glucose metabolism; improved quality of life; reduced risk of some chronic diseases. Greater amounts of activity can help prevent weight gain and promote weight loss.	All the benefits of lifestyle physical activity, plus improved physical fitness (increased cardiorespiratory endurance, muscular strength and endurance, and flexibility) and even greater improvements in health and quality of life and reductions in chronic disease risk.	All the benefits of lifestyle physical activity and a moderate exercise program, with greater increases in fitness and somewhat greater reductions in chronic disease risk. Participating in a vigorous exercise program may increase risk of injury and overtraining.

FIGURE 10.2   Health and fitness benefits of different amounts of physical activity and exercise.

Basic Principles of Physical Training   To put together an effective exercise program, you should first understand the basic principles of physical training.

SPECIFICITY   To develop a fitness component, you must perform exercises that are specifically designed for that component. This is the principle of **specificity.** Weight training, for example, develops muscular strength but is less effective for developing flexibility or cardiorespiratory endurance. A well-rounded exercise program includes exercises geared to each component of fitness, to different parts of the body, and to specific activities or sports.

PROGRESSIVE OVERLOAD   When the amount of exercise, or overload, is progressively increased, fitness continues to improve. This training principle is called **progressive overload.** Too little exercise has no effect on fitness; too much may cause injury. The appropriate amount depends on your current level of fitness, your genetic capacity to adapt to exercise, your fitness goals, and the fitness components being developed.

The amount of overload needed to maintain or improve a particular level of fitness is determined in four dimensions, represented by the acronym FITT: Frequency, Intensity, Time and Type. These dimensions are described individually for each of the components of fitness in the sections that follow.

REST AND RECUPERATION   Fitness gains occur following exercise as the body adapts to the stress of training. Adequate rest is as important to this process as training. Overtraining—an imbalance between training and recovery—leads to injury, illness, and excessive fatigue.

REVERSIBILITY   The body adjusts to lower levels of physical activity in the same way it adjusts to higher levels—this is the principle of **reversibility.** When you stop exercising, you can lose up to 50% of fitness improvements within two months. Try to exercise consistently, and don't quit if you miss a few workouts.

INDIVIDUAL DIFFERENCES   There are genetic limits to how much a person can improve fitness, as well as large individuals differences between people in their ability to improve fitness, achieve a desirable body composition, and perform and learn sports skills. In studies, some people on a diet and exercise program improve fitness by 50%, while others on the same program improve by only 2-3%. It is more difficult for those whose bodies don't respond as well to exercise to make changes in fitness or body fat levels. Elite athletes start out with a genetic advantage over the average person. However, everyone has the capacity to improve fitness and reap the health benefits of exercise.

Selecting Activities   If you have been inactive, begin by gradually increasing the amount of moderate physical activity in your life (the bottom of the activity pyramid). Once your body adjusts to your new level of activity, you can choose additional activities for your exercise program.

Be sure the activities you choose contribute to your overall wellness and make sense for you. Are you competitive? If so, try racquetball, basketball, or squash. Do you prefer to exercise alone? Then consider cross-country skiing or road running. Have you been sedentary? A walking program may be a good place to start. If you think you may have trouble sticking with an exercise program, find a structured activity that you can do with a friend, a personal trainer, or a group. Be realistic about the constraints presented by some sports, such as accessibility, expense, and time.

Cardiorespiratory Endurance Exercise

Exercises that condition your heart and lungs and improve your metabolism should have a central role in your fitness program.

Frequency   The optimal workout schedule for endurance training is 3–5 days per week. Beginners should start with 3 days and work up to 5 days. Training more than 5 days a week often leads to injury for recreational athletes.

Intensity   Intensity is the crucial factor in attaining a significant training effect—that is, in increasing the body's cardiorespiratory capacity. A primary purpose of endurance training is to increase **maximal oxygen consumption ($\dot{V}O_{2max}$).** $\dot{V}O_{2max}$ represents the cells' maximum ability to use oxygen and is considered the best measure of cardiorespiratory capacity. Intensity of training is the crucial factor in improving $\dot{V}O_{2max}$.

One of the easiest ways to determine exactly how intensely you should work involves measuring your heart rate. It is not necessary or desirable to exercise at your maximum heart rate—the fastest heart rate possible before exhaustion sets in—to improve your cardiorespiratory capacity. Beneficial effects occur at lower heart rates with a much lower risk of injury. **Target heart rate range** is the range of rates within which you should exercise to obtain cardiorespiratory benefits. To determine the intensity at which you should exercise, see the box "Determining Your Target Heart Rate Range".

Heart rate monitors make it easy to monitor your heart rate before, during, and after exercise. Some include global positioning system (GPS) receivers that help you determine your location and track the distance you walk, run, or bike.

Your target heart rate is the range of rates at which you should exercise to experience cardiorespiratory benefits. Your target heart rate range is based on your maximum heart rate, which can be estimated from your age. If you are a serious athlete or face possible cardiovascular risks from exercise, you may want to have your maximum heart rate determined more accurately through a treadmill test in a physician's office, hospital, or sports medicine laboratory. Your target heart rate is a range: the lower value corresponds to moderate-intensity exercise, and the higher value is associated with high-intensity exercise. Target heart rate ranges are shown in the accompanying table.

You can monitor the intensity of your workouts by measuring your pulse either at your wrist or at one of your carotid arteries, located on either side of your Adam's apple. Your pulse rate drops rapidly after exercise, so begin counting immediately after you have finished exercising. You will get the most accurate results by counting beats for 10 seconds and then multiplying by 6 to get your heart rate in beats per minute (bpm). The 10-second counts corresponding to each target heart rate range are also shown in the table.

COUNT AGE (YEARS)	TARGET HEART RATE RANGE (BPM)*	10-SECOND (BEATS)*
20–24	127–180	21–30
25–29	124–176	20–29
30–34	121–171	20–28
35–39	118–167	19–27
40–44	114–162	19–27
45–49	111–158	18–26
50–54	108–153	18–25
55–59	105–149	17–24
60–64	101–144	16–24
65+	97–140	16–23

*Target heart rates lower than those shown here are appropriate for individuals with a very low initial level of fitness. Ranges based on the following formula: Target heart rate = 0.65 to 0.90 of maximum heart rate, assuming maximum heart rate = 220 − age.

Time (Duration) A total time of 20–60 minutes per workout is recommended for cardiorespiratory endurance training. Exercise can be done in a single session or several sessions lasting 10 or more minutes. The total duration of exercise depends on its intensity. To improve cardiorespiratory endurance during a moderate-intensity activity such as walking or slow swimming, you should exercise for 45–60 minutes. For high-intensity exercise performed at the top of your target heart rate zone, a duration of 20 minutes is sufficient. Start with less vigorous activities and gradually increase intensity.

Type The best exercises for developing cardiorespiratory endurance stress a large portion of the body's muscle mass for a prolonged period of time. These include walking, jogging, running, swimming, bicycling, and aerobic dance. Many popular sports and recreational activities, such as racquetball, tennis, basketball, and soccer, are also good if the skill level and intensity or the game are sufficient to provide a vigorous workout.

The Warm-Up and Cool-Down It is always important to warm up before you exercise and to cool down afterward. Warming up enhances your performance and decreases your chances of injury. A warm-up session should include low-intensity movements similar to those in the activity that will follow. For example, hit forehands and backhands before a tennis game or jog slowly for 400 meters before progressing to an 8-minute mile.

Some people like to include stretching exercises in their warm-up, but experts recommend stretching *after* the active part of your warm-up, when your body temperature is elevated. Studies have found that stretching prior to exercise can temporarily decrease muscle strength and power.

Cooling down after exercise is important to restore the body's circulation to its normal resting condition. When you are at rest, a relatively small percentage of your total blood volume is directed to muscles, but during exercise, as much as 90% of the heart's output is directed to them. Cooling down helps regulate the return of blood to your heart. During recovery from exercise, it is important to continue exercising at a low level to provide a smooth transition to the resting state. After exercising, avoid taking a hot shower until you have cooled down.

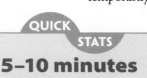

QUICK STATS

5–10 minutes
of warming up and cooling down are adequate for a 30-minute workout of brisk walking.
—CDC, 2011

Exercises for Muscular Strength and Endurance

Any program designed to promote health should include exercises that develop muscular strength and endurance.

Types of Strength Training Exercises Muscular strength and endurance can be developed in many ways, from weight training to calisthenics. Common exercises such as curl-ups, push-ups, pull-ups, and nonweighted squats maintain the muscular strength of most people if they practice them several times a week. To condition and tone your whole body, choose exercises that work the major muscles of the shoulders, chest, back, arms, abdomen, and legs.

To increase muscular strength and endurance, you must do **resistance exercise**—exercises in which your muscles must exert force against a significant amount of resistance. Resistance can be provided by weights, exercise machines, your own body weight, or even objects such as rocks.

Isometric (static) exercises involve applying force without movement, such as when you contract your abdominal muscles. This type of exercise is valuable for toning and strengthening muscles. Isometrics can be practiced anywhere and do not require any equipment. For maximum strength gains, hold an isometric contraction maximally for 6 seconds, and do 5–10 repetitions. Don't hold your breath: doing so can restrict blood flow to your heart and brain. Within a few weeks, you will notice the effect of this exercise. Isometrics are particularly useful when recovering from an injury.

Isotonic (dynamic) exercises involve applying force with movement, as in weight training exercises such as the bench press. These are the most popular type of exercises for increasing muscle strength and seem to be most valuable for

developing strength that can be transferred to other forms of physical activity. They include exercises using barbells, dumbbells, kettlebells, weight machines, and body weight (as in push-ups or curl-ups).

Core Training The core muscles include those in the abdomen, pelvic floor, sides of the trunk, back, buttocks, hips, and pelvis. They stabilize the spine and the midsection when you sit, stand, reach, walk, jump, twist, squat, throw, or bend. Strong core muscles make movements more forceful and help prevent back pain. The best exercises for low-back health are whole-body exercises that force the core muscles to stabilize the spine in many different directions.

Gender Differences in Muscular Strength Men are generally stronger than women because their bodies are typically larger overall and a larger proportion of their total body mass is made up of muscle. But when strength is expressed per unit of muscle tissue, men are only 1–2% stronger than women in the upper body and about equal to women in the lower body.

Men also have more testosterone than women. Testosterone promotes the growth of muscle tissue in both males and females, but testosterone levels are about 6–10 times higher in men than in women, so men develop larger muscles. Most women will not develop large muscles from strength training. Resistance exercise helps women reduce their overall body fat levels and reduce fat in the midsection. It also helps them preserve muscle mass as they age. Because men start out with more muscle when they are young, older women often have greater impairment of muscle function than older men.

Choosing Equipment Many people prefer weight machines to free weights because they are safe, convenient, and easy to use. You set the resistance, sit down at the machine, and start working. Free weights require more care, balance, and coordination to use, but they strengthen your body in ways that are more adaptable to real life. When using free weights, you need to use a *spotter*—someone who stands by to assist in case you lose control of a weight.

Choosing Exercises A complete weight training program works all the major muscle groups: neck, upper back, shoulders, arms, chest, abdomen, lower back, thighs, buttocks, and calves. Different exercises work different muscles,

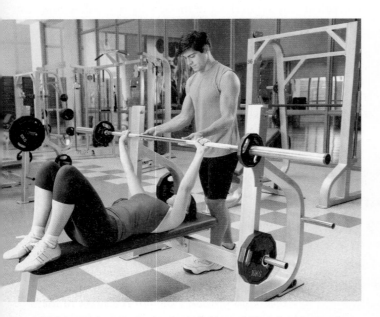

Weight training exercises are isotonic (dynamic) exercises that involve applying force with movement.

TERMS

resistance exercise Exercise that forces muscles to contract against increased resistance; also called *strength training*.

isometric (static) exercise The application of force without movement.

isotonic (dynamic) exercise The application of force with movement.

so it usually takes about 8–10 exercises to get a complete workout for general fitness. For example, you can do bench presses to develop the chest, shoulders, and upper arms; pull-ups to work the biceps and upper back; squats to develop the legs and buttocks; toe raises to work the calves; and so on.

Frequency   For general fitness, the American College of Sports Medicine recommends a workout frequency of at least two nonconsecutive days per week. This allows your muscles one or more days of rest between workouts to avoid soreness and injury. If you enjoy weight training and would like to train more often, try working different muscle groups on alternate days.

Intensity and Time   The amount of weight (resistance) you lift in weight training exercises is equivalent to intensity in cardiorespiratory endurance training, and the number of repetitions of each exercise is equivalent to time. To improve fitness, you must do enough repetitions of each exercise to temporarily fatigue your muscles. The number of repetitions needed to cause fatigue depends on the amount of resistance: the heavier the weight, the fewer repetitions to reach fatigue. In general, a heavy weight and a low number of repetitions (1–5) build strength, whereas a light weight and a high number of repetitions (10–25) build endurance. For a general fitness program to build both strength and endurance, try to do 8–12 repetitions of each exercise. For people who are over 50 years of age, 10–15 repetitions of each exercise using a lighter weight is recommended.

To start, choose a weight that you can move easily through 8–12 repetitions. Add weight when you can do more than 12 repetitions of an exercise. If adding weight means you can do only 7 or 8 repetitions before your muscles fatigue, stay with that weight until you can again complete 12 repetitions. If you can do only 4–6 repetitions after adding weight, or if you can't maintain good form, you've added too much and should take some off.

For developing strength and endurance for general fitness, a single set (a group of repetitions) of each exercise is sufficient, provided you use enough weight to fatigue your muscles. Doing more than one set of each exercise may increase strength development further, and most serious weight trainers do at least three sets of each exercise. If you do more than one set of an exercise, rest long enough between sets (1–5 minutes) to allow your muscles to recover. You should warm up before every weight training session and cool down afterward.

A Caution about Supplements   No nutritional supplement or drug will change a weak person into a strong person. Those changes require regular training that stresses the body and causes physiological adaptations. Supplements or drugs that promise quick, large gains in strength usually don't work and are often dangerous, expensive, or illegal. Over-the-counter supplements are not carefully regulated, and their long-term effects have not been systematically studied.

Flexibility Exercises

Flexibility, or stretching, exercises are important for maintaining the normal range of motion in the major joints of the body. Some exercises, such as running, can decrease flexibility because they require only a partial range of motion. Like a good weight training program, a good stretching program includes exercises for all the major muscle groups and joints of the body: neck, shoulders, back, hips, thighs, hamstrings, and calves. In tandem with core training, flexibility training is important for preventing lower back injuries and maintaining lower back health.

Proper Stretching Technique   Timing determines the best stretching technique: in general, do static stretching after a workout and dynamic or active stretching before a workout. *Static stretching* involves extending to a certain position, then holding it. *Dynamic stretching* is done by actively moving through the joints' ranges of motion. *Ballistic stretching* (known as "bouncing") is dangerous and counterproductive. The safest and most convenient technique for increasing flexibility may be active static stretching with a passive assist. For example, you might do a seated stretch of your calf muscles by contracting the muscles on the top of your shin and by grabbing your feet and pulling them toward you.

Frequency   Do stretching exercises at least 2–3 days per week (but 5–7 days is optimal). If you stretch after cardiorespiratory endurance exercise or strength training, during your cool-down, you may develop more flexibility because your muscles are warmer then and can be stretched farther.

Intensity and Time   For each exercise, stretch to the point of tightness in the muscle, then hold the position for 15–30 seconds. Rest for 30–60 seconds, then repeat, trying to stretch a bit farther. Relax and breathe easily as you stretch. You should feel a pleasant, mild stretch as you let the muscles relax; stretching should not be painful. Do 2–4 repetitions of each exercise. A complete flexibility workout usually takes about 20–30 minutes.

Increase your intensity gradually over time. Improved flexibility takes many months to develop. There are large individual differences in joint flexibility. Don't feel you have to compete with others during stretching workouts.

Training in Specific Skills

The final component in your fitness program is learning the skills required for the sports or activities in which you choose to participate. The first step in learning a new skill is getting help. Sports like tennis, golf, and skiing require mastery of basic movements and techniques, so instruction from a qualified teacher or coach can save you hours of frustration and increase your enjoyment. Skill is also important in conditioning activities such as jogging, swimming, and cycling. Even if you learned a sport as a child, additional instruction now can help you refine your technique.

	Cardiorespiratory Endurance Training	Strength Training	Flexibility Training
Frequency	3–5 days per week	2–3 nonconsecutive days per week	2–3 days per week (minimum); 5–7 days per week (ideal)
Intensity	55/65–90% of maximum heart rate	Sufficient resistance to fatigue muscles	Stretch to the point of tension
Time	20–60 minutes in sessions lasting 10 minutes or more	8–12 repetitions of each exercise, 1 or more sets	2–4 repetitions of each exercise, held for 15–30 seconds
Type	Continuous rhythmic activities using large muscle groups	Resistance exercises for all major muscle groups	Stretching exercises for all major joints

FIGURE 10.3 A summary of the FITT principle for the health-related components of fitness.

Putting It All Together

Now that you know the basic components of a fitness program, you can put them all together in a program that works for you. See Figure 10.3 for a summary of the FITT principle for the health-related components of fitness.

GETTING STARTED AND STAYING ON TRACK

Once you have a program that fulfills your basic fitness needs and suits your personal tastes, adhering to a few basic principles will help you improve quickly, have fun, and minimize the risk of injury.

Selecting Instructors, Equipment, and Facilities

One of the best places to get help is an exercise class, where an expert instructor can teach you the basics of training and answer your questions. A qualified personal trainer can also get you started on an exercise program or a new form of training. Make sure that your instructor or trainer has proper qualifications, such as a college degree in exercise physiology, kinesiology, or physical education and certification by the American College of Sports Medicine (ACSM), National Strength and Conditioning Association (NSCA), International Sports Science Association (ISSA), or another professional organization.

Many websites provide fitness programs, including ongoing support and feedback via e-mail. Many of these sites charge fees, so it is important to review the sites, decide which ones seem most appropriate, and if possible go through a free trial period before subscribing. Also remember to consider the reliability of the information at fitness websites, especially those that also advertise or sell products.

If you plan to purchase equipment, try to buy the best you can afford. Good equipment will enhance your enjoyment and decrease your risk of injury. Appropriate safety equipment, such as pads and helmets for skateboarding, is particularly important. Before you invest in a new piece of equipment, try it out at a local gym to make sure that you'll use it regularly. Footwear is an important piece of equipment for almost any activity; see the box "What to Wear" for shopping strategies.

If you are thinking of joining a health club or fitness center, be sure to choose one that has the right programs and equipment available at the times you will use them. Also make sure the facility is certified. Look for the displayed names American College of Sports Medicine (ACSM), National Strength and Conditioning Association (NSCA), American Council on Exercise (ACE), or Aerobics and Fitness Association of America (AFAA). These trade associations have established standards to help protect consumer health, safety, and rights.

QUICK STATS

Only 16% of the U.S. population belongs to a health club, but membership has increased more than 10% over the past three years to over 50.2 million members.

—IHRSA, 2012

Eating and Drinking for Exercise

Most people do not need to change their eating habits when they begin a fitness program. In most cases a well-balanced diet contains all the energy and nutrients needed to sustain an exercise program. A balanced diet is also the key to improving body composition when you begin to exercise more. One of the promises of a fitness program is a decrease in body fat and an increase in muscle mass. The best way to control body fat is to follow a reduced-calorie diet and to be physically active.

One of the most important principles to follow when exercising is to drink enough water. Sweating during exercise depletes the

Clothing

Modern exercise clothing is attractive, comfortable, and functional. Shorts made of elastic material, such as spandex, hug the body, supplying support. If you prefer, you can wear running shorts and a T-shirt. The main requirement for workout clothes is that they let you move easily but are not so loose that they get caught in the exercise machines or on fences when running outside. Don't wear street clothes when exercising because they can interfere with movement, and sweat, oil, and dirt can ruin them. If you run or cycle on the street, wear bright-colored clothing so motorists can see you.

Breast Support for Women

Breast support is important when running, playing volleyball, or weight training. A good sports bra should support the breasts in all directions, contain little elastic material, absorb moisture freely, and be easily laundered. Seams, hooks, and catches should not irritate the skin.

Footwear

Footwear is perhaps the most important item of equipment for almost any activity. Shoes protect and support your feet and improve your traction. They also help cushion your lower legs against the stress of running or jumping, thereby preventing injuries.

When choosing athletic shoes, first consider the activity you've chosen for your exercise program. Shoes appropriate for different activities have different characteristics. Foot type is another important consideration. If your feet tend to roll inward excessively, you may need additional stability features on the inner side of the shoe to counteract this movement. If your feet tend to roll outward excessively, you may need highly flexible and cushioned shoes that promote foot motion. Most women will get a better fit if they choose shoes that are specially designed for women's feet rather than downsized versions of men's shoes.

Successful Shoe Shopping

For successful shoe shopping, keep the following strategies in mind:

- Shop late in the day or, ideally, following a workout. Your foot size increases during the day and after exercise.

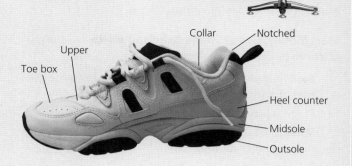

- Wear socks like those you plan to wear during exercise.

- Try on both shoes and wear them around for 10 minutes or more. Try walking on a noncarpeted surface. Approximate the movements of your activity: walk, jog, run, jump, and so on.

- Check the fit and style carefully:

  - Is the toe box roomy enough? Your toes will spread out when your foot hits the ground or you push off. There should be at least one thumb's width of space from the longest toe to the end of the toe box.
  - Do the shoes have enough cushioning? Do your feet feel supported when you bounce up and down? Try bouncing on your toes and on your heels.
  - Do your heels fit snugly in the shoe? Do they stay put when you walk, or do they slide up?
  - Are the arches of your feet on top of the shoes' arch supports?
  - Do the shoes feel stable when you twist and turn on the balls of your feet? Try twisting from side to side while standing on one foot.
  - Do you feel any pressure points?

- If you exercise at dawn or dusk, choose shoes with reflective sections for added visibility and safety.

- Replace athletic shoes about every three months or 300–500 miles of jogging or walking.

body's water supply and can lead to dehydration if fluids are not replaced. Serious dehydration can cause reduced blood volume, accelerated heart rate, elevated body temperature, muscle cramps, heat stroke, and other serious problems.

Thirst receptors in the brain make you want to drink fluids, but during heavy or prolonged exercise or exercise in hot weather, thirst alone isn't a good indication of how much fluid you need to drink. As a rule of thumb, drink at least 16 ounces of fluid two hours before exercise and then drink enough during exercise to prevent significant fluid

loss in sweat. After exercise, let thirst be your guide to your fluid needs.

Bring a bottle of water when you exercise so you can replace your fluids when they're depleted. For exercise sessions lasting less than 60–90 minutes, cool water is an excellent fluid replacement. For longer workouts, a sports drink that contains water and small amounts of electrolytes (sodium, potassium, and magnesium) and simple carbohydrates (sugar, usually in the form of sucrose or glucose) is recommended.

Managing Your Fitness Program

How can you tell when you're in shape? When do you stop improving and start maintaining? How can you stay motivated? If your program is going to become an integral part of your life, these are key questions.

Start Slowly, Get in Shape Gradually An exercise program can be divided into three phases:

- *Beginning phase.* The body adjusts to the new type and level of activity.
- *Progress phase.* Fitness increases.
- *Maintenance phase.* The targeted level of fitness is sustained over the long term.

When beginning a program, start slowly to give your body time to adapt to the stress of exercise. Choose activities carefully, according to your fitness status.

Exercising Consistently Steady fitness improvement comes when you overload your body consistently over time. The best way to ensure consistency is to record the details of your workouts in a journal: how far you ran, how much weight you lifted, and so on. This record will help you evaluate your progress and plan workout sessions intelligently. Don't increase your exercise volume by more than 5–10% per week.

Assessing Your Fitness When are you in shape? It depends. One person may be out of shape running a mile in 5 minutes, but another may be in shape running a mile in 12 minutes. Your ultimate level of fitness depends on your goals, your program, and your natural ability. The important thing is to set goals that make sense for you. If you are interested in finding out exactly how fit you are before starting a program, the best approach is to get an assessment from a sports medicine laboratory.

Preventing and Managing Athletic Injuries It is important to learn how to deal with injuries so they don't derail your fitness program or escalate into chronic problems (Table 10.1). Some injuries require medical attention. See a physician right away if you suffer a head or eye injury, a possible ligament injury, a broken bone, or an internal disorder such as chest pain, fainting, or intolerance to heat. Also seek medical attention for apparently minor injuries that do not get better within a reasonable amount of time.

Table 10.1	Care of Common Exercise Injuries and Discomforts	
INJURY	SYMPTOMS	TREATMENT
Blister	Accumulation of fluid in one spot under the skin	Don't pop or drain it unless it interferes too much with your daily activities. If it does pop, clean the area with antiseptic and cover with a bandage. Do not remove the skin covering the blister.
Bruise (contusion)	Pain, swelling, and discoloration	R-I-C-E: rest, ice, compression, elevation.
Fracture and/or dislocation	Pain, swelling, tenderness, loss of function, and deformity	Seek medical attention, immobilize the affected area, and apply cold.
Joint sprain	Pain, tenderness, swelling, discoloration, and loss of function	R-I-C-E. Apply heat when swelling has disappeared. Stretch and strengthen affected area.
Muscle cramp	Painful, spasmodic muscle contractions	Gently stretch for 15–30 seconds at a time and/or massage the cramped area. Drink fluids and increase dietary salt intake if exercising in hot weather.
Muscle soreness or stiffness	Pain and tenderness in the affected muscle	Stretch the affected muscle gently; exercise at a low intensity; apply heat. Nonsteroidal anti-inflammatory drugs, such as ibuprofen, help some people.
Muscle strain	Pain, tenderness, swelling, and loss of strength in the affected muscle	R-I-C-E; apply heat when swelling has disappeared. Stretch and strengthen the affected area.
Plantar fasciitis	Pain and tenderness in the connective tissue on the bottom of your feet	Apply ice, take nonsteroidal anti-inflammatory drugs, and stretch. Wear night splints when sleeping.
Shin splint	Pain and tenderness on the front of the lower leg; sometimes also pain in the calf muscle	Rest; apply ice to the affected area several times a day and before exercise; wrap with tape for support. Stretch and strengthen muscles in the lower legs. Purchase good-quality footwear and run on soft surfaces.
Side stitch	Pain on the side of the abdomen	Stretch the arm on the affected side as high as possible; if that doesn't help, try bending forward while tightening the abdominal muscles.
Tendinitis	Pain, swelling, and tenderness of the affected area	R-I-C-E; apply heat when swelling has disappeared. Stretch and strengthen the affected area.

- *Set realistic goals.* Unrealistically high goals will discourage you.

- *Sign a contract and keep a fitness journal.* A journal can help keep your program on track, identify problems, and give you a continuing sense of accomplishment.

- *Start slowly and increase your intensity and duration gradually.* Overzealous exercising can result in discouraging discomfort and injuries. Your program is meant to last a lifetime. The important first step is to break your established pattern of inactivity.

- *Make your program fun.* Participate in a variety of different activities that you enjoy. Vary the routes you take when walking, running, or biking.

- *Exercise with a friend.* The social side of exercise is important to many people.

- *Focus on the positive.* Concentrate on the improvements you get from your program, and how good you feel during and after exercise.

- *Revisit and revise.* If your program turns out to be unrealistic, revise it. Expect to make many adjustments in your program along the way.

- *Expect fluctuation.* On some days your progress will be excellent, but on others you'll barely be able to drag yourself through your scheduled activities.

- *Expect lapses.* Don't let lapses discourage you or make you feel guilty. Instead make a renewed commitment to your exercise program.

- *Plan ahead for difficult situations.* Think about what circumstances might make it tough to keep up with your fitness routine, and develop strategies for sticking with your program. For example, devise a plan for your program during vacation, travel, bad weather, and so on.

- *Reward yourself.* Give yourself frequent rewards for sticking with your program.

- *Renew your attitude.* If you notice you're slacking off, try to list the negative thoughts and behaviors that are causing you to lose interest. Devise a strategy to reduce negative thoughts and behaviors. Make changes in your program plan and reward system to help renew your enthusiasm and commitment.

- *Review your goals.* Visualize what it will be like to reach them, and keep these pictures in your mind as an incentive to stick to your program.

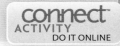

connect ACTIVITY DO IT ONLINE

For minor cuts and scrapes, stop the bleeding and clean the wound with soap and water. Treat soft tissue injuries (muscles and joints) with the R-I-C-E principle:

Rest: Stop using the injured tissue as soon as you experience pain, protect it from further injury, and avoid any activity that causes pain.

Ice: Apply ice to the injured tissue to reduce swelling and alleviate pain. Apply ice immediately for 10–20 minutes, and repeat every few hours until the swelling disappears. Let the injured part return to normal temperature between icings, and do not apply ice to one area for more than 20 minutes (10 minutes if you are using a cold gel pack).

Compression: Wrap the injured area with an elastic or compression bandage between icings. If the area starts throbbing or begins to change color, the bandage may be wrapped too tightly. Do not sleep with the bandage on.

Elevation: Raise the injured area above heart level to decrease the blood supply and reduce swelling.

After 36–48 hours, if the swelling has disappeared, apply heat to relieve pain, relax muscles, and reduce stiffness. Immerse the affected area in warm water or apply warm compresses, a hot water bottle, or a heating pad.

To prevent injuries, follow a few basic guidelines:

- Stay in condition: haphazard exercise programs invite injury.
- Warm up thoroughly before exercising.
- Use proper body mechanics when lifting objects or executing sports skills.
- Don't exercise when you're ill or overtrained (experiencing extreme fatigue due to overexercising).
- Use the proper equipment.
- Don't return to your normal exercise program until athletic injuries have healed.

You can minimize the risk of injury by following safety guidelines, respecting signals from your body that something may be wrong, and treating injuries promptly. Use special caution in heat or humidity (over 80°F and/or 60% humidity): Exercise slowly, rest frequently in the shade, wear clothing that breathes, and drink plenty of fluids. Slow down or stop if you begin to feel uncomfortable. During hot weather, exercise in the early morning or evening when temperatures are lowest.

Staying with Your Program   Once you have attained your desired level of fitness, you can maintain it by exercising regularly at a consistent intensity, 3–5 days a week. In general, if you exercise at the same intensity over a long period, your fitness will level out and can be maintained easily.

Adapt your program to changes in environment or schedule. Don't use wet weather or a new job as an excuse to give up your fitness program. If you walk in the summer, dress appropriately and walk in the winter as well. If you can't go out because of darkness or an unsafe neighborhood, walk in a local shopping mall or on campus or join a gym and walk on a treadmill.

What if you run out of steam? Although good health is an important *reason* to exercise, it's a poor *motivator*. It's a good idea to have a meaningful goal, anything from fitting into a new pair of jeans to skiing down a new slope. For more pecific suggestions for staying with your program, see the box "Maintaining Your Exercise Program" and the "Behavior Change Strategy" section at the end of the chapter.

Varying your program is another key strategy. Some people alternate two or more activities—swimming and jogging, for example—to improve a particular component of fitness. The practice, called **cross-training,** can help prevent boredom and overuse injuries. Try new activities, especially ones that you will be able to do for the rest of your life.

Connect to Your Choices

connect™

Have you ever thought about how you came to have the physical activity patterns you have? Many factors can influence our physical activity and exercise choices, some not as obvious as others. Was your family physically active when you were growing up? Do you have access to a fitness center or facilities and equipment for working out? Do you hang out with people who make physical activity part of their daily lives—or with couch potatoes?

What are the external factors that influence your choices about exercise? What are your inner motivations and core values, and how do they affect your choices? Based on what you learned in this chapter, will you make some different choices in the future? If so, what will they be?

Go online to Connect to complete this activity:
www.mcgraw-hillconnect.com

TIPS FOR TODAY AND THE FUTURE

Physical activity and exercise offer benefits in nearly every area of wellness. Even a low to moderate level of activity provides valuable health benefits.

RIGHT NOW YOU CAN:
- Go outside and take a brisk 15-minute walk.
- Look at your calendar for the rest of the week and write in some physical activity—such as walking, running, or playing Frisbee—on as many days as you can. Schedule the activity for a specific time and stick to it.
- Call a friend and invite him or her to start planning a regular exercise program with you.

IN THE FUTURE YOU CAN:
- Schedule a session with a qualified personal trainer who can evaluate your current fitness level and help you set personalized fitness goals.
- Create seasonal workout programs for the summer, spring, fall, and winter. Develop programs that are varied but consistent with your overall fitness goals.

SUMMARY

- The five components of physical fitness most important to health are cardiorespiratory endurance, muscular strength, muscular endurance, flexibility, and body composition.

- Exercise improves the functioning of the heart and the ability of the cardiorespiratory system to carry oxygen to the body's tissues. It also increases metabolic efficiency and improves body composition.

- Exercise lowers the risk of cardiovascular disease, cancer, osteoporosis, and diabetes. It improves immune function and psychological health and helps prevent injuries and low-back pain.

- Most people should accumulate at least 150 minutes per week of moderate-intensity or 75 minutes of vigorous-intensity physical activity. Longer-duration or more vigorous activity produces additional health and fitness benefits.

- Cardiorespiratory endurance exercises stress a large portion of the body's muscle mass. Endurance exercise should be performed 3–5 days per week for a total of 20–60 minutes per day. Intensity can be evaluated by measuring the heart rate.

- Warming up before exercising and cooling down afterward improve your performance and decrease your chances of injury.

- Exercises that develop muscular strength and endurance involve exerting force against a significant resistance. A strength training program for general fitness typically involves one or more sets of 8–12 repetitions of 8–10 exercises performed on at least 2 nonconsecutive days per week.

- A good stretching program includes exercises for all the major muscle groups and joints of the body. Do a series of active, static stretches at least 2–3 days per week. Hold each stretch for 15–30 seconds and do 2–4 repetitions. Stretch when muscles are warm.

- Instructors, equipment, and facilities should be chosen carefully to enhance enjoyment and prevent injuries.

- A well-balanced diet contains all the energy and nutrients needed to sustain a fitness program. When exercising, remember to drink enough fluids.

- Rest, ice, compression, and elevation (R-I-C-E) are treatments for minor muscle and joint injuries.

FOR MORE INFORMATION

BOOKS

Fahey, T. 2013. *Basic Weight Training for Men and Women*, 8th ed. New York: McGraw-Hill. *Weight training and plyometric exercises for fitness, weight control, and improved sports performance.*

Fahey, T., P. Insel, and W. Roth. 2013. *Fit and Well: Core Concepts and Labs in Physical Fitness and Wellness*, 10th ed. New York: McGraw-Hill. *A comprehensive guide to developing a complete fitness program.*

Fenton, M. 2008. *The Complete Guide to Walking, New and Revised: For Health, Weight Loss, and Fitness.* Guildford, CT: Lyons Press. *Discusses walking as a fitness method and a way to avoid diseases such as diabetes.*

Nieman, D. C. 2010. *Exercise Testing and Prescription: A Health-Related Approach*, 7th ed. New York: McGraw-Hill. *A comprehensive discussion of the effect of exercise and exercise testing and prescription.*

Richmond, M. 2011. *The Physiology Storybook: An Owner's Manual for the Human Body.* Monterey, CA: Healthy Learning. *A discussion of human physiology and wellness written for the average person.*

Woods, R., and C. Jordon. 2010. *Energy Every Day.* Champaign, IL: Human Kinetics. *A sensible guide to fitness and nutrition that will help you attain your fitness goals.*

ORGANIZATIONS, HOTLINES, AND WEBSITES

American Alliance for Health, Physical Education, Recreation, and Dance (AAHPERD). A professional organization dedicated to promoting quality health and physical education programs.

http://www.aahperd.org

American College of Sports Medicine (ACSM). The principal professional organization for sports medicine and exercise science. Provides brochures, publications, and audio- and videotapes.

http://www.acsm.org

American Council on Exercise (ACE). Promotes exercise and fitness; the website features fact sheets on many consumer topics, including choosing shoes, cross-training, and steroids.

http://www.acefitness.org

American Heart Association: Start! Walking for a Healthier Lifestyle. Provides practical advice for people of all fitness levels plus an online fitness diary.

http://www.startwalkingnow.org/about_start.jsp

CDC Physical Activity Information. Provides information about the benefits of physical activity and suggestions for incorporating moderate physical activity into daily life.

http://www.cdc.gov/physicalactivity/

Disabled Sports USA. Provides sports and recreation services to people with physical or mobility disorders.

http://www.dsusa.org

MedlinePlus: Exercise and Physical Fitness. Provides links to news and reliable information about fitness and exercise from government agencies and professional associations.

http://www.nlm.nih.gov/medlineplus/exerciseandphysicalfitness.html

President's Council on Physical Fitness and Sports (PCPFS). Provides information about PCPFS programs and publications, including fitness guides and fact sheets.

http://www.fitness.gov

http://www.presidentschallenge.org

Shape Up America! A nonprofit organization that provides information and resources for exercise, nutrition, and weight loss.

http://www.shapeup.org

SELECTED BIBLIOGRAPHY

American College of Sports Medicine. 2009. *ACSM's Guidelines for Exercise Testing and Prescription*, 8th ed. Philadelphia: Lippincott Williams & Wilkins.

American College of Sports Medicine. 2009. *ACSM's Resource Manual for Guidelines for Exercise Testing and Prescription*, 6th ed. Philadelphia: Lippincott Williams & Wilkins.

American College of Sports Medicine. 2011. Quantity and quality of exercise for developing and maintaining cardiorespiratory, musculoskeletal, and neuromotor fitness in apparently healthy adults: Guidance for prescribing exercise. *Medicine and Science in Sports and Exercise.* 43(7):1334–1359.

American Heart Association. 2010. *Heart Disease and Stroke Statistics—2010 Update.* Dallas: American Heart Association.

Blair, S. N., and J. N. Morris. 2009. Healthy hearts—and the universal benefits of being physically active: Physical activity and health. *Annals of Epidemiology* 19(4): 253–256.

Burns, R. W. 2010. Exercise guidelines for adults: Past, present & future. *Missouri Medical Journal* 107(1): 65–68.

Centers for Disease Control and Prevention. 2008. Prevalence of self-reported physically active adults—United States, 2007. *Morbidity and Mortality Weekly Report* 57(48): 1297–1300.

Deusinger, S. S. 2012. Exercise intervention for management of obesity. *Pediatric Blood Cancer* 58(1): 135–139.

Garber, C.E., et al. 2011. Quantity and quality of exercise for developing and maintaining cardiorespiratory, musculoskeletal, and neuromotor fitness in apparently healthy adults: Guidance for prescribing exercise. *Medicine and Science in Sports and Exercise* 43(7):1334–1359.

Hamer, M., and G. O'Donovan. 2010. Cardiorespiratory fitness and metabolic risk factors in obesity. *Current Opinion in Lipidology* 21(1): 1–7.

Janiszewski, P. M., and R. Ross. 2009. The utility of physical activity in the management of global cardiometabolic risk. *Obesity* 17: supplement 3: s3–s14.

Keller, P., et al. 2011. A transcriptional map of the impact of endurance exercise training on skeletal muscle phenotype. *Journal of Applied Physiology* 110 (1): 46–59.

Kloubec, J. A. 2010. Pilates for improvement of muscle endurance, flexibility, balance, and posture. *Journal of Strength Conditioning Research.* 24(3): 661–667.

Lanza, I. R., and K. S. Nair. 2010. Mitochondrial function as a determinant of life span. *Pflugers Archives* 459(2): 277–289.

Larson-Meyer, D. E., et al. 2010. Caloric restriction with or without exercise: The fitness versus fatness debate. *Medicine and Science in Sports Exercise* 42(1): 152–159.

Lum, D., G. Landers, and P. Peeling. 2010. Effects of a recovery swim on subsequent running performance. *International Journal of Sports Medicine*. 31(1): 26–30.

McGill, S. M. 2010. Core training: Evidence translating to better performance and injury prevention. *Strength and Conditioning Journal* 32(3): 33–46.

McGill, S. M., and A. Karpowicz. 2009. Exercises for spine stabilization: Motion/motor patterns, stability progressions and clinical technique. *Archives of Physical Medicine and Rehabilitation* 90: 118–126.

Nelson, M. E., et al. 2007. Physical activity and public health in older adults: Recommendations from the American College of Sports Medicine and the American Heart Association. *Medicine and Science in Sports and Exercise* 39(8): 1435–1445.

Norton, K., et al. 2009. Position statement on physical activity and exercise intensity terminology. *Journal of Science and Medicine in Sport* 13(5): 496–502.

Sawka, M. N., et al. 2007. American College of Sports Medicine position stand: Exercise and fluid replacement. *Medicine and Science in Sports and Exercise* 39(2): 377–390.

Shehab, R., et al. 2006. Pre-exercise stretching and sports-related injuries: Knowledge, attitudes and practices. *Clinical Journal of Sports Medicine* 16(3): 228–231.

U.S. Department of Health and Human Services. 2008. *2008 Physical Activity Guidelines for Americans*. Hyattsville, MD: U.S. Department of Health and Human Services. ODPHP Publication U0036.

U.S. Department of Health and Human Services. 2010. *The Surgeon General's Vision for a Healthy and Fit Nation*. Rockville, MD: U.S. Department of Health and Human Services, Office of the Surgeon General.

Warner, S. O., et al. 2010. The effects of resistance training on metabolic health with weight regain. *Journal of Clinical Hypertension* 12(1): 64–72.

Willis, F. B. 2009. Frequency of exercise for body fat loss: A controlled cohort study. *Journal of Strength Conditioning Research* 23(8): 2377–2380

Ylinen, J. 2009. Effect of stretching on hamstring muscle compliance. *Journal of Rehabilitation Medicine* 41(1): 80–84.

Although most people recognize the importance of incorporating exercise into their lives, many find it difficult to do. No single strategy will work for everyone, but the general steps outlined here should help you create an exercise program that fits your goals, preferences, and lifestyle. A carefully designed contract and program plan can help you convert your vague wishes into a detailed plan of action. And the strategies for program compliance outlined here and in Chapter 1 can help you enjoy and stick with your program for the rest of your life.

Step 1: Set Goals

Setting specific goals to accomplish by exercising is an important first step in a successful fitness program because it establishes the direction you want to take. Your goals might be specifically related to health, such as lowering your blood pressure and risk of heart disease, or they might relate to other aspects of your life, such as improving your tennis game or the fit of your clothes. If you can decide why you're starting to exercise, it can help you keep going.

Step 2: Select Activities

As discussed in the chapter, the success of your fitness program depends on the consistency of your involvement. Select activities that encourage your commitment: the right program will be its own incentive to continue, but poor activity choices provide obstacles and can turn exercise into a chore.

When choosing activities for your fitness program, consider the following:

- Is this activity fun? Will it hold my interest over time?

- Will this activity help me reach the goals I have set?

- Will my current fitness and skill level enable me to participate fully in this activity?

- Can I easily fit this activity into my daily schedule? Are there any special requirements (facilities, partners, equipment, etc.) that I must plan for?

- Can I afford any special costs required for equipment or facilities?

- If I have special exercise needs due to a particular health problem, does this activity conform to those exercise needs? Will it enhance my ability to cope with my specific health problem?

Using these guidelines listed, select a number of sports and activities.

Step 3: Make a Commitment

By completing a contract, you make a firm commitment and will be more likely to follow through until you meet your goals.

Step 4: Begin and Maintain Your Program

Start slowly to allow your body time to adjust. Be realistic and patient—meeting your goals will take time. The following guidelines may help you start and stick with your program:

- Set aside regular periods for exercise. Choose times that fit in best with your schedule, and stick to them. Allow an adequate amount of time for warm-up, cool-down, and a shower.

- Take advantage of any opportunity for exercise that presents itself (for example, walk to class or take stairs instead of an elevator).

- Do what you can to avoid boredom. Do stretching exercises or jumping jacks to music, or watch the evening news while riding your stationary bicycle.

- Exercise with a group that shares your goals and general level of competence.

- Vary the program. Change your activities periodically. Alter your route or distance if biking or jogging. Change racquetball partners, or find a new volleyball court.

- Establish minigoals or a point system, and work rewards into your program. Until you reach your main goals, a series of small rewards will help you stick with your program. Rewards should be things you enjoy that are easily obtainable.

Step 5: Record and Assess Your Progress

Keeping a record that notes the daily results of your program will help remind you of your ongoing commitment to your program and give you a sense of accomplishment. Create daily and weekly program logs that you can use to track your progress. Record the activity frequency, intensity, time, and type. Keep your log handy, and fill it in immediately after each exercise session. Post it in a visible place to remind you of your activity schedule and to provide incentive for improvement.

SOURCE: Adapted from Kusinitz, I., and M. Fine. 1995. *Your Guide to Getting Fit*, 3rd ed. Mountain View, CA: Mayfield.

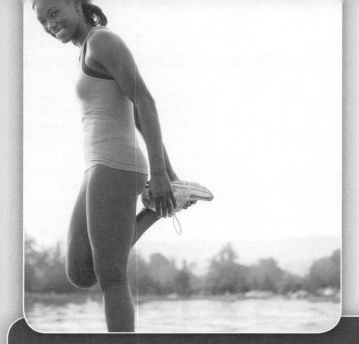

LOOKING AHEAD...

After reading this chapter, you should be able to

- Discuss different methods for assessing body weight and body composition
- Explain the health risks associated with overweight and obesity
- Explain factors that may contribute to a weight problem, includin genetic, physiological, lifestyle, and psychosocial factors
- Describe lifestyle factors that contribute to weight gain and loss including the roles of diet, exercise, and emotions
- Identify and describe the symptoms of eating disorders and the health risks associated with them
- Design a personal plan for successfully managing body weight

Weight Management

11

Achieving and maintaining a healthy body weight is a public health priority and a serious challenge for many Americans. By the standards developed by the National Institutes of Health (NIH), 68.8% of American adults are overweight, including 35.7% who are obese (Table 11.1). Of adult men, an estimated 35.5% are obese, and of adult women, an estimated 35.8%. One study predicted that at current rates, 42% of Americans will be obese by 2050. And while millions struggle to lose weight, others fall into dangerous eating patterns such as binge eating or self-starvation.

Although not completely understood, managing body weight is not a mysterious process. It's basically a matter of balancing the calories you take in with calories you expend in daily activities—in other words, eating a moderate diet and being physically active. To manage your weight successfully, you must coordinate many aspects of your life—including nutrition, physical activity, and stress control—over the long term.

BASIC CONCEPTS OF WEIGHT MANAGEMENT

Many people are concerned about their weight, but they may not know whether they are overweight or whether it is something they need to address.

What Is Body Composition, and Why Is It Important?

The human body can be divided into fat-free mass and body fat. Fat-free mass is composed of all the body's nonfat tissues: bone, water, muscle, connective tissue, organ tissues, and teeth. A certain amount of body fat is necessary for the body to function. Fat is incorporated into the nerves, brain, heart, lungs, liver, mammary glands, and other body organs and tissues. It is the main source of stored energy in the body; it also cushions body organs and helps regulate body temperature. This **essential fat** makes up about 3–5% of total body weight in men and about 8–12% in women. The percentage is higher in women due to fat deposits in the breasts, uterus, and other sex-specific sites.

Most of the fat in the body is stored in fat cells, or **adipose tissue,** located under the skin (**subcutaneous fat**) and around major organs (**visceral** or *intra-abdominal* **fat**). People have a genetically determined number of fat cells, but these cells can increase or decrease in size depending on how much fat is being stored, which in turn depends on several factors, including age, sex, metabolism, diet, and activity level. The primary source of excess body fat is excess calories consumed in the diet—that is, calories consumed in excess of calories expended in metabolism, physical activity, and exercise.

Table 11.1	Weight of Americans Aged 20 and Older, 2009–2010	
GROUP	PERCENT OVERWEIGHT*	PERCENT OBESE
Both sexes	68.8	35.7
All races, male	74.1	35.5
All races, female	64.5	35.8
White, male	74.0	36.2
White, female	59.5	32.2
African American, male	69.9	38.8
African American, female	82.1	58.5
Latino, male	81.7	37.0
Latino, female	75.7	41.4

*Includes obesity

SOURCE: Flegal, K. M., et al. 2012. Prevalence of Obesity and Trends in the Distribution of Body Mass Index among U.S. Adults, 1999–2010. *Journal of the American Medical Association* 307(5): 491–497.

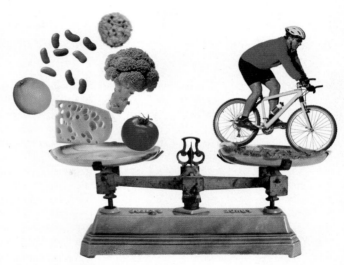

ENERGY IN
Food calories

ENERGY OUT
Physical activity 20–30%
Food digestion ±10%
Resting metabolism 65–70%

FIGURE 11.1 The energy balance equation.

A pound of body fat is equal to 3500 calories. If you take in 100 calories per day in excess of the calories you expend, you will gain 10 pounds in a year. Excess stored body fat is associated with increased risk of chronic diseases like arthritis, diabetes, and cardiovascular disease.

Overweight and Obesity Defined

Some methods of assessing and clarifying body composition are based on body weight and others on body fat. Methods based on body weight are less accurate than those based on body fat, but they are commonly used because body weight is easier to measure than body fat.

In the past, many people relied on height/weight tables (which were based on insurance company mortality statistics) to determine whether they were at a healthy weight. Such tables can be very inaccurate for some people. Because muscle tissue is denser and heavier than fat, a fit person can easily weigh more that the recommended weight on a height/weight table, and an unfit person may weigh less.

When looking at body composition, the most important consideration is the proportion of the body's total weight that is fat—the **percent body fat.** For example, two women may both be 5 feet, 5 inches tall and weigh 130 pounds. But one woman may have only 15% of her body weight as fat, whereas the other woman could have 34% body fat. Although neither woman is overweight by most standards, the second woman is overfat. Too much body fat can have a negative effect on health and well-being. Just as the amount of body fat is important, so is its distribution in your body. Visceral fat is more harmful to health than subcutaneous fat.

Overweight is usually defined as total body weight above the recommended range for good health, as determined by large-scale population surveys. **Obesity** is defined as a more serious degree of overweight that carries multiple health

risks. Both terms are used to identify weight ranges that are associated with increased likelihood of certain diseases and health problems. Cutoff points for defining overweight and obesity vary with the method used to measure and evaluate body weight and percent body fat.

Energy Balance

The key to achieving and maintaining a healthy body weight and keeping a healthy ratio of fat to fat-free mass across the lifespan is energy balance (Figure 11.1). You take in energy (calories) from the food you eat. Your body uses energy (calories) to maintain vital body functions (resting metabolism), to digest food, and to fuel physical activity. When energy in equals energy out, you maintain your current weight. To change your weight and body composition, you must tip the energy balance equation in a particular direction. If you take

essential fat Fat incorporated in various tissues of the body; critical for normal body functioning.

adipose tissue Connective tissue in which fat is stored.

subcutaneous fat Fat located under the skin.

visceral fat Fat located around major organs; also called *intra-abdominal fat.*

percent body fat The percentage of total body weight that is composed of fat.

overweight Body weight above the recommended range for good health.

obesity Severe overweight, characterized by an excessive accumulation of body fat; may also be defined in terms of some measure of total body weight.

TERMS

	<18.5 Underweight		18.5–24.9 Normal						25–29.9 Overweight					30–34.9 Obesity (Class I)					35–39.9 Obesity (Class II)					≥40 Extreme obesity
BMI	17	18	19	20	21	22	23	24	25	26	27	28	29	30	31	32	33	34	35	36	37	38	39	40
Height													Body Weight (pounds)											
4' 10"	81	86	91	96	101	105	110	115	120	124	129	134	139	144	148	153	158	163	168	172	177	182	187	192
4' 11"	84	89	94	99	104	109	114	119	124	129	134	139	144	149	154	159	163	168	173	178	183	188	193	198
5'	87	92	97	102	108	113	118	123	128	133	138	143	149	154	159	164	169	174	179	184	190	195	200	205
5' 1"	90	95	101	106	111	117	122	127	132	138	143	148	154	159	164	169	175	180	185	191	196	201	207	212
5' 2"	93	98	104	109	115	120	126	131	137	142	148	153	159	164	170	175	181	186	191	197	202	208	213	219
5' 3"	96	102	107	113	119	124	130	136	141	147	153	158	164	169	175	181	186	192	198	203	209	215	220	226
5' 4"	99	105	111	117	122	128	134	140	146	152	157	163	169	175	181	187	192	198	204	210	216	222	227	233
5' 5"	102	108	114	120	126	132	138	144	150	156	162	168	174	180	186	192	198	204	210	216	222	229	235	241
5' 6"	105	112	118	124	130	136	143	149	155	161	167	174	180	186	192	198	205	211	217	223	229	236	242	248
5' 7"	109	115	121	128	134	141	147	153	160	166	173	179	185	192	198	204	211	217	224	230	236	243	249	256
5' 8"	112	118	125	132	138	145	151	158	165	171	178	184	191	197	204	211	217	224	230	237	244	250	257	263
5' 9"	115	122	129	136	142	149	156	163	169	176	183	190	197	203	210	217	224	230	237	244	251	258	264	271
5' 10"	119	126	133	139	146	153	160	167	174	181	188	195	202	209	216	223	230	237	244	251	258	265	272	279
5' 11"	122	129	136	143	151	158	165	172	179	187	194	201	208	215	222	230	237	244	251	258	265	273	280	287
6'	125	133	140	148	155	162	170	177	184	192	199	207	214	221	229	236	243	251	258	266	273	280	288	295
6' 1"	129	137	144	152	159	167	174	182	190	197	205	212	220	228	235	243	250	258	265	273	281	288	296	303
6' 2"	132	140	148	156	164	171	179	187	195	203	210	218	226	234	242	249	257	265	273	281	288	296	304	312
6' 3"	136	144	152	160	168	176	184	192	200	208	216	224	232	240	248	256	264	272	280	288	296	304	312	320
6' 4"	140	148	156	164	173	181	189	197	206	214	222	230	238	247	255	263	271	280	288	296	304	312	321	329

FIGURE 11.2 Body mass index (BMI). To determine your BMI, find your height in the left column. Move across the appropriate row until you find the weight closest to your own. The number at the top of the column is the BMI at that height and weight.

SOURCE: Ratings from National Heart, Lung, and Blood Institute. 1998. *Clinical Guidelines on the Identification, Evaluation, and Treatment of Overweight and Obesity in Adults: The Evidence Report*. Bethesda, Md.: National Institutes of Health

in more calories daily than your body burns (a *positive* energy balance), the excess calories will be stored as fat and you will gain weight over time. If you eat fewer calories than you burn each day (a *negative* energy balance), you will lose some of the stored fat and probably lose weight.

If we look at the energy balance equation today as expressed for the general American population, the equation is tipped heavily toward the energy-in side. Our environment is rich in large portion sizes; high-fat, high-calorie foods; and palatable, easily available, and inexpensive foods. Unfortunately the energy-out side of the equation has not compensated for increased energy intake; instead we've decreased work-related physical activity, decreased activity associated with daily living, and increased time spent in sedentary pastimes like TV watching and computer use. The good news, however, is that you control both parts of the energy balance equation.

Evaluating Body Weight and Body Composition

Several methods can be used to measure and evaluate body weight and percent body fat, some of them simple and inexpensive. These assessments can help you establish reasonable goals and set a starting point for current and future decisions about weight loss and weight gain.

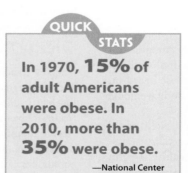

QUICK STATS

In 1970, **15%** of adult Americans were obese. In 2010, more than **35%** were obese.

—National Center for Health Statistics

Body Mass Index Body mass index (**BMI**) is a measure of body weight that is useful for estimating a person's weight status and for classifying the health risks of body weight if more sophisticated methods aren't available. BMI is based on the concept that weight should be proportional to height. Easy to calculate and rate, BMI is a fairly accurate measure of the health risks of body weight for most average (nonathletic) people. BMI is correlated with body fat, but it does not directly measure body fat.

BMI is calculated by dividing your body weight (expressed in kilograms or pounds) by the square of your height (expressed in meters or inches). You can look up your BMI in the chart in Figure 11.2, or you can use the following formula to calculate it more precisely:

$$\text{BMI} = \frac{\text{weight in kg}}{(\text{height in meters})^2}$$

$$\text{OR} \quad \frac{\text{weight in pounds}}{(\text{height in inches})^2} \times 703 \text{ (conversion factor)}$$

body mass index (BMI)   A measure of relative body weight that takes height into account and is highly correlated with more direct measures of body fat; calculated by dividing total body weight (in kilograms) by the square of height (in meters).

TERMS

Body weight status is categorized as underweight, healthy weight, overweight, or obese in comparison with what is considered healthy for a given height. Under standards issued by the National Institutes of Health and adopted by the Dietary Guidelines for Americans, a BMI between 18.5 and 24.9 is considered healthy, a BMI of 25 or above is classified as overweight, and a BMI of 30 or above is classified as obese. A person with a BMI below 18.5 is classified as underweight, although low BMI values may be healthy in some cases if they are not the result of smoking, an eating disorder, or an underlying disease.

BMI is a valuable tool for assessing weight, but it is not such a good tool for determining body composition. Like height–weight tables, it does not distinguish between fat weight and fat-free weight. It can also be inaccurate for some groups, including short people (under 5 feet tall), muscular athletes, and older adults with little muscle mass due to inactivity or an underlying disease. People in these groups should use one of the methods described in the next section for estimating percent body fat to assess whether their weight and body composition are healthy.

Body Composition Analysis   The most accurate and direct way to evaluate body composition is to determine percent body fat, and there are several methods to do so. However, specific guidelines for healthy body fat ranges have not been established. A healthy body fat range for men is usually considered to be about 12–20%, and for women, about 20–30%. Men with more than 25% body fat are considered obese, as are women with more than 33% body fat. No matter which method of body composition analysis is used, the measurements must be performed by someone with appropriate training to ensure accuracy.

SKINFOLD MEASUREMENT   Skinfold measurement is a simple and practical way to assess body composition based on amount of subcutaneous fat. A practitioner measures the thickness of skinfolds at several different sites on the body with special calipers, and the measurements are plugged into formulas that calculate body fat percentages. The accuracy of this method is highly dependent on the expertise of the practitioner.

BIOELECTRICAL IMPEDANCE ANALYSIS (BIA)   In this method, electrodes are attached to the body, and a harmless electrical current is transmitted from electrode to electrode. The electrical conduction through the body favors the path of the fat-free tissues over the fat tissues, so the amount of resistance to the current is related to the amount of fat-free tissue in the body. A computer then calculates fat percentages from measurements of the resistance to the current.

HYDROSTATIC WEIGHING AND THE BOD POD   In hydrostatic (underwater) weighing, a person is submerged and weighed under water. Percent body fat can be calculated from body

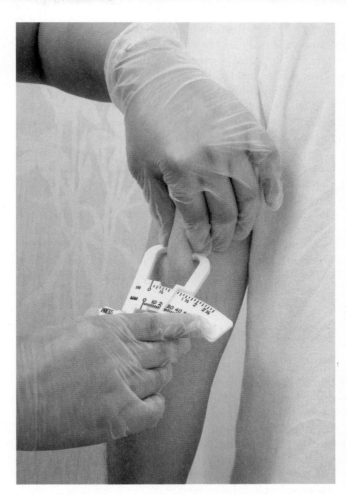

Skinfold measurements are a simple and inexpensive way to determine body fat levels. This method requires a caliper designed for this purpose and a practitioner trained in its use.

density. Muscle has a higher density and fat a lower density than water, so people with more fat tend to float and weigh less under water, while lean people tend to sink and weigh more under water.

A specialized body composition analysis device called the Bod Pod uses air instead of water. A person sits in a chamber, and computerized pressure sensors determine the amount of air displaced by the person's body to determine percentage of body fat.

To ensure accuracy, body composition measurements must be performed by **someone with appropriate training**.

SCANNING PROCEDURES   High-tech scanning procedures are very accurate means of assessing body composition, but they require expensive equipment. These procedures include computed tomography (CT), magnetic resonance imaging (MRI), dual-energy X-ray absorptiometry (DEXA), and dual-photon absorptiometry. Other procedures include infrared reactance (Futrex 1100) and total body electrical conductivity (TOBEC). These techniques are generally offered only at medical or research facilities.

Body Fat Distribution   As noted earlier, the location of fat on your body also has implications for health, with abdominal fat posing a greater risk than fat located in other places. Abdominal fat appears to be an independent risk factor regardless of BMI.

Two of the simplest methods for measuring body fat distribution are waist circumference measurement and waist-to-hip ratio calculation. In the first method, you measure your waist circumference using a tape measure placed around your abdomen at the top of your hip bone. A waist circumference of ≥40 inches (102 cm) for men or ≥35 in (88 cm) for women is associated with an increased risk for chronic disease for most adults. In the second method, you divide your waist circumference by your hip circumference (measured around the widest part of the buttocks). A waist-to-hip ratio above 0.94 for young men and above 0.82 for young women is associated with an increased risk of heart disease and diabetes.

EXCESS BODY FAT AND WELLNESS

The amount and distribution of fat in the body can have profound effects on health. Obesity doubles mortality rates and can reduce life expectancy by 10–20 years. In fact, if the current trends in overweight and obesity (and their related health problems) continue, some experts predict that the average American's life expectancy will soon decline by 5 years.

Obese people have an increased risk of death from all causes compared with people of normal weight. Obesity is associated with diabetes, cardiovascular diseases, many kinds of cancer, impaired immune function, gallbladder and kidney diseases, skin problems, impotence, sleep and breathing disorders, back pain, arthritis, and other bone and joint disorders. Obesity is also associated with complications of pregnancy, menstrual irregularities, urine leakage (stress incontinence), increased surgical risk, and psychological disorders and problems (such as depression, low self-esteem, and body dissatisfaction).

There is debate over the health risks for people who are overweight but not obese (BMI of 25 to 29), particularly for people who are overweight and physically active. These risks depend in part on an individual's overall health and other risk factors, such as blood pressure, cholesterol levels, body fat distribution, tobacco use, and level of physical activity. Some research has indicated that subjects who were even slightly overweight were up to 40% more likely to die within the next decade, compared to age-matched people who had a desirable weight. But it is also important to realize that small weight losses—5% to 10% of total body weight—can lead to significant health improvements.

Diabetes

About 26 million Americans have one of the two major types of **diabetes mellitus,** a disease that disrupts normal metabolism. About 5–10% of people with diabetes have a form known as type 1 diabetes, a disease that usually begins in childhood or adolescence and is not related to obesity. The remaining 90–95% of people with diabetes have type 2 diabetes, a disease that is strongly associated with excess body fat. The prevalence of type 2 diabetes has been rising dramatically in parallel with the increase in prevalence of obesity. In 2010 almost 2 million new cases of diabetes were diagnosed in adults over the age of 20.

Diabetes involves the production of the hormone insulin by the pancreas. In normal metabolism, the pancreas secretes insulin, which stimulates cells to take up blood sugar (glucose) to produce energy. In diabetes, this process is disrupted, causing a buildup of glucose in the bloodstream. In type 1 diabetes, the body's immune system, triggered by a viral infection or some other environmental factor, destroys the insulin-producing cells in the pancreas. Little or no insulin is produced, so daily doses of insulin are required. In type 2 diabetes, the pancreas doesn't produce enough insulin, or body cells are resistant to insulin (called *insulin resistance*), or both. This condition can develop slowly, and about 25% of type 2 diabetics are unaware of their condition. About one-third of people with type 2 diabetes must take insulin; others may take medications that increase insulin production or stimulate the cells to take up glucose.

A third type of diabetes, called *gestational diabetes*, occurs in about 7% of women during pregnancy. The condition usually disappears after pregnancy, but about half of women who experience it eventually develop type 2 diabetes. *Prediabetes* is a condition in which blood sugar levels are higher than normal but not high enough for a diagnosis of full-blown diabetes. About 57 million Americans have prediabetes, and most will develop type 2 diabetes unless they adopt preventive lifestyle measures. The warning signs of diabetes include frequent urination, extreme hunger or thirst, unexplained weight loss, extreme fatigue, blurred vision, frequent infections, tingling or numbness in the hands or feet, and generalized itching with no rash.

Complications of diabetes include kidney failure; nerve damage; circulation problems and amputations; retinal damage and blindness; and increased rates of heart attack, stroke, and hypertension. Diabetes is currently the seventh leading cause of death in the United States.

The major risk factors for diabetes are age, obesity, physical inactivity, a family history of diabetes, and lifestyle. Ethnicity also plays a role, with Native Americans, Alaska Natives, African Americans, and Hispanics having higher rates than Asian Americans and white Americans. Excess body fat reduces cell sensitivity to insulin, and insulin resistance is almost always a precursor of type 2 diabetes. Nearly 90% of people with type 2 diabetes are overweight when diagnosed, including 55% who are obese.

diabetes mellitus   A disease that disrupts normal metabolism, interfering with cells' ability to take in glucose for energy production.

TERMS

It is estimated that 90% of cases of type 2 diabetes could be prevented if people adopted healthy lifestyle behaviors, including regular physical activity, a moderate diet to control body fat, and modest weight loss. Even a small amount of weight loss can be beneficial. For people with prediabetes, lifestyle measures are more effective than medication for delaying or preventing the development of diabetes. Exercise (endurance and/or strength training) makes cells more sensitive to insulin and helps stabilize blood glucose levels; it also helps keep body fat at healthy levels. Regular exercise and a healthy diet are often sufficient to control type 2 diabetes. There is no cure for diabetes, but it can be successfully managed by keeping blood sugar levels within safe limits through diet, exercise, and, if necessary, medication.

Diabetes is one of the six major controllable risk factors for heart disease, and obesity is another. Excess body fat is strongly associated with hypertension, unhealthy cholesterol and triglyceride levels, and impaired heart function. Many overweight and obese people—especially those who are sedentary and eat a poor diet—also suffer from a group of symptoms called *metabolic syndrome*. Symptoms include insulin resistance, high blood pressure, high blood glucose, unhealthy cholesterol levels, chronic inflammation, and abdominal fat. Metabolic syndrome increases the risk of heart disease.

Body Fat Distribution and Health

Men and postmenopausal women tend to store fat in the upper regions of their bodies, particularly in the abdominal area, as visceral fat. People with this pattern of fat distribution, called *android obesity*, are said to be apple-shaped. Premenopausal women usually store fat in the hips, buttocks, and thighs, as subcutaneous fat. People with this pattern, called *gynoid obesity*, are said to be pear-shaped.

Abdominal obesity increases the risk of high blood pressure, diabetes, early-onset heart disease, stroke, certain types of cancer, and mortality. This risk is independent of a person's BMI. Even people who have a BMI in the normal range may be at increased risk of diabetes, high blood pressure, and CVD if they have a large waist circumference, particularly if they have additional risk factors.

The reason for the increased risk associated with abdominal obesity appears to be that visceral fat is more easily mobilized and sent into the bloodstream, increasing disease-related blood fat levels. Subcutaneous fat is not metabolically active the way visceral fat is.

Body Image

The collective picture of the body as seen through the mind's eye, **body image** consists of perceptions, images, thoughts, attitudes, and emotions. A negative body image is characterized by dissatisfaction with the body in general or some part of the body in particular. People may be dissatisfied with their bodies for a variety of reasons, including sociocultural forces and factors that are specific to life stages.

Losing weight or getting cosmetic surgery does not necessarily improve body image. However, improvements in body image may occur in the absence of changes in weight or appearance. Many experts now believe that body image issues must be dealt with as part of treating obesity and eating disorders.

Problems Associated with Very Low Levels of Body Fat

Health experts have generally viewed very low levels of body fat—less than 8–12% for women and 3–5% for men—as a threat to wellness. Extreme leanness has been linked with reproductive, circulatory, and immune system disorders. Extremely lean people may experience muscle wasting and fatigue; they are also more likely to suffer from dangerous eating disorders.

In physically active women and girls, particularly those involved in sports where weight and appearance are important (ballet, gymnastics, skating, and distance running, for example), a condition called the **female athlete triad** may develop. The triad consists of three interrelated disorders: abnormal eating patterns (and excessive exercising), followed by **amenorrhea** (absence of menstruation), followed by decreased bone density (premature osteoporosis). Prolonged amenorrhea can cause bone density to erode to a point that a woman in her twenties

Ask Yourself

QUESTIONS FOR CRITICAL THINKING AND REFLECTION

Calculate your BMI using the formula given in this chapter; then compare it with the BMIs of some classmates. Do the results surprise you? How well do you think BMI reflects body composition? Why do you think it is such a commonly used measure?

TERMS

body image The mental representation a person holds about his or her body at any given time, consisting of perceptions, images, thoughts, attitudes, and emotions about the body.

female athlete triad A condition consisting of three interrelated disorders: abnormal eating patterns (and excessive exercising) followed by lack of menstrual periods (amenorrhea) and decreased bone density (premature osteoporosis).

amenorrhea The absence of menstruation.

According to popular belief, college students typically gain 15 pounds in their first year at school—the infamous "freshman 15." Is this the fate of all college students, or is it a myth that adds stress for body-conscious young adults?

Research indicates that the truth lies somewhere between these two scenarios. While many people do gain weight in the first year at college, the weight gain tends to be less than 5 pounds. A 2011 study found that freshmen gain between 2.5 and 3.5 pounds, on average, during their first year. This is only half a pound more than is gained by individuals of the same age who are not attending college. Reasons for the weight gain include newfound food independence, changes in eating habits, stress, and social comparison and the influence of roommates and friends.

Although 5 pounds may not seem like a lot of weight, it still can pose a health risk or contribute to lower self-esteem. Changes in body composition—specifically, increased body fat—can begin a troublesome pattern for students. Even if they don't have a spike in weight during their first year, college-educated individuals tend to experience a moderate but steady weight gain during and after college.

More importantly, whether the weight gain is 5 pounds, 15 pounds, or even more, freshman weight gain is avoidable! In addition to the healthy eating strategies for college students described in Chapter 12, try following these tips and guidelines for avoiding freshman weight gain:

- Listen to your hunger cues.
- Watch portion sizes, and avoid second and third servings.
- Follow a daily schedule for your meals and snack times.
- Don't skip meals—especially breakfast.
- Plan ahead so you have healthy snacks in your room.
- Eat when you are hungry—not for emotional reasons.
- If you cook, try to shop at a regular grocery store and not a campus convenience store.
- Avoid late-night eating.
- Be more physically active: walk to and from class, use the campus fitness facility, and consider taking a sports class for credit (tennis, dance, aerobics, weight training).

SOURCES: Zagorsky, J. L., and P. K. Smith. 2011. The freshman 15: Critical time for obesity intervention or media myth? *Social Science Quarterly*, 92(5): 1389–1407; Smith-Jackson, T., and J. J. Reed. 2012. Freshman women and the "Freshman 15": Perspectives on prevalence and causes of college weight gain. *Journal of American College Health*, 60(1): 14–20; Yakusheva, O., K. Kapinos, and M. Weiss. 2011. Peer effects and the freshman 15: Evidence from a natural experiment. *Economics & Human Biology* 9(2):119–132.

will have the bone density of a woman in her sixties. Left untreated, the triad can lead to decreased physical performance, increased incidence of bone fractures, disturbances of heart rhythm and metabolism, and even death.

What Is the Right Weight for You?

To answer the question of what you should weigh, let your lifestyle be your guide. Don't focus on a particular weight as your goal. Instead focus on living a lifestyle that includes eating moderate amounts of healthful foods, getting plenty of exercise, thinking positively, and learning to cope with stress. Then let the pounds fall where they may. For most people, the result will be close to the recommended weight ranges discussed earlier. For some, their weight will be somewhat higher than societal standards—but right for them. By letting a healthy lifestyle determine your weight, you can avoid developing unhealthy patterns of eating and a negative body image (see the box "The Freshman 15: Fact or Myth").

FACTORS CONTRIBUTING TO EXCESS BODY FAT

Body weight and body composition may be determined by multiple factors that may vary with each individual.

Genetic Factors

Estimates of the genetic contribution to obesity vary widely, from about 25% to 40% of an individual's body fat. Scientists have so far identified more than 600 genes associated with obesity. Genes influence body size and shape, body fat distribution, and metabolic rate. Genetic factors also affect the ease with which weight is gained as a result of overeating and where on the body extra weight is added.

If both parents are obese, their children have an 80% risk of being obese; children with only one obese parent face a 50% risk of becoming obese. In studies that compared adoptees and their biological parents, the weights of the adoptees were found to be more like those of the biological parents than those of the adoptive parents, again indicating a strong genetic link.

Hereditary influences, however, must be balanced against the contribution of environmental factors. Not all children of obese parents become obese, and normal-weight parents may have overweight children. Environmental factors like diet and exercise are probably responsible for such differences. Thus the *tendency* to develop obesity may be inherited, but the expression of this tendency is affected by environmental influences.

It is true that some people have a harder time losing weight and maintaining weight loss than others. However, with increased exercise and attention to diet, even those with a genetic tendency toward obesity can maintain a healthy body weight.

Physiological Factors

Metabolism is a key physiological factor in the regulation of body fat and body weight; hormones and fat cell types also play a role.

Metabolism   Metabolism is the sum of all the vital processes by which food energy and nutrients are made available to and used by the body. The largest component of metabolism, **resting metabolic rate (RMR),** is the energy required to maintain vital body functions, including respiration, heart rate, body temperature, and blood pressure, while the body is at rest. As shown in Figure 11.1, RMR accounts for about 65–70% of daily energy expenditure. The energy required to digest food accounts for as much as 10% of daily energy expenditure. The remaining 20–30% is expended during physical activity.

Both genetics and behavior affect metabolic rate. Men, who have a higher proportion of muscle mass than women, have a higher RMR because muscle tissue is more metabolically active than fat. Also, some individuals inherit a higher or lower RMR than others. A higher RMR means that a person burns more calories while at rest and can therefore take in more calories without gaining weight.

Weight loss or gain also affects metabolic rate. When a person loses weight, both RMR and the energy required to perform physical tasks decrease. The reverse occurs when weight is gained. One of the reasons why exercise is so important during a weight loss program is that exercise, especially resistance training, helps maintain muscle mass and metabolic rate.

Hormones   Hormones clearly play a role in the accumulation of body fat, especially for females. Hormonal changes at puberty, during pregnancy, and at menopause contribute to the amount and location of fat accumulation. One hormone thought to be linked to obesity is *leptin*. Secreted by the body's fat cells, leptin is carried to the brain, where it appears to let the brain know how big or small the body's fat stores are. With this information, the brain can regulate appetite and metabolic rate accordingly. However, as most of us will admit, hunger is often *not* the primary reason we overeat. Cases of obesity based solely or primarily on hormone abnormalities do exist, but they are rare.

Fat Cells   The amount of fat (adipose tissue) the body can store is a function of the number and size of fat (adipose) cells.

Some people are born with an above-average number of fat cells and thus have the potential for storing more energy as body fat. Overeating at critical times, such as in childhood, can cause the body to create more fat cells. If a person loses weight, fat cell content is depleted, but it is unclear whether the number of fat cells can be decreased.

Lifestyle Factors

Although genetic and physiological factors may increase the risk for excess body fat, they are not sufficient to explain the increasingly high rate of obesity seen in the United States. The gene pool has not changed dramatically in the past 60 years, but the rate of obesity among Americans has more than doubled. Clearly, other factors are at work—particularly lifestyle factors such as increased eating and decreased physical activity.

Eating   Americans have access to plenty of calorie-dense foods, and many have eating habits that contribute to weight gain. Most overweight adults admit to eating more than they should of high-fat, high-sugar, high-calorie foods. Americans eat out more frequently now than in the past and rely more heavily on fast food and packaged convenience foods. Restaurant and convenience food portion sizes tend to be large, and the foods themselves are likely to be high in fat, sugar, and calories and low in nutrients. Many people underestimate the actual number of calories they eat.

The popularity of sugar-free soft drinks does not appear to be helping people lose weight, though it is not yet clear why this may be the case. Compared to people who don't drink soda, people who drink more than one soda per day, either regular or diet, are more likely to be obese, develop metabolic syndrome, and have high blood pressure.

Physical Activity   Activity levels among Americans are declining, beginning in childhood and continuing throughout life. Many schools have cut back on physical education classes and recess. Most adults drive to work, sit all day, and then relax in front of the TV at night. Incidence of overweight is consistently linked to excessive screen time—whether time spent watching TV, playing video games, or using computers.

An "Obesogenic" Environment   The 2010 Dietary Guidelines for Americans focused attention on the "obesogenic" environment in which most Americans live. This environment promotes overconsumption of calories while at the same time discouraging physical activity. Food and activity choices are influenced by the communities in which individuals live, their socioeconomic status, religion and culture, and geographic location. People living in areas with limited access to healthy foods and opportunities for physical activity do not have the same options for choosing a healthy lifestyle as do people living in more enriched environments.

Psychosocial Factors

Many people have learned to use food as a means of coping with stress and negative emotions. Eating can provide a powerful distraction from difficult feelings—loneliness, anger,

---

resting metabolic rate (RMR)   The energy required to maintain vital body functions, including respiration, heart rate, body temperature, and blood pressure, while the body is at rest.

TERMS

boredom, anxiety, shame, sadness, inadequacy. It can be used to combat low moods, low energy levels, and low self-esteem. When food and eating become the primary means of regulating emotions, binge eating or other disturbed eating patterns can develop.

Obesity is strongly associated with socioeconomic status. The prevalence of obesity in women and children tends to go down as income level goes up, though it stays the same in men. These differences may reflect the greater sensitivity and concern for a slim physical appearance among upper-income women, as well as greater access to information about nutrition, to low-fat and low-calorie foods, and to opportunities for physical activity. It may also reflect the greater acceptance of obesity among certain ethnic groups, as well as different cultural values related to food choices.

In some families and cultures, food is used as a symbol of love and caring. It is an integral part of social gatherings and celebrations. In such cases, it may be difficult to change established eating patterns because they are linked to cultural and family values.

ADOPTING A HEALTHY LIFESTYLE FOR SUCCESSFUL WEIGHT MANAGEMENT

A good time to develop a lifestyle for successful weight management is during early adulthood, when healthy behavior patterns have a better chance of taking a firm hold.

Diet and Eating Habits

In contrast to dieting, which involves some form of food restriction, the term *diet* refers to your daily food choices. Everyone has a diet, but not everyone is dieting. You need to develop a diet that you enjoy and that enables you to maintain a healthy body composition. Use MyPlate or the DASH Eating Plan as the basis for a healthy diet. For weight management, pay special attention to total calories, portion sizes, energy density, fat and carbohydrate intake, and eating habits.

Total Calories MyPlate suggests approximate daily energy needs based on gender, age, and activity level. However, energy balance may be a more important consideration for weight management than total calories consumed. To maintain your current weight, you have to burn the same number of calories that you take in. To lose weight, you must decrease your calorie intake and/or increase the number of calories you burn; to gain weight, the reverse is true.

The best approach for weight loss is combining an increase in physical activity with moderate calorie restriction. Don't go on a crash diet. To maintain weight loss, you may need to maintain some degree of the calorie

restriction you used to lose the weight. Therefore, you need to adopt a level of food intake that provides all the essential nutrients that you can live with over the long term. For most people, maintaining weight loss is more difficult than losing the weight in the first place.

Portion Sizes Overconsumption of total calories is closely tied to portion sizes. Many Americans are unaware that the portions of packaged foods and of foods served at restaurants have increased in size, and most of us significantly underestimate the amount of food we eat. Studies have found that the larger the meal, the more calories people tend to eat. Portion size is associated with body weight, so limiting portion sizes is critical for maintaining a healthy body weight.

Energy (Calorie) Density Experts also recommend that you pay attention to *energy density*—the number of calories per ounce or gram of weight in a food. Studies suggest that it isn't consumption of a certain amount of fat or calories in food that reduces hunger and leads to feelings of fullness and satisfaction; rather, it is consumption of a certain weight of food. Foods that are low in energy density have more volume and bulk—that is, they are relatively heavy but have few calories. Examples include air-poppd popcorn, fat-free yogurt with fruit, and fresh fruits and vegetables.

As you decrease foods high in energy density, increase foods high in nutrient density—foods that are low in calories and high in nutrients. Strategies for lowering the energy density of your diet while at the same time increasing its nutrient density include the following:

- Eat fruit with breakfast and for dessert.
- Add extra vegetables to sandwiches, casseroles, stir-fry dishes, pizza, pasta dishes, and fajitas.
- Start meals with a bowl of broth-based soup; include a green salad or fruit salad.
- Snack on fresh fruits and vegetables rather than crackers, chips, or other energy-dense snack foods.

Limit serving sizes of energy-dense foods such as butter, mayonnaise, cheese, chocolate, fatty meats, croissants, and snack foods that are fried, are high in added sugars (including reduced-fat products), or contain trans fats.

Eating Habits Equally important to weight management is the habit of eating regular meals daily, including breakfast and snacks. Skipping meals leads to excessive hunger, feelings of deprivation, and increased vulnerability to binge eating or unhealthy snacking. In addition to establishing a regular pattern of eating, set some rules to govern your food choices. Rules for breakfast might be these, for example: Choose a high-fiber cereal that is low in added sugar with fat-free milk on most days; save pancakes and waffles for special occasions unless they are whole-grain. For effective weight management, it is better to consume the majority of calories

> For weight management, it's **better to have the majority of calories during the day** rather than in the evening.

during the day when your activity levels are higher rather than in the evening.

Physical Activity and Exercise

Physical activity and exercise burn calories and keep the metabolism geared to using food for energy instead of storing it as fat. Making significant cuts in food intake to lose weight is a difficult strategy to maintain; increasing your physical activity is a better approach. Regular physical activity protects against weight gain, is essential for maintaining weight loss, and improves quality of life.

Thinking and Emotions

The way you think about yourself and your world influences, and is influenced by, how you feel and how you act. Often people with low self-esteem mentally compare the actual self to an internally held picture of an "ideal self," an image based on perfectionistic goals and beliefs about how they and others should be. The more these two pictures differ, the larger the impact on self-esteem and the more likely the presence of negative emotions.

Besides the internal picture we carry of ourselves, all of us carry on an internal dialogue about events happening to us and around us. This *self-talk* can be self-deprecating or positively motivating, depending on our beliefs and attitudes. Having realistic beliefs and goals, and practicing positive self-talk and problem solving, support a healthy lifestyle.

Coping Strategies

Appropriate coping strategies help you deal with the stresses of life; they are also an important lifestyle factor in weight management. Those who overeat might use food to alleviate loneliness or to serve as a pickup for fatigue, as an antidote to boredom, or as a distraction from problems.

Those who recognize that they are misusing food in such ways can consciously attempt to find new coping strategies and begin to use food appropriately—to fuel life's activities, to foster growth, and to bring pleasure, but *not* as a way to manage stress.

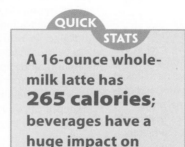

QUICK STATS

A 16-ounce whole-milk latte has **265 calories;** beverages have a huge impact on calorie intake.

—CDC, 2011

APPROACHES TO OVERCOMING A WEIGHT PROBLEM

Americans spend approximately $62 billion on weight loss efforts every year, including diet plans, diet products, and health club memberships. If you are overweight, you may already be creating a plan to lose weight and keep it off. You have many options.

Doing It Yourself

If you need to lose weight, focus on adopting the healthy lifestyle described throughout this book. The right weight for you will naturally evolve, and you won't have to diet. Combine modest cuts in energy intake with exercise, and avoid very low-calorie diets. (In general, a low-calorie diet should provide 1200–1500 calories per day.) By producing a negative energy balance of 250–1000 calories per day, you will produce the recommended weight loss of 0.5–2.0 pounds per week.

Most low-calorie diets cause a rapid loss of body water at first. When this phase passes, weight loss declines. As a result, dieters are often misled into believing that their efforts are not working. They then give up, not realizing that smaller, mostly fat, losses later in the diet are actually better than the initial larger, mostly fluid losses. Reasonable weight loss is 8–10% of body weight over six months.

Many diets can cause weight loss if the diet is maintained; however, the real difficulty is finding a safe and healthy pattern of food choices and physical activity that results in long-term maintenance of a healthy body weight and reduced risk of chronic disease (see the box "Is Any Diet Best for Weight Loss?"). A registered dietitian or nutritionist can recommend an appropriate plan for you when you want to lose weight on your own.

Dietary Supplements and Diet Aids

Dietary supplements marketed for weight loss so are subject to fewer regulations than over-the-counter (OTC) medications. According to the Federal Trade Commission, more than half of advertisements for weight loss products make representations that were likely to be false. And although the FTC will order companies to stop making baseless and bogus product claims when monitors become aware of them, consumers are urged to critically evaluate any product that sounds too good to be true.

Formula Drinks and Food Bars Canned diet drinks, powders used to make shakes, and diet food bars and snacks are designed to achieve weight loss by substituting for some or all of a person's daily food intake. However, most people find

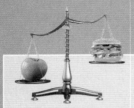

CRITICAL CONSUMER
Is Any Diet Best for Weight Loss?

Many popular weight loss plans promote specific food choices and macronutrient combinations. Research findings have been mixed, but two points are clear: total calorie intake matters, and the best diet is probably the one you can stick with.

Low-Carbohydrate Diets

Some low-carb diets advocate fewer than 10% of total calories from carbohydrates, compared to the 45–65% recommended by the Food and Nutrition Board. Some suggest daily carbohydrate intake below the 130 grams needed to provide essential carbohydrates in the diet. Low-carb diets that advocate switching to "healthy carbs" are better for you than the more extreme versions.

Low-Fat Diets

Many experts advocate diets that are relatively low in fat, high in carbohydrates, and moderate in protein. If you try a low-fat diet, high-carb diet, you still need to pay attention to the quality of the carbohydrates you consume, focusing on whole grains and your total calorie intake. A low-fat diet is not a license to consume excess calories, even in low-fat foods.

High-Protein Diets

High-protein diets advocate high protein intake, moderate fat intake, and low carbohydrate intakes. These diets can be low in fiber, whole grains, vegetables, and fruits and so may lack some essential nutrients. Diets high in protein and saturated fat have been linked to an increased risk of heart disease, high blood pressure, and cancer. One study found that following a diet with a normal protein-to-carbohydrate ratio (1 gram of protein to 2 grams of carbohydrate) promoted more improvements in body fat, waist circumference, and waist-to-hip ratio than following either a low-protein diet (1 gram of protein to 4 grams of carbohydrate) or a high-protein diet (1 gram of protein to 1 gram of carbohydrate) and was probably superior in reducing long-term chronic disease risk.

How Do Different Diets Measure Up?

A study comparing weight loss among adults assigned to one of four reduced-calorie diets differing in percentages of protein, carbohydrate, and fat found that weight loss at two years was similar for all four diets (about 9 pounds). Weight loss was strongly associated with attendance at group sessions. Other studies have also found little difference in weight loss among popular reduced-calorie diets; most resulted in modest weight loss and reduced heart disease risk factors. The more closely people adhered to each diet, the more weight they lost.

Adding exercise helps people lose weight and improve disease risk factors. A study found that when overweight and obese people added exercise and weight loss to the DASH Eating Plan, they experienced greater reductions in blood pressure and greater improvements in insulin sensitivity and lipid levels than those who follow the DASH diet alone or regular diet plans.

Energy Balance Counts: The National Weight Control Registry

Future research may determine that certain macronutrient patterns are somewhat more helpful for disease reduction in people with particular risk profiles. In terms of weight loss, however, such differences among diets are likely overshadowed by the importance of total calorie intake and physical activity. Important lessons about energy balance can be drawn from the National Weight Control Registry—an ongoing study of people who have lost significant amounts of weight and kept it off. The average participant in the registry has lost 71 pounds and kept the weight off for more than five years. Nearly all participants use a combination of diet and exercise to manage their weight. This study illustrates that to lose weight and keep it off, you must decrease daily calorie intake and/or increase daily physical activity—and continue to do so over your lifetime.

SOURCES: Campbell, D. D., and K. A. Meckling. 2012. Effect of the protein:carbohydrate ratio in hypenergetic diets on metabolic syndrome risk factors in exercising overweight and obese women. *British Journal of Nutrition,* Jan 16: 1–14; Sacks, F. M., et al. 2009. Comparison of weight loss diets with different compositions of fat, protein, and carbohydrates. *The New England Journal of Medicine* 360: 859–873; Blumenthal, J. A., et al. 2010. Effects of the dietary approaches to stop hypertension diet alone and in combination with exercise and caloric restriction on insulin sensitivity and lipids. *Hypertension* 55(5): 1199–1205; Hill, J., and R. Wing. 2003. The National Weight Control Registry. *Permanente Journal* 7(3): 34–37.

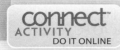

connect
ACTIVITY
DO IT ONLINE

it difficult to use these products for long periods, and muscle loss and other serious health problems may result if they are used as the sole source of nutrition for an extended period. Use of such products sometimes results in rapid short-term weight loss, but the weight is typically regained because users don't learn to change their eating and lifestyle behaviors.

Herbal Supplements Most herbal weight loss products work by increasing urination (causing water loss); by stimulating the central nervous system (causing the body's activities to speed up or increasing metabolism); or by affecting levels of brain chemicals (causing appetite suppression). Herbs are marketed as dietary supplements, so there is little information about effectiveness, proper dosage, drug interactions, or side effects. In addition, labels may not accurately reflect the ingredients and dosages present, and safe manufacturing practices are not guaranteed. Weight loss occurs only while the product is being taken.

The FDA has banned the sale of ephedra (*ma huang* in Chinese medicine), stating that it presented a significant and unreasonable risk to human health. Ephedrine, the active ingredient in ephedra, is structurally similar to amphetamine and was widely used in weight loss supplements. It may suppress appetite, but adverse effects have included elevated blood pressure, panic attacks, seizures, insomnia, and increased risk of heart attack or stroke, particularly when combined with another stimulant such as caffeine. The FDA banned the synthetic stimulant phenylpropanolamine for similar reasons.

Other Supplements   Fiber is another common ingredient in OTC diet aids, promoted for appetite control. Many diet aids contain only 3 or fewer grams of fiber, which does not contribute much toward the recommended daily intake of 25–38 grams. Other popular dietary supplements include conjugated linoleic acid, carnitine, chromium, pyruvate, calcium, B vitamins, chitosan, and a number of products labeled "fat absorbers," "fat blockers," and "starch blockers." Research has not found these products to be effective, and many have potentially adverse side effects.

Weight Loss Programs

Weight loss programs come in a variety of types, including noncommercial support organizations, commercial programs, websites, and clinical programs. According to the NIH, safe and effective weight loss programs should include

- Healthy eating plans that reduce calories but do not exclude specific foods or food groups.

- Tips on ways to increase moderate-intensity physical activity.

- Tips on healthy habits that also keep your cultural needs in mind, such as lower-fat versions of your favorite foods.

- Slow and steady weight loss. Depending on your starting weight, experts recommend losing weight at a rate of ½ to 2 pounds per week.

- A recommendation for medical evaluation and care if you have health problems, are taking medication, or are planning to follow a special formula diet that requires monitoring by a doctor.

- A plan to keep the weight off after you have lost it.

Noncommercial Weight Loss Programs   Noncommercial programs such as TOPS (Take Off Pounds Sensibly) and Overeaters Anonymous (OA) mainly provide group support. They do not advocate any particular diet but do recommend seeking professional advice for creating an individualized plan. These types of programs are generally free. Your physician or a registered dietitian can also provide information and support for weight loss.

Commercial Weight Loss Programs   Commercial weight loss programs typically provide group support, nutrition education, physical activity recommendations, and behavior modification advice. Some also make available packaged foods to assist in following dietary advice.

In addition to the features of a safe and effective program outlined earlier, commercial weight loss programs should provide information about all fees and costs, including those of supplements and prepackaged foods, as well as data on risks and expected outcomes of participating in the program. They should also have a registered dietitian on staff along with qualified counselors and health professionals.

A strong commitment and a plan for maintenance are especially important because only about 10–15% of program participants maintain their weight loss—the rest gain back all or more than they had lost. One study found that important predictors of weight loss and maintenance of weight loss in commercial programs include an increased intake of vegetables, fruit, and low-fat dairy products; decreased intake of sweets; and regular exercise.

> All prescription weight loss medications have potential side effects, ranging from diarrhea to elevated blood pressure.

Online Weight Loss Programs   Most weight loss websites combine self-help with group support through chat rooms, bulletin boards, and e-newsletters. Many sites offer online self-assessment for diet and physical activity habits as well as a meal plan; some provide access to a staff professional for individualized help. Many are free, but some charge a weekly or monthly fee. Research suggests that this type of program provides an alternative to in-person diet counseling and can lead to weight loss for some people.

Clinical Weight Loss Programs   Medically supervised clinical programs are usually located in a hospital or other medical setting. Designed to help those who are severely obese, these programs typically involve a closely monitored very low-calorie diet. The cost of a clinical program is usually high, but insurance may cover part of the fee for those with obesity-related health problems.

Prescription Drugs

The medications most often prescribed for weight loss are appetite suppressants that reduce feelings of hunger or increase feelings of fullness. Appetite suppressants usually work by increasing levels of brain chemicals that affect mood and appetite. Most appetite suppressants are approved by the FDA only for short-term use, but one, sibutramine (Meridia), is approved for longer-term use. All prescription weight loss drugs have potential side effects, including sleeplessness, nervousness, euphoria, increases in blood pressure and heart, headaches, constipation or diarrhea, dry mouth, and insomnia. Sibutramine's safety and efficacy record is good, but regular monitoring of blood pressure is required during therapy.

Another type of weight loss drug works by blocking fat absorption in the intestines. Orlistat (Xenical) prevents about 30% of the fat in food from being digested. Similar to the fat substitute olestra, orlistat reduces the absorption of fat-soluble vitamins and antioxidants. Therefore, taking a vitamin supplement is highly recommended for people taking orlistat. Side effects include diarrhea, cramping, and other gastrointestinal problems if users do not follow a low-fat diet. Alli is an FDA-approved, a lower-dose version of orlistat that is sold over the counter.

These medications work best in conjunction with behavior modification. Studies have generally found that appetite suppressants produce modest weight loss—about 5–22 pounds above the loss expected with nondrug obesity treatments. Unfortunately weight loss tends to level off or reverse after 4–6 months on a medication, and many people regain the weight they've lost when they stop taking the drug.

Prescription drugs are recommended only for people who have been unable to lose weight with nondrug options and who have a BMI over 30 (or over 27 if two or more additional risk factors such as diabetes and high blood pressure are present).

Surgery

It is estimated that 5.7% of adult Americans have a BMI greater than 40, qualifying them as extremely or "morbidly" obese. Extreme obesity is a serious medical condition that is often complicated by other health problems such as diabetes, heart disease, arthritis, and sleep disorders. Surgical intervention may be necessary as a treatment of last resort. According to the NIH, weight loss (bariatric) surgery is recommended for patients with a BMI greater than 40, or greater than 35 with obesity-related illnesses.

Bariatric surgery modifies the gastrointestinal tract by changing either the size of the stomach or how the intestine drains, thereby reducing food intake. The keys to success with surgical weight loss procedures are adequate follow-up and continued motivation so that eating patterns and lifestyle behaviors are permanently changed.

> **QUICK STATS**
>
> **Most bariatric surgery patients can expect to lose 50% or more of their excess weight within two years of the procedure.**
>
> —Mayo Clinic, 2011

BODY IMAGE

Developing a positive body image is an important aspect of psychological wellness and an important component of successful weight management.

Severe Body Image Problems

A person can become preoccupied with a perceived defect in appearance, thereby damaging self-esteem and interfering with relationships. Adolescents and adults who have a negative body image are more likely to diet restrictively, eat compulsively, or develop some other form of disordered eating.

When dissatisfaction becomes extreme, the condition is called *body dysmorphic disorder (BDD)*. BDD affects about 2% of Americans, males and females in equal numbers; BDD usually begins before age 18 but can begin in adulthood. Sufferers are overly concerned with physical appearance, often focusing on slight flaws that are not obvious to others. Low self-esteem is common. Individuals with BDD may spend hours every day thinking about their flaws and looking at themselves in mirrors; they may desire and seek repeated cosmetic surgeries. BDD is related to obsessive-compulsive disorder and can lead to depression, social phobia, and suicide if left untreated. An individual with BDD needs to get professional evaluation and treatment. Medication and therapy can help people with BDD.

In some cases, body image may bear little resemblance to fact. A person suffering from the eating disorder anorexia nervosa typically has a severely distorted body image—she believes herself to be fat even when she has become emaciated. Distorted body image is also a hallmark of *muscle dysmorphia*, a disorder experienced by some bodybuilders and other active people who see themselves as small and out of shape despite being very muscular. Those who suffer from muscle dysmorphia

Ask Yourself

QUESTIONS FOR CRITICAL THINKING AND REFLECTION

Why do you think people continue to buy into fad diets and weight loss gimmicks, even though they are constantly reminded that the key to weight management is lifestyle change? Have you ever tried a fad diet or weight loss supplement? If so, what were your reasons for trying it? What were the results?

Ask Yourself

QUESTIONS FOR CRITICAL THINKING AND REFLECTION

Describe your own body image in the fewest words possible. What satisfies you most and least about your body? Do you think your self-image is in line with the way others see you?

may let obsessive exercise—interfere with their work and relationships. They may also use steroids and other potentially dangerous muscle-building drugs.

Acceptance and Change

There are limits to the changes that can be made to body weight and body shape, both of which are influenced by heredity. The changes that can and should be made are lifestyle changes, as described throughout this chapter.

Knowing when you've reached the limits of healthy change—and learning to accept those limits—is crucial for overall wellness. Obesity is a serious health risk, but weight management needs to take place in a positive and realistic atmosphere. For an obese person, losing as few as 10 pounds can improve blood glucose control, reduce blood pressure and improve mood. The hazards of excessive dieting and

Knowing when you've **reached the limits of healthy change,** and accepting those limits, are crucial for overall wellness.

overconcern about body weight need to be countered by a change in attitude. A reasonable weight must take into account a person's weight history, social circumstances, metabolic profile, and psychological well-being.

EATING DISORDERS

Problems with body weight and weight control are not limited to excessive body fat. A growing number of people, especially adolescent girls and young women, experience **eating disorders**—psychological disorders characterized by severe disturbances in body image, eating patterns, and eating-related behaviors. The major eating disorders are anorexia nervosa, bulimia nervosa, and binge-eating disorder. In the United States, almost 10 million females and 1 million males suffer from anorexia and bulimia, and millions more suffer from binge eating disorder. Many more people have abnormal eating habits and attitudes about food that disrupt their lives, even though these habits do not meet the criteria for a major eating disorder.

Anorexia Nervosa

A person with **anorexia nervosa** does not eat enough food to maintain a reasonable body weight. Anorexia affects 0.6% of Americans, only one-third of whom are receiving treatment. Although it can occur earlier or later, anorexia typically develops during puberty and the late teenage years, with an average age of onset of about 19 years.

Characteristics of Anorexia Nervosa   People with anorexia have an intense fear of gaining weight or becoming fat. Their body image is so distorted that even when emaciated they think they are fat. People with anorexia may engage in compulsive behaviors or rituals that help keep them from eating, though some may also binge and **purge.** They often use vigorous and prolonged exercise to reduce body weight as well. Although they may express a great interest in food, even taking over the cooking responsibilities for the

Exercise is a healthy practice, but people with eating disorders sometimes exercise compulsively, building their lives around their workouts. Compulsive exercise can lead to injuries, low body fat, and other health problems.

> **eating disorder**   A serious disturbance in eating patterns or eating-related behavior, characterized by a negative body image and concerns about body weight or body fat.
>
> **anorexia nervosa**   An eating disorder characterized by a refusal to maintain body weight at a minimally healthy level and an intense fear of gaining weight or becoming fat; self-starvation.
>
> **purging**   The use of vomiting, laxatives, excessive exercise, restrictive dieting, enemas, diuretics, or diet pills to compensate for food that has been eaten and that the person fears will produce weight gain.

TERMS

rest of the family, their own diet becomes more and more restricted. People with anorexia often hide or hoard food without eating it.

People with anorexia are typically introverted, emotionally reserved, and socially insecure. They are often model children who rarely complain and are anxious to please others and win their approval. Although school performance is typically above average, they are often critical of themselves and not satisfied with their accomplishments. For people with anorexia nervosa, their entire sense of self-esteem may be tied up in their evaluation of their body shape and weight.

Health Risks of Anorexia Nervosa   Because of extreme weight loss, females with anorexia often stop menstruating, become intolerant of cold, and develop low blood pressure and heart rate. They develop dry skin that is often covered by fine body hair like that of a newborn. Their hands and feet may swell and take on a blue tinge.

Anorexia nervosa has been linked to a variety of medical complications, including disorders of the cardiovascular, gastrointestinal, endocrine, and skeletal systems. When body fat is virtually gone and muscles are severely wasted, the body turns to its own organs in a desperate search for protein. Death can occur from heart failure caused by electrolyte imbalances. About 1 in 10 women with anorexia dies of starvation, cardiac arrest, or other medical complications—the highest death rate for any psychiatric disorder. Depression is also a serious risk: about half the fatalities related to anorexia are suicides.

Bulimia Nervosa

A person suffering from **bulimia nervosa** engages in recurrent episodes of binge eating followed by purging. Bulimia is often difficult to recognize because sufferers conceal their eating habits and usually maintain a normal weight, although they may experience weight fluctuations of 10–15 pounds. Although bulimia usually begins in adolescence or young adulthood, it has begun to emerge at increasingly younger (11–12 years) and older (40–60 years) ages; the average age of onset is about 20 years.

Characteristics of Bulimia Nervosa   During a binge, a bulimic person may rapidly consume thousands of calories. This is followed by an attempt to get rid of the food by purging, usually by vomiting or using laxatives or diuretics. During a binge, bulimics feel as though they have lost control and cannot stop or limit how much they eat. Some binge and purge only occasionally; others do so many times every day.

People with bulimia may appear to eat normally, but they are rarely comfortable around food. Binges usually occur in secret and can become nightmarish—uncontrollably raiding the kitchen for food, going from one grocery store to another to buy food, or stealing food. During the binge, food acts as an anesthetic, blocking out feelings. Afterward, bulimics feel physically drained and emotionally spent. They usually feel deeply ashamed and disgusted with both themselves and their behavior and terrified that they will gain weight from the binge.

Major life changes such as leaving for college, getting married, having a baby, or losing a job can trigger a binge-purge cycle. At such times, stress is high and the person may have no good outlet for emotional conflict or tension. As with anorexia, bulimia sufferers are often insecure and depend on others for approval and self-esteem. They may hide difficult emotions such as anger and disappointment from themselves and others. Binge eating and purging become a way of dealing with feelings.

Health Risks of Bulimia Nervosa   The binge-purge cycle of bulimia places a tremendous strain on the body and can have serious health effects. Contact with vomited stomach acids erodes tooth enamel. Repeated vomiting or the use of laxatives, in combination with deficient calorie intake, can damage the liver and kidneys and cause cardiac arrhythmia. Chronic hoarseness and esophageal tearing with bleeding may also result from vomiting. More rarely, binge eating can lead to rupture of the stomach. Although less often associated with suicide or premature death than anorexia, bulimia is associated with increased depression, excessive preoccupation with food and body image, and sometimes disturbances in cognitive functioning.

Binge-Eating Disorder

Binge-eating disorder (BED) affects almost 3% of American adults. It is characterized by uncontrollable eating, usually followed by feelings of guilt and shame about weight gain. Common eating patterns are eating more rapidly than normal, eating until uncomfortably full, eating when not hungry, and preferring to eat alone. Binge eaters may eat large amounts of food throughout the day, with no planned mealtimes. Many people with binge-eating disorder mistakenly see rigid dieting as the only solution to their problem. However, rigid dieting usually causes feelings of deprivation and a return to overeating.

> ## QUICK STATS
>
> Only about **34%** of people with anorexia, **43%** of those with bulimia, and **44%** of those with binge-eating disorders receive treatment.
>
> —National Institutes of Mental Health Statistics

> **TERMS**
>
> **bulimia nervosa**   An eating disorder characterized by recurrent episodes of binge eating and purging—overeating and then using compensatory behaviors such as vomiting, laxatives, and excessive exercise to prevent weight gain.
>
> **binge-eating disorder**   An eating disorder characterized by binge eating and a lack of control over eating behavior in general.

Compulsive overeaters rarely eat because of hunger. Instead food is used as a means of coping with stress, conflict, and other difficult emotions or to provide solace and entertainment. People who do not have the resources to deal effectively with stress may be more vulnerable to binge-eating disorder. Inappropriate overeating often begins during childhood. In some families, eating may be used as an activity to fill otherwise empty time. Parents may reward children with food for good behavior or withhold food as a means of punishment, thereby creating distorted feelings about the use of food.

Binge eaters are almost always obese, so they face all the health risks associated with obesity. In addition, binge eaters may have higher rates of depression and anxiety.

Borderline Disordered Eating

People with borderline disordered eating have some symptoms of eating disorders but do not meet the full diagnostic criteria for anorexia, bulimia, or binge-eating disorder. Behaviors such as excessive dieting, occasional bingeing or purging, or the inability to control eating turn food into the enemy and create havoc in the lives of millions of Americans.

How do you know if you have disordered eating habits? When thoughts about food and weight dominate your life, you have a problem. If you're convinced that your worth as a person hinges on how you look and how much you weigh, it's time to get help. Other danger signs include frequent feelings of guilt after a meal or snack, any use of vomiting or laxatives after meals, or overexercising or severely restricting your food intake to compensate for what you've already eaten.

If you suspect you have an eating problem, don't go it alone or delay getting help, because disordered eating habits can develop into a full-blown eating disorder. Check with your student health or counseling center—nearly all colleges have counselors and medical personnel who can help you or refer you to a specialist if needed.

Treating Eating Disorders

Anorexia nervosa treatment first involves averting a medical crisis by restoring adequate body weight; then the psychological aspects of the disorder can be addressed. The treatment of bulimia nervosa or binge-eating disorder involves first stabilizing the eating patterns, then identifying and changing the patterns of thinking that led to disordered eating, and then improving coping skills. Concurrent problems, such as depression, anxiety, and other mental disorders, must also be addressed.

Treatment of eating disorders usually involves a combination of psychotherapy and medical management. The therapy may be done individually or in a group; sessions involving the entire family may be recommended. A support or self-help group can be a useful adjunct to such treatment.

Connect to Your Choices

Have you ever thought about how you came to have the body weight and body composition you have? Many factors can influence our weight management choices, some not as obvious as others. Do you have easy access to high-calorie, high-fat snacks in your dorm or dining hall? Does your school provide transportation around campus, making it less appealing to walk to class? Does your TV or computer lure you into hours of sedentary entertainment?

What are the external factors that influence your choices about weight management? What are your inner motivations and core values, and how do they affect your choices? Based on what you learned in this chapter, will you make some different choices in the future? If so, what will they be?

Go online to Connect to complete this activity: www.mcgraw-hillconnect.com

TIPS FOR TODAY AND THE FUTURE

Many approaches work, but the simplest formula for weight management is moderate food intake coupled with regular exercise.

RIGHT NOW YOU CAN:
- Assess your weight management needs. Do you need to gain weight, lose weight, or stay at your current weight?
- List five things you can do to add more physical activity (not exercise) to your daily routine.
- Identify the foods you regularly eat that may be sabotaging your ability to manage your weight.

IN THE FUTURE YOU CAN:
- Make an honest assessment of your current body image. Is it accurate and fair, or is it unduly negative and unhealthy? If your body image presents a problem, consider getting professional advice on how to view yourself realistically.
- Keep track of your energy needs to determine whether your energy balance equation is correct. Use this information as part of your long-term weight management efforts.

SUMMARY

- Body composition is the relative amounts of fat-free mass and fat in the body. *Overweight* and *obesity* refer to body weight or the percentage of body fat that exceeds what is associated with good health.

- The key to weight management is maintaining a balance of calories in (food) and calories out (resting metabolism, food digestion, and physical activity).

- Standards for assessing body weight and body composition include body mass index (BMI) and percent body fat.

- Too much or too little body fat is linked to health problems; the distribution of body fat can also be a significant risk factor for many kinds of health problems.

- Genetic factors help determine a person's weight, but the influence of heredity can be overcome with attention to lifestyle factors. Physiological factors involved in the regulation of body weight and body fat include metabolic rate, hormonal influences, and the size and number of fat cells.

- Nutritional guidelines for weight management include consuming a moderate number of calories; limiting portion sizes, energy density, and the intake of fat, simple sugars, refined carbohydrates, and protein to recommended levels; and developing an eating schedule and rules for food choices.

- Activity guidelines for weight management emphasize daily physical activity and regular sessions of cardiorespiratory endurance exercise and strength training.

- Weight management requires developing positive self-talk and self-esteem, realistic weight and body composition goals, and a repertoire of appropriate techniques for handling stress and other emotional and physical challenges.

- People can be successful at long-term weight loss on their own by combining diet and exercise. Diet aids and supplements should be assessed for safety and efficacy, as should formal weight loss programs.

- Professional help is needed in cases of severe obesity; medical treatments include prescription drugs, surgery, and psychological therapy.

- Dissatisfaction with weight and shape are common to all eating disorders. Anorexia nervosa is characterized by self-starvation, distorted body image, and an intense fear of gaining weight. Bulimia nervosa is characterized by recurrent episodes of uncontrolled binge eating and frequent purging. Binge-eating disorder involves binge eating without regular use of compensatory purging.

- Treatment of eating disorders usually involves a combination of psychotherapy and medical management.

FOR MORE INFORMATION

BOOKS

American Heart Association. 2011. *American Heart Association No-Fad Diet, 2nd Edition: A Personal Plan for Healthy Weight Loss*. New York: Clarkson Potter. *Provides guidelines for successful weight management.*

Costin, C., and G. S. Grabb. 2011. *8 Keys to Recovery from an Eating Disorder: Effective Strategies from Therapeutic Practice and Personal Experience*. New York: Norton. *A motivating description of the recovery process, written by two therapists who interweave their personal narratives with clinical strategies.*

Dillon, E. 2009. *Issues That Concern You: Obesity*. New York: Greenhaven Press. *A collection of perspectives on the causes of obesity, its management, and its impact on individuals and society.*

Fulda, J. 2008. *Half-Assed: A Weight-Loss Memoir*. Berkeley, CA: Seal Press. *A funny, inspiring memoir detailing how the author lost half her body weight, 186 pounds, while struggling with issues of identity, self-acceptance, and change.*

Mayo Clinic. 2012. *Mayo Clinic's Essential Diabetes Book*, 2nd ed. Rochester, MN: Mayo Clinic. *A user-friendly guide to diabetes.*

Samuelson, D. A., and A. D. Salzburg. 2011. *The Weight Loss Surgery Workbook: Deciding on Bariatric Surgery, Preparing for the Procedure, and Changing Habits for Post-Surgery Success*. Oakland, CA: New Harbinger Publications. *A step-by-step workbook that guides patients through the process of weight loss surgery; written by a psychologist and a physician.*

ORGANIZATIONS, HOTLINES, AND WEBSITES

American Diabetes Association. Provides information, a free newsletter, and referrals to local support groups; the website includes an online diabetes risk assessment.

   http://www.diabetes.org

Centers for Disease Control and Prevention: Obesity. The home page for accessing all the CDC's information about overweight and obesity, their health risks, statistics, and diet and exercise.

   http://www.cdc.gov/obesity/index.html

FDA Center for Food Safety and Applied Nutrition: Dietary Supplements. Provides background facts and information on the current regulatory status of dietary supplements, including compounds marketed for weight loss.

   http://www.fda.gov/Food/DietarySupplements/default.htm

National Heart, Lung, and Blood Institute (NHLBI): Aim for a Healthy Weight. Provides information and tips on diet and physical activity, as well as a BMI calculator.

   http://www.nhlbi.nih.gov/health/public/heart/obesity/lose_wt

National Institute of Diabetes and Digestive and Kidney Diseases (NIDDK): Weight-Control Information Network. Provides information and referrals for problems related to obesity, weight control, and nutritional disorders.

   http://win.niddk.nih.gov

RESOURCES FOR PEOPLE CONCERNED ABOUT EATING DISORDERS

Eating Disorder Referral and Information Center
   http://www.edreferral.com

Eating Disorders Coalition for Research, Policy and Action
   http://www.something-fishy.org

MedlinePlus: Eating Disorders
   http://www.nlm.nih.gov/medlineplus/eatingdisorders.html

National Association of Anorexia Nervosa and Associated Eating Disorders
   630-577-1330 (help line)
   http://www.anad.org

National Eating Disorders Association
   http://www.nationaleatingdisorders.org

National Institute of Mental Health: Eating Disorders
   http://www.nimh.nih.gov/health/topics/eating-disorders/index
      .shtml

American Academy of Child and Adolescent Psychiatry. 2011. *Obesity in Children and Teens* (http://www.aacap.org/cs/root/facts_for_families/obesity_in_children_and_teens).

American Diabetes Association. 2011. *Diabetes Statistics* (http://www.diabetes.org/diabetes-basics/diabetes-statistics/).

Anderson, S. E., and R. C. Whitaker. 2009. Prevalence of obesity among US preschool children in different racial and ethnic groups. *Archives of Pediatrics and Adolescent Medicine*, 163(4): 344–348.

Campbell, I. C., J. Miller, R. Uher, and U. Schmidt. 2011. Eating disorders, gene–environment interactions, and epigenetics. *Neuroscience & Biobehavioral Reviews*, 35(3): 784–793.

Canfi, A., et al. 2011. Effect of changes in the intake of weight of specific food groups on successful body weight loss during a multi-dietary strategy intervention trial. *Journal of the American College of Nutrition*, 30(6): 491–501.

Centers for Disease Control and Prevention. 2011. *National Diabetes Fact Sheet: General Information and National Estimates on Diabetes and Prediabetes in the United States, 2011*. Atlanta: Centers for Disease Control and Prevention.

Centers for Disease Control and Prevention. 2012. *Genomics and Health: Genes and Obesity* (http://www.cdc.gov/genomics/resources/diseases/obesity/obesedit.htm).

Centers for Disease Control and Prevention. 2011. *Rethink Your Drink. Healthy Weight: It's Not a Diet, It's a Lifestyle* (http://www.cdc.gov/healthyweight/healthy_eating/drinks.html).

Champagne, C. M., et al. 2011. Dietary intakes associated with successful weight loss and maintenance during the Weight Loss Maintenance trial. *Journal of the American Dietetic Association*, 111(12): 1826–1835.

Dingemans, A. E., Y. R. van Rood, I. de Groot, and E. F. van Furth. 2012. Body dysmorphic disorder in patients with an eating disorder: Prevalence and characteristics. *International Journal of Eating Disorders*, 45(4): 562–569.

Drewnowski, A., and P. Eichelsdoerfer. 2010. Can low-income Americans afford a healthy diet? *Nutrition Today* 44(6): 246–249.

Federal Trade Commission. 2011. *Facts for Consumers: Dietary Supplements* (http://www.ftc.gov/bcp/edu/pubs/consumer/health/hea11.shtm).

Federal Trade Commission. 2011. *Facts for Consumers: Weighing the Evidence in Diet Ads* (http://www.ftc.gov/bcp/edu/pubs/consumer/health/hea03.shtm).

Flegal, K., et al. 2012. Prevalence of obesity and trends in the distribution of body mass index among U.S. adults, 1999–2010. *Journal of the American Medical Association*, 307(5): 491–497.

Fleischhacker, S. E., et al. 2011. A systematic review of fast food access studies. *Obesity Reviews*, 12(5): e460–471.

Mayo Clinic. 2011. *Gastric Bypass Surgery* (http://www.mayoclinic.com/health/g.astric-bypass/MY00825/DSECTION=results).

Hudson, J. I., E. Hiripi, H. G. Pope, and R. C. Kessler. 2007. The prevalence and correlates of eating disorders in the National Comorbidity Survey Replication. *Biological Psychiatry*, 61:348–358.

Mata, J., et al. 2010. When weight management lasts: Lower perceived rule complexity increases adherence. *Appetite* 54(1): 37–43.

Medscape. 2008. *Gastric Bypass Surgery May Be Effective for Weight Loss in Most Patients* (http://www.medscape.org/viewarticle/580560).

Ogden, C. L., et. 2010. Obesity and socioeconomic status in adults: United States, 2005–2008. *NCHIS Data Brief* 50: 1–8. (http://www.ncbi.nlm.nih.gov/pubmed/21211165).

Ogden, C. L., et al. 2010. Prevalence of high body mass index in US children and adolescents, 2007–2008. *Journal of the American Medical Association* 303(3): 242–249.

Ogden, C. L., et al. 2012. Prevalence of obesity in the United States, 2009–2010. NCHS Data Brief, No. 82 (http://www.cdc.gov/nchs/data/databriefs/db82.pdf).

Olshansky, S. J., et al. 2005. A potential decline in life expectancy in the United States in the 21st century. *New England Journal of Medicine* 352(11): 1138–1145.

Sax, H. C. 2011. Selecting the "best" weight loss procedure: More may be better. *Archives of Surgery* 146(2): 155.

Schmidt, M. E., et al. 2012. Systematic review of effective strategies for reducing screen time among young children. *Obesity*, 20(7): 1338–1354.

Slevec, J. H., and M. Tiggerman. 2011. Predictors of body dissatisfaction and disordered eating in middle-aged women. *Clinical Psychology Review*, 31(4): 515–524.

Tsai, A. G., and T. A. Wadden. 2005. Systematic review: An evaluation of major commercial weight loss programs in the United States. *Annals of Internal Medicine* 142(1): 56–66.

Urquhart, C. S., and T. V. Mihalynuk. 2011. Disordered eating in women: Implications for the obesity pandemic. *Canadian Journal of Dietetic Practice and Research* 72(1): e115–125.

U.S. Department of Health and Human Services and U.S. Department of Agriculture. 2011. *Dietary Guidelines for Americans, 2010*. 7th ed. Washington, DC: U.S. Government Printing Office.

U.S. Department of Health and Human Services. 2012. *Healthy People 2020: Nutrition and Weight Status* (http://healthypeople.gov/2020/topicsobjectives2020/overview.aspx?topicid=29).

BEHAVIOR CHANGE STRATEGY
Creating a Personal Weight Management Plan

The behavior management plan described in Chapter 1 provides an excellent framework for a weight management program. Following are some suggestions about specific ways you can adapt that general plan to controlling your weight.

Motivation and Commitment

Make sure you are motivated and committed before you begin. Failure at weight loss is a frustrating experience that can make it more difficult to lose weight in the future. Think about why you want to lose weight. Make a list of your reasons for wanting to lose weight, and post it in a prominent place.

Setting Goals

Choose a reasonable weight you think you would like to reach over the long term, and be willing to renegotiate it as you get further along. Break down your long-term weight and behavioral goals into a series of short-term action-oriented goals.

Creating a Negative Energy Balance

When your weight is constant, you are burning approximately the same number of calories as you are taking in. To tip the energy balance toward weight loss, you must consume fewer calories, or burn more calories through physical activity, or both. To generate a negative energy balance, it's usually best to begin by increasing activity level rather than decreasing your calorie consumption.

Physical Activity

Consider how you can increase your energy output simply by increasing routine physical activity, such as walking or taking the stairs. If you are not already involved in a regular exercise routine aimed at increasing endurance and building or maintaining muscle mass, seek help from someone who is competent to help you plan and start an appropriate exercise routine. If you are already doing regular physical exercise, evaluate your program according to the guidelines in Chapter 10.

Diet and Eating Habits

If you can't generate a large enough negative energy balance solely by increasing physical activity, you may want to supplement exercise with modest cuts in your calorie intake. Your goal is to make small changes in your diet that you can maintain for a lifetime. Focus on cutting your intake of saturated and trans fats and added sugars and on eating a variety of nutritious foods in moderation. Don't skip meals, fast, or go on a very low-calorie diet or a diet that is unbalanced.

Self-Monitoring

Keep a record of your weight and behavior change progress. Try keeping a record of everything you eat. Write down what you plan to eat, in what quantity, *before* you eat. You'll find that just having to record something that is not OK to eat is likely to stop you from eating it. Also, keep track of your daily activities and your formal exercise program so you can monitor increases in physical activity.

Putting Your Plan into Action

- Examine the environmental cues that trigger poor eating and exercise habits, and devise strategies for dealing with them. Anticipate problem situations, and plan ways to handle them more effectively.

- Create new environmental cues that will support your new healthy behaviors. Move fruits and vegetables to the front of the refrigerator.

- Get others to help. Talk to friends and family members about what they can do to support your efforts. Find a buddy to join you in your exercise program.

- Give yourself lots of praise and rewards. Focus attention to your accomplishments and achievements and congratulate yourself. Plan special nonfood treats for yourself, such as a walk or a movie. Reward yourself often and for anything that counts toward success.

- If you slip, don't waste time on self-criticism. Think positively instead of getting into a cycle of guilt and self-blame.

- Don't get discouraged. Be aware that although weight loss is bound to slow down after the first loss of body fluid, the weight loss at this slower rate is more permanent than earlier, more dramatic, losses.

- Remember that weight management is a lifelong project. You need to adopt reasonable goals and strategies that you can maintain over the long term.

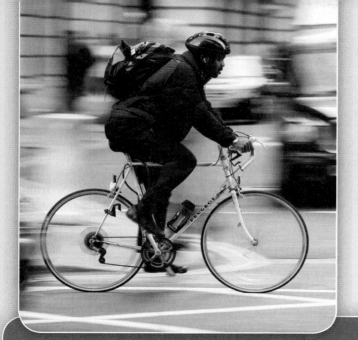

LOOKING AHEAD...

After reading this chapter, you should be able to

- List the major components of the cardiovascular system and describe how blood is pumped and circulated throughout the body

- Describe the controllable and uncontrollable risk factors associated with cardiovascular disease

- Discuss the major forms of cardiovascular disease and how they develop

- Explain what cancer is and how it spreads

- List and describe common cancers—their risk factors, signs and symptoms, and treatments, and approaches to prevention

- List the steps you can take to lower your personal risk of developing cardiovascular disease and cancer

Cardiovascular Disease and Cancer

12

Cardiovascular disease (CVD) affects more than 81 million Americans and is the leading cause of death in the United States, claiming one life every 38 seconds—nearly 2300 Americans every day. Heart attacks and strokes are the number-one and number-three causes of death, respectively, making them the most common life-threatening manifestations of CVD. Cancer is the second leading cause of death in the United States, claiming over 570,000 lives annually—more than 1500 each day.

Although genes, age, and environmental factors play roles in the development of these diseases, CVD and cancer are primarily lifestyle diseases, linked to many lifestyle factors. This chapter describes the features and causes of these diseases and provides information about how you can reduce your risk of developing them.

THE CARDIOVASCULAR SYSTEM

The **cardiovascular system** consists of the heart and blood vessels. Together they move blood throughout the body (see page T2-2 of the color transparency insert "Touring the Cardiorespiratory System"). When the lungs are included, the system is known as the *cardiorespiratory* or *cardiopulmonary system*.

The heart is a four-chambered, fist-sized muscle located just beneath the sternum (breastbone). It pumps deoxygenated (oxygen-poor) blood to the lungs and delivers oxygenated (oxygen-rich) blood to the rest of the body. Blood actually travels through two separate circulatory systems. The right side of the heart pumps blood to the lungs in what is called **pulmonary circulation,** and the left side pumps blood through the rest of the body in the **systemic circulation.** The path of blood flow through the heart and cardiorespiratory system is illustrated on page T2-3 of the color transparency insert "Touring the Cardiorespiratory System."

Oxygen-poor blood travels through large vessels, the **venae cavae,** into the heart's right upper chamber, the right **atrium.** After the right atrium fills, it contracts and pumps blood into the heart's right lower chamber, the right **ventricle.** When the right ventricle is full, it contracts and pumps blood through the pulmonary artery into the lungs. In the lungs, blood picks up oxygen and discards carbon dioxide. The oxygenated blood then flows from the lungs through the pulmonary veins into the heart's left atrium. After the left atrium fills, it contracts and pumps blood into the left ventricle. When the left ventricle is full, it pumps blood through the **aorta**—the body's largest artery—for distribution to the rest of the body's blood vessels. The period of the heart's contraction is called **systole;** the period of relaxation is called **diastole.** The heartbeat—the sequence of contractions of the heart's four chambers—is controlled by nerve impulses. These signals originate in a bundle of specialized cells in the right atrium called the *sinoatrial node* or *pacemaker.*

Blood vessels are classified by size and function. **Veins** carry blood to the heart. **Arteries** carry blood away from the heart. Veins have thin walls, but arteries have thick elastic walls that enable them to expand and relax with the volume of blood being pumped through them.

After leaving the heart, the aorta branches into smaller and smaller vessels. The smallest arteries branch still further into **capillaries**—tiny vessels with walls only one cell thick. The capillaries deliver oxygen- and nutrient-rich

blood to the tissues and pick up oxygen-poor, carbon dioxide–laden blood. From the capillaries, this blood empties into small veins (*venules*) and then into larger veins that return it to the heart to repeat the cycle.

Two large vessels, the right and left **coronary arteries,** branch off the aorta and supply the heart muscle with oxygenated blood. (The coronary arteries are shown on page T2-3 of the color transparency insert "Touring the Cardiorespiratory System.") Blockage of a coronary artery is the leading cause of heart attacks.

RISK FACTORS FOR CARDIOVASCULAR DISEASE

Researchers have identified a variety of factors associated with an increased risk of developing CVD. They are grouped into two categories: major risk factors and contributing risk factors. Some risk factors are linked to controllable aspects of lifestyle and can therefore be changed. Others are beyond our control.

Monitoring blood pressure is a key strategy for the prevention of CVD. Blood pressure can be measured during a health care visit or at home with a home blood pressure monitor.

TERMS

cardiovascular disease (CVD) The collective term for various diseases of the heart and blood vessels.

cardiovascular system The system that circulates blood through the body; consists of the heart and blood vessels.

pulmonary circulation The part of the circulatory system controlled by the right side of the heart: the circulation of blood between the heart and the lungs.

systemic circulation The part of the circulatory system controlled by the left side of the heart: the circulation of blood between the heart and the rest of the body.

vena cava Either of two large veins through which blood is returned to the right atrium of the heart (plural, *venae cavae*).

atrium Either of the two upper chambers of the heart in which blood collects before passing to the ventricles (plural, *atria*).

ventricle Either of the two lower chambers of the heart that pump blood to the lungs and other parts of the body.

aorta The large artery that receives blood from the left ventricle and distributes it to the body.

diastole The relaxation phase of the heart.

systole The contraction phase of the heart.

vein A vessel that carries blood to the heart.

artery A vessel that carries blood away from the heart.

capillary A small blood vessel that exchanges oxygen and nutrients between the blood and the tissues.

coronary artery One of the system of arteries branching from the aorta that provides blood to the heart muscle.

Major Risk Factors That Can Be Changed

The American Heart Association (AHA) has identified six major risk factors for CVD that can be changed: tobacco use, high blood pressure, unhealthy blood cholesterol levels, physical inactivity, overweight and obesity, and diabetes.

Tobacco Use   Nearly one in five deaths is attributable to smoking. People who smoke a pack of cigarettes a day have twice the risk of heart attack as nonsmokers; smoking two or more packs a day triples the risk. When smokers have heart attacks, they are two to three times more likely than nonsmokers to die from them. Cigarette smoking also doubles the risk of stroke.

Smoking harms the cardiovascular system in several ways. It damages the lining of arteries. It reduces the level of high-density lipoproteins (HDL), or "good" cholesterol and raises the levels of triglycerides and low-density lipoproteins (LDL), or "bad" cholesterol. Nicotine increases blood pressure and heart rate. The carbon monoxide in cigarette smoke displaces oxygen in the blood, reducing the amount of oxygen available to the body. Smoking causes **platelets** to stick together in the bloodstream, leading to clotting, and it speeds the development of fatty deposits in the arteries.

You don't have to smoke to be affected. The risk of developing heart disease increases up to 30% among those exposed to environmental tobacco smoke (ETS) at home or at work. Researchers estimate that about 46,000 nonsmokers die from heart disease each year as a result of exposure to ETS.

High Blood Pressure   High blood pressure, or **hypertension,** is a risk factor for many forms of cardiovascular disease, including heart attacks and strokes, and is itself the most prevalent form of CVD.

Blood pressure, the force exerted by the blood on the vessel walls, is created by the pumping action of the heart. High blood pressure occurs when too much force is exerted against the walls of the arteries. Many factors affect blood pressure, such as exercise or excitement. Short periods of high blood pressure are normal, but chronic high blood pressure is a health risk.

Health care professionals measure blood pressure with a stethoscope and an instrument called a *sphygmomanometer*. Blood pressure is expressed as two numbers—for example, 120 over 80—and measured in millimeters of mercury (mm Hg). The first number is the *systolic* blood pressure; the second is the *diastolic* blood pressure. A normal blood pressure reading for a healthy adult is below 120 systolic and below 80 diastolic, and CVD risk increases when blood pressure rises above that level. High blood pressure in adults is defined as equal to or greater than 140 over 90 (Table 12.1).

CAUSES   High blood pressure results from an increased output of blood by the heart or from increased resistance to

---

Table 12.1	Blood Pressure Classification for Healthy Adults		
CATEGORY[a]	SYSTOLIC (mm Hg)		DIASTOLIC (mm Hg)
Normal[b]	below 120	and	below 80
Prehypertension	120–139	or	80–89
Hypertension[c]			
Stage 1	140–159	or	90–99
Stage 2	160 and above	or	100 and above

[a]When systolic and diastolic pressure fall into different categories, the higher category should be used to classify blood pressure status.

[b]The risk of death from heart attack and stroke begins to rise when blood pressure is above 115/75.

[c]Based on the average of two or more readings taken at different physician visits. In people older than 50, systolic blood pressure greater than 140 is a much more significant CVD risk factor than diastolic blood pressure.

SOURCE: *The Seventh Report of the Joint National Committee on Prevention, Detection, Evaluation, and Treatment of High Blood Pressure.* 2003. Bethesda, MD: National Heart, Lung, and Blood Institute. National Institutes of Health (NIH Publication No. 03-5233).

---

blood flow in the arteries. The latter condition can be caused by constriction of smooth muscle surrounding the arteries or by **atherosclerosis,** a disease process that causes arteries to become clogged and narrowed. Atherosclerosis also scars and hardens arteries, making them less elastic and further increasing blood pressure. When a person has high blood pressure, the heart must work harder than normal to force blood through the narrowed and stiffened arteries, straining both the heart and the arteries.

High blood pressure is often called a silent killer because it usually has no symptoms. A person may have high blood pressure for years without realizing it. But during that time, it damages vital organs and increases the risk of heart attack, congestive heart failure, stroke, kidney failure, and blindness.

Recent research has shed new light on the importance of lowering blood pressure to improve cardiovascular health. The risk of death from heart attack or stroke begin to rise when blood pressure is above 115 over 75, well below the traditional 140 over 90 cutoff for a diagnosis of hypertension. People with blood pressure in the

---

QUICK STATS

33% of Americans have high blood pressure; **20%** of them aren't aware of their condition.

—CDC, 2010

TERMS

platelets   Cells in the blood that are necessary for the formation of blood clots.

hypertension   Sustained abnormally high blood pressure.

atherosclerosis   A form of CVD in which the inner layers of artery walls are made thick and irregular by plaque deposits; arteries become narrow, and blood supply is reduced.

prehypertension range are at increased risk of heart attack and stroke as well as at significant risk of developing full-blown hypertension.

PREVALENCE Hypertension is common. About 30% of adults have hypertension, and 37% have prehypertension (defined as systolic pressure of 120–139 and/or diastolic pressure of 80–89). The incidence of high blood pressure increases with age, but it can occur among children and young adults, and women sometimes develop hypertension during pregnancy (blood pressure usually returns to normal following pregnancy). The rate of hypertension is highest in African Americans (41%). Among African Americans, compared with other groups, the disorder is often more severe, more resistant to treatment, and more likely to be fatal at an early age.

TREATMENT Hypertension cannot be cured, but it can be controlled. Because hypertension has no early warning signs, it's crucial to have your blood pressure tested at least once every two years (more often if you have other CVD risk factors). In fact, experts now advise that anyone with hypertension or prehypertension monitor their own blood pressure several times each week.

Lifestyle changes are recommended for everyone with prehypertension and hypertension. These changes include weight reduction, regular exercise, a healthy diet, and moderation of alcohol use. The DASH diet is recommended specifically for people with high blood pressure.

Sodium restriction is also helpful for most people with hypertension. The 2010 Dietary Guidelines for Americans recommend restricting sodium consumption to less than 2,300 mg per day and to less than 1500 mg per day for people with hypertension, African Americans, and middle-aged and older adults. For people whose blood pressure isn't adequately controlled with lifestyle changes, medication is prescribed.

High Cholesterol   *Cholesterol* is a fatty, waxlike substance that circulates through the bloodstream. It is an important component of cell membranes, sex hormones, vitamin D, the fluid that coats the lungs, and the protective sheaths around nerves. Adequate cholesterol is essential for the proper functioning of the body. Excess cholesterol, however, can clog arteries and increase the risk of CVD. There are two sources of cholesterol: your liver manufactures it, and you get it from the foods you eat.

GOOD VERSUS BAD CHOLESTEROL Cholesterol is carried in the blood in protein-and-lipid packages called **lipoproteins. Low-density lipoproteins (LDLs)** shuttle cholesterol from the liver to the organs and tissues that require it. LDL is known as "bad" cholesterol because if there is more than the body can use, the excess is deposited in the blood vessels. If coronary arteries are blocked, the result may be a heart attack; if an artery carrying blood to the brain is blocked, a stroke may occur. **High-density lipoproteins (HDLs),** or

Table 12.2	Cholesterol Guidelines
TOTAL CHOLESTEROL (mg/dl)	
Less than 200	Desirable
200–239	Borderline high
240 or more	High
LDL CHOLESTEROL (mg/dl)	
Less than 100	Optimal
100–129	Near optimal/above optimal
130–159	Borderline high
160–189	High
190 or more	Very high
HDL CHOLESTEROL (mg/dl)	
Less than 40	Low (undesirable)
60 or more	High (desirable)
TRIGLYCERIDES (mg/dl)	
Less than 150	Normal
150–199	Borderline high
200–499	High
500 or more	Very high

SOURCE: Expert Panel on Detection, Evaluation, and Treatment of High Blood Cholesterol in Adults. 2001. Executive Summary of the Third Report of the National Cholesterol Education Program (NCEP) Expert Panel on Detection, Evaluation, and Treatment of High Blood Cholesterol in Adults (Adult Treatment Panel III). *Journal of the American Medical Association* 285(19).

"good" cholesterol, shuttle unused cholesterol back to the liver for recycling. By removing cholesterol from blood vessels, HDL helps protect against atherosclerosis.

RECOMMENDED BLOOD CHOLESTEROL LEVELS The risk for cardiovascular disease increases with higher blood cholesterol levels, especially LDL (Table 12.2). The National Cholesterol Education Program (NCEP) recommends lipoprotein testing at least once every five years for all adults, beginning at age 20. The recommended test measures total cholesterol, LDL cholesterol, HDL cholesterol, and triglycerides (another blood fat). In general, high LDL, total cholesterol, and triglyceride levels, combined with low HDL levels, are associated with a higher risk for CVD. You can reduce this risk by lowering LDL, total cholesterol, and triglycerides. Raising HDL is important because a high HDL level seems to offer protection

TERMS

lipoproteins   Protein-and-lipid substances in the blood that carry fats and cholesterol; classified according to size, density, and chemical composition.

low-density lipoprotein (LDL)   A lipoprotein containing a moderate amount of protein and a large amount of cholesterol, which tends to become deposited on artery walls and increase the risk of heart disease; "bad" cholesterol.

high-density lipoprotein (HDL)   A lipoprotein containing relatively little cholesterol that helps transport cholesterol out of the arteries and thus protects against heart diseases; "good" cholesterol.

from CVD even in cases where total cholesterol is high. This appears to be especially true for women.

As shown in Table 12.2, LDL levels below 100 mg/dl (milligrams per deciliter) and total cholesterol levels below 200 mg/dl are desirable. An estimated 102 million American adults have total cholesterol levels of 200 mg/dl or higher. Research now shows that levels of cholestrol as low as 60 mg/dl have even better outcomes. The CVD risk associated with elevated cholesterol levels also depends on how many other risk factors a person has.

BENEFITS OF CONTROLLING CHOLESTEROL People can cut their heart attack risk by about 2% for every 1% that they reduce their total blood cholesterol levels. People who lower their total cholesterol from 250 to 200 mg/dl, for example, reduce their risk of heart attack by 40%. Your primary goal should be to reduce your LDL to healthy levels.

Important dietary changes for reducing LDL levels include increasing fiber intake and substituting unsaturated for saturated and trans fats. Exercising regularly and eating more fruits, vegetables, fish, and whole grains also help. In recent years, a group of medications called statins have been shown to reduce total cholestrol levels and LDL.

Physical Inactivity An estimated 40–60 million Americans are so sedentary that they are at high risk for developing CVD. Exercise is thought to be the closest thing we have to a magic bullet against heart disease. It lowers CVD risk by helping to decrease blood pressure and resting heart rate, increase HDL levels, maintain desirable weight, improve the condition of blood vessels, and prevent or control diabetes. One study found that women who accumulated at least three hours of brisk walking each week cut their risk of heart attack and stroke by more than 50%.

Obesity Death from CVD is two to three times more likely in obese people (BMI ≥ 30) than it is in lean people (BMI 18.5–24.9), and for every 5-unit increase in BMI, a person's risk of death from coronary heart disease increases by 30%.

Excess body fat is strongly associated with hypertension, high cholesterol levels, insulin resistance, diabetes, physical inactivity, and increasing age. With excess weight, there is also more blood to pump and the heart has to work harder. This causes chronically elevated pressures within the heart chambers that can lead to ventricular **hypertrophy** (enlargement). Eventually the heart muscle can start to fail.

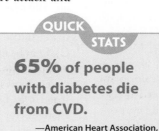

Exercise is thought to be **the closest thing we have to a magic bullet** against heart disease.

QUICK STATS

65% of people with diabetes die from CVD.
—American Heart Association, 2012

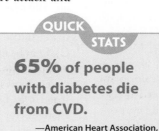

Overweight and obesity are major risk factors for cardiovascular disease, but physical activity, including walking, can lower that risk. Modest weight loss can also reduce CVD risk.

Physical activity and fitness have a strong positive influence on cardiovascular health in those who are overweight and obese. People who are obese but have at least moderate cardiorespiratory fitness may have lower rates of cardiovascular disease than their normal-weight but unfit peers. For someone who is overweight, even modest weight reduction—5–10% of body weight—can reduce CVD risk.

Diabetes As described in Chapter 11, *diabetes* is a disorder characterized by elevated blood glucose levels due to an insufficient supply or inadequate action of insulin. (See page T2-5 of the color transparency insert "Touring the Cardiorespiratory System" in this chapter.) Diabetes doubles the risk of CVD for men and triples the risk for women. The most common cause of death in adults with diabetes is CVD.

People with diabetes have higher rates of other CVD risk factors, including hypertension, obesity, and unhealthy blood lipid levels (typically, high triglyceride levels and low HDL levels). The elevated blood glucose and insulin levels that occur in diabetes can damage the endothelial cells that line the arteries, making them more vulnerable to atherosclerosis. People with prediabetes also face a significantly increased risk of CVD.

In people with prediabetes, a healthy diet and exercise are more effective than medication at preventing diabetes. For people with diabetes, a healthy diet, exercise, and careful control of glucose levels are recommended to reduce the chances of developing complications. Even people whose diabetes is under control face a high risk of CVD, so control of other risk factors is critical.

| **hypertrophy** | Abnormal enlargement of an organ. | **TERMS** |

Contributing Risk Factors That Can Be Changed

Other CVD risk factors that can be changed include triglyceride levels and psychological and social factors, among others.

High Triglyceride Levels   Like cholesterol, **triglycerides** are blood fats that are obtained from food and manufactured by the body. High triglyceride levels are a reliable predictor of heart disease, especially if associated with other risk factors. Factors contributing to elevated triglyceride levels include excess body fat, physical inactivity, cigarette smoking, type 2 diabetes, excessive alcohol intake, very high-carbohydrate diets, and certain diseases and medications.

A full lipid profile should include testing and evaluation of triglyceride levels (see Table 12.2). For people with borderline high triglyceride levels, increased physical activity, reduced intake of added sugars, and weight reduction can help bring levels down into the healthy range. For people with high triglyceride levels, drug therapy may be recommended. Being moderate in the use of alcohol and quitting smoking are also important.

Insulin Resistance and Metabolic Syndrome   As people gain weight and become less active, their muscles, fat, and liver become less sensitive to t1he effect of insulin—a condition known as *insulin resistance* (or prediabetes). As the body becomes increasingly insulin resistant, the pancreas must secrete more and more insulin (hyperinsulinemia) to keep glucose levels within a normal range. Eventually even high levels of insulin may become insufficient, and blood glucose levels start to rise (hyperglycemia), resulting in type 2 diabetes.

Those who have insulin resistance tend to have several other related risk factors. This cluster of abnormalities is called *metabolic syndrome* or *insulin resistance syndrome* (Table 12.3). Metabolic syndrome significantly increases the risk of CVD. It is estimated that about 34% of the adult U.S. population have metabolic syndrome.

To reduce your risk of metabolic syndrome, choose a healthy diet and get plenty of exercise. Reducing calorie intake to prevent weight gain or losing weight if needed also reduces insulin resistance. Eating more unsaturated fats, protein, vegetables, and fiber while limiting simple carbohydrates and added sugars may be beneficial.

Psychological and Social Factors   Many of the psychological and social factors that influence other areas of wellness are also important risk factors for CVD.

STRESS   Excessive stress can strain the heart and blood vessels over time and contribute to CVD. If you are healthy, you can tolerate the cardiovascular responses that take place during stress; but if you already have CVD, stress can lead to adverse outcomes such as abnormal heart rhythms (arrhythmias) and heart attacks.

CHRONIC HOSTILITY AND ANGER   Certain traits in the hard-driving Type A personality—hostility, cynicism, and anger—are associated with increased risk of heart disease. See the box "Anger, Hostility, and Heart Disease" for more information.

SUPPRESSING PSYCHOLOGICAL DISTRESS   Consistently suppressing anger and other negative emotions may also be hazardous to a healthy heart. People who hide psychological distress appear to have higher rates of heart disease than people who experience similar distress but share it with others.

DEPRESSION   Depression appears to increase the risk of CVD in healthy people and the risk of adverse cardiac events in those who already have heart disease. The relationship between depression and CHD is complex and not fully understood. One factor may be that depression causes physiological changes; for example, it elevates basal levels of stress hormones, which induce a variety of stress-related responses.

ANXIETY   Chronic anxiety and anxiety disorders (such as phobias and panic disorder) are associated with up to a threefold increased risk of coronary heart disease, heart attack, and sudden cardiac death. People with anxiety are more likely to have a subsequent adverse cardiac event after having a heart attack.

SOCIAL ISOLATION   Social isolation and low social support (living alone, or having few friends or family members) are associated with an increased incidence of CHD and poorer outcomes after the first diagnosis of CHD. A strong social support network is a major antidote to stress. Friends and family members can also promote and support a healthy lifestyle.

Table 12.3	Defining Characteristics of Metabolic Syndrome*	
Abdominal obesity (waist circumference)		
Men	>40 in (>102 cm)	
Women	>35 in (>88 cm)	
Triglycerides	≥150 mg/dl	
HDL cholesterol		
Men	<40 mg/dl or drug-treated	
Women	<50 mg/dl or drug-treated	
Blood pressure	≥130/≥85 mmHg or drug-treated	
Fasting glucose	≥100 mg/dl or drug-treated	

*A person is diagnosed with metabolic syndrome if she or he has three or more of the risk factors listed here.

SOURCE: Adapted with permission of the American Heart Association from Table 2. Grundy, S. M., et al. 2005. Diagnosis and management of the metabolic syndrome: An American Heart Association/National Heart, Lung, and Blood Institute Scientific Statement. *Circulation* 112: 2735.

triglyceride   A type of blood fat that can be a predictor of heart disease.

TERMS

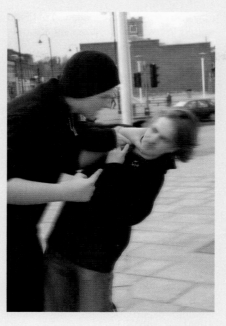

People with a quick temper, a persistently hostile outlook, and a cynical, mistrusting attitude toward life are more likely to develop heart disease than those with a calmer, more trusting attitude. People who are angry frequently and for long periods experience the stress response much more often than more relaxed individuals. Over the long term, the effects of stress may damage arteries and promote CVD.

Are You Too Hostile?

To help answer that question, Duke University researcher Redford Williams, M.D., has devised a short self-test. It's not a scientific evaluation, but it offers a rough measure of hostility. Are the following statements true or false for you?

1. I often get annoyed at checkout cashiers or the people in front of me when I'm waiting in line.
2. I usually keep an eye on the people I work or live with to make sure they do what they should.
3. I often wonder how homeless people can have so little respect for themselves.
4. I believe that most people will take advantage of you if you let them.
5. The habits of friends or family members often annoy me.
6. When I'm stuck in traffic, I often start breathing faster and my heart pounds.
7. When I'm annoyed with people, I really want to let them know it.
8. If someone does me wrong, I want to get even.
9. I'd like to have the last word in any argument.
10. At least once a week, I have the urge to yell at or even hit someone.

According to Williams, five or more "true" statements suggest that you're excessively hostile and should consider taking steps to mellow out.

Managing Your Anger

Begin by monitoring your angry responses and looking for triggers—people or situations that typically make you angry. Familiarize yourself with the patterns of thinking that lead to angry or hostile feelings, and then try to head them off before they develop into full-blown anger. If you feel your anger starting to build, try reasoning with yourself by asking the following questions:

1. *Is this really important enough to get angry about?*
2. *Am I really justified in getting angry?*
3. *Is getting angry going to make a real and positive difference in this situation?*

If you answer yes to all three questions, then calm but assertive communication may be an appropriate response. If your anger isn't reasonable, try distracting yourself or removing yourself from the situation. Exercise, humor, social support, and other stress management techniques can also help. Your heart—and the people around you—will benefit from your calmer, more positive outlook.

SOURCE: From Virginia Williams and Redford Williams, 1999, *Lifeskills: 8 Simple Ways to Build Stronger Relationships, Communicate More Clearly, and Improve Your Health,* New York: Times Books. Reprinted by permission.

LOW SOCIOECONOMIC STATUS Low socioeconomic status and low educational attainment are also associated with an increased risk of CVD. These associations are probably due to a variety of factors, including lifestyle and access to health care.

Alcohol and Drugs Although moderate drinking may have health benefits for some people, drinking too much alcohol raises blood pressure and can increase the risk of stroke and heart failure. Stimulant drugs, particularly cocaine and methamphetamines, can also cause serious cardiac problems, including heart attack, stroke, and sudden cardiac death. Injection drug use can cause heart infections and stroke.

Major Risk Factors That Can't Be Changed

A number of major risk factors for CVD cannot be changed. These include family history of CVD (heredity), aging, gender, and ethnicity.

Heredity Multiple genes contribute to the development of CVD and its associated risk factors, such as high cholesterol, hypertension, diabetes, and obesity. Having a favorable set of genes decreases your risk of developing CVD; having an unfavorable set of genes increases your risk. Risk, however, may be modified by lifestyle factors.

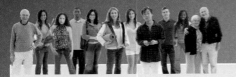

DIVERSITY MATTERS
Ethnicity and CVD

African Americans are at substantially higher risk of death from CVD than other groups. The rate of hypertension among African Americans is among the highest of any group in the world. Blacks tend to develop hypertension at an earlier age than whites, and their average blood pressures are much higher. African Americans have a higher risk of stroke, have strokes at younger ages, and if they survive, have more significant stroke-related disabilities. Some experts recommend that blacks be treated with antihypertensive drugs when blood pressure reaches 130/80 rather than the typical 140/90 cutoff for hypertension.

A number of genetic and biological factors may contribute to CVD in African Americans. They may be more sensitive to dietary sodium, leading to greater blood pressure elevation in response to a given amount of sodium. African Americans

may also experience less dilation of blood vessels in response to stress, an attribute that also raises blood pressure.

Heredity also plays a large role in the tendency to develop diabetes, another important CVD risk factor that is more common in blacks than whites. However, Latinos are even more likely to develop diabetes and insulin resistance, and at a younger age, than African Americans. There is variation within the Latino population, however: a higher prevalence of diabetes occurs among Mexican Americans and Puerto Ricans and a relatively lower prevalence among Cuban Americans.

Another factor that likely contributes to the high incidence of CVD among ethnic minority groups is low income, which usually means reduced access to health care. Also associated with low income is low educational attainment, which often means less information about preventive health measures, such as diet and stress management. People with low incomes tend to

smoke more, use more salt, and exercise less than those with higher incomes.

Discrimination may also play a role in CVD. Physicians and hospitals may treat the medical problems of ethnic minorities differently than those of whites. Discrimination, low income, and other forms of deprivation may also increase stress, which is linked with hypertension and CVD. Lack of access to care, such as insurance coverage and availability of high-tech cardiac equipment in hospitals that serve minorities, may also play a role.

All Americans are advised to have their blood pressure checked regularly, exercise, eat a healthy diet, manage stress, and avoid smoking. These general preventive strategies may be particularly helpful for ethnic minorities. Tailoring your lifestyle to your particular ethnic risk may also be helpful in some cases. Discuss your particular risk profile with your physician to help identify the lifestyle changes most appropriate for you.

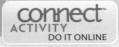
connect
ACTIVITY
DO IT ONLINE

Aging About 70% of all heart attack victims are age 65 or older, and about 75% who suffer fatal heart attacks are over 65. For people over 55, the incidence of stroke more than doubles in each successive decade. However, even people in their thirties and forties, especially men, can have heart attacks.

Gender Although CVD is the leading killer of both men and women in the United States, men face a greater risk of heart attack than women, especially earlier in life. Until age 55, men also have a greater risk of hypertension. The incidence of stroke is higher for males than females until age 65. By age 75 this gender gap nearly disappears. Women who have heart attacks are more likely than men to die within a year.

Ethnicity Rates of heart disease vary among ethnic groups in the United States, with African Americans having much higher rates of hypertension, heart disease, and stroke than other groups (see the box "Ethnicity and CVD"). Puerto Rican Americans, Cuban Americans, and Mexican Americans are also more likely to suffer from high blood pressure and angina (a warning sign of blocked coronary arteries) than non-Hispanic white Americans. Asian Americans historically have had far lower rates of CVD than white Americans.

> In general, men face **a greater risk of heart attack, hypertension, and stroke** than women.

Inflammation and C-Reactive Protein Inflammation plays a key role in the development of CVD. When an artery is injured by smoking, cholesterol, hypertension, or other factors, the body's response is to produce inflammation. A substance called *C-reactive protein (CRP)* is released into the bloodstream during the inflammatory response, and high levels of CRP indicate a substantially elevated risk of heart attack and stroke. CRP may also harm the coronary arteries themselves. Lifestyle changes and certain drugs can reduce CRP levels.

Ask Yourself

QUESTIONS FOR CRITICAL THINKING AND REFLECTION

What risk factors do you have for cardiovascular disease? Which ones are factors you have control over, and which are factors you can't change? If you have risk factors you cannot change (such as a family history of CVD), were you aware that you can make lifestyle adjustments to reduce your risk? Do you think you will make them?

Possible Risk Factors Currently Being Studied

In recent years other possible risk factors for cardiovascular disease have been identified. For example elevated levels of homocysteine, an amino acid circulating in the blood, are associated with an increased risk of CVD. Homocysteine appears to damage the lining of blood vessels, resulting in inflammation and the development of fatty deposits in artery walls. These changes can lead to the formation of clots and blockages in arteries, which in turn can cause heart attacks and strokes.

Several infectious agents have been identified as possible culprits in the development of CVD. *Chlamydia pneumoniae*, a common cause of flulike respiratory infections, has been found in sections of clogged, damaged arteries but not in sections of healthy arteries. This effect may be secondary to the inflammation that many of these infectious agents produce in the body.

Other factors currently under investigation include a particular type of LDL called lipoprotein(a), blood levels of iron, and blood levels of uric acid.

MAJOR FORMS OF CARDIOVASCULAR DISEASE

According to the CDC, heart diseases killed nearly 616,000 Americans in 2008. Figure 12.1 shows the death rates among various ethnic groups due to heart disease in 2008, the most recent year for which data are available.

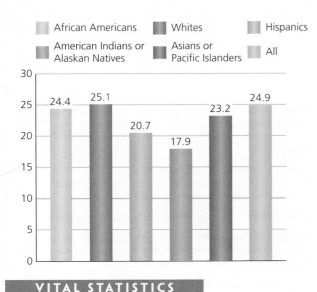

VITAL STATISTICS

FIGURE 12.1   Percentage of deaths due to heart disease, by ethnic group.

SOURCE: Miniño, A. M., et al. 2011. Deaths: final data for 2008. *National Vital Statistics Reports* 59(10). Hyattsville, MD: National Center for Health Statistics.

The main forms of CVD are atherosclerosis, coronary artery disease and heart attack, stroke, peripheral arterial disease (PAD), congestive heart failure, congenital heart disease, rheumatic heart disease, and heart valve problems. Many forms are interrelated and have elements in common; we treat them separately here for the sake of clarity. Hypertension, which is both a major risk factor and a form of CVD, was described earlier in the chapter.

Atherosclerosis

Atherosclerosis is a form of arteriosclerosis, or thickening and hardening of the arteries. In atherosclerosis, arteries become narrowed by deposits of fat, cholesterol, and other substances (see page T2-4 of the color transparency insert "Touring the Cardiorespiratory System"). The process begins when the endothelial cells (cells that line the arteries) become damaged, most likely through a combination of factors such as smoking, high blood pressure, high insulin or glucose levels, and deposits of oxidized LDL particles. The body's response to this damage results in inflammation and changes in the artery lining that create a magnet for LDL, platelets, and other cells. These cells build up and cause a bulge in the wall of the artery. As these deposits, called **plaques,** accumulate in artery walls, the arteries lose their elasticity and their ability to expand and contract, restricting blood flow. Once narrowed by a plaque, an artery is vulnerable to blockage by blood clots.

If the heart, brain, or other organs are deprived of blood and the oxygen it carries, the effects of atherosclerosis can be deadly. Coronary arteries, which supply the heart with blood, are particularly susceptible to plaque buildup, a condition called **coronary heart disease** (**CHD**) or *coronary artery disease (CAD)*. The blockage of a coronary artery causes a heart attack, and blockage of a cerebral artery (leading to the brain) causes a stroke. Blockage of an artery in a limb causes *peripheral arterial disease*, a condition that causes pain and sometimes amputation of the affected limb.

The main risk factors for atherosclerosis are cigarette smoking, physical inactivity, high blood cholesterol levels, high blood pressure, and diabetes. Atherosclerosis often begins in childhood: autopsy studies of young trauma victims have revealed atherosclerosis of the coronary arteries in adolescents.

Coronary Artery Disease and Heart Attack

The most common form of heart disease is coronary artery disease caused by atherosclerosis. When one of the coronary

> **plaque**   A deposit of fatty (and other) substances on the inner wall of an artery.
>
> **coronary heart disease (CHD)**   Heart disease caused by atherosclerosis in the arteries that supply blood to the heart muscle; also called *coronary artery disease*.
>
> TERMS

arteries becomes blocked, the result is a **heart attack,** or *myocardial infarction (MI)*. Although a heart attack may come without warning, it usually results from a chronic disease process.

Heart attack symptoms may include chest pain or pressure; arm, neck, or jaw pain; difficulty breathing; excessive sweating; nausea and vomiting; and loss of consciousness. Most people having a heart attack suffer chest pain, but about one-third of heart attack victims do not. Women, ethnic minorities, older adults, and people with diabetes are the most likely groups to experience heart attacks without chest pain.

Angina Arteries narrowed by disease may still be open enough to deliver blood to the heart. At times, however—during stress or exertion, for example—the heart needs more oxygen than can flow through narrowed arteries. When the need for oxygen exceeds the supply, chest pain, called **angina pectoris,** may occur. Angina pain is usually felt as an extreme tightness in the chest and heavy pressure behind the breastbone or in the shoulder, neck, arm, hand, or back. Angina may be controlled in a number of ways (with drugs and surgical or nonsurgical procedures), but its course is unpredictable. Over a period ranging from hours to years, the narrowing may go on to full blockage and a heart attack.

Arrhythmias and Sudden Cardiac Death The pumping of the heart is controlled by electrical impulses from the sinus node, located in the right atrium that maintain a regular heartbeat of 60–100 beats per minute. If this electrical conduction system is disrupted, the heart may beat too quickly, too slowly, or in an irregular fashion—a condition known as an **arrhythmia.** Arrhythmias can cause symptoms ranging from imperceptible to severe and even fatal.

Sudden cardiac death, also called *cardiac arrest,* is most often caused by an arrhythmia called *ventricular fibrillation,* a kind of quivering of the ventricle that makes it ineffective in pumping blood. If ventricular fibrillation continues for more than a few minutes, it is generally fatal. Cardiac defibrillation, in which an electrical shock is delivered to the heart, can be effective in jolting the heart into a more efficient rhythm. Emergency personnel typically carry defibrillators, and automated external defibrillators (AEDs) are becoming increasingly available in public places for use by the general public. Training in the use of AEDs is available from organizations such as the American Red Cross and the American Heart Association.

Helping a Heart Attack Victim Most deaths from heart attacks occur within two hours of the first symptoms. If you or someone you are with has any of the warning signs of heart attack listed in the box "What to Do in Case of a Heart Attack, Stroke, or Cardiac Arrest," take immediate action. Many experts also suggest that the heart attack victim chew and swallow one adult aspirin tablet (325 mg) as soon as possible after symptoms begin. Aspirin has an immediate anticlotting effect.

If the victim loses consciousness, a qualified person should immediately start administering emergency **cardiopulmonary resuscitation (CPR).** Damage to the heart muscle increases with time. If the person receives emergency care quickly enough, a clot-dissolving agent or emergency surgical procedure can be used to break up the clot in the coronary artery.

Detecting and Treating Heart Disease Currently the most common initial screening tool for CAD is the stress, or exercise, test. During an exercise stress test, a patient runs or walks on a treadmill or pedals a stationary cycle while being monitored for abnormalities with an **electrocardiogram (ECG or EKG).** Certain characteristic changes in the heart's electrical activity while under stress can reveal particular

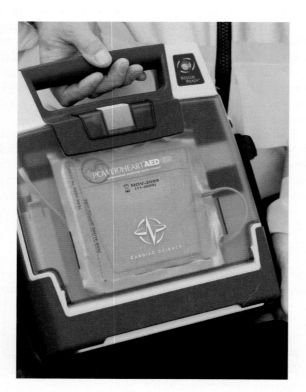

Automated external defibrillators can save the lives of individuals experiencing sudden cardiac arrest. AEDs are becoming more common in public places.

What to Do in Case of a Heart Attack, Stroke, or Cardiac Arrest

Warning Signs of Heart Attack

Some heart attacks are sudden and intense—the "movie heart attack," where no one doubts what's happening. But most heart attacks start slowly with mild pain or discomfort. Often people affected aren't sure what's wrong and wait too long before getting help. Here are signs that can mean a heart attack is happening:

- **Chest discomfort.** Heart attacks often involve discomfort in the chest that lasts more than a few minutes, or that goes away and comes back. It can feel like uncomfortable pressure, squeezing, fullness, or pain.

- **Discomfort in other areas of the upper body.** Symptoms can include pain or discomfort in one or both arms, the back, neck, jaw, or stomach.

- **Shortness of breath.** May occur with or without chest discomfort.

- **Other signs:** These may include breaking out in a cold sweat, nausea, vomiting, or lightheadedness.

Not all the signs occur in every heart attack. As with men, women's most common heart attack symptom is chest pain or discomfort, but women are somewhat more likely than men to experience some of the other symptoms, particularly shortness of beath, nausea/vomiting, and back or jaw pain.

If you or someone you're with has chest discomfort, especially with one or more of the other signs, don't wait longer than a few minutes (no more than five) before calling for help.

Calling 911 is almost always the fastest way to get lifesaving treatment. Emergency medical services staff can begin treatment when they arrive—up to an hour sooner than if someone gets to the hospital by car. The staff are also trained to revive someone whose heart has stopped. Patients with chest pain who arrive by ambulance usually receive faster treatment at the hospital, too. Today medications and treatments are available that weren't available in the past, but they must be given relatively quickly after the heart attack to be effective.

If you can't access emergency medical services (EMS), have someone drive you to the hospital right away. If you're the one having symptoms, don't drive yourself unless you have absolutely no other option.

Warning Signs of Stroke

- Sudden numbness or weakness of the face, arm, or leg, especially on one side of the body.

- Sudden confusion or trouble speaking or understanding.

- Sudden trouble seeing in one or both eyes.

- Sudden trouble walking, dizziness, or loss of balance or coordination.

- Sudden severe headache with no known cause.

If you or someone with you has one or more of these signs, call 911 immediately. If given within three hours of the start of symptoms, a clot-busting drug called tissue plasminogen activator (tPA) can reduce long-term disability for the most common type of stroke. tPA is the only FDA-approved medication for the treatment of stroke within three hours of symptom onset.

Signs of Cardiac Arrest

Cardiac arrest strikes immediately and without warning. Here are the signs:

- Sudden loss of responsiveness.

- No response to tapping on the shoulders.

- No normal breathing. The victim does not take a normal breath when you tilt the head up and check for at least five seconds.

If these signs of cardiac arrest are present, tell someone to call 911 and to get an automated external defibrillator (AED) if one is available before you begin CPR. Use the AED as soon as it arrives.

SOURCE: Adapted from American Heart Association, 2005, *Heart Attack, Stroke, and Cardiac Arrest Warning Signs.* (http://www.heart.org/HEARTORG /General/Heart-Attack-Stroke-and-Cardiac-Arrest-Signs_UCM-303977 _SubHomePage.jsp). Copyright © 2007, American Heart Association.

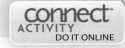

connect ACTIVITY DO IT ONLINE

heart problems, such as restricted blood flow. Exercise testing can also be performed in conjunction with imaging techniques that provide pictures of the heart, which can help pinpoint abnormal areas of the heart. Imaging techniques include echocardiography, **magnetic resonance imaging (MRI)**, and positron emission tomography (PET), among others.

If symptoms or imaging tests suggest coronary artery disease, the next step is usually a coronary **angiogram**, a test that can identify arterial narrowing or blockages. If a problem is found, it is usually treated with a **balloon angioplasty**, a

TERMS

magnetic resonance imaging (MRI) A computerized imaging technique that uses a strong magnetic field to create detailed pictures of body structures.

angiogram A picture of the arterial system taken after injecting a dye that is opaque to X-rays.

balloon angioplasty A technique in which a catheter with a deflated balloon on the tip is inserted into an artery; the balloon is then inflated at the point of obstruction in the artery, pressing the plaque against the artery wall to improve blood supply.

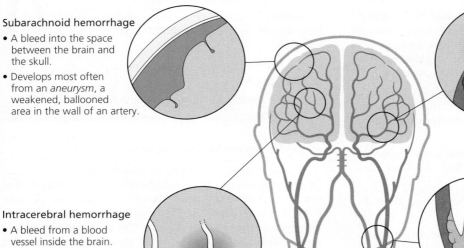

HEMORRHAGIC STROKE

- 13% of strokes.
- Caused by ruptured blood vessels followed by blood leaking into tissue.
- Usually more serious than ischemic stroke.

Subarachnoid hemorrhage

- A bleed into the space between the brain and the skull.
- Develops most often from an *aneurysm*, a weakened, ballooned area in the wall of an artery.

Intracerebral hemorrhage

- A bleed from a blood vessel inside the brain.
- Often caused by high blood pressure and the damage it does to arteries.

ISCHEMIC STROKE

- 87% of strokes.
- Caused by blockages in brain blood vessels; potentially treatable with clot-busting drugs.
- Brain tissue dies when blood flow is blocked.

Embolic stroke

- Caused by *emboli*, blood clots that travel from elsewhere in the body to the brain blood vessels.
- 25% of embolic strokes are related to atrial fibrillation.

Thrombotic stroke

- Caused by *thrombi*, blood clots that form where an artery has been narrowed by atherosclerosis.
- Most often develops when part of a thrombus breaks away and causes a blockage in a downstream artery.

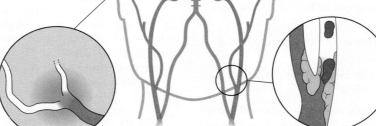

FIGURE 12.2 Types of stroke.

SOURCE: Excerpted from *Harvard Health Letter,* April 2000. © 2000 Harvard University. Reprinted with permission. For more information visit health.harvard.edu.

procedure that opens the blocked artery. In more serious cases, surgeons may perform **coronary bypass surgery,** in which a healthy blood vessel, usually a vein from the patient's leg, is grafted from the aorta to one or more coronary arteries to bypass a blockage.

Other treatments, ranging from medication to major surgery, are also available. Along with a low-fat diet, regular exercise, and smoking cessation, one frequent recommendation is to take a low-dose aspirin tablet every day. Aspirin helps prevent platelets in the blood from sticking to arterial plaques and forming clots, and it also reduces inflammation. Prescription drugs can help control heart rate, dilate arteries, lower blood pressure, and reduce the strain on the heart. In patients with coronary artery disease, cholesterol-lowering statins are effective in preventing heart attacks; statins also have beneficial anti-inflammatory effects.

Stroke

A **stroke,** also called a *cerebrovascular accident (CVA),* occurs when the blood supply to the brain is cut off.

Types of Strokes There are two major types of strokes (Figure 12.2).

ISCHEMIC STROKE An **ischemic stroke** is caused by a blockage in a blood vessel. There are two types of ischemic strokes.

A *thrombotic stroke* is caused by a **thrombus,** a blood clot that forms in a cerebral or carotid artery that has been narrowed or damaged by atherosclerosis. An *embolic stroke* is caused by an **embolus,** which is a wandering blood clot that is carried in the bloodstream and may become wedged in a cerebral artery. Ischemic strokes account for 87% of all strokes.

HEMORRHAGIC STROKE A **hemorrhagic stroke** occurs when a blood vessel in the brain bursts, spilling blood into the

---

TERMS

coronary bypass surgery Surgery in which a blood vessel is grafted from the aorta to a point below an obstruction in a coronary artery, improving the blood supply to the heart.

stroke Impeded blood supply to some part of the brain resulting in the destruction of brain cells; also called a *cerebrovascular accident.*

ischemic stroke Impeded blood supply to the brain caused by the obstruction of a blood vessel by a clot.

thrombus A blood clot in a blood vessel that usually remains at the point of its formation.

embolus A blood clot that breaks off from its place of origin in a blood vessel and travels through the bloodstream.

hemorrhagic stroke Impeded blood supply to the brain caused by the rupture of a blood vessel.

surrounding tissue. Cells normally nourished by the vessel are deprived of blood and cannot function. In addition, accumulated blood from the burst vessel may put pressure on surrounding brain tissue, causing damage and even death. There are two types of hemorrhagic strokes. In an *intracerebral hemorrhage*, a blood vessel ruptures within the brain. About 10% of strokes are caused by intracerebral hemorrhages. In a *subarachnoid hemorrhage*, a blood vessel on the brain's surface ruptures and bleeds into the space between the brain and the skull. About 3% of strokes are of this type.

Hemorrhages can be caused by head injuries or the bursting of a malformed blood vessel or **aneurysm,** which is a blood-filled pocket that bulges out from a weak spot in the artery wall. Aneurysms in the brain may remain stable and never break. But when they do, the result is a stroke. Aneurysms may be caused or worsened by hypertension.

The Effects of a Stroke   The interruption of the blood supply to any area of the brain prevents the nerve cells there from functioning—in some cases causing death. Stroke survivors usually have some lasting disability. A stroke may cause paralysis, walking disability, speech impairment, memory loss, or changes in behavior. The severity of the stroke and how long the effects last depend on which brain cells have been injured, how widespread the damage is, how effectively the body can restore the blood supply, and how rapidly other areas of the brain can take over the functions of the damaged areas.

Detecting and Treating Stroke   Effective treatment requires the prompt recognition of symptoms and correct diagnosis of the type of stroke. Many people have strokes without knowing it. These "silent strokes" do not cause any noticeable symptoms while they are occurring. Although they may be mild, silent strokes leave their victims at a higher risk for subsequent and more serious strokes. They also contribute to loss of mental and cognitive skills.

Some stroke victims have a **transient ischemic attack (TIA),** or "ministroke," days, weeks, or months before they have a full-blown stroke. A TIA produces temporary stroke-like symptoms, such as weakness or numbness in an arm or a leg, speech difficulty, or dizziness. These symptoms are brief, often lasting just a few minutes, and do not cause permanent damage. TIAs should be taken as warning signs of a stroke, however, and anyone with a suspected TIA should get immediate medical attention.

A person with stroke symptoms should be rushed to the hospital. A **computed tomography (CT)** scan, which uses a computer to construct an image of the brain from X-rays, can assess brain damage and determine the type of stroke. Newer techniques using MRI and ultrasound are becoming increasingly available and should improve the speed and accuracy of stroke diagnosis.

If tests reveal that a stroke is caused by a blood clot—and if help is sought within a few hours of the onset of symptoms—the person can be treated with the same kind of clot-dissolving drugs that are used to treat coronary artery blockages. If the clot is dissolved quickly enough, brain damage is minimized and symptoms may disappear.

If tests reveal that a stroke was caused by a cerebral hemorrhage, drugs may be prescribed to lower the blood pressure, which will usually be high. Careful diagnosis is crucial, because administering clot-dissolving drugs to a person suffering a hemorrhagic stroke could cause more bleeding and potentially more brain damage.

If detection and treatment of stroke come too late, rehabilitation is the only treatment. Although damaged or destroyed brain tissue does not normally regenerate, nerve cells in the brain can make new pathways, and some functions can be taken over by other parts of the brain.

Some people recover completely in a matter of days or weeks, but most stroke victims who survive must adapt to some disability.

Peripheral Arterial Disease

Peripheral arterial disease (PAD) refers to atherosclerosis in the arteries of the arm or leg, a process that can eventually limit or completely obstruct blood flow. The same process that occurs in the coronary arteries can occur in any artery of the body. The risk of PAD is significantly increased in people with diabetes and people who smoke. The likelihood of needing an amputation is increased in those who continue to smoke, and PAD in people with diabetes tends to be extensive and severe.

Symptoms of PAD include claudication and rest pain. *Claudication* is aching or fatigue in the affected leg with exertion, particularly walking, which resolves with rest. Claudication occurs when leg muscles do

QUICK STATS

795,000 Americans suffer strokes each year.
—American Heart Association, 2011

The same disease process that occurs in the heart arteries **can occur in any artery of the body.**

TERMS

aneurysm   A sac formed by a distention or dilation of the artery wall.

transient ischemic attack (TIA)   A small stroke; usually a temporary interruption of blood supply to the brain, causing numbness or difficulty with speech.

computed tomography (CT)   The use of computerized X-ray images to create a cross-sectional depiction (scan) of tissue density.

peripheral arterial disease (PAD)   Atherosclerosis in the arteries in the legs (or less commonly, the arms) that can impede blood flow and lead to pain, infection, and loss of the affected limb.

not get adequate blood and oxygen supply. *Rest pain* occurs when the artery is unable to supply adequate blood and oxygen even when the body is not physically active. This occurs when the artery is significantly narrowed or completely blocked. PAD is the leading cause of amputation in people over age 50.

Congestive Heart Failure

When the heart has been damaged by high blood pressure or other disease conditions and cannot maintain its regular pumping rate and force, fluid begins to back up. When extra fluid seeps through capillary walls, edema (swelling) results, usually in the legs and ankles, but sometimes in other parts of the body as well. Fluid can collect in the lungs and interfere with breathing, particularly when a person is lying down. This condition is called **pulmonary edema,** and the entire process is known as **congestive heart failure**.

Treatment includes reducing the workload on the heart, modifying salt intake, and using drugs that help the body eliminate excess fluid. The risk of heart failure increases with age, and being overweight is a significant independent risk factor.

Other Forms of Heart Disease

Other, less common, disorders and diseases also affect the heart.

Congenital Heart Defects   About 36,000 children born each year in the United States have a defect or malformation of the heart or major blood vessels. These conditions are collectively referred to as **congenital heart defects,** and they cause about 3600 deaths a year. The most common congenital defects are holes in the wall that divides the chambers of the heart and *coarctation of the aorta*, a narrowing, or constriction, of the aorta. Most of the common congenital defects can now be accurately diagnosed and treated with medication or surgery.

Hypertrophic cardiomyopathy (HCM) occurs in 1 out of every 600 people in the United States and is the most common cause of sudden death among athletes younger than age 35. The disease causes the heart muscle to become hypertrophic (enlarged). People with hypertrophic cardiomyopathy are at high risk for sudden death, mainly due to serious arrhythmias. Hypertrophic cardiomyopathy may be identified by a **murmur** and diagnosed using echocardiography. Possible

treatments include medication and a pacemaker or an internal defibrillator.

Rheumatic Heart Disease   **Rheumatic fever,** a consequence of certain types of untreated streptococcal throat infections, is a leading cause of heart disease worldwide. Rheumatic fever can permanently damage the heart muscle and heart valves, a condition called *rheumatic heart disease (RHD)*. Symptoms of strep throat include the sudden onset of a sore throat, painful swallowing, fever, swollen glands, headache, nausea, and vomiting. If left untreated, up to 3% of strep infections progress into rheumatic fever.

Heart Valve Disorders   Age, previous heart attacks, congenital defects, and certain types of infections can cause abnormalities in the valves between the chambers of the heart.

The most common heart valve disorder is **mitral valve prolapse (MVP),** which occurs in about 3% of the population. MVP is characterized by a billowing of the mitral valve, which separates the left ventricle and left atrium, during ventricular contraction. Most people with MVP have no symptoms and do not need treatment. They have the same ability to exercise and live as long as people without MVP.

PROTECTING YOURSELF AGAINST CARDIOVASCULAR DISEASE

CVD can begin very early in life. Reducing CVD risk factors when you are young can pay off with many extra years of life and health.

TERMS

pulmonary edema   The accumulation of fluid in the lungs.

congestive heart failure   A condition resulting from the heart's inability to pump enough blood to keep up with the body's metabolic needs: blood backs up in the veins leading to the heart, causing an accumulation of fluid in various parts of the body.

congenital heart defect   A defect or malformation of the heart or its major blood vessels, present at birth.

hypertrophic cardiomyopathy (HCM)   An inherited condition in which there is an enlargement of the heart muscle, especially the muscle between the two ventricles.

murmur   An abnormal heart sound indicating turbulent blood flow through a valve or hole in the heart.

rheumatic fever   A disease, mainly of children, characterized by fever, inflammation, and pain in the joints. It often damages the heart valves and muscle, a condition called rheumatic heart disease.

mitral valve prolapse (MVP)   A condition in which the mitral valve billows out during ventricular contraction, allowing leakage of blood from the left ventricle into the left atrium.

Ask Yourself

QUESTIONS FOR CRITICAL THINKING AND REFLECTION

Has anyone you know ever had a heart attack? If so, was the onset gradual or sudden? Were appropriate steps taken to help the person (for example, did anyone call 911, give CPR, or use an AED)? Do you feel comfortable dealing with a cardiac emergency? If not, what can you do to improve your readiness?

Eat Heart-Healthy

For most Americans, eating a heart-healthy diet involves decreasing fat and cholesterol intake, eating a high-fiber diet, reducing sodium intake and increase potassium intake, avoiding excessive alcohol consumption, and eating foods rich in omega-3 fatty acids. In addition to these familiar guidelines, a few specifics pertain to heart health:

• *Plant stanols and sterols.* Plant stanols and sterols, found in some types of trans-fat–free margarines and other products, reduce the absorption of cholesterol in the body and help lower LDL levels.

• *Folic acid, vitamin B-6, and vitamin B-12.* These vitamins lower homocysteine levels, and folic acid has also been found to reduce the risk of hypertension.

• *Calcium.* Diets rich in calcium may help prevent hypertension and possibly stroke by reducing insulin resistance and platelet aggegration.

• *Soy protein.* Replacing some animal proteins with soy protein (such as tofu) may help lower LDL cholesterol.

• *Healthy carbohydrates.* Healthy carbohydrates are important for people with insulin resistance, prediabetes, or diabetes.

• *Total calories.* Reducing energy intake can improve cholesterol and triglyceride levels as much as reducing fat intake does. Reduced calorie intake also helps control body weight.

A diet plan that reflects many of the recommendations is the DASH diet. The DASH study found that a diet low in fat and high in fruits, vegetables, and low-fat dairy products reduces blood pressure. It is one of the eating patterns recommended in the 2010 Dietary Guidelines for Americans.

Exercise Regularly

You can significantly reduce your risk of CVD with a moderate amount of physical activity. In addition to aerobic exercise for building and maintaining cardiovascular health, strength training helps reduce body fat and improves lipid levels and glucose metabolism. The more exercise you get, the less likely you are to develop or die from CVD.

Avoid Tobacco

The number-one risk factor for CVD that you can control is smoking. If you smoke, quit. If you don't, don't start. If you live or work with people who smoke, take steps to prevent or stop the exposure.

Know and Manage Your Blood Pressure and Cholesterol Levels

If you have no CVD risk factors, have your blood pressure measured by a trained professional at least once every two years. Yearly tests are recommended if you have risk factors. If your blood pressure is high, follow your physician's advice on how to lower it. All people aged 20 and over should have their cholesterol checked at least once every five years.

Develop Effective Ways to Handle Stress and Anger

To reduce the psychological and social risk factors for CVD, develop effective strategies for handling the stress in your life. Shore up your social support network, and try some of the techniques described in Chapter 2 for managing stress.

WHAT IS CANCER?

Cancer is the abnormal, uncontrolled multiplication of cells, which can ultimately cause death if left untreated.

Tumors

Most cancers take the form of tumors, although not all tumors are cancerous. A **tumor** (or *neoplasm*) is a mass of tissue that serves no physiological purpose.

Benign (noncancerous) **tumors** are made up of cells similar to the surrounding normal cells and are enclosed in a membrane that prevents them from penetrating neighboring tissues. They are dangerous only if their physical presence interferes with body functions. A benign brain tumor, for example, can cause death if it blocks the blood supply to the brain.

TERMS

cancer The abnormal, uncontrolled multiplication of cells.

tumor A mass of tissue that serves no physiological purpose; also called a *neoplasm*.

benign tumor A tumor that is not cancerous.

The term **malignant tumor** is synonymous with cancer. A malignant tumor can invade surrounding structures, including blood vessels, the **lymphatic system,** and nerves. It can also spread to distant sites via the blood and lymphatic circulation, producing invasive tumors in almost any part of the body. A few cancers, like leukemia (cancer of the blood), do not produce a mass but still have the fundamental property of rapid, uncontrolled cell proliferation. For this reason, such diseases are malignant and are considered to be a form of cancer.

Cancer begins when a change (or mutation) in a cell occurs that allows the cell to grow and divide when it should not. Normally (in adults) cells multiply at a rate just sufficient to replace dying cells. In contrast, a malignant cell divides into new cells without regard for normal control mechanisms and gradually produces a mass of abnormal cells, or a tumor. A pea-sized mass is made up of about a billion cells, so a single tumor cell must go through many divisions, often taking years, before the tumor grows to a noticeable size.

Eventually a tumor becomes large enough to cause symptoms or to be directly detected. In the breast, for example, a tumor may be felt as a lump or diagnosed as cancer by an X-ray or **biopsy.** In less accessible locations, like the lung, a tumor may be noticed only after it has grown considerably and may then be detected only by an indirect symptom, such as a persistent cough or unexplained bleeding. In the case of leukemia, changes in the blood are eventually noticed as increasing fatigue, infection, or abnormal bleeding.

Metastasis

Metastasis is the spread of cancer cells from one part of the body to another. Metastasis occurs because cancer cells do not stick to each other as strongly as normal cells do and therefore may move away from the site of the *primary tumor* (the cancer's original location). After cancer cells break away, they can pass through the lining of lymph or blood vessels to invade nearby tissue. They can also travel to different parts of the body where they eatablish new cancer cells. This traveling and seeding process is called *metastasizing,* and the new tumors are called *secondary tumors* or *metastases.* The ability of cancer cells to metastasize makes early cancer detection critical. To control the cancer, every cancerous cell must be removed. Once cancer cells enter either the lymphatic system or the bloodstream, it is extremely difficult to stop their spread to other organs of the body.

Remission

A significant number of cancer cases go into **remission,** which in some cases lasts for years. In remission, signs and symptoms of cancer disappear, and the disease is considered to be under control. Remission typically results from treatment, but some cancer patients enter remission spontaneously.

QUICK STATS
The overall cost of cancer in the United States is projected to reach at least **$158 billion** in 2020.
—National Cancer Institute, 2011

THE CAUSES OF CANCER

Although scientists do not know everything about what causes cancer, they have identified genetic, environmental, and lifestyle factors that increase the risk of developing the disease.

The Role of DNA

Heredity and genetics are important factors in a person's risk of cancer. Certain genes may predispose some people to cancer, and specific genetic mutations—changes in the normal makeup of a gene—have been associated with cancer.

Some mutations are inherited, and others are caused by environmental agents, including radiation, certain viruses, and chemical substances in air pollution. An example of an inherited mutation is BRCA1 (breast cancer gene 1). Women who inherit an altered copy of this gene face a significantly increased risk of breast and ovarian cancer. Testing and identification of hereditary cancer risks can be helpful for some people, especially if it leads to increased attention to controllable risk factors and better medical screening. The result of copying errors that occur when DNA replicates.

Tobacco Use

Smoking is responsible for at least 80% of lung cancers and 30% of all cancer deaths. Overall, tobacco use is responsible for nearly one in five American deaths—approximately 443,000 premature deaths each year. The U.S. Surgeon General has reported that tobacco use is a direct cause of several types of cancer besides lung and bronchial cancer, including cancer of the larynx, mouth, pharynx, esophagus, stomach, pancreas, kidneys, bladder, and cervix.

Dietary Factors

Food contains many biologically active compounds, and your food choices affect your cancer risk by both exposing

TERMS

malignant tumor   A tumor that is capable of spreading and thus is cancerous.

lymphatic system   A system of vessels that returns proteins, lipids, and other substances from fluid in the tissues to the circulatory system.

biopsy   The removal of a small piece of body tissue; a needle biopsy uses a needle to remove a small sample of tissue, but some biopsies require surgery.

metastasis   The spread of cancer cells from one part of the body to another.

remission   A period during the course of cancer in which there are no symptoms or other evidence of disease.

you to potentially dangerous compounds and depriving you of potentially protective ones.

The following foods and beverages may affect cancer risk:

- *Dietary fat and meat:* Diets high in fat and meat may contribute to certain cancers, including colon, stomach, and prostate cancer. Certain types of fats may be riskier than others. Omega-6 polyunsaturated fats are associated with a higher risk of certain cancers; omega-3 fats are not.

- *Alcohol:* Alcohol is associated with an increased incidence of several cancers. Women who have two to five drinks daily have about 1.5 times the cancer risk of women who drink no alcohol. Alcohol and tobacco interact as risk factors for oral cancer.

- *Fried foods:* High levels of the chemical acrylamide (a probable human carcinogen) are found in starch-based foods that have been fried or baked at high temperatures, especially french fries and certain types of snack chips and crackers.

- *Fiber:* Further study is needed to clarify the relationship between fiber intake and cancer risk, but experts recommend a high-fiber diet for its overall positive effect on health.

- *Fruits and vegetables:* Researchers have identified many mechanisms by which food components may act against cancer. Some may prevent carcinogens from forming in the first place or block them from reaching or acting on target cells. Others boost enzymes that detoxify carcinogens and render them harmless. Some essential nutrients act as **anticarcinogens.** For example, vitamin C, vitamin E, selenium, and the **carotenoids** (vitamin A precursors) may help block cancer by acting as antioxidants.

Many other anti-cancer agents in the diet fall under the broader heading of **phytochemicals,** which are substances in plants that help protect against chronic diseases. One of the first to be identified was sulforaphane, a potent anticarcinogen found in broccoli and other cruciferous vegetables, such as cauliflower, Brussels sprouts, and cabbage. Most fruits and vegetables contain beneficial phytochemicals, and researchers are just beginning to identify them.

Inactivity and Obesity

The American Cancer Society (ACS) recommends maintaining a healthy weight throughout life by balancing caloric intake with physical activity, and by achieving and maintaining a healthy weight if you are currently overweight or obese. Being overweight or obese is linked with increased risk mortality from several kinds of cancer, including breast and colon cancer.

Carcinogens in the Environment

Some carcinogens occur naturally in the environment, like viruses and the sun's UV rays. Others are manufactured or synthetic substances that show up occasionally in the general environment but more often in the work environments of specific industries.

Microbes It is estimated that about 15–20% of the world's cancers are caused by microbes, including viruses, bacteria, and parasites. Certain types of human papillomavirus are known to cause oropharyngeal cancer, cervical cancer, and other cancers, and the Helicobacter pylori bacterium has been linked to stomach cancer. Hepatitis viruses B and C together cause as many as 80% of the world's liver cancers.

Ingested Chemicals Some of the compounds added to foods are potentially dangerous, including the nitrates and nitrites found in processed meat. While nitrates and nitrites are not themselves carcinogenic, they can combine with substances in the stomach and be converted to nitrosamines, which are highly potent carcinogens. Foods cured with nitrites, as well as those cured by salt or smoke, have been linked to esophageal and stomach cancer, and they should be eaten only in modest amounts.

Environmental and Industrial Pollution Pollutants in the air have long been suspected of contributing to the incidence of lung cancer. Although fewer than 2% of cancer deaths are probably caused by general environmental pollution, such as substances in our air and water, exposure to carcinogenic materials in the workplace is a more serious problem. Occupational exposure to specific carcinogens may account for about 4% of cancer deaths. With increasing industry and government regulation, we can anticipate that the industrial sources of cancer risk will continue to diminish, at least in the United States.

Ask Yourself
QUESTIONS FOR CRITICAL THINKING AND REFLECTION

What do you think your risks for cancer are? Do you have a family history of cancer, or have you been exposed to carcinogens? How about your diet and exercise habits? What can you do to reduce your risks?

TERMS

anticarcinogen   An agent that destroys or otherwise blocks the action of carcinogens.

carotenoid   Any of a group of yellow-to-red plant pigments that can be converted to vitamin A by the liver; many act as antioxidants or have other anti-cancer effects. The carotenoids include beta-carotene, lutein, lycopene, and zeaxanthin.

phytochemical   A naturally occurring substance found in plant foods that may help prevent chronic diseases such as cancer and heart disease; *phyto* means "plant."

Table 12.4		Screening Guidelines for the Early Detection of Cancer in Average-Risk Asymptomatic People	

CANCER SITE	POPULATION	TEST OR PROCEDURE	FREQUENCY
Breast	Women, age 20+	Breast self-examination	Beginning in their early 20s, women should be told about the benefits and limitations of breast self-examination (BSE). The importance of prompt reporting of any new breast symptoms to a health professional should be emphasized. Women who choose to do BSE should receive instruction and have their technique reviewed on the occasion of a periodic health examination. It is acceptable for women to choose not to do BSE or to do BSE irregularly.
		Clinical breast examination	For women in their 20s and 30s, it is recommended that clinical breast examination (CBE) be part of a periodic health examination, preferably at least every three years. Asymptomatic women aged 40 and over should continue to receive a clinical breast examination as part of a periodic health examination, preferably annually.
		Mammography	Begin annual mammography at age 40.*
Colorectalâ	Men and women, age 50+	*Tests that find polyps and cancer:*	
		Flexible sigmoidoscopy[‡], or	Every five years, starting at age 50
		Colonoscopy, or	Every 10 years, starting at age 50
		Double-contrast barium enema (DCBE)[‡], or	Every five years, starting at age 50
		CT colonography (virtual colonoscopy)[‡]	Every five years, starting at age 50
		Tests that mainly find cancer:	Annual, starting at age 50
		Fecal occult blood test (FOBT) with at least 50% test sensitivity for cancer, or fecal immunochemical test (FIT) with at least 50% test sensitivity for cancer[‡§] or	Annual starting at age 50. Testing at home with adherence to manufacturer's recommendation for collection techniques and number of samples is recommended. FOBT with a single stool sample collected on the clinician's fingertip during a digital rectal examination in the health care setting is not recommended. Guaiac based toilet bowl FOBT tests also are not recommended. In comparison with guaiac-based tests for the detection of occult blood, immunochemical tests are more patient-friendly, and are likely to be equal or better in sensitivity and specificity. There is no justification for repeating FOBT in response to an initial positive finding.
		Stool DNA test (sDNA)[‡]	Interval uncertain, starting at age 50
Prostate	Men, age 50+	Prostate-specific antigen test (PSA) with or without digital rectal examination (DRE)	Men who have at least a 10-year life expectancy should have an opportunity to make an informed decision with their health care provider about screening for prostate cancer after receiving information about the uncertainties, risks, and potential benefits associated with prostrate cancer screening screening. Prostrate cancer screening should not occur without an informed decision-making process.
Cervix	Women, age 21+	Pap test HPV DNA test	Cervical cancer screening should begin approximately three years after a woman begins having vaginal intercourse, but no later than 21 years of age. Screening should be done every year with conventional Pap tests or every two years using liquid-based Pap tests. At or after age 30, women who have had three normal test results in a row may get screened every two to three years with cervical cytology (either conventional or liquid-based Pap test) alone, or every three years with an HPV DNA test plus cervical cytology. Women 70 years of age and older who have had three or more normal Pap tests and no abnormal Pap tests in the past 10 years and women who have had a total hysterectomy may choose to stop cervical cancer screening.
Endometrial	Women, at menopause	At the time of menopause, women at average risk should be informed about risks and symptoms of endometrial cancer and strongly encouraged to report any unexpected bleeding or spotting to their physicians.	
Cancer-related checkup	Men and women, age 20+	During a periodic health examination, the cancer-related checkup should include examination for cancers of the thyroid, testicles, ovaries, lymph nodes, oral cavity, and skin, as well as health counseling about tobacco, sun exposure, diet and nutrition, risk factors, sexual practices, and environmental and occupational exposures.	

*Beginning at age 40, annual clinical breast examination should be performed prior to mammography.

†Individuals with a personal or family history of colorectal cancer or adenomas, inflammatory bowel disease, or high-risk genetic syndromes should continue to follow the most recent recommendations for individuals at increased or high risk.

‡Colonoscopy should be done if test results are positive.

SOURCE: American Cancer Society. *Cancer Facts and Figures, 2010.* Atlanta: American Cancer Society, Inc. Reprinted by the permission of the American Cancer Society, Inc., from www.cancer.org. All rights reserved.

Radiation All sources of radiation are potentially carcinogenic, including medical X-rays, radioactive substances (radioisotopes), and **ultraviolet (UV) radiation** from the sun. Successful efforts have been made to reduce the amount of radiation needed for mammograms, dental X-rays, and medical X-rays. Sunlight is also a potential carcinogen, and care should be taken to avoid excessive exposure.

DETECTING, DIAGNOSING, AND TREATING CANCER

Early cancer detection often depends on your awareness of changes in your own body and on keeping up with recommended screening tests.

Detecting Cancer

Self-monitoring is the first line of defense against cancer. By being aware of the risk factors in your own life, your immediate family's cancer history, and your own history, you may bring a problem to the attention of a physician long before it would have been detected at a routine physical. In addition to self-monitoring, the ACS recommends routine cancer checkups, as well as specific screening tests for certain cancers (Table 12.4).

Diagnosing and Treating Cancer

Methods for determining the exact location, type, and extent of a cancer continue to improve. A biopsy may be performed to confirm the type of tumor. Several diagnostic imaging techniques have replaced exploratory surgery for some patients. They include MRIs, CT scanning, and ultrasonography.

For most cancers, surgery is the most useful treatment. **Chemotherapy,** or the use of targeted drugs that destroy rapidly growing cancer cells, works by interfering with DNA synthesis and replication in rapidly dividing cells. Normal cells, which usually grow slowly, are not significantly destroyed by these drugs. However, some normal tissues such as intestinal, hair, and blood-forming cells are always growing, and damage to these tissues produces the unpleasant side effects of nausea, vomiting, diarrhea, and hair loss. Radiation therapy uses a beam of X-rays or gamma rays directed at the tumor to kill tumor cells. Occasionally, when an organ is small enough, radioactive seeds are surgically placed inside the cancerous organ to destroy the tumor and then removed later if necessary. Radiation destroys both normal and cancerous cells, but because it can be precisely directed at the tumor, it is usually less toxic for the patient than either surgery or chemotherapy.

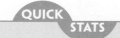

QUICK STATS

Worldwide, **7.6 million** people died of cancer in 2008.
—World Health Organization, 2012

QUICK STATS

Nearly **12 million Americans** with a history of cancer were alive in January 2008.
—American Cancer Society, 2012

TYPES AND INCIDENCE OF CANCER

Figure 12.3 shows the most common types of cancer and the incidence of each type. Cancers are classified according to the types of cells that give rise to them:

- **Carcinomas** arise from *epithelia*—tissues that cover external body surfaces, line internal tubes and cavities, and form the secreting portion of glands. This is the most common type of cancer. Major sites include the skin, breast, uterus, prostate, lungs, and gastrointestinal tract.

- **Sarcomas** arise from connective and fibrous tissues such as muscle, bone, cartilage, and the membranes covering muscles and fat.

- **Lymphomas** are cancers of the lymph nodes, part of the body's infection-fighting system.

- **Leukemias** are cancers of the blood-forming cells, which reside chiefly in the bone marrow.

Cancers vary greatly in how easily they can be detected and how well they respond to treatment. For example, certain types of skin cancer are easily detected, grow slowly, and are easy to remove; virtually all of these cancers are cured. Cancer of the pancreas, on the other hand, is difficult to detect or treat, and few patients survive the disease.

Most of the more than 1.5 million people in the United States who are diagnosed with cancer each year will be cured or live many years past their initial cancer diagnosis. In fact, the American Cancer Society (ACS) estimates that the **five-year relative survival rate** for all cancers diagnosed between 2001 and 2007 is 67%. These statistics exclude more than 1 million cases of the curable types of skin cancer.

TERMS

ultraviolet (UV) radiation Light rays of a specific wavelength emitted by the sun; most UV rays are blocked by the ozone layer in the upper atmosphere.

chemotherapy The treatment of cancer with chemicals that selectively destroy cancerous cells.

carcinoma Cancer that originates in epithelial tissue (skin, glands, and lining of internal organs).

sarcoma Cancer arising from bone, cartilage, or striated muscle.

lymphoma A tumor originating from lymphatic tissue.

leukemia Cancer of the blood or the blood-forming cells.

five-year relative survival rate The percentage of patients diagnosed with a certain disease who will be alive five years after the date of diagnosis; used to estimate the prognosis of a particular disease.

New cases	Deaths	Male	Female	New cases	Deaths
28,540	5,440	Oral cavity and pharynx	Brain and other nervous system	10,280	5,980
44,250	9,180	Melanoma of the skin	Thyroid	43,210	1,000
116,470	87,750	Lung and bronchus	Melanoma of the skin	32,000	3,120
13,950	12,040	Esophagus	Lung and bronchus	109,690	72,590
21,370	13,980	Liver and intrahepatic bile duct	Breast	226,870	39,510
22,090	18,850	Pancreas	Liver and intrahepatic bile duct	7,350	6,570
40,250	8,650	Kidney and renal pelvis	Kidney and renal pelvis	24,520	4,920
73,420	26,470	Colon and rectum	Pancreas	21,830	18,540
55,600	10,510	Urinary bladder	Colon and rectum	70,040	25,220
241,740	28,170	Prostate	Ovary	22,280	15,500
26,830	13,500	Leukemia	Uterine corpus	47,130	8,010
38,160	10,320	Non-Hodgkin lymphoma	Leukemia	20,320	10,040
			Non-Hodgkin lymphoma	31,970	8,620
848,170	301,820	All sites	All sites	790,740	275,370

VITAL STATISTICS

FIGURE 12.3   Cancer cases and deaths by site and sex. The *new cases* columns indicate the number of cancers that occur annually in each site; the *deaths* columns indicate the number of cancer deaths that are annually attributed to each type.

SOURCE: American Cancer Society. 2012. *Cancer Facts and Figures, 2012.* Atlanta: American Cancer Society.

At current U.S. rates, however, nearly one in two men and slightly more than one in three women will develop cancer at some point in their lives.

Death rates from cancer are not declining as fast as those from heart disease, in large part because of the differing effects that quitting smoking has on disease risk. Heart-related damage of smoking reverses more quickly and more significantly than the cancer-related damage from smoking. Smoking-related gene mutations cannot be reversed, although other mechanisms can sometimes control cellular changes. If heart disease death rates continue to decline faster than cancer death rates, cancer may overtake heart disease as the leading cause of death among Americans of all ages.

Still, many more people could be saved from cancer. The overwhelming majority of skin cancers could be prevented by protecting the skin from excessive sun exposure, and the majority of lung cancer could be prevented by avoiding exposure to tobacco smoke. Thousands of cases of colon, breast, and uterine cancer could be prevented by improving the diet and controlling body weight. Regular screenings and self-examinations have the potential to save an additional 100,000 lives per year.

COMMON CANCERS

In this section we look at some of the most common cancers and their causes, prevention, and treatment.

Lung Cancer

Lung cancer accounts for about 14% of all new cancer diagnoses and is the most common cause of cancer death in the United States: it is responsible for about 160,000 deaths each year. Since 1987 lung cancer has surpassed breast cancer as the leading cause of cancer death in women.

Ask Yourself

QUESTIONS FOR CRITICAL THINKING AND REFLECTION

Most people think of cancer as a death sentence, but is that necessarily true? Have you or has anyone you know had an experience with cancer? If so, what was the outcome? Have you ever considered whether you might be at increased risk for some types of cancer? Have you taken any steps to reduce your risk?

Risk Factors The chief risk factor for lung cancer is tobacco smoke, which currently accounts for 30% of all cancer deaths and 90% of lung cancer deaths. When smoking is combined with exposure to other carcinogens, such as asbestos particles or certain pollutants, the risk of cancer can be multiplied by a factor of 10 or more. Exposure to environmental tobacco smoke (ETS) increases the risk of lung cancer.

Detection and Treatment Lung cancer is difficult to detect at an early stage and hard to cure even when detected early. Symptoms of lung cancer do not usually appear until the disease has advanced to the invasive stage. Signs and symptoms such as a persistent cough, chest pain, or recurring bronchitis may be the first indication of a tumor's presence. A diagnosis can usually be made by CT scanning, chest X rays, or analysis of the cells in sputum. If caught early, localized cancers can be treated with surgery alone. The majority of patients are diagnosed with advanced disease, however, and radiation and chemotherapy are often used in addition to surgery. The five-year survival rate for all stages combined is only 16%. Phototherapy, gene therapy, and immunotherapy (vaccines) are being studied in the hope of improving these statistics.

Colon and Rectal Cancer

Another common cancer in the United States is colon and rectal cancer. Although there are effective screening methods for colorectal cancer, it is the third most common type of cancer.

Risk Factors Age is a key risk factor for colon and rectal cancer, (also called *colorectal cancer*), with more than 91% of cases diagnosed in people aged 50 and older. Heredity also plays a role. Many cancers arise from preexisting **polyps,** which are small growths on the wall of the colon that may gradually develop into malignancies. The tendency to form colon polyps appears to be determined by specific genes, so many colon cancers may be due to inherited gene mutations.

Excessive alcohol use and smoking may increase the risk of colorectal cancer. Regular physical activity appears to reduce a person's risk, whereas obesity increases risk. A diet rich in red and processed meats increases risk, whereas eating fruits, vegetables, and whole grains is associated with lower risk. However, research findings on whether dietary fiber prevents colon cancer have been mixed. Studies have suggested a protective role for folic acid, magnesium, vitamin D, and calcium; in contrast, high intake of refined carbohydrates, simple sugars, and smoked meats and fish may increase risk.

> **polyp** A small, usually harmless, mass of tissue that projects from the inner surface of the colon or rectum.
>
> TERMS

Use of oral contraceptives or hormone replacement therapy may reduce risk in women. Regular use of nonsteroidal anti-inflammatory drugs such as aspirin and ibuprofen may decrease the risk of colon cancer and other cancers of the digestive tract. However, these agents are not recommended for colorectal cancer prevention, given that they can have other negative health effects.

Detection and Treatment If identified early, precancerous polyps and early-stage cancers can be removed before they become malignant or spread. Because polyps may bleed as they progress, common warning signs of colon cancer are bleeding from the rectum and a change in bowel habits.

Regular screening tests are recommended beginning at age 50 (earlier for people with a family history of the disease or who are otherwise at high risk). A yearly stool blood test can detect small amounts of blood in the stool long before obvious bleeding would be noticed. More involved screening tests are recommended at 5- or 10-year intervals.

Surgery is the primary treatment for colon and rectal cancer. Radiation and chemotherapy may be used before surgery to shrink a tumor or after surgery to destroy any remaining cancerous cells. The five-year survival rate is 90% for colon and rectal cancers detected early and 64% overall.

Breast Cancer

Breast cancer is the most common cancer in women. In the United States, about one woman in eight will develop breast cancer during her lifetime. About 227,000 American women are diagnosed with breast cancer each year. About 40,000 women die from breast cancer each year.

Fewer than 2% of breast cancer cases occur in women under age 35, but incidence rates increase quickly with age. About 50% of cases are diagnosed in women age 45–65.

Risk Factors There is a strong genetic factor in breast cancer. A woman who has two close relatives with breast cancer is more than four times more likely to develop the disease than a woman who has no close relatives with it. However, even though genetic factors are important, inherited mutations in breast cancer susceptibility genes account for only approximately 5–10% of all breast cancer cases.

Other risk factors include early onset of menstruation, late onset of menopause, having no children or having a first child after age 30, current use of hormone replacement therapy, obesity, and alcohol use. Estrogen may be a unifying element for many of these risk factors. Estrogen circulates in a woman's body in high concentrations between puberty and menopause. Fat cells also produce estrogen, and estrogen levels are higher in obese women. Alcohol can interfere with estrogen metabolism in the liver and increase estrogen levels in the blood. Estrogen promotes the growth of cells in responsive sites, including the breast and the uterus, so any factor that increases estrogen exposure may raise breast cancer risk.

A dramatic drop in rates of breast cancer from 2001 to 2004 was attributed in part to reduced use of hormone

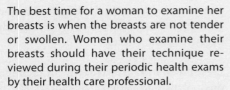

TAKE CHARGE
How to Perform a Breast Self-Exam

The best time for a woman to examine her breasts is when the breasts are not tender or swollen. Women who examine their breasts should have their technique reviewed during their periodic health exams by their health care professional.

Women with breast implants can do BSE. It may be helpful to have the surgeon help identify the edges of the implant so that you know what you are feeling. There is some thought that the implants push out the breast tissue and may actually make it easier to examine. Women who are pregnant or breast-feeding can also choose to examine their breasts regularly.

It is acceptable for women to choose not to do BSE or to do BSE once in a while. Women who choose not to do BSE should still be aware of the normal look and feel of their breasts and report any changes to their doctor right away.

How to Examine Your Breasts

• Lie down and place your right arm behind your head. The exam is done while lying down, not standing up. This is because when lying down the breast tissue spreads evenly over the chest wall and is as thin as possible, making it much easier to feel all the breast tissue.

• Use the finger pads of the three middle fingers on your left hand to feel for lumps in the right breast. Use overlapping dime-sized circular motions of the finger pads to feel the breast tissue.

• Use three different levels of pressure to feel all the breast tissue. Light pressure is needed to feel the tissue closest to the skin;

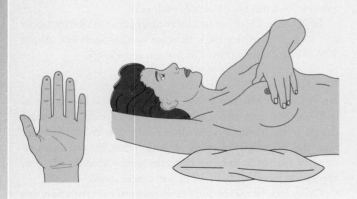

medium pressure to feel a little deeper; and firm pressure to feel the tissue closest to the chest and ribs. It is normal to feel a firm ridge in the lower curve of each breast but you should tell your doctor if you feel anything else out of the ordinary. If you're not sure how hard to press, talk with your doctor or nurse. Use each pressure level to feel the breast tissue before moving on to the next spot.

• Move around the breast in an up and down pattern starting at an imaginary line drawn straight down your side from the underarm and moving across the breast to the middle of the chest bone (sternum or breastbone). Be sure to check the entire breast area going down until you feel only ribs and up to the neck or collar bone (clavicle).

• There is some evidence to suggest that the up-and-down pattern (sometimes called the vertical pattern) is the most effective pattern for covering the entire breast, without missing any breast tissue.

• Repeat the exam on your left breast, putting your left arm behind your head and using the finger pads of your right hand to do the exam.

• While standing in front of a mirror with your hands pressing firmly down on your hips, look at your breasts for any changes of size, shape, contour, or dimpling, or redness or scaliness of the nipple or breast skin. (The pressing down on the hips position contracts the chest wall muscles and enhances any breast changes.)

• Examine each underarm while sitting up or standing and with your arm only slightly raised so you can easily feel in this area. Raising your arm straight up tightens the tissue in this area and makes it harder to examine.

This procedure for doing breast self-exam is different from previous recommendations. These changes represent an extensive review of the medical literature and input from an expert advisory group. There is evidence that this position (lying down), the area felt, pattern of coverage of the breast, and use of different amounts of pressure increase a woman's ability to find abnormal areas.

---

replacement therapy (HT) by women over 50 beginning in July 2002. Millions of women stopped taking the hormones after research linked HT with an increased risk of breast cancer and heart disease.

Eating a low-fat, vegetable-rich diet, exercising regularly, limiting alcohol intake, and maintaining a healthy body weight can minimize the chance of developing breast cancer, even for women at risk from family history or other factors. Despite some popular myths, studies have shown that breast cancer incidence is not increased by underwire bras, antiperspirants, breast implants, or abortions.

Early Detection A cure is most likely if breast cancer is detected early, so regular screening is a good investment, even for younger women. The ACS advises a three-part personal program for the early detection of breast cancer:

• *Mammography:* The ACS recommends a **mammogram** (low-dose breast X-ray) every year for women over 40.

> **mammogram** A low-dose X-ray of the breasts used to check for early signs of breast cancer. **TERMS**

Some groups have argued that between ages 40 and 50 the rates of false positive mammograms are higher and thus women should not begin receiving mammograms until age 50. However, most organizations in the United States still recommend beginning screening with mammograms at age 40.

Studies show that magnetic resonance imaging (MRI) may be better than mammography at detecting breast abnormalities in some women. The ACS recommends both an annual mammogram and an annual MRI for women who are at high risk for breast cancer. **Ultrasonography** is sometimes used as a follow-up investigational tool if a mammogram reveals an abnormality in breast tissue.

• *Clinical breast exam:* Women between ages 20 and 39 should have a clinical breast exam every three years, and women aged 40 and older should have one every year before their scheduled mammogram.

• *Breast self-exams:* Breast self-exam (BSE) allows a woman to become familiar with her breasts, so she can alert her health care provider to any changes. Women who choose to do breast self-exams should begin at age 20 (see the box "How to Perform a Breast Self-Exam").

Breast pain or tenderness is usually associated with benign conditions such as menstruation rather than breast cancer. The first physical signs of breast cancer are more likely to be a lump, swelling, or thickening; skin irritation or dimpling; or nipple pain, scaliness, or retraction. Although most breast lumps are benign, any breast lump should be brought to the attention of a health care provider.

Treatment   If a lump is detected, it may be scanned by ultrasonography and biopsied to see if it is cancerous. In most cases, the lump is found to be a cyst or other harmless growth, and no further treatment is needed. If the lump contains cancer cells, a variety of surgeries may be indicated, ranging from a lumpectomy (removal of the lump and surrounding tissue) to a mastectomy (removal of the breast).

If the tumor is discovered before it has spread to the adjacent lymph nodes or outside the breast, the patient has about a 99% chance of surviving more than five years. The relative survival rate for all stages is 90% at five years.

New Strategies for Treatment and Prevention   A number of drugs have been developed for the treatment or prevention of breast cancer. A family of drugs called *selective estrogen receptor modulators (SERMs)* act like estrogen in some tissues of the body but block estrogen's effects in others. One SERM, tamoxifen, has long been used in breast cancer treatment because it blocks the action of estrogen in breast tissue. In 1998 the FDA approved the use of tamoxifen to reduce the risk of breast cancer in healthy women who are at high risk for the disease. Another SERM, raloxifene, was approved in 2007 for the reduction of invasive breast cancer risk in postmenopausal women at high risk for breast cancer. Compared to tamoxifen, raloxifene has been shown to pose a slightly lower risk of blood clots and uterine cancer, but the

risk is still higher than that of a placebo. Raloxifene has also been shown to improve bone mineral density.

Treatment with the **monoclonal antibodies** trastuzumab or lapatinib is an option for some women. A monoclonal antibody is a special type of antibody that is produced in a laboratory and designed to bind to a specific cancer-related target. Many other monoclonal antibodies are currently in development for breast cancer.

Prostate Cancer

The prostate gland is located at the base of the bladder in men and completely surrounds the male's urethra; if enlarged, it can block the flow of urine. Prostate cancer is the most common cancer in men and the second leading cause of cancer death in men. Nearly 242,000 new cases are diagnosed each year, and more than 28,000 American men die from the disease each year.

Risk Factors   Age is the strongest predictor of risk, with approximately 60% of cases of prostate cancer diagnosed in men over age 65. Inherited genetic predisposition may be responsible for 5–10% of cases, and men with a family history of the disease should be particularly vigilant about screening. African American men and Jamaican men of African descent have the highest rates of prostate cancer of any groups in the world. Both genetic and lifestyle factors may be involved.

Diets high in calories, dairy products, and animal fats and low in plant foods have also been implicated as possible culprits, as have obesity, inactivity, and a history of sexually transmitted diseases. Type 2 diabetes and insulin resistance are also associated with prostate cancer. Soy foods, tomatoes, and cruciferous vegetables are being investigated for their possible protective effects.

Detection   Warning signs of prostate cancer can include changes in urinary frequency, weak or interrupted urine flow, painful urination, and blood in the urine. Techniques for early detection include a digital rectal examination and the **prostate-specific antigen (PSA) test.** Currently there is insufficient data in support of or against routine screening with the PSA test. The ACS recommends that men be provided information about the benefits and limitations of the tests and that both the exam and the PSA test be offered annually, beginning at age 50, for men who are at average risk of prostate

---

TERMS

ultrasonography   An imaging method in which sound waves are bounced off body structures to create an image on a TV monitor; also called *ultrasound.*

monoclonal antibody   An antibody designed to bind to a specific cancer-related target.

prostate-specific antigen (PSA) test   A screening test for prostate cancer that measures blood levels of prostate-specific antigen (PSA).

cancer, do not have any major medical problems, and have a life expectancy of at least 10 years. Men at high risk, including African Americans and those with a family history of the disease, should consider beginning screening at age 45. Men with multiple family members who have been diagnosed with the disease should begin screening at age 40.

PSA testing has been a subject of controversy among experts for several years because of its tendency to yield misleading results, leading to further testing, including biopsies, that can potentially cause harm. In older men, most prostate cancers are not deadly, making treatments pointless and potentially harmful.

Treatment Treatments vary based on the stage of the cancer and the age of the patient. A small, slow-growing tumor in an older man may be treated with watchful waiting and no initial therapy because he is more likely to die from another cause before his cancer becomes life-threatening. More aggressive treatment would be indicated for younger men or those with more advanced cancers. Treatment may involve *radical prostatectomy* (surgical removal of the prostate). Although radical surgery has an excellent cure rate, it is major surgery and often results in **incontinence** and/or erectile dysfunction. Minimally invasive surgery, which utilizes a laparoscopic or robotic approach, can sometimes be performed with fewer complications and quicker recovery.

A less invasive alternative involves surgical implantation of radioactive seeds that destroy the tumor and much of the normal prostate tissue but leave surrounding tissue relatively untouched. Several new treatments for advanced prostate cancer have recently been approved by the U.S. Food and Drug Administration (FDA). A cancer vaccine, known as sipuleucel-T, was approved for some men. Another option is Abiraterone, which was approved for the treatment of metastatic prostate cancer that is resistant to hormonal therapy and chemotherapy. Survival rates for all stages of this cancer have improved steadily since 1940; the five-year survival rate is now nearly 100%.

Cancers of the Female Reproductive Tract

Several types of cancer can affect the female reproductive tract, and a few of these cancers are relatively common.

Cervical Cancer Cancer of the cervix occurs in women in their twenties and thirties. Virtually all cases of cervical cancer stem from infection by the human papillomavirus (HPV), a group of about 100 related viruses that also cause common warts and genital warts. When certain types of HPV are introduced into the cervix, usually by an infected sex partner,

the virus infects cervical cells, causing them to divide and grow. If unchecked, this growth can develop into cervical cancer. Cervical cancer is associated with multiple sex partners and is extremely rare in women who have not had heterosexual intercourse. Smoking, immunosuppression, and prolonged use of oral contraceptives also have been associated with increased risk.

Screening for the changes in cervical cells that precede cancer is done chiefly by means of the **Pap test.** During a pelvic exam, loose cells are scraped from the cervix and examined under a microscope to see whether they are normal. If cells are abnormal but not yet cancerous, the patient has a condition commonly referred to as *cervical dysplasia*. Sometimes such abnormal cells spontaneously return to normal, but in about one-third of cases the cellular changes progress toward malignancy. If this happens, the abnormal cells must be removed, either surgically or with a cryoscopic (ultracold) probe or localized laser treatment. Without timely surgery, the malignant cells invade the cervical wall and spread to the uterus and adjacent lymph nodes. At this stage, chemotherapy may be used with radiation to kill the cancer cells, but chances for a complete cure are reduced.

> ### QUICK STATS
> **55 million** Pap tests are performed each year in the United States; about 6% are abnormal and require medical follow-up.
> —National Cancer Institute, 2009

Because the Pap test is highly effective, all sexually active women and women between ages 18 and 70 should be tested. The recommended schedule for testing depends on risk factors, the type of Pap test performed, and whether the Pap test is combined with HPV testing. Two HPV vaccines have been approved by the FDA for the prevention of cervical cancer. Women who receive one of the vaccines should continue to receive routine Pap tests because the vaccines do not protect against all types of the virus (see the box "HPV and Cancer").

Uterine, or Endometrial, Cancer Cancer of the lining of the uterus (the *endometrium*) most often occurs after the age of 55. The risk factors are similar to those for breast cancer, including prolonged exposure to estrogen, early onset of menstruation, late menopause, never having been pregnant, and obesity. Type 2 diabetes is also associated with increased risk. The use of oral contraceptives and hormone therapy that contain estrogen plus progestin do not appear to increase risk.

Endometrical cancer often presents with abnormal vaginal bleeding in a postmenopausal woman. It is treated surgically, commonly by *hysterectomy*, or removal of the uterus.

> **TERMS**
>
> **incontinence** The inability to control the flow of urine.
>
> **Pap test** A scraping of cells from the cervix for examination under a microscope to detect cancer.

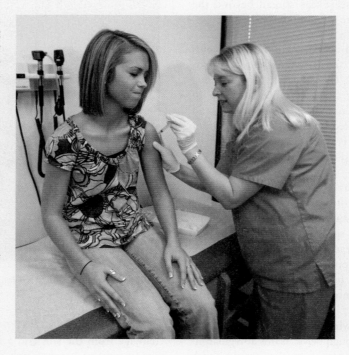

Human papillomavirus (HPV), the virus that causes the most commonly diagnosed sexually transmitted disease in the United States, is linked to several types of cancer. About 75–80% of sexually active adults will acquire HPV before the age of 50. Much of the time, the infection clears and the person may never know that he or she was infected. People with persistent HPV infection are at the highest risk of developing precancerous or cancerous lesions, a process that can take months or years. The regular use of condoms can reduce the risk of transmitting HPV.

HPV may be best known for causing genital warts, which usually appear as pink or gray bumps on the skin of the penis, vulva, cervix, vagina, or anal region. Two types of HPV (genotypes 6 and 11) cause approximately 90% of all cases of genital warts. For some people, infections are asymptomatic, but others require treatment with chemical agents, immunotherapy, or surgery. Several types of cancer are linked to HPV infection. These include the following:

- *Cervical cancer:* HPV is thought to be responsible for more than 99% of all cervical cancers. Each year in the United States, approximately 12,000 women develop cervical cancer, and over 4,200 die from it. In developing countries, cervical cancer is the second most common cause of cancer-related deaths. On average, it takes 15 years from the time of initial HPV infection for invasive cervical cancer to develop.

- *Oropharyngeal cancer:* Nearly 50% of all cancers of the oropharynx (mouth and throat), particularly the tonsils and base of tongue, are related to HPV infection. Patients require aggressive therapy with combined chemotherapy and radiation, which have severe side effects of their own.

- *Other cancers:* Up to 70% of cancers of the vulva, vagina, and penis and approximately 90% of anal cancers have been linked to HPV infection. Even when they can be treated locally, such cancers can cause significant compromise of sexual function and lead to long-term illness.

Currently two commercially available HPV vaccines are approved by the FDA. Gardasil targets four types of HPV (genotypes 6, 11, 16, 18). Cervarix targets genotypes 16 and 18 only. Both vaccines are administered in three doses. In 2007 the Advisory Committee on Immunization Practices recommended that all girls be vaccinated at age 11–12 with Gardasil and that females aged 13–26 who had not been previously vaccinated receive catch-up vaccinations. In 2009 the committee added Cervarix to the list of approved vaccines for the prevention of cervical cancer, and an FDA panel expanded the recommendation for Gardasil vaccination to males age 9–26 for the prevention of genital warts and anal cancer.

Young girls are targeted for vaccination because the greatest benefits are experienced by those who are not yet sexually active. However, it is likely that young sexually active individuals will not have been exposed to all HPV genotypes targeted by the vaccines. Thus individuals who have already been infected with one or more HPV types will still derive protection from the vaccine types they have not acquired. Women who are vaccinated still need to receive regular Pap tests for cervical cancer screening because not all of the HPV genotypes responsible for cervical cancer are covered by the vaccine.

Data from the National Immunization Survey of Teens demonstrated that among girls aged 13 to 17, initiation of the HPV vaccine (at least one of the three-dose HPV vaccination series) increased from 25.1% in 2007 to 44.3% in 2009. Nearly one-third (26.7%) of girls had the complete three-shot vaccine series in 2009. As more educational programs are launched, experts hope that vaccination rates will increase, leading to associated declines in the rates of HPV-related cancers discusses HPV and other sexually transmitted diseases in detail.

SOURCES: Slade, B. A., et al. 2009. Postlicensure safety surveillance for quadrivalent human papillomavirus recombinant vaccine. *Journal of the American Medical Association* 302(7): 750–757; Ryerson, A. B., et al. 2008. Burden of potentially human papillomavirus-associated cancers of the oropharynx and oral cavity in the U.S., 1998–2003. *Cancer* 113(10 Suppl.): 2901–2909; Broomall, E. M., et al. 2010. Epidemiology, clinical manifestations, and recent advances in vaccination against human papillomavirus. *Postgraduate Medicine* 122(2): 121–129; Wong, C., et al. 2010. *National HPV Vaccine Uptake and Vaccination Predictors and Barriers for Girls 8–17 Years Old.* Oral Presentation at the National STD Prevention Conference, March 8–11, 2010, Atlanta; Centers for Disease Control and Prevention. 2011. National and state vaccination coverage among adolescents aged 13 through 17 years—United States, 2010. *Morbidity and Mortality Weekly Reports,* August 26, 60(33):1117–1123.

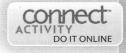

Radiation treatment, hormones, and chemotherapy may be used in addition to surgery. When the tumor is detected at an early stage, about 96% of patients are alive and disease-free five years later. When the disease has spread beyond the uterus, the five-year survival rate is less than 67%.

Ovarian Cancer   Although ovarian cancer is rare compared with cervical or uterine cancer, it causes more deaths than the other two combined. There are often no warning signs of ovarian cancer. Early symptoms may include increased abdominal size and bloating, urinary urgency, and pelvic pain. It cannot be detected by Pap tests or any other simple screening method and is often diagnosed late in its development, when surgery and other therapies are unlikely to be successful.

The risk factors are similar to those for breast and endometrial cancer: increasing age (most ovarian cancer occurs after age 60), never having been pregnant, a family history of breast or ovarian cancer, obesity, and specific genetic mutations. A high number of ovulations appears to increase the chance that a cancer-causing genetic mutation will occur, so anything that lowers the number of lifetime ovulation cycles—pregnancy, breastfeeding, or use of oral contraceptives—reduces a woman's risk of ovarian cancer.

Women with symptoms or who are at high risk because of family history should have thorough pelvic exams at regular intervals. Ovarian cancer is treated by surgical removal of both ovaries, the fallopian tubes, and the uterus. Radiation and chemotherapy are sometimes used in addition to surgery. When the tumor is localized to the ovary, the five-year survival rate is 93%. For all stages, the five-year survival rate is only 44%, reflecting the difficulty of early detection.

Skin Cancer

Skin cancer is the most common type of cancer, but it is often not included in cancer statistics because many types of skin cancer are easily curable. Of the approximate 3.5 million cases of skin cancer diagnosed each year, about 76,000 are of the most serious type, **melanoma.**

Risk Factors   Almost all cases of skin cancer can be traced to excessive exposure to ultraviolet radiation from the sun, including longer-wavelength ultraviolet A (UVA) and shorter-wavelength ultraviolet B (UVB) radiation. UVB radiation causes sunburns and can damage the eyes and the immune system. UVA is less likely to cause an immediate sunburn, but it damages connective tissue and leads to premature aging of the skin, giving it a wrinkled, leathery appearance. (Tanning lamps and tanning salon beds emit mostly UVA radiation.) Both UVA and UVB radiation have been linked to the development of skin cancer, and the National Toxicology Program has declared both solar and artificial sources of UV radiation, including sunlamps and tanning beds, to be known human carcinogens.

Both severe, acute sun reactions (sunburns) and chronic low-level sun reactions (suntans) can lead to skin cancer. People with fair skin have less natural protection against skin

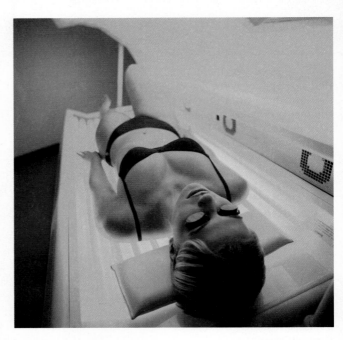

Tanning, either under direct sunlight or in a tanning bed, is a known cause of skin cancer.

damage from the sun and a higher risk of developing skin cancer, whereas people with naturally dark skin have a considerable degree of protection. Caucasians are about 10 times more likely than African Americans to develop melanoma, but African Americans and Latinos are still at risk.

Severe sunburns in childhood have been linked to a significantly increased risk of skin cancer in later life, so children in particular should be protected. According to the Skin Cancer Foundation, the risk of skin cancer doubles in people who have had five or more sunburns in their lifetime. Because of damage to the ozone layer of the atmosphere, there is a chance that we may all be exposed to increasing amounts of UV radiation in the future. Other risk factors for skin cancer include having many moles (particularly large ones), spending time at high altitudes, and a family history of the disease.

Types of Skin Cancer   There are three main types of skin cancer, named for the types of skin cells from which they develop. **Basal cell** and **squamous cell carcinomas** together account for about 95% of the skin cancers diagnosed each year. They are usually found in chronically sun-exposed areas, such as the face, neck, hands, and arms. They usually appear as pale, waxlike, pearly nodules or red, scaly, sharply outlined

---

TERMS

melanoma   A malignant tumor of the skin that arises from pigmented cells, usually a mole.

basal cell carcinoma   Cancer of the deepest layers of the skin.

squamous cell carcinoma   Cancer of the surface layers of the skin.

CRITICAL CONSUMER
Sunscreens and Sun-Protective Clothing

If you consistently use sun-protective clothing, sunscreen, and common sense, you can lead an active outdoor life *and* protect your skin against most sun-induced damage.

Clothing

• Wear long-sleeved shirts and long pants. Consider clothing made from special sun-protective fabrics; these garments have an ultraviolet protection factor (UPF) rating, similar to the SPF for sunscreens.

• Wear a hat. A good choice is a broad-brimmed hat or a legion-naire-style cap that covers the ears and neck. Wear sunscreen on your face even if you are wearing a hat.

• Wear sunglasses. Exposure to UV rays can damage the eyes and cause cataracts.

Sunscreen

• Use a sunscreen and lip balm with a sun protection factor (SPF) of 15 or higher. An SPF rating refers to the amount of time you can stay out in the sun before you burn, compared with not using sunscreen. For example, a product with an SPF of 15 would allow you to remain in the sun without burning 15 times longer, on average, than if you didn't apply sunscreen.

• Shake sunscreen before applying. Apply it 30 minutes before exposure to allow it time to bond to the skin. Reapply sunscreen frequently and generously to all sun-exposed areas. Reapply sunscreen 15–30 minutes after sun exposure begins and then every two hours after that and/or following activities, such as swimming, that could remove sunscreen.

Time of Day and Location

• Avoid sun exposure between 10 a.m. and 4 p.m., when the sun's rays are most intense.

• Consult the day's UV index, which predicts UV levels on a 0–11+ scale, to get a sense of the amount of sun protection you'll need. UV index ratings are available in local newspapers, from the weather bureau, or from certain websites.

Tanning Salons

• Avoid tanning salons. Tanning beds and lamps emit mostly UVA radiation, increasing your risk of premature skin aging (such as wrinkles) and skin cancer.

• If you really want a tan, consider using a sunless tanning product. Lotions, creams, and sprays containing the color additive dihydroxyacetone (DHA) are approved by the FDA for tanning.

---

patches. These cancers are often painless, although they may bleed, crust, and form an open sore on the skin.

Melanoma is by far the most dangerous skin cancer because it spreads so rapidly. It can occur anywhere on the body, but the most common sites are the back, chest, abdomen, and lower legs. A melanoma usually appears at the site of a preexisting mole. The mole may begin to enlarge, become mottled or varied in color (colors can include blue, pink, and white), or develop an irregular surface or irregular borders. Tissue invaded by melanoma may also itch, burn, or bleed easily.

Prevention   One of the major steps you can take to protect yourself against all forms of skin cancer is to avoid life-long overexposure to sunlight. Blistering, peeling sunburns from unprotected sun exposure are particularly dangerous, but suntans—whether from sunlight or from tanning lamps—also increase your risk of developing skin cancer later in life. People of every age, especially babies and children, need to be protected from the sun with **sunscreens** and protective clothing (see the box "Sunscreens and Sun-Protective Clothing").

Detection and Treatment   Make it a habit to examine your skin regularly. Most of the spots, freckles, moles, and blemishes on your body are normal; you were born with some of them, and others appear and disappear throughout your life. But if you notice an unusual growth, discoloration, sore that does not heal, or mole that undergoes a sudden or progressive change, see your physician or dermatologist immediately.

Figure 12.4 illustrates the characteristics that may signal a melanoma—asymmetry, border irregularity, color change, and a diameter greater than $1/4$ inch. If you have an unusual skin lesion, your physician will examine it and possibly perform a biopsy. If the lesion is cancerous, it is usually removed surgically, a procedure that can almost always be performed in the physician's office using a local anesthetic.

In 2011 the FDA approved two new therapies for metastatic melanoma: ipilimumab (Yervoy), a monoclonal antibody that activates the body's anticancer immune response, and vemurafenib (Zelboraf), which targets a specific gene mutation in melanoma. For melanoma, the five-year survival rate is 98% if the tumor is localized but only 62% if the cancer has spread to adjacent lymph nodes. Improvements in

---

sunscreen   A substance used to protect the skin from UV rays; usually applied as a lotion, cream, or spray.

TERMS

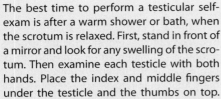
The best time to perform a testicular self-exam is after a warm shower or bath, when the scrotum is relaxed. First, stand in front of a mirror and look for any swelling of the scrotum. Then examine each testicle with both hands. Place the index and middle fingers under the testicle and the thumbs on top. Roll the testicle gently between the fingers and thumbs. Don't worry if one testicle seems slightly larger than the other; that's common. Also, expect to feel the epididymis, which is the soft, sperm-carrying tube at the rear of the testicle.

Perform a self-exam each month. If you find a lump, swelling, or nodule, see a physician right away. The abnormality may not be cancer, but only a physician can make a diagnosis.

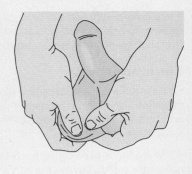

Other possible signs of testicular cancer include a change in the way a testicle feels, a sudden collection of fluid in the scrotum, a dull ache in the lower abdomen or groin, a feeling of heaviness in the scrotum, or pain in a testicle or the scrotum.

SOURCES: Testicular Cancer Resource Center. 2009. *How to Do a Testicular Self Examination* (http://tcrc.acor.org/tcexam.html); National Cancer Institute. 2005. *Questions and Answers about Testicular Cancer* (http://www.cancer.gov/cancertopics/factsheet/sites-types/testicular).

---

survival are anticipated with the use of these new targeted treatments.

Head and Neck Cancers

Head and neck cancers—cancers of the oral cavity, pharynx, larynx, and nasal cavity—can be traced principally to cigarette, cigar, or pipe smoking, the use of spit tobacco, and the excessive consumption of alcohol. The incidence of head and neck cancer is twice as great in men as in women, and the disease is most frequent in men over 40.

A—Asymmetry: Is one half unlike the other?

B—Border irregularity: Does it have an uneven, scalloped edge rather than a clearly defined border?

C—Color variation: Is the color uniform, or does it vary from one area to another, from tan to brown to black, or from white to red to blue?

¼ in.

D—Diameter larger than ¼ inch: At its widest point, is the growth as large as, or larger than, a pencil eraser?

FIGURE 12.4   The ABCD test for melanoma. To see a variety of photos of melanoma and benign moles, visit the National Cancer Institute's Visuals Online site (http://visualsonline.cancer.gov).

Chemotherapy, radiation, and surgery are the primary methods of treatment for head and neck cancers. Patients often endure intense mouth and throat inflammation and some require disfiguring surgeries, but many can be cured. Among those who survive, a significant number will develop another primary cancer of the head and neck. The five-year survival rate is about 61%.

Testicular Cancer

Testicular cancer is relatively rare, accounting for only 1% of cancer in men (about 8,590 cases per year), but it is the most common cancer in men aged 20–35. It is much more common among white Americans than among Latinos, Asian Americans, or African Americans and among men whose fathers had testicular cancer. Men with undescended testicles are at increased risk for testicular cancer, and for this reason that condition should be corrected in early childhood. Self-examination may help in the early detection of testicular cancer (see the box "Testicle Self-Examination"). Tumors are treated by surgical removal of the testicle and, if the tumor has spread, by chemotherapy; radiation treatment is used only rarely. The five-year survival rate for testicular cancer is 95%.

Ask Yourself
QUESTIONS FOR CRITICAL THINKING AND REFLECTION

Has anyone you know had cancer? If so, what type of cancer was it? What were its symptoms? Based on the information presented so far in this chapter, did the person have any of the known risk factors for the disease?

Connect to Your Choices

Have you ever thought about where you get your behaviors and habits related to CVD and cancer? Many factors can influence our behaviors and habits, some not as obvious as others. When you were growing up, did your family avoid risk-increasing behaviors like smoking and being physically inactive? Currently, do you live on a campus or in a community where smoking is discouraged and physical activity is encouraged? Does your health clinic offer programs to facilitate physical activity or help smokers quit? Does your clinic discourage tanning and offer free blood pressure and cholesterol checks?

What are the external factors that influence your choices about cancer-related behaviors? What are your inner motivations and core values, and how do they affect your choices? Based on what you learned in this chapter, will you make some different choices in the future? If so, what will they be?

Go online to Connect to complete this activity: www.mcgraw-hillconnect.com

TIPS FOR TODAY AND THE FUTURE

A growing body of research suggests that we can take an active role in preventing CVD and many cancers by adopting a wellness lifestyle.

RIGHT NOW YOU CAN:
- Plan to replace one high-fat item in your diet with one that is high in fiber. For example, replace a doughnut with a bowl of whole-grain cereal.
- Check the cancer screening guidelines in this chapter and make sure you are up-to-date on your screenings.

IN THE FUTURE YOU CAN:
- Sign up for a class in cardiopulmonary resuscitation (CPR).
- Learn where to find information about daily UV radiation levels in your area, and learn how to interpret the information.
- Gradually add foods with abundant phytochemicals to your diet.

SUMMARY

- The cardiovascular system circulates blood throughout the body. The heart pumps blood to the lungs via the pulmonary artery and to the body via the aorta.

- The six major risk factors for CVD that can be changed or controlled are smoking, high blood pressure, unhealthy cholesterol levels, inactivity, overweight and obesity, and diabetes.

- Hypertension occurs when blood pressure exceeds normal levels most of the time. It weakens the heart, scars and hardens arteries, and can damage the eyes and kidneys.

- Physical inactivity, obesity, and diabetes are interrelated and are associated with high blood pressure and unhealthy cholesterol levels.

- Contributing risk factors that can be changed include high triglyceride levels, insulin resistance and metabolic syndrome, and psychological and social factors.

- Risk factors for CVD that can't be changed include being over 65, being male, being African American, and having a family history of CVD.

- Atherosclerosis is a progressive hardening and narrowing of arteries that can lead to restricted blood flow and even complete blockage.

- Heart attacks are usually the result of a long-term disease process. Warning signs of a heart attack include chest discomfort, shortness of breath, nausea, and sweating.

- A stroke occurs when the blood supply to the brain is cut off by a blood clot or hemorrhage. A transient ischemic attack (TIA) may be a warning sign of an impending stroke.

- Congestive heart failure occurs when the heart's pumping action becomes less efficient and fluid collects in the lungs or in other parts of the body.

- CVD risk can also be reduced by eating a heart-healthy diet, exercising regularly, avoiding tobacco and environmental tobacco smoke, knowing and managing your blood pressure and cholesterol levels, and developing effective ways of handling stress and anger.

- Cancer is the abnormal, uncontrolled multiplication of cells; it can cause death if untreated.

- One in two men and one in three women will develop cancer.

- Mutational damage to a cell's DNA can lead to rapid and uncontrolled growth of cells; mutagens include radiation, viral infection, and chemical substances in food and air.

- Other possible causes of cancer include tobacco use, dietary factors, inactivity and obesity, certain types of infections and chemicals, and radiation.

- Self-monitoring and regular screening tests are essential to early cancer detection. Methods of cancer diagnosis include biopsy and imaging techniques like MRI scanning, CT scanning, and ultrasound.

- Treatment methods usually consist of some combination of surgery, chemotherapy, and radiation. Research continues to show promise with newer therapies.

- Lung cancer kills more people than any other type of cancer. Tobacco smoke is the primary cause.

- Colon and rectal cancer is linked to age, heredity, obesity, and a diet rich in red meat and low in fruits and vegetables. Most colon cancers arise from preexisting polyps.

- Breast cancer affects about one in eight women in the United States. Although there is a genetic component to breast cancer, diet and hormones are also risk factors.

- Prostate cancer is chiefly a disease of aging; diet and lifestyle probably are factors in its occurrence. Early detection is possible through rectal examinations and PSA blood tests.

- Cancers of the female reproductive tract include cervical, uterine, and ovarian cancer. The Pap test is an effective screening test for cervical cancer.

- Abnormal cellular changes in the epidermis, often a result of exposure to the sun, cause skin cancer, as does chronic exposure to certain chemicals. Skin cancers include basal cell carcinoma, squamous cell carcinoma, and melanoma.

- Head and neck cancers are caused primarily by smoking, excess alcohol consumption, and use of smokeless tobacco.

- Testicular cancer can be detected early through self-examination.

FOR MORE INFORMATION

BOOKS

American Cancer Society. 2009. *The American Cancer Society Complete Guide to Complementary & Alternative Cancer Therapies.* Atlanta: American Cancer Society. *Provides in-depth information about cancer therapies being used alongside traditional Western medicine in treating cancer.*

Hartmann, L. C., C. L. Loprinzi, and B. S. Gostout. 2008. *Mayo Clinic: Guide to Women's Cancers.* New York: Kensington. *Provides information about a variety of women's cancers.*

Heller, M. 2005. *The DASH Diet Action Plan, Based on the National Institutes of Health Research: Dietary Approaches to Stop Hypertension.* Northbrook, IL: Amidon Press. *Provides background information and guidelines for adopting the DASH diet; also includes meal plans to suit differing caloric needs and recipes.*

Lipsky, M. S., et al. 2008. *American Medical Association Guide to Preventing and Treating Heart Disease.* New York: Wiley. *A team of doctors provides advice for heart health to consumers.*

Mukherjee, S. 2011. *The Emperor of All Maladies: A Biography of Cancer.* New York: Scribner. *The author, a practicing physician and award-winning science writer, traces the history of humankind's battle with cancer, interweaving stories of cancer patients and meditations on mortality and medical ethics.*

Rosenbaum, E., et al. 2008. *Everyone's Guide to Cancer Therapy,* rev. 5th ed. Riverside, NJ: Andrews McMeel. *Reviewed by a panel of more than 100 oncologists; provides articles on the known causes, diagnoses, and treatments for many types of cancer.*

ORGANIZATIONS, HOTLINES, AND WEBSITES

American Academy of Dermatology. Provides information about skin cancer prevention.

http://www.aad.org

American Cancer Society. Provides a wide range of free materials on the prevention and treatment of cancer.

http://www.cancer.org

American Heart Association. Provides information about hundreds of topics relating to cardiovascular disease; the AHA's website links to several sites focusing on specific heart-related topics.

http://www.heart.org (general information)

Clinical Trials. Information about clinical trials for new cancer treatments can be accessed at the following sites:

http://www.cancer.gov/clinicaltrials

http://www.centerwatch.com

Dietary Approaches to Stop Hypertension (DASH). Provides information about the design, diets, and results of the DASH study, including tips on how to follow the DASH diet at home.

http://www.nhlbi.nih.gov/health/public/heart/hbp/dash

EPA/Sunwise. Information about the UV index and the effects of sun exposure, with links to sites with daily UV index ratings for cities in the United States and other countries.

http://www.epa.gov/sunwise/uvindex.html

Harvard School of Public Health: Disease Risk Index. Includes interactive risk assessments as well as tips for preventing common cancers.

http://www.diseaseriskindex.harvard.edu/update

MedlinePlus: Blood, Heart, and Circulation Topics. Provides links to reliable sources of information on many topics relating to cardiovascular health.

http://www.nlm.nih.gov/medlineplus/bloodheartandcirculation.html

National Cancer Institute. Provides information about treatment options, screening, and clinical trials.

http://www.cancer.gov

National Cholesterol Education Program (NCEP): Cholesterol Counts for Everyone. Provides information about cholesterol for people with heart disease and people who want to avoid it.

http://www.nhlbi.nih.gov/about/ncep/index.htm

National Heart, Lung, and Blood Institute. Provides information about and interactive applications for a variety of topics relating to cardiovascular health and disease, including cholesterol, smoking, obesity, hypertension, and the DASH diet.

http:// http://www.nhlbi.nih.gov/

National Stroke Association. Provides information and referrals for stroke victims and their families as well as a stroke risk assessment.

http://www.stroke.org

SELECTED BIBLIOGRAPHY

American Cancer Society. 2012. *Breast Cancer Facts & Figures 2012.* Atlanta: American Cancer Society.

American Cancer Society. 2012. *Cancer Facts and Figures 2012.* Atlanta: American Cancer Society.

American Cancer Society. 2012. *Colorectal Cancer Facts & Figures 2012.* Atlanta: American Cancer Society.

American Heart Association. 2012. *Heart Disease and Stroke Statistics—2012 Update.* Dallas: American Heart Association.

Artero, E. G., et al. 2012. Effects of muscular strength on cardiovascular risk factors and prognosis. *Journal of Cardiopulmonary Rehabilitation and Prevention,* August 17 (Epub ahead of print).

Bibbins-Doming, K., et al. 2010. Projected Effect of Dietary Salt Reductions on Future Cardiovascular Disease. *New England Journal of Medicine* 362(7): 590–599.

Broomall, E. M., et al. 2010. Epidemiology, clinical manifestations, and recent advances in vaccination against human papillomavirus. *Postgraduate Medicine* 122(2): 121–129.

Centers for Disease Control and Prevention. 2009. Application of lower sodium intake recommendations to adults—United States, 1999–2006. *Morbidity and Mortality Weekly Report* 58(11): 281–283.

Centers for Disease Control and Prevention. 2011. Vital signs: Current cigarette smoking among adults aged ≥18 years—United States, 2005–2010. *Morbidity and Mortality Weekly Report* (60)35: 1207–1212.

Centers for Disease Control and Prevention. 2011. National and state vaccination coverage among adolescents aged 13 through 17 years—United States, 2010. *Morbidity and Mortality Weekly Reports.* August 26, 60(33):1117–1123.

Chapman, P. B., et al. 2011. Improved survival with Vemurafenib in melanoma with BRAF V600E mutation. *New England Journal of Medicine* 364: 2507–2516.

Danaei, G., et al. 2005. Causes of cancer in the world: Comparative risk assessment of nine behavioral and environmental risk factors. *Lancet* 2005(366): 1784–1793.

Finn, O. J., 2008. Cancer immunology. *New England Journal of Medicine* 358(25): 2704–2715.

Gommans, J., et al. 2009. Preventing strokes: The assessment and management of people with transient ischemic attack. *New Zealand Medical Journal* 122(1293): 50–60.

Harvard Medical School. 2008. The status of statins. *Harvard Women's Health Watch* 15(6): 1–3.

Hodis, H. N., et al. 2012. The timing hypothesis for coronary heart disease prevention with hormone therapy: Past, present, and future in perspective. *Climacteric* 15(3): 217–228.

Hu, J. C., et al. 2008. Patterns of care for radical prostatectomy in the United States from 2003 to 2005. *Journal of Urology* 180(5): 1969–1974.

Jacobs, et al. 2012. Coronary artery calcium can predict all-cause mortality and cardiovascular events on low-dose CT screening for lung cancer. *AJR American Journal of Roentgenology* 198(3): 505–511.

Kauff, N. D., et al. 2008. Risk-reducing salpingo-oophorectomy for the prevention of BRCA1- and BRCA2-associated breast and gynecologic cancer: A multicenter, prospective study. *Journal of Clinical Oncology* 26(8): 1331–1337.

Marshall, D. A., et al. 2009. Achievement of heart health characteristics through participation in an intensive lifestyle change program (Coronary Artery Disease Reversal Study). *Journal of Cardiopulmonary Rehabilitation and Prevention* 29(2): 84–94.

Mirmiran, P., et al. 2009. Fruit and vegetable consumption and risk factors for cardiovascular disease. *Metabolism* 58(4): 460–468.

Müller, D., et al. 2006. How sudden is sudden cardiac death? *Circulation* 114(11): 1146–1150.

National Center for Health Statistics. 2012. Deaths: final data for 2008. *National Vital Statistics Reports* 58(19): 1–73.

Park, Y., et al. 2009. Dairy food, calcium, and risk of cancer in the NIH-AARP diet and health study. *Archives of Internal Medicine* 169(4): 391–401.

Pickering, T. G., et al. 2008. Call to action on use and reimbursement for home blood pressure monitoring: A joint scientific statement from the American Heart Association, American Society of Hypertension, and Preventive Cardiovascular Nurses Association. *Hypertension* 52(1): 10–29.

Raman, K., et al. 2012. Genetic markers of inflammation and their role in cardiovascular disease. *The Canadian Journal of Cardiology*, Sept. 19 (Epub ahead of print).

Robert, C., et al. 2011. Ipilimumab plus dacarbazine for previously untreated metastatic melanoma. *New England Journal of Medicine* 364: 2517–2526.

Samet, J., et al. 2009. Lung cancer in never smokers: Clinical epidemiology and environmental risk factors. *Clinical Cancer Research* 15(18): 5626–5645.

Schiller, J.S., et al. 2012. Summary health statistics for U.S. adults: National Health Interview Survey, 2010. National Center for Health Statistics. *Vital Health Stat* 10(252).

Schnell, O., M. Erbach, and M. Hummel. 2012. Primary and secondary prevention of cardiovascular disease in diabetes with aspirin. *Diabetes and Vascular Disease Research* 9(4): 245–255.

Slade, B. A., et al. 2009. Postlicensure safety surveillance for quadrivalent human papillomavirus recombinant vaccine. *Journal of the American Medical Association* 302(7): 750–757.

Stokes, N. A. 2012. The effect of the AED and AED programs on survival or individuals, groups, and populations. *Prehospital and Disaster Medicine*, August 21 (Epub ahead of print).

U.S. Department of Health and Human Services, Public Health Service, National Toxicology Program. 2005. *Report on Carcinogens*, 11th ed. Washington, DC.

U.S. Preventive Services Task Force. 2008. Screening for prostate cancer: U.S. Preventive Services Task Force recommendation statement. *Annals of Internal Medicine* 149(3): 185–191.

Vogel, V. G., et al. 2006. Effects of tamoxifen vs. raloxifene on the risk of developing invasive breast cancer and other disease outcomes: The NSABP Study of Tamoxifen and Raloxifene (STAR) P-2 Trial. *Journal of the American Medical Association* 295(23): 2727–2741.

BEHAVIOR CHANGE STRATEGY
Modifying Your Diet for Heart Health and Cancer Prevention

Gradually modifying your diet to include less saturated and trans fat and more fruits and vegetables can help you avoid both CVD and cancer in the future. Begin by assessing your current diet. Keep a record of everything you eat for a week. At the end of the week you can evaluate your diet and start taking steps to modify it.

Reducing Saturated and Trans Fat in Your Diet

The American Heart Association recommends that no more than 7% of the calories in your diet come from saturated fats and no more than 1% from trans fats. Similarly, the report of the 2010 Dietary Guidelines Advisory Committee recommends that Americans limit saturated fat intake to no more than 7% of daily calories and that they avoid trans fat from industrial sources completely and consume only small amounts (less than 0.5% of calories) of trans fat from natural sources. Foods high in these fats include red meat, poultry skin, full-fat dairy products, coconut and palm oils, and products made with hydrogenated vegetable oils, such as deep-fried fast food and packaged baked goods. Although food manufacturers are phasing out trans fats, it's important to read labels to see how much trans fat a product contains. If a product contains less than 0.5% trans fat, the manufacturer is allowed to list trans fat content as 0%.

To see if you are within the 7% and 1% limits, record the calories and the grams of fat next to the foods you've eaten during the week. This information is available on many food labels, in books, and on the Internet. Determine the percentage of daily calories as fat that you consumed for each day: multiply grams of saturated and trans fats by 9 (fat has 9 calories per gram)

and then divide by total calories. For example, if you consumed 30 grams of saturated and trans fats and 2100 calories on a particular day, then your saturated and trans fat consumption as a percentage of total calories would be calculated as $30 \times 9 = 270$ calories of fat $\div$ 2100 total calories = 0.13, or 13%.

To plan healthy changes, take a close look at your food record and try making healthy substitutions. Instead of a grilled cheese sandwich, try turkey, or substitute a plain baked potato for french fries. If you frequently eat in fast-food restaurants, try finding an appealing alternative—and recruit some friends to join you. When you choose foods that are rich in saturated fats, *watch your portion sizes carefully* and try to balance your choices throughout the day.

Many fruits and vegetables contain phytochemicals, compounds that help slow, stop, or even reverse the process of cancer. The National Cancer Institute (NCI) reports that people who eat five or more servings a day of fruits and vegetables have half the risk of cancer of those who eat fewer than two; according to the NCI, seven to nine servings or more per day are optimal.

Most Americans need to double the amount of fruits and vegetables they eat every day. After you have monitored your diet to assess your current intake, look for ways to incorporate more fruits and vegetables into your diet. Here are some tips to get you started.

Breakfast
- Drink fruit juice every morning.
- Add raisins, berries, or sliced fruit to cereal, pancakes, or waffles.
- Try a fruit smoothie made from fresh or frozen fruit and orange juice or low-fat yogurt.

Lunch
- Choose vegetable soup or salad with your meal.
- Replace potato chips or french fries with cut-up vegetables.
- Add vegetables such as roasted peppers, cucumber slices, shredded carrots, avocado, or salsa to sandwiches.

Dinner
- Choose a vegetarian main course, such as stir-fry or vegetable stew. Have at least two servings of vegetables with every dinner.
- Substitute vegetables for meat in casseroles and pasta and chili recipes.
- At the salad bar, pile your plate with healthful vegetables and use low-fat or nonfat dressing.

Snacks and On the Go
- Keep ready-to-eat-fruits and vegetables on hand (apples, plums, pears, and carrots).
- Keep small packages of dried fruit in the car (try dried apples, apricots, peaches, pears, and raisins).

The All-Stars
Different fruits and vegetables contribute different vitamins, phytochemicals, and other nutrients, so be sure to get a variety. The following types of produce are particularly rich in nutrients and phytochemicals:
- Cruciferous vegetables (broccoli, cauliflower, cabbage, bok choy, brussels sprouts, kohlrabi, turnips, etc.).
- Citrus fruits
- Berries
- Dark green leafy vegetables
- Deep yellow, orange, and red fruits and vegetables

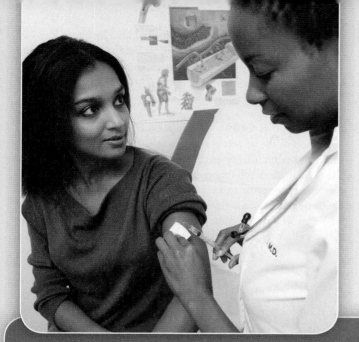

Immunity and Infection

13

Countless microscopic organisms live around, on, and in us. Although most microbes are beneficial, many of them can cause **infections** and infectious diseases, including sexually transmitted diseases. For the most part, the vigilance of our immune system keeps them at bay and our bodies healthy. The immune system protects us not just from **pathogens** but also from cancer.

This chapter introduces you to the mechanisms of immunity and infection, as well as strategies for keeping yourself well in a world of disease-causing microorganisms.

THE BODY'S DEFENSE SYSTEM

Our bodies have very effective ways of protecting themselves against invasion by foreign organisms. The **immune system** is the body's collective set of defenses that includes surface barriers as well as the specialized cells, tissues, and organs that carry out the immune reponse. The first line of defense is a formidable array of physical and chemical barriers. When these barriers are breached, cellular processes of the immune system come into play. Together these defenses provide an effective response to nearly all the invasions our bodies experience.

Physical and Chemical Barriers

The skin, the body's largest organ, prevents many microorganisms from entering the body. Although many bacterial and fungal organisms live on the surface of the skin, few can penetrate it except through a cut or break.

Wherever there is an opening in the body, or an area without skin, other barriers exist. All body cavities and passages that are exposed to the external environment are lined with mucous membranes, which secrete mucus and contain cells designed to prevent the passage of unwanted organisms and particles. This includes the mouth, nostrils, eyelids, bronchioles, vagina, and other organs of the respiratory, digestive, and urogenital tracts. The surface of both skin and mucous membranes is made of epithelial tissue, which consists of one or more layers of closely packed cells with almost no space between cells. The fluids that cover epithelial tissue, such as tears, saliva, and vaginal secretions, are rich in enzymes and other proteins that break down and destroy many microorganisms.

The respiratory tract is lined not only with mucous membranes but also with cells having hairlike protrusions called *cilia*. The cilia sweep foreign matter up and out of the respiratory tract. Particles that are not caught by this mechanism may be expelled from the system by a cough.

The Immune System: Cells, Tissues, and Organs

Beyond surface barriers, the immune system operates through a remarkable information network involving billions of cellular defenders that rush to protect the body when a threat arises. The immune system can be thought of as two systems—the innate immune system, which you are born with, and the adaptive immune system, which you acquire over time as you are exposed to microorgansms. The innate immune system is nonspecific; that is, it launches the same kind of defense regardless of the type of invading micoror- ganism. The adaptive immune system is very specific, operat- ing through mechanisms that work like a lock and key. The complete elimination of a pathogen involves the coordinated activities of both systems.

The immune system works through the action of different types of white blood cells, which are continuously produced in the bone marrow. A key feature of these cells is that they can distinguish foreign cells from the body's own cells.

Cells of the Innate Immune System
The cells of the innate immune system rec- ognize pathogens as "foreign" and kill them, but they cannot develop a memory of these pathogens. Thus they respond the same way no matter how many times a pathogen invades. *Neutrophils*, one type of white blood cell, travel in the bloodstream to ar- eas of invasion, attacking and ingesting pathogens. *Eosino- phils*, white blood cells that occur in mucosal tissues such as those in the gastrointestinal tract and the mammary glands, provide innate immunity to certain microbes. *Macrophages*, or "big eaters," act as scavengers, devouring pathogens and worn-out cells. *Natural killer cells* directly destroy virus-infected cells and cells that have turned cancerous. *Dendritic cells*, which reside in tissues, engulf pathogens and activate lymphocytes.

Cells of the Adaptive Immune System
The cells of the adaptive immune system are white blood cells called **lym- phocytes**. The two main types of lymphocytes are **T cells** and **B cells**, which differ in function. Whereas cells of the innate immune system can recognize a cell as foreign, lymphocytes are capable of exquisite specificity and of immunological memory.

Antigens and Antibodies
All of your body cells display markers on their surface that identify them as "self" to lym- phocytes. Invading microbes also display markers, and these markers identify them as foreign, or "nonself," to lymphocytes. Nonself markers that trigger an immune response are known as **antigens**.

Antibodies are specialized proteins that circulate in your bloodstream and are present in most body fluids. Produced by white blood cells, they have complementary markers on their surface that work with antigens like a lock and key, al- lowing them to recognize and neutralize specific microbes. When an antibody encounters an antigen with a complemen- tary pattern, it locks onto it and neutralizes it or tags it for attack by immune system cells.

T Cells and B Cells
When a B cell or T cell encounters the antigen for which it is specific, it proliferates, producing many more lymphocytes that are specific to the same antigen. These daughter cells then differentiate into cells with specific immune functions and attack the invading organisms. B cells become plasma cells that secrete antibodies. T cells differen- tiate into helper T cells, killer T cells, or suppressor T cells (also called regulatory T cells.) Some B and T cells become memory B and T cells, which can mount a rapid and power- ful response should they encounter the same invader months or even years in the future.

The Inflammatory Response
When injured or infected, the body reacts by pro- ducing an inflammatory response. Macro- phages, dendritic cells, and other specialized cells in the area of invasion or injury release **histamine** and other substances that cause blood vessels to dilate and fluid to flow out of capillaries into the injured tissue. This produces increased heat, swelling, and red- ness in the affected area. White blood cells are drawn to the area and attack the invaders, in many cases destroying them. At the site of infection there may be *pus*—a collection of dead white blood cells and debris resulting from the encounter.

> The immune system has a remarkable ability: it can **distinguish foreign cells from the body's own cells**.

TERMS

infection   Invasion of the body by a microorganism.

pathogen   A microorganism that causes disease.

immune system   The body's collective system of defenses that includes surface barriers as well as the specialized cells, tissues, and organs that carry out the immune reponse.

lymphocyte   A type of white blood cell that carries out important functions in the immune system.

T cell   A type of lymphocyte with specific immune system functions; T cells arise in bone marrow and mature in the thymus (thus the name).

B cell   A type of lymphocyte with specific immune system functions; B cells mature in the bone marrow and produce antibodies.

antigen   A marker on the surface of a foreign substance that immune system cells recognize as nonself; a foreign antigen's presence in the body triggers the immune response.

antibody   A specialized protein, produced by white blood cells, that can recognize and neutralize specific microbes.

histamine   A chemical responsible for the dilation and increased permeability of blood vessels in the inflammatory response.

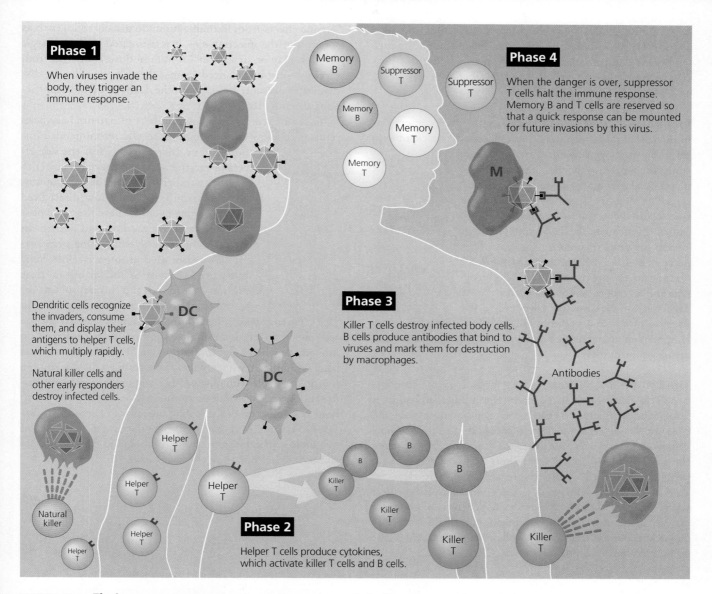

Phase 1

When viruses invade the body, they trigger an immune response.

Memory B

Suppressor T

Memory B

Memory T

Suppressor T

Memory T

Phase 4

When the danger is over, suppressor T cells halt the immune response. Memory B and T cells are reserved so that a quick response can be mounted for future invasions by this virus.

M

Dendritic cells recognize the invaders, consume them, and display their antigens to helper T cells, which multiply rapidly.

Natural killer cells and other early responders destroy infected cells.

DC

DC

Phase 3

Killer T cells destroy infected body cells. B cells produce antibodies that bind to viruses and mark them for destruction by macrophages.

Antibodies

Helper T

Helper T

Helper T

Helper T

Helper T

Natural killer

Killer T

B

B

B

Killer T

Killer T

Killer T

Killer T

Phase 2

Helper T cells produce cytokines, which activate killer T cells and B cells.

FIGURE 13.1 The immune response. Once invaded by a pathogen, the body mounts a complex series of reactions to destroy the invader. Pictured here are the phases of the immune response as the body responds to a virus.

The Immune Response   The immune response can be thought of as happening in four phases (Figure 13.1).

•   *Phase 1: Recognition.* Dendritic cells are drawn to the site of the injury and consume the foreign cells. They then migrate to nearby lymphoid tissue, where they activate T cells by displaying the foreign cells' antigen on their surfaces. Natural killer cells and other early responders destroy infected cells.

•   *Phase 2: Proliferation.* Helper T cells specific to the antigen multiply rapidly and stimulate the proliferation of killer T cells and B cells. Cytokines, which are chemical messengers secreted by lymphocytes and other cells of the immune system, help regulate and coordinate the immune response.

•   *Phase 3: Elimination.* Killer T cells strike at foreign cells and infected body cells, identifying them by the antigens displayed on the cell surfaces. Puncturing the cell membrane, they sacrifice body cells in order to destroy the foreign organism within. This type of action is known as a *cell-mediated immune response* because the attack is carried out by cells. Killer T cells also recruit more macrophages to help clean up the site.

B cells work in a different way. They produce large quantities of antibody molecules, which are released in the bloodstream and tissues. Antibodies bind to antigen-bearing targets and mark them for destruction by macrophages. This type of response is known as an *antibody-mediated immune response*. Cells of the innate immune system then eliminate the antibody-marked pathogens.

- **Phase 4: Slowdown.** Regulatory molecules and suppressor T cells inhibit lymphocyte proliferation and induce lymphocyte death, causing a slowdown of activity; this process restores "resting" levels of B and T cells. Some memory T and B cells remain in the body.

Immunity   After an infection, survival often confers **immunity**; that is, an infected person will not be susceptible to the same pathogen again. This is because some of the lymphocytes created during phase 2 of the immune response are reserved as memory T and B cells. As part of the acquired immune response, they continue to circulate in the blood and lymphatic system for years or even for the rest of the person's life. If the same antigen enters the body again, the memory T and B cells recognize and destroy it before it can cause illness. This subsequent response takes only a few days to initiate and prevents illness. The ability of memory lymphocytes to remember previous infections is known as **acquired immunity.**

The Lymphatic System   The lymphatic system consists of a network of vessels that carry a clear fluid called lymph; it also includes organs and structures, including the spleen and the lymph nodes, that function as part of the immune system. The lymphatic vessels pick up excess fluid from body tissues; the fluid passes through the lymph nodes, where macrophages and dendritic cells congregate. They help clear the fluid of debris and pathogens. Lymph nodes are also the sites where T cells and B cells are activated. When these nodes are actively involved in fighting an infection, they fill with cells. Physicians use the location of swollen lymph nodes as a clue to an infection's location and cause.

Immunization

The ability of the immune system to remember previously encountered organisms and retain its strength against them is the basis for **immunization.** When a person is immunized, the immune system is primed with an antigen similar to the pathogenic organism but not as dangerous. The body responds by producing antibodies, which prevent serious infection if the person is exposed to the disease organism itself. The preparations used to manipulate the immune system are known as **vaccines.**

Vaccines confer *active immunity*, meaning that the vaccinated person produces his or her own antibodies to the microorganism. This contrasts with *passive immunity*, which is conferred by injecting antibodies produced by other human beings or animals who have recovered from a given disease. Gamma globulin, a product made from the blood plasma of many individuals containing all the antibodies they have ever made, can provide a rapid but temporary immunity to a particular disease, or it can be used to treat antibody deficiency syndromes.

QUICK STATS

27 common diseases can be prevented by vaccines.

—CDC, 2012

Side effects from immunization are usually mild, such as soreness at the injection site. It is estimated that an allergic reaction may occur in 1 in 1.5 million doses. Any risk from vaccines must be balanced against the risk posed by the diseases they prevent; for example, the death rate from diphtheria is about 5–10%.

In recent years, increasing numbers of parents have been refusing to allow their children to receive recommended immunizations. Many parents fear the side effects of vaccinations, and they also object to the large number of recommended immunizations. Because of some now-discredited research, some people believe there is a possible link between vaccines and autism. In addition, the mercury-containing preservative thimerosol used in some vaccines came under fire as a cause of autism, but no clear link was ever found, and thimerosol was removed from pediatric vaccines beginning in 1999. Parents who refuse immunization for their children are relying on **herd immunity,** the immunity conferred on individuals when a significant portion of the community has been immunized, which makes it harder for a disease to get a foothold. People who rely on herd immunity are actually undermining it. With fewer immunizations in a community, herd immunity erodes, allowing outbreaks of infectious diseases to occur. This is believed to be the case in outbreaks of meningitis, measles, mumps, and whooping cough (pertussis) across the country in the last decade.

Ask Yourself

QUESTIONS FOR CRITICAL THINKING AND REFLECTION

What are your views on government-required child vaccinations? What has shaped your views on this issue?

TERMS

immunity   Resistance to infection.

acquired immunity   The body's ability to mobilize the cellular memory of an attack by a pathogen to prevent subsequent illness; acquired through the normal immune response and through vaccination.

immunization   The process of conferring immunity to a pathogen by administering a vaccine.

vaccine   A preparation of killed or weakened microorganisms, inactivated toxins, or components of microorganisms that is administered to stimulate an immune response; a vaccine protects against future infection by the pathogen.

herd immunity   A type of immunity that occurs when a significant proportion of a community has been vaccinated against a disease and that immunity confers protection on unvaccinated individuals.

Touring the Cardiorespiratory System

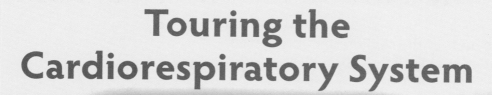

The Cardiorespiratory System

The Heart and Lungs

Atherosclerosis: The Process of Cardiovascular Disease

Diabetes: A Disorder of Metabolism

GOALS OF THE TOUR

1. **The Cardiorespiratory System.** Identify the parts of the cardiorespiratory system and the pattern of blood flow through the body.

2. **The Heart and Lungs.** Identify the chambers of the heart and describe the flow of blood through the right side of the heart to the lungs (pulmonary circulation) and through the left side of the heart to the body (systemic circulation).

3. **Atherosclerosis.** Explain the process of cardiovascular disease and compare and contrast the outcomes affecting the heart and the brain.

4. **Diabetes.** Describe how the body uses digested food for energy and growth and how this process is disrupted when a person has diabetes.

The Cardiorespiratory System

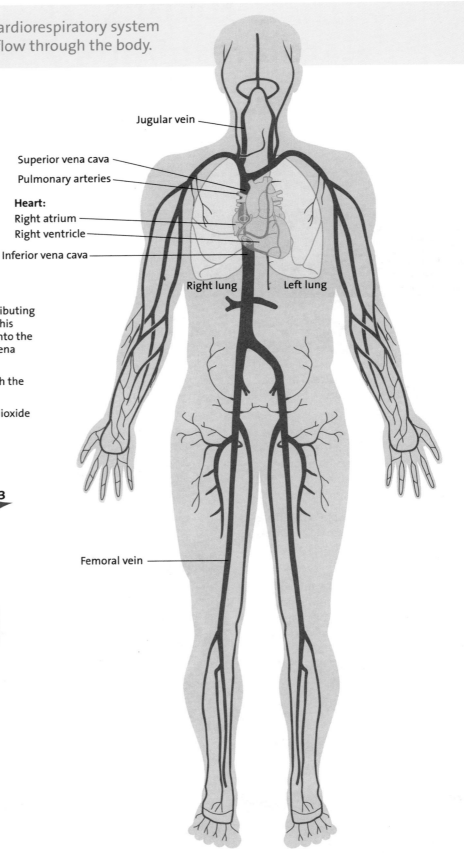

Jugular vein

Superior vena cava

Pulmonary arteries

Heart:
Right atrium
Right ventricle

Inferior vena cava

Right lung   Left lung

Femoral vein

Return of deoxygenated blood to the heart

1. Blood travels through the body, distributing oxygen and picking up carbon dioxide. This waste-laden, oxygen-poor blood flows into the right side of the heart via the superior vena cava and the inferior vena cava.

2. From there, blood is pumped through the pulmonary arteries into the lungs.

3. In the lungs, blood discards carbon dioxide and picks up oxygen.

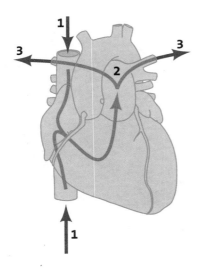

The Heart and Lungs

Identify the chambers of the heart and describe the flow of blood through the right side of the heart to the lungs (pulmonary circulation) and through the left side of the heart to the body (systemic circulation).

2

Blood is supplied to the heart muscle by the right and left coronary arteries, which branch off the aorta.

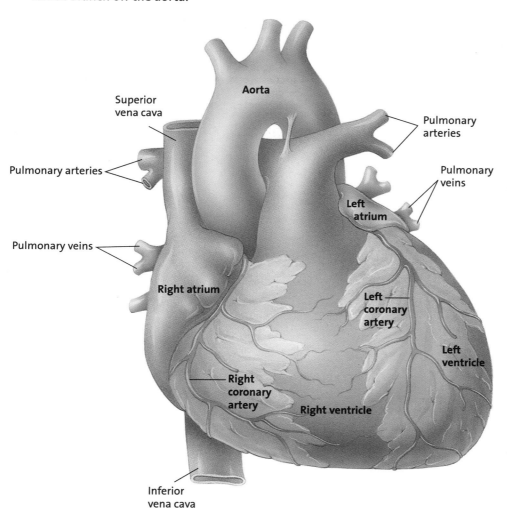

Atherosclerosis: The Process of Cardiovascular Disease

3 Explain the process of cardiovascular disease and compare and contrast the outcomes affecting the heart and the brain.

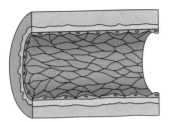

1. A healthy artery allows blood to flow through freely.

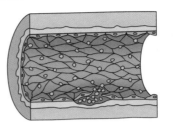 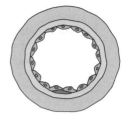

2. Plaque buildup begins when endothelial cells lining the arteries are damaged by smoking, high blood pressure, oxidized LDL cholesterol, and other causes. Excess cholesterol particles collect beneath these cells.

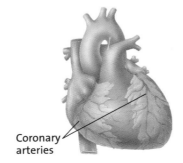

Coronary arteries

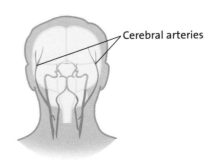

Cerebral arteries

Diabetes: A Disorder of Metabolism

Describe how the body uses digested food for energy and growth and how this process is disrupted when a person has diabetes.

Normal metabolism

1. When a meal is consumed, food is broken down into nutrients that the body can use to produce energy and build and nourish cells. Carbohydrates are broken down into glucose, which is the body's primary source of energy.

2. When glucose enters the bloodstream, the pancreas secretes the hormone insulin, which allows glucose to enter body cells.

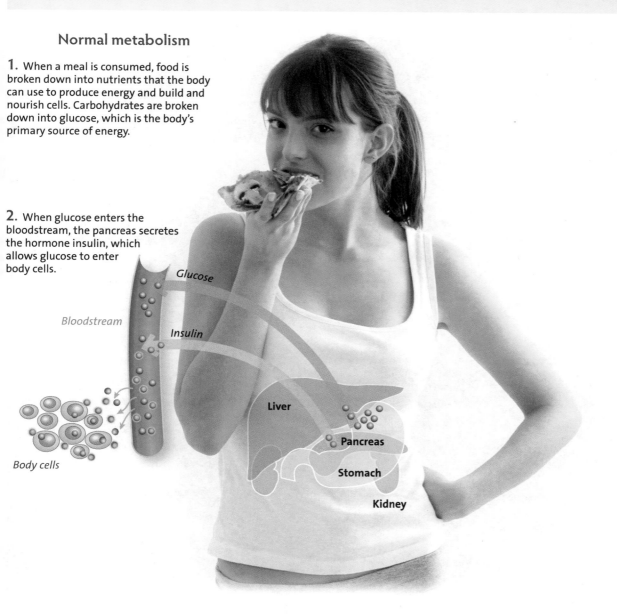

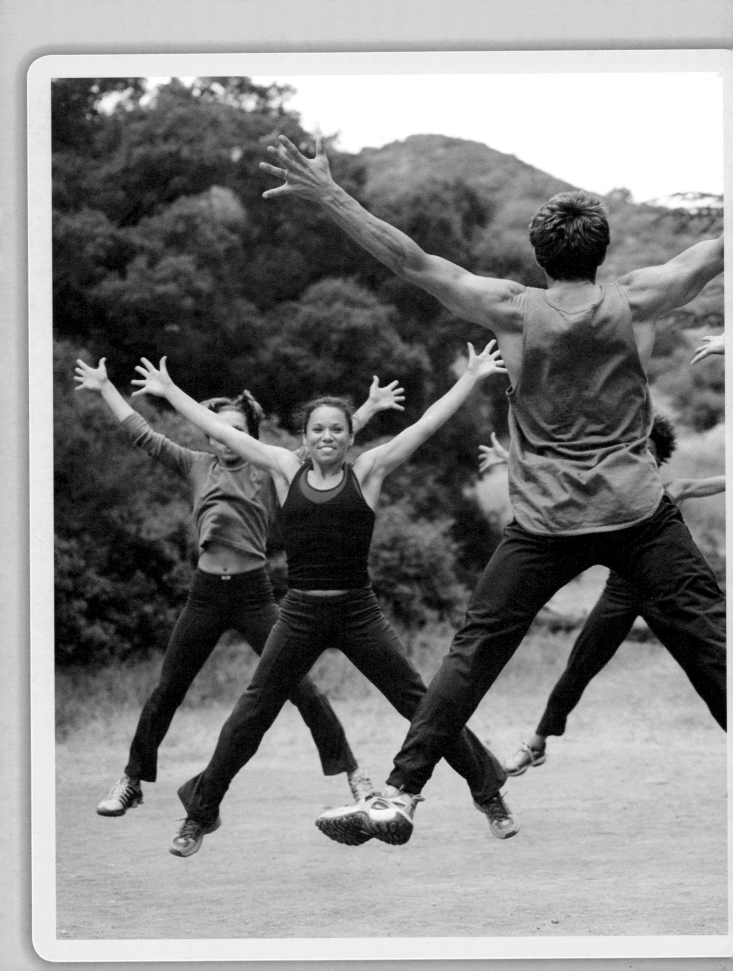

Allergy: The Body's Defense System Gone Haywire

Allergies result from a hypersensitive and overactive immune system. The immune system reacts to a harmless substance such as pollen or animal dander as if it were a harmful pathogen. For the most part, allergy symptoms—stuffy nose, sneezing, wheezing, skin rashes, and so on—are the result of the immune response.

Substances that provoke allergies are known as **allergens**. Common allergens include pollen, animal dander, dust mites and cockroaches, mold and mildew, insect stings, and some foods.

The Allergic Response   Most allergic reactions are due to an immune response that causes the release of large amounts of *histamine* and other compounds into surrounding tissues. Histamine has many effects, including increasing the inflammatory response and stimulating mucus production. In the nose, histamine may cause congestion and sneezing; in the eyes, itchiness and tearing; in the skin, redness, swelling, and itching; in the intestines, bloating and cramping; and in the lungs, coughing, wheezing, and shortness of breath. In some people, an allergen can trigger an **asthma** attack. Symptoms often occur immediately, within minutes of exposure.

The most serious, but rare, kind of allergic reaction is **anaphylaxis,** which results from a release of histamine throughout the body. Anaphylactic reactions can be life-threatening because symptoms may include swelling of the throat, extremely low blood pressure, fainting, heart arrhythmia, and seizures. Anaphylaxis is a medical emergency, and treatment requires immediate injection of epinephrine.

Dealing with Allergies   If you suspect you might have an allergy, visit your physician or an allergy specialist. You may be able to avoid or minimize exposure to allergens by changing your environment or behavior. For example, removing carpets from the bedroom and using special bedding can reduce dust mite contact. There are also medications available for allergy sufferers. Many over-the-counter antihistamines are effective at controlling symptoms, and prescription corticosteroids delivered by aerosol markedly reduce allergy symptoms. A third approach is immunotherapy, in which a person is desensitized to a particular allergen through the administration of gradually increasing doses of the allergen over a period of months or years.

THE SPREAD OF DISEASE

The immune system is operating at the cellular level at all times, maintaining its vigilance when you're well and fighting invaders when you're sick.

Symptoms and Contagion

The symptoms you experience during an illness are related to the phase of infection and the actions of your immune system. During the first phase of infection, **incubation,** when viruses or bacteria are actively multiplying before the immune system has gathered momentum, you may not have any symptoms of the illness, but you may be contagious. Symptoms first appear during the *prodromal period*, which follows incubation. If you have acquired immunity, the infection may be eradicated during the incubation period or the prodromal period. In this case it does not develop into a full-blown illness.

Many symptoms of an illness are actually due to the body's immune response rather than to the actions or products of the invading organism. For example, fever is caused by the release of certain cytokines during the immune response that cause the body's thermostat to be reset to a higher level. The resulting elevated temperature helps the body fight against pathogens by enhancing immune responses.

You may be contagious before you experience any symptoms, which means that you can transmit an illness without knowing you're infected or catch an illness from someone who doesn't appear to be sick. On the other hand, your symptoms may continue after the pathogens have been mostly destroyed, when you are no longer infectious.

The Chain of Infection

Infectious diseases are transmitted from one person to another through a series of steps—a chain of infection. The cycle begins with a *pathogen*, which has a natural environment—called a **reservoir**—in which it typically lives. This reservoir can be a person, an animal, or an environmental space like soil or water. To transmit infection, the pathogen must leave the reservoir through some *portal of exit*. In the case of a human reservoir, portals of exit include saliva, the mucous membranes, blood, feces, and nose and throat discharges. Next, there has to be a *means of transmission:* Transmission can

---

TERMS

allergy   A disorder caused by the body's exaggerated response to foreign chemicals and proteins; also called *hypersensitivity*.

allergen   A substance that triggers an allergic reaction.

asthma   A disease in which chronic inflammation and periodic constriction of the airways cause wheezing, shortness of breath, and coughing.

anaphylaxis   A severe systemic hypersensitive reaction to an allergen characterized by difficulty breathing, low blood pressure, heart arrhythmia, seizure, and sometimes death.

incubation   The period when bacteria or viruses are actively multiplying inside the body's cells; usually a period without symptoms of illness.

reservoir   A natural environment in which a pathogen typically lives.

occur directly or indirectly. In *direct transmission*, the pathogen is passed from one person to another without an intermediary. In *indirect transmission*, animals or insects such as rats, ticks, and mosquitoes serve as **vectors,** carrying the pathogen from one host to another. Pathogens can also be transmitted via contaminated soil, food, or water or from inanimate objects, such as eating utensils, doorknobs, and handkerchiefs.

To infect a new host, a pathogen must have a *portal of entry* into the body. Pathogens can enter through direct contact with or penetration of the skin or mucous membranes, inhalation, or ingestion. Pathogens that enter the skin or mucous membranes can cause a local infection of the tissue, or they may penetrate into the bloodstream or lymphatic system, thereby causing a **systemic infection**. Once in the *new host*, a variety of factors determine whether the pathogen will be able to establish itself and cause infection. If conditions are right, the pathogen will multiply and produce disease in the new host, who then becomes a reservoir from which a new chain of infection can be started.

Interrupting the chain of infection at any point can prevent disease. Strategies for breaking the chain include both public health measures and individual action. For example, a pathogen's reservoir can be isolated or destroyed, as when a sick individual is placed under quarantine or when insects or animals carrying pathogens are killed. Public sanitation practices, such as sewage treatment and the chlorination of drinking water, can also kill pathogens. Transmission can be disrupted through strategies like hand washing and the use of face masks. Immunization and the treatment of infected hosts can stop the pathogen from multiplying, producing a serious disease, and being passed on to a new host.

Epidemics and Pandemics

The rapid spread of a disease or health condition is called an **epidemic.** Although the word is usually used with reference to infectious diseases, it is also used for health conditions that are not caused by an infectious organism. For example, it is often said that obesity and diabetes have reached epidemic proportions in the United States.

> In an epidemic, the occurrence of the disease is greater than normally expected. Because the common cold occurs very frequently, it is **never classified as an epidemic**.

In an epidemic, the occurrence of the disease is greater than what is expected normally. Thus the common cold, which occurs with great frequency, is never classified as an epidemic. Conversely, the term *epidemic* is used to refer to outbreaks of diseases that are not widespread. For example, outbreaks of Ebola virus, which causes highly lethal hemorrhagic fever, are referred to as epidemics even though they have never been widespread.

A **pandemic** is an epidemic that has spread across a large area, such as an entire nation, a continent, or even the world. In contrast to the term *epidemic*, the term *pandemic* refers exclusively to infectious disease. Human history has been punctuated by numerous pandemics of various diseases, including bubonic plague, smallpox, and influenza. One of the most severe influenza pandemics occurred in 1918–1919, following World War 1, when 20–40% of the world's population became ill and as many as 40 million people died.

Not all widespread infectious diseases are pandemics. An infectious disease that is maintained in a human population or in a particular area in the absence of the introduction of an external infectious agent is said to be *endemic*. Endemic diseases generally occur at low frequency in particular populations or regions. For example, malaria is endemic to low-altitude areas of northern and eastern South Africa.

H1N1 Influenza   In 2009 an outbreak of influenza caused by a virus never before identified as a cause of human illness sparked fears of a worldwide influenza pandemic. Most people had no immunity to this new strain, initially called swine flu and subsequently labeled H1N1 influenza A virus. This strain resulted from a combination of genes from four different viruses: two from swine flu viruses, one from an avian (bird) flu virus, and one from a human flu virus. The addition of the gene from a human virus meant that humans could be infected with it, and, because it was new, they would have no prior immunity. In June 2009, the World Health Organization declared that a pandemic was under way. By February 2010, the WHO reported up to 86 million cases and up to nearly 18,000 deaths. By May of that year, flu activity had tapered off and declined to normal levels, but the WHO

TERMS

vector   An insect, rodent, or other organism that carries and transmits a pathogen from one host to another.

systemic infection   An infection spread by the blood or lymphatic system to large portions of the body.

epidemic   A rapidly spreading disease or health-related condition.

pandemic   A widespread epidemic.

continues to track trends globally, and the CDC continues to recommend H1N1 vaccination for persons aged 6 months to 24 years and people aged 25–64 years who are at high risk.

H5N1 Influenza Since 1998 scientists have been monitoring the progress of another influenza A virus known as H5N1, or avian (bird) influenza. This strain infects chickens, ducks, and geese as well as wild birds; it doesn't pass easily to humans or among humans, but when it does, it is deadly. According to recent WHO reports, more than 600 people worldwide have been infected with H5N1, and 350 of them have died.

Scientists studying the virus have been investigating how many mutations would be needed for H5N1 to pass easily among humans. In 2011 reports came that a lab in the Netherlands and another at the University of Wisconsin had succeeded in creating an airborne version of H5N1 with just four mutations. Before the studies could be published, the U.S. National Science Advisory Board on Biosafety requested that sensitive information about how the virus was created be withheld out of fear it could be used in a bioterrorist attack. By March 2012, however, public health officials decided that concerns were overblown, and the advisory board recommended that these studies be published in full.

PATHOGENS AND DISEASE

The pathogens that cause infectious diseases include bacteria, viruses, fungi, protozoa, parasitic worms, and prions (Figure 13.2).

Bacteria

The most abundant living things on earth are **bacteria,** which are single-celled organisms that usually reproduce by splitting in two to create a pair of identical cells. Bacteria are often classified by their shape: bacilli (rod-shaped), cocci (spherical), spirochete (spiral-chaped), or vibrios (comma-shaped).

Many species of bacteria are beneficial, but some are pathogenic, causing disease in their hosts. About 100 species of bacteria can cause disease in humans. We harbor both helpful and harmful bacteria on our skin and in our gastrointestinal and reproductive tracts. The human colon contains helpful bacteria that produce certain vitamins and help digest nutrients. Helpful bacteria also keep harmful bacteria in check by competing for food and resources and secreting substances toxic to pathogenic bacteria.

Pneumonia Inflammation of the lungs, called **pneumonia,** may be caused by infection with bacteria, viruses, or fungi or by contact with chemical toxins or irritants. Pneumonia can be serious if the alveoli (air sacs) become clogged with fluid, thus preventing oxygen from reaching the bloodstream. Pneumonia often follows another illness, such as a cold or the flu, but the symptoms are typically more severe—fever, chills, shortness of breath, increased mucus production, and cough. Pneumonia is one of the 10 leading causes of

death for Americans; people most at risk for severe infection include those under age 2 and over age 75 and those with chronic health problems such as heart disease, asthma, or HIV. Worldwide, pneumonia is the leading cause of death for children under 5 years of age.

The most common cause of bacterial pneumonia is *Streptococcus pneumoniae*, or pneumococcus. A vaccine is available for pneumoccocal pneumonia and is recommended for all adults aged 65 and older and others at risk. Mycoplasma is a very small bacterium; *M. pneumoniae* causes a mild form of pneumonia often called "walking pneumonia." Outbreaks of infection with mycoplasmas are relatively common among young adults, especially in crowded settings such as dormitories. Bacterial pneumonia can be treated with antibiotics.

Meningitis Inflammation of the *meninges*, the protective membranes covering the brain and spinal cord, is called **meningitis.** Most cases of meningitis are viral; they are usually mild and go away on their own. Bacterial meningitis, however, can be life-threatening and requires immediate treatment with antibiotics. Symptoms of meningitis include fever, a severe headache, stiff neck, sensitivity to light, and confusion. Immediate treatment is needed because death can occur within hours. The disease is fatal in about 10% of cases, and about 10–20% of people who recover have permanent disabilities, including brain damage, seizures, and hearing loss. Today *Neisseria meningitidis* (meningococcus) and *Streptococcus pneumoniae* (pneumococcus) are the leading causes of bacterial meningitis, particularly in adolescents and young adults (see the box "Meningococcal Meningitis and College Students").

Strep Throat and Other Streptococcal Infections The **streptococcus** bacterium can cause streptococcal pharyngitis, or strep throat, characterized by a red, sore throat with white patches on the tonsils, swollen lymph nodes, fever, and headache. It is typically spread through close contact with an infected person via respiratory droplets (sneezing or coughing). If left untreated, strep throat can develop into the more serious rheumatic fever. A particularly virulent type of streptococcus can invade the bloodstream, spread to other parts of the body, and produce dangerous systemic illness. It can also cause a serious but rare infection of the deeper layers

---

TERMS

bacterium (plural, bacteria) A microscopic single-celled organism that may be helpful or harmful to humans.

pneumonia Inflammation of the lungs, typically caused by infection or exposure to chemical toxins or irritants.

meningitis Infection of the meninges (membranes covering the brain and spinal cord).

streptococcus Any of a genus (*Streptococcus*) of spherical bacteria; streptococcal species can cause skin infections, strep throat, rheumatic fever, pneumonia, scarlet fever, and other diseases.

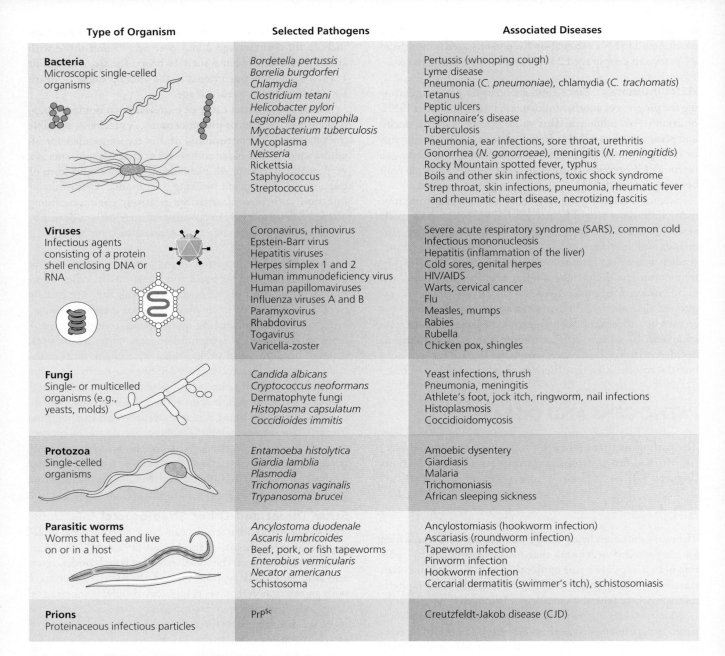

Type of Organism	Selected Pathogens	Associated Diseases
Bacteria Microscopic single-celled organisms	*Bordetella pertussis* *Borrelia burgdorferi* *Chlamydia* *Clostridium tetani* *Helicobacter pylori* *Legionella pneumophila* *Mycobacterium tuberculosis* Mycoplasma *Neisseria* Rickettsia Staphylococcus Streptococcus	Pertussis (whooping cough) Lyme disease Pneumonia (*C. pneumoniae*), chlamydia (*C. trachomatis*) Tetanus Peptic ulcers Legionnaire's disease Tuberculosis Pneumonia, ear infections, sore throat, urethritis Gonorrhea (*N. gonorroeae*), meningitis (*N. meningitidis*) Rocky Mountain spotted fever, typhus Boils and other skin infections, toxic shock syndrome Strep throat, skin infections, pneumonia, rheumatic fever and rheumatic heart disease, necrotizing fascitis
Viruses Infectious agents consisting of a protein shell enclosing DNA or RNA	Coronavirus, rhinovirus Epstein-Barr virus Hepatitis viruses Herpes simplex 1 and 2 Human immunodeficiency virus Human papillomaviruses Influenza viruses A and B Paramyxovirus Rhabdovirus Togavirus Varicella-zoster	Severe acute respiratory syndrome (SARS), common cold Infectious mononucleosis Hepatitis (inflammation of the liver) Cold sores, genital herpes HIV/AIDS Warts, cervical cancer Flu Measles, mumps Rabies Rubella Chicken pox, shingles
Fungi Single- or multicelled organisms (e.g., yeasts, molds)	*Candida albicans* *Cryptococcus neoformans* Dermatophyte fungi *Histoplasma capsulatum* *Coccidioides immitis*	Yeast infections, thrush Pneumonia, meningitis Athlete's foot, jock itch, ringworm, nail infections Histoplasmosis Coccidioidomycosis
Protozoa Single-celled organisms	*Entamoeba histolytica* *Giardia lamblia* *Plasmodia* *Trichomonas vaginalis* *Trypanosoma brucei*	Amoebic dysentery Giardiasis Malaria Trichomoniasis African sleeping sickness
Parasitic worms Worms that feed and live on or in a host	*Ancylostoma duodenale* *Ascaris lumbricoides* Beef, pork, or fish tapeworms *Enterobius vermicularis* *Necator americanus* Schistosoma	Ancylostomiasis (hookworm infection) Ascariasis (roundworm infection) Tapeworm infection Pinworm infection Hookworm infection Cercarial dermatitis (swimmer's itch), schistosomiasis
Prions Proteinaceous infectious particles	PrP^{Sc}	Creutzfeldt-Jakob disease (CJD)

FIGURE 13.2 Pathogens and associated infectious diseases.

of the skin, a condition called necrotizing fascitis or "flesh-eating strep."

Toxic Shock Syndrome and Other Staphylococcal Infections

The spherical-shaped **staphylococcus** bacterium can cause infections ranging from minor skin infections such as boils to very serious conditions such as blood infections and pneumonia. *Staphylococcus aureus* is responsible for many cases of toxic shock syndrome (TSS). The bacteria produce a toxin that results in tissue damage, widespread coagulation of blood in the blood vessels, and ultimately organ failure.

A very serious antibiotic-resistant infection is caused by a staphylococcus bacterium known as methicillin-resistant *Staphylococcus aureus* (MRSA). Many cases of MRSA infection occur in hospitalized patients, and these infections tend

When meningitis is caused by the bacterium *Neisseria meningitidis*, it is called meningococcal meningitis. Although rates of this disease have been declining since the 1990s, it still causes deaths. The disease is spread by the exchange of respiratory and throat secretions (as in coughing and sneezing) and through person-to-person contact (as in kissing); it can readily spread among people living in close quarters.

In the United States nearly 30% of meningitis cases occur in adolescents and young adults, and there is an increased risk in college students. Lifestyle factors, such as crowded living situations, irregular sleep patterns, sharing of personal items, bar patronage, and smoking (active or passive) all increase the risk for meningococcal miningitis.

A vaccine is available that protects agains four of the five most common strains of *N. meningiditis*. Because rates of the disease rise beginning in early adolescence and peak between ages 15 and 20, the CDC and the American College Health Association recommend vaccination for all unvaccinated first-year college students living in dormitories, and some schools require it. In 2012 Texas became the first state to require all college students, even those living off campus, to be vaccinated against meningitis.

A person diagnosed with meningococcal meningitis is treated with antibiotics, and often those who have direct contact with the patient, such as housemates, roommates, and romantic partners, are also given antibiotics. Besides being vaccinated, you can protect yourself against meningococcal meningitis by getting enough sleep, not smoking and not being around tobacco smoke, and avoiding people who are sick.

SOURCES: Centers for Disease Control and Prevention. 2012. *Meningitis* (http://www.cdc.gov/meningitis/index.html); American College Health Association. 2009. *Meningitis on Campus* (http://www.acha.org/projects_programs/meningitis/disease_info.cfm).

---

to be severe. MRSA is also common in the community (outside hospital settings), where it usually infects the skin, causing painful lesions that resemble infected spider bites. The spread of MRSA infection is associated with places where people are in close contact with one another, such as locker rooms and playing fields; athletes are particularly at risk and should keep any cuts or abrasions covered.

Tuberculosis   Caused by the bacterium *Mycobacterium tuberculosis*, **tuberculosis (TB)** is a chronic bacterial infection that usually affects the lungs, though it can affect other organs as well. Symptoms include coughing, fatigue, night sweats, weight loss, and fever. Between 10 and 15 million Americans have been infected with *M. tuberculosis* and continue to carry it. Only about 10% of people with latent TB infections actually develop an active case of the disease; the immune system usually prevents the disease from becoming active. In the United States, active TB is most common among people infected with HIV, recent immigrants from countries where TB is endemic, and those who live in inner cities.

Many strains of tuberculosis respond to antibiotics, but only over a course of treatment lasting 6–12 months. Failure to complete treatment can lead to relapse and the development of strains of antibiotic-resistant bacteria. Multidrug-resistant TB (MDR TB) is resistant to at least two of the best anti-TB drugs. Extensively drug-resistant TB (XDR TB) is resistant to those drugs as well as some second-line drugs. TB is a leading cause of death in people with HIV infection.

Tickborne Infections   Lyme disease is spread by the bite of a tick that is infected with the spiral-shaped bacterium *Borrelia burgdorferi*. The deer tick is responsible for transmitting Lyme disease bacteria to humans in the northeastern and north-central United States; on the Pacific Coast, the culprit is the western black-legged tick.

Symptoms of Lyme disease vary but typically occur in three stages. In the first stage, about 80% of victims develop a bull's-eye-shaped red rash expanding from the area of the bite, usually about two weeks after the bite occurs. The second stage occurs weeks to months later in 10–20% of untreated patients; symptoms can include impaired coordination, partial facial paralysis, and heart rhythm abnormalities. The third stage, which occurs in about half of untreated people, can develop months or years after the tick bite and usually consists of chronic or recurring arthritis. Lyme disease is preventable by avoiding contact with ticks or by removing a tick before it has had the chance to transmit the infection.

Rocky Mountain spotted fever is also transmitted via a tick bite; it is characterized by sudden onset of fever, headache, and muscle pain, followed by development of a spotted rash.

Other Bacterial Infections   The following are a few of the many other infections caused by bacteria:

- *Ulcers:* Up to 90% of ulcers are caused by infection with the bacterium *Helicobacter pylori*. If tests show the presence of *H. pylori*, antibiotics often cure the infection and the ulcers.

> **QUICK STATS**
>
> **One-third** of the world's population is infected with tuberculosis.
>
> —CDC, 2012

> **TERMS**
>
> **tuberculosis (TB)**   A chronic bacterial infection that usually affects the lungs.

• **Tetanus:** Also known as lockjaw, tetanus is caused by the bacterium *Clostridium tetani*, which thrives in deep puncture wounds and produces a deadly toxin. Due to widespread vaccination, tetanus is rare in the United States, but worldwide, more than 200,000 people die from tetanus each year.

• **C. diff:** Another type of *Clostridium* bacteria, called *Clostridium difficile* (*C. diff*), has joined MRSA as a major emerging threat in American health care settings, particularly hospitals. It causes inflammation of the colon, resulting in diarrhea, fever, and nausea. The CDC recommends that doctors, nurses, and other health care providers wash their hands frequently to reduce the spread of the bacterium.

• **Pertussis:** Also known as whooping cough, pertussis is a highly contagious respiratory illness caused by the bacterium *Bordetella pertussis*. Those at high risk include infants and children who are too young to be fully vaccinated. Adolescents and adults become susceptible when immunity from vaccination wanes, so a booster shot is recommended at 11–12 years and thereafter every 10 years.

• **Urinary tract infections (UTIs):** Infection of the bladder and urethra is most common among sexually active women, but UTIs can occur in anyone. The bacterium *Escherichi coli* is the most common infectious agent, responsible for about 80% of all UTIs.

Antibiotic Treatments   **Antibiotics** are both naturally occurring and synthetic substances that can kill bacteria. Most antibiotics work in a similar fashion: they interfere with the reproduction of bacteria. Antibiotics are among the most widely prescribed and most effective drugs. Overuse of antibiotics has led to an increase in bacterial resistance to their effects. When exposed to antibiotics, resistant bacteria can grow and flourish while the antibiotic-sensitive bacteria die off. Antibiotic-resistant strains of many common bacteria have developed, including strains of gonorrhea, salmonella, and tuberculosis. Antibiotic resistance is a major factor contributing to the rise in problematic infectious diseases.

Resistance is promoted when people fail to take the full course of an antibiotic or when they inappropriately take antibiotics for viral infections. Another possible source of resistance is the use of antibiotics in agriculture, which is estimated to account for 50–80% of the 25,000 tons of antibiotics used annually in the United States. You can help prevent the development of antibiotic-resistant strains of bacteria by using antibiotics properly. Don't ask your doctor for an antibiotic every time you get sick. Antibiotics are helpful for bacterial infections but are ineffective against viruses. Use antibiotics as directed, and finish the full course of medication even if you begin to feel better. Never take an antibiotic without a prescription.

Viruses

A **virus** is a microscopic organism consisting of genetic material covered by a protein coat. Viruses lack the enzymes essential to energy production and protein synthesis in normal animal cells, and they can replicate only inside the cells of another organism. Once a virus is inside the host cell, it sheds its protein covering and exploits the host's cellular machinery to produce more viruses like itself. Most contagious diseases are caused by viruses.

The Common Cold   A cold may be caused by any of more than 200 different viruses that attack the lining of the nasal passages. Cold viruses are almost always transmitted by hand-to-hand contact. To lessen your risk of contracting a cold, wash your hands frequently; if you touch someone else, avoid touching your face until after you've washed your hands. If you catch a cold, over-the-counter cold remedies like decongestants and antihistamines may relieve your symptoms and make you more comfortable, but they do not eliminate the virus. The jury is still out on whether other remedies, including zinc gluconate lozenges, Echinacea, and vitamin C, relieve symptoms or shorten the duration of a cold. Antibiotics will not help a cold, unless a bacterial infection is also present, such as a sinus infection.

Influenza   Commonly called the flu, **influenza** is an infection of the respiratory tract caused by the influenza virus. Compared to the common cold, influenza is a more serious illness, usually including a fever and extreme fatigue. Most people who get the flu recover within 1–2 weeks, but some develop potentially life-threatening complications, such as pneumonia. The highest rates of infection occur in children. Influenza is highly contagious and is spread via respiratory droplets. The most effective way of preventing the flu is through annual vaccination. The CDC recommends vaccination for all people aged 6 months and older.

Chicken Pox, Cold Sores, and Other Herpesvirus Infections   The **herpesviruses** are a large group of viruses. Once infected, the host is never free of the virus. The virus lies latent within certain cells and becomes active periodically, producing symptoms. The family of herpesviruses includes varicella-zoster virus, which causes chicken pox and shingles;

> **Antibiotics are not effective against viral illnesses.** Talk to your doctor before taking antibiotics.

> **TERMS**
>
> **antibiotics**   Synthetic or naturally occurring substances used as drugs to kill bacteria.
>
> **virus**   A very small infectious agent composed of nucleic acid (DNA or RNA) surrounded by a protein coat; lacks an independent metabolism and reproduces only within a host cell.
>
> **influenza**   Infection of the respiratory tract by the influenza virus, which is highly infectious and prone to variation; the form changes so rapidly that every year new strains arise; commonly known as the flu.
>
> **herpesvirus**   A large family of viruses responsible for cold sores, mononucleosis, chicken pox, shingles, and the STD herpes; causes latent infections.

herpes simplex virus (HSV) types 1 and 2, which cause cold sores and the STD herpes; and epstein-Barr virus (EBV), which causes infectious mononucleosis. Two herpesviruses that can cause severe infections in people who have a suppressed immune system are cytomegalovirus (CMV), which infects the lungs, brain, colon, and eyes, and human herpesvirus 8 (HHV-8), which has been linked to Kaposi's sarcoma, a cancer of the connective tissue.

Viral Hepatitis   Viral **hepatitis** is a term used to describe several different infections that cause inflammation of the liver. Hepatitis is usually caused by one of the three most common hepatitis viruses. Hepatitis A virus (HAV) causes the mildest form of the disease and is usually transmitted by food or water contaminated by sewage or an infected person. Hepatitis B virus (HBV) is usually transmitted sexually Hepatitis C virus (HCV) can also be transmitted sexually, but it is much more commonly passed through direct contact with infected blood via injection drug use or, prior to the development of screening tests, blood transfusions. HBV and, to a lesser extent, HCV can also be passed from a pregnant woman to her child.

There are effective vaccines for hepatitis A and B. Symptoms of acute hepatitis infection can include fatigue, **jaundice,** abdominal pain, loss of appetite, nausea, and diarrhea. Most people recover from hepatitis A within a month or so. However, 5–10% of people infected with HBV and 85–90% of people infected with HCV become chronic carriers of the virus, capable of infecting others for the rest of their lives. Some chronic carriers remain asymptomatic, while others slowly develop chronic liver disease, cirrhosis, or liver cancer. The extent of HCV infection has only recently been recognized, and most infected people are unaware of their condition. To ensure proper treatment and prevention, testing for HCV may be recommended for people at risk, including people who have ever injected drugs (even once), who received a blood transfusion or a donated organ prior to July 1992, who have engaged in high-risk sexual behavior, or who have had body piercing, tattoos, or acupuncture involving unsterile equipment. If you are thinking of getting a tattoo or body piercing, choose the artist carefully and follow aftercare directions.

Human Papillomavirus (HPV)   The more than 100 different types of HPV cause a variety of warts, including common warts on the hands, plantar warts on the soles of the feet, and genital warts around the genitalia. Depending on their location, warts may be removed using over-the-counter preparations or professional methods such as laser surgery or cryosurgery. Because HPV infection is chronic, warts can reappear despite treatment. HPV causes the majority of cases of cervical cancer. Two HPV vaccines are available and recommended for girls age 9–12, but may also be taken up to age 26. Experts now advise that boys receive HPV vaccine to protect them against genital warts and prevent certain cancers later in life.

Treating Viral Illnesses   Antiviral drugs typically work by interfering with some part of the viral life cycle; for example,

they may prevent a virus from entering body cells or from successfully reproducing within cells. Antivirals are currently available to fight infections caused by HIV, influenza, herpes simplex, varicella-zoster, HBV, and HVC. Most other viral diseases must simply run their course.

Fungi

A **fungus** is an organism that reproduces by spores and feeds on organic matter. Only about 50 of the many thousands of species of fungi cause disease in humans, and these diseases are usually restricted to the skin, mucous membranes, and lungs. Some fungal diseases are extremely difficult to treat because spores are an especially resistant dormant stage of the organism.

Candida albicans is a common fungus found naturally in the vagina of most women. When excessive growth occurs, the result is itching and discomfort, commonly known as a yeast infection. Other common fungal conditions, including athlete's foot, jock itch, and ringworm, affect the skin. These three conditions are usually mild and easy to cure. Fungi can also cause systemic diseases that are severe, life-threatening, and extremely difficult to treat. Fungal infections can be especially deadly in people with impaired immune systems.

Protozoa

Protozoa are single-celled organisms that can cause a range of diseases in humans. Millions of people in developing countries suffer from protozoal infections. **Malaria,** caused by a parasitic protozoan of the genus *Plasmodium*, is a major killer worldwide; each year there are 350–500 million new cases of malaria globally and more than 1 million deaths, mostly among infants and children. Drug-resistant strains of malaria have emerged, requiring new medicines.

Giardiasis is caused by *Giardia lamblia*, a single-celled parasite that lives in the intestines of humans and animals. Giardiasis is characterized by nausea, diarrhea, bloating, and abdominal cramps, and it is among the most common waterborne diseases in the United States. People may become infected with *Giardia* if they consume contaminated food or water.

TERMS

hepatitis   Inflammation of the liver, which can be caused by infection, drugs, or toxins.

jaundice   Increased bile pigment levels in the blood, characterized by yellowing of the skin and the whites of the eyes.

fungus   A single-celled or multicelled organism that reproduces by spores and feeds on organic matter; examples include molds, mushrooms, and yeasts. Fungal diseases include yeast infections, athlete's foot, and ringworm.

protozoan (plural, protozoa)   A microscopic single-celled organism that often produces recurrent, cyclical attacks of disease.

malaria   A severe, recurrent, mosquito-borne infection caused by the parasitic protozoan *Plasmodium*.

giardiasis   An intestinal disease caused by the parasitic protozoan *Giardia lamblia*.

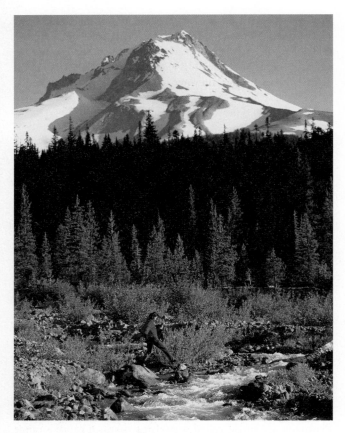

Even seemingly pristine mountain streams can be contaminated with the protozoan Giardia lamblia, as many unwary hikers and campers have discovered. Symptoms of giardiasis include abdominal pain, bloating, and diarrhea.

Parasitic Worms

The **parasitic worms** are the largest organisms that can enter the body to cause infection. They include tapeworms, hookworms, pinworms, and flukes. They cause a variety of relatively mild infections, primarily of the intestines. Worm infections generally originate from contaminated food or drink and can be prevented by careful attention to hygiene.

Prions

In recent years, several fatal degenerative disorders of the central nervous system have been linked to **prions,** or *proteinaceous infectious particles.* Unlike all other infectious agents, prions appear to lack DNA or RNA and to consist only of

protein; their presence in the body does not trigger an immune response. Prions are associated with a class of diseases known as *transmissible spongiform encephalopathies (TSEs),* which are characterized by spongelike holes in the brain. Symptoms of TSEs include loss of coordination, weakness, dementia, and death. Known prion diseases include Creutzfeldt-Jakob disease (CJD) in humans; bovine spongiform encephalopathy (BSE), or mad cow disease, in cattle; and scrapie in sheep. Some prion diseases are inherited or the result of spontaneous genetic mutations, whereas others are the result of eating infected tissue or being exposed to prions during medical procedures such as organ transplants.

Emerging Infectious Diseases

Emerging infectious diseases are infections whose incidence in humans has increased or threatens to increase in the near future. They include both known diseases that have experienced a resurgence, such as tuberculosis and cholera, and diseases that were previously unknown or confined to specific areas, such as the Ebola and West Nile viruses.

Selected Infections of Concern   Although the chances of the average American contracting an exotic infection are very low, emerging infections are a concern to public health officials and represent a challenge to all nations in the future.

WEST NILE VIRUS   A mini-outbreak of encephalitis in New York in 1999 led to identification of this virus, which had previously been restricted to Africa, the Middle East, and parts of Europe. Between 1999 and 2007 the virus spread across the United States and caused more than 27,605 cases of human illness and 1086 deaths. West Nile virus is carried by birds and then passed to humans when mosquitoes bite first an infected bird and then a person. Most people who are bitten have few or no symptoms, but the virus can cause permanent brain damage or death in some.

SEVERE ACUTE RESPIRATORY SYNDROME (SARS)   In February 2003 SARS appeared in southern China and quickly spread to more than 15 countries; it is a form of pneumonia that is fatal in 5–15% of cases. SARS is caused by a type of coronavirus found in wildlife that may have crossed the species barrier. By 2004 SARS had been responsible for more than 8000 illnesses and 800 deaths, but there have been no new cases reported since 2004.

ROTAVIRUS   The leading viral cause of gastroenteritis, an intestinal inflammation that results in vomiting and diarrhea, rotavirus infects almost every child at one time or another. Worldwide, the virus kills about 600,000 children each year, mostly in developing countries. Left untreated, rotavirus-induced diarrhea can become severe and lead to dehydration, which can be fatal. Rotavirus spreads through poor hygiene and sanitation practices.

ESCHERICHIA COLI O157:H7   This potentially deadly strain of *E. coli,* transmitted in contaminated food, can cause bloody diarrhea and kidney damage. In 2012 an outbreak reported

> **TERMS**
>
> **parasitic worm**   A pathogen that causes intestinal and other infections; includes tapeworms, hookworms, pinworms, and flukes.
>
> **prions**   Proteinaceous infectious particles; infectious agents thought to be responsible for a class of neurodegenerative diseases known as transmissible spongiform encephalopathies.

in nine states was traced to contaminated romaine lettuce. Other outbreaks have been linked to ground beef, alfalfa sprouts, unpasteurized juice, petting zoos, and contaminated public swimming pools. An estimated 70,000 cases and 61 deaths occur in the United States each year.

HANTAVIRUS Since hantavirus pulmonary syndrome (HPS) was first recognized in 1993, over 300 cases have been reported in the United States. HPS is caused by the rodent-borne Sin Nombre virus (SNV) and is spread primarily through airborne viral particles from rodent urine, droppings, or saliva. It is characterized by a dangerous fluid buildup in the lungs and is fatal in about 45% of cases. In 2012, an outbreak of hantvirus caused the death of at least three campers in Yosemite National Park.

EBOLA Outbreaks of the often fatal Ebola hemorrhagic fever (EHF) have occurred only in Africa. The Ebola virus is transmitted by contact with infected blood or other body secretions. Because symptoms appear quickly and 70% of victims die, usually within a few days, the virus tends not to spread widely.

Factors Contributing to Emerging Infections What's behind this rising tide of infectious diseases? One factor is drug resistance. New or increasing drug resistance has been found in organisms that cause malaria, tuberculosis, gonorrhea, influenza, AIDS, and pneumococcal and staphylococcal infections. Some bacterial strains now appear to be resistant to all available antibiotics.

Another factor is poverty. More than 1 billion people live in extreme poverty, and half the world's population has no regular access to essential drugs. Population growth, urbanization, overcrowding, and migration (including the movement of refugees) also spread infectious diseases. A poor public health infrastructure is often associated with poverty and social upheaval, but problems such as contaminated water supplies can occur even in industrial countries. Inadequate vaccination has led to the reemergence of diseases such as diphtheria and pertussis. Natural disasters such as hurricanes also disrupt the public health infrastructure, leaving survivors with contaminated water and food supplies and no shelter from disease-carrying insects.

Travel, commerce, and mass food production and distribution also contribute, as do human behaviors. More than 500 million travelers cross national borders each year, and international tourism and trade open the world to infectious agents. SARS was quickly spread throughout the world by infected air travelers. Food now travels long distances to our table, and microbes are transmitted along with it. Mass production of food increases the likelihood that a chance contamination can lead to mass illness. The widespread use of injectable drugs rapidly transmits HIV infection and hepatitis. Changes in sexual behavior over the past 40 years have led to a proliferation of old and new STDs. The use of day care facilities for children has led to increases in the incidence of several infections that cause diarrhea. Finally, the deliberate release of deadly infectious agents is an ongoing concern. Potential bioterrorism agents that the CDC categorizes as a highest concern are those that can be easily disseminated or transmitted from person to person and that have a high mortality rate and the potential for a major public health impact. These include anthrax, smallpox, plague, botulism, and viral hemorrhagic fevers such as Ebola.

Immune Disorders

Considering the compexity of the immune system, it is not surprising that some disorders and diseases occur when the system fails to operate properly. When the immune system loses the ability to recognize body cells and tissues as "self," the result is an autoimmune disease. In most autoimmune diseases, the immune system targets or destroys specific tissues. For example, in type 1 diabetes, the insulin-producing cells of the pancreas are destroyed. In multiple sclerosis, the protective coating around nerves is targeted and destroyed. In rheumatoid arthritis, the membranes lining the joints are destroyed. The causes of autoimmune diseases are not well understood, but the rates of many of these diseases are much higher in women than in men. The role of estrogen is under investigation as a contributing factor in this discrepancy, as is the somewhat enhanced immunity of women compared to men.

Sometimes the immune system loses its ability to detect and destroy cells that have become abnormal, as in the case of cancerous mutations. This can happen when people get older, when they have certain immune disorders (like HIV infection), or when the immune system is suppressed by chemotherapy or other drugs. Cancer cells may multiply uncontrollably before the immune system is able to respond sufficiently. In recent years, conventional cancer treatments have been augmented with a treatment known as immunotherapy. The goal of immunotherapy is to stimulate the patient's immune system to attack tumor cells. Cancer-specific vaccines are also under development.

> Some bacterial strains now appear to be **resistant to all available antibiotics**.

SUPPORTING YOUR IMMUNE SYSTEM

You can help ensure the optimal functioning of your immune system by choosing healthy behaviors. Here are some general guidelines for supporting your immune system:

- Eat a balanced diet and maintain a healthy weight.

- Get enough sleep. Most people need about eight hours every night.

- Exercise, but not when you're sick.

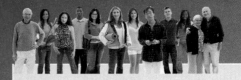

In 2011 the world marked the 30th year since AIDS was diagnosed in five young gay men in Los Angeles. HIV is now a worldwide scourge, with 65 million people infected and more than 25 million deaths since the epidemic began.

The vast majority of cases—95%—have occurred in developing countries, where heterosexual contact is the primary means of transmission, responsible for 85% of all adult infections. HIV continues to be a disease that disproportionately affects ethnic minorities and the poor. Worldwide, women are the fastest-growing group of newly infected people; half of adults living with HIV in 2010 were women. In sub-Saharan Africa, the region most heavily burdened with HIV, 59% of adults living with HIV were women. About 3.4 million children were living with HIV in 2010, and more than 90% of these children were living in sub-Saharan Africa.

Despite the ongoing tragedy of the HIV epidemic, strides have been made in treatment and prevention measures. In 2003 only 7% of HIV-infected individuals in low- and middle-income countries were receiving antiretroviral treatment; by the end of 2010 that percentage had increased to 47%. In 2010, 67% of pregnant women received treatment to prevent transmission of HIV to their babies, up from just 10% in 2004. Treating HIV with effective drugs not only prolongs life and decreases suffering—it also has a major impact in reducing the spread of the virus because treated individuals are generally much less infectious than untreated people.

The HIV epidemic seems to have stabilized in many parts of the world. Rates of new infections have remained steady or have even dropped in a few regions. Though sub-Saharan Africa remains the hardest-hit area of the world, the number of new infections dropped from 2.2 million in 2001 to 1.8 million in 2009. The expanded availability of antiretroviral medications to this region has contributed significantly to this decline, with a 20% drop in AIDS-related deaths between 2004 and 2009 alone. Still, two-thirds of all HIV-infected people in the world live in sub-Saharan Africa, and nearly three-quarters of all deaths due to AIDS in 2009 occurred there.

Eastern Europe and parts of Asia have also been hit hard by HIV. In many of these areas, HIV infection is seen in intravenous drug users and their sexual partners.

Efforts to combat AIDS are complicated by political, economic, and cultural barriers. Education and prevention programs are often hampered by resistance from social and religious institutions and by the taboo on openly discussing sexual issues. Condoms are not commonly used in many countries, and women in many societies do not have sufficient control over their lives to demand that men use condoms during sex. Empowering women is a crucial priority in reducing the spread of HIV. In particular, reducing sexual violence against women, promoting financial independence, and increasing women's education and employment opportunities are essential.

Successful prevention approaches include STD treatment and education, public education campaigns about safer sex, and syringe exchange programs for injection drug users. Efforts are ongoing to improve access to barrier protective devices such as condoms. Other measures have included male circumcision, which has been shown to reduce HIV transmission in some studies.

In developed nations such as the United States, new drugs are easing AIDS symptoms and lowering viral levels dramatically for some patients. In the past few years, a growing number of people in poor countries have gained access to antiviral drugs because of the introduction of inexpensive generic drugs and increased international funding for HIV treatment. Still, far too many people with HIV remain untreated, and far too many new infections are occurring.

- Don't smoke.

- If you drink alcohol, do so only in moderation.

- Make sure that you have sufficient vitamin D in your diet. Vitamin D deficiency has been implicated in several allergic and autoimmune disorders.

- Wash your hands frequently. Use hand sanitizer not antibacterial soap—when soap and water aren't available.

- Avoid contact with people who are contagious with an infectious disease.

- Make sure you drink water only from clean sources.

- Avoid contact with disease carriers such as rodents, mosquitoes, and ticks.

- Practice safer sex, and don't use injectable drugs.

- Make sure you have received all your recommended vaccinations, and keep them up-to-date.

THE MAJOR STDs

Sexually transmitted diseases (STDs)—also called sexually transmitted infections (STIs)—spread from person to person mainly through sexual activity. STDs are a particularly

> **sexually transmitted disease (STD) or sexually transmitted infection (STI)**   A disease that is mainly transmitted by sexual contact; some can also be transmitted by other means.
>
> **TERMS**

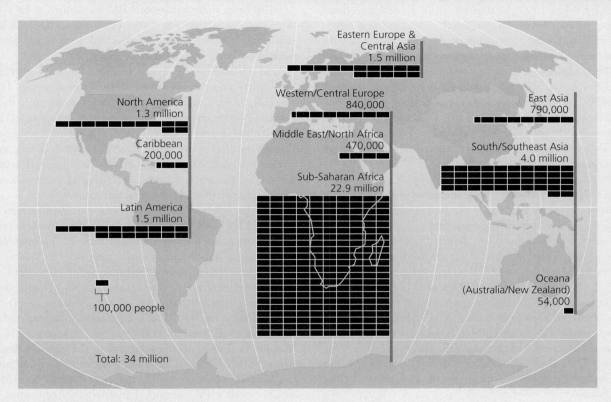

North America
1.3 million

Caribbean
200,000

Latin America
1.5 million

Eastern Europe &
Central Asia
1.5 million

Western/Central Europe
840,000

Middle East/North Africa
470,000

Sub-Saharan Africa
22.9 million

East Asia
790,000

South/Southeast Asia
4.0 million

Oceana
(Australia/New Zealand)
54,000

100,000 people

Total: 34 million

Approximate number of people living with HIV/AIDS in 2010.

SOURCE: Joint United Nations Programme on HIV/AIDS. 2011. *UNAIDS Report on the Global AIDS Epidemic, 2010.* Geneva: UNAIDS.

insidious group of illnesses because a person can be infected and able to transmit the disease, yet not look or feel sick; this is why the term *sexually transmitted infection (STI)* is coming into common use. The following seven STDs pose a major health threat:

+ HIV/AIDS
+ Chlamydia
+ Gonorrhea
+ Human papillomavirus (HPV)
+ Herpes
+ Hepatitis
+ Syphilis

These diseases are considered major threats because they are serious in themselves, cause grave complications if left untreated, and pose risks to a fetus or newborn. STDs often result in severe long-term consequences, including chronic pain, infertility, stillbirths, genital cancers, and death.

The United States has the highest rate of STDs of any developed nation; at current rates, half of all young people will acquire an STD by age 25. About 19 million Americans become newly infected with an STD each year.

HIV Infection and AIDS

The **human immunodeficiency virus (HIV)** causes **acquired immunodeficiency syndrome (AIDS)**, a disease that without treatment ultimately kills nearly all of its victims. An estimated total of 65 million people have been infected since the HIV/AIDS epidemic began—nearly 1% of the world's population—and tens of millions of those people have died (see the box "HIV/AIDS around the World").

> **TERMS**
>
> **human immunodeficiency virus (HIV)** The virus that causes HIV infection and AIDS.
>
> **acquired immunodeficiency syndrome (AIDS)** A generally fatal, incurable, sexually transmitted viral disease.

Currently about 34 million people are infected with HIV worldwide.

Many experts believe that the global HIV epidemic peaked in the late 1990s, at about 3.5 million new infections per year, compared with an estimated 2.7 million new infections in 2010. Despite a slowing of the epidemic, however, AIDS remains a primary cause of death in Africa and continues to be a major cause of mortality around the world. In the United States about 1.2 million people have been infected with HIV. The incidence of HIV has leveled off at about 50,000 new infections annually. More than 619,000 Americans have died from AIDS since the start of the epidemic in 1981. Today about 20% of HIV-infected Americans are unaware of their condition.

What Is HIV Infection?   **HIV infection** is a chronic disease that progressively damages the body's immune system, making an otherwise healthy person less able to resist a variety of infections and disorders. Normally, when a virus or other pathogen enters the body, it is targeted and destroyed by the immune system. But HIV attacks the immune system itself, invading and taking over **CD4 T cells** (a type of helper T cell), macrophages, and other essential elements of the immune system. HIV enters a human cell and converts its own genetic material, RNA, into DNA. It then inserts this DNA into the chromosomes of the host cell. The viral DNA takes over the CD4 cell, causing it to produce new copies of HIV; it also makes the CD4 cell incapable of performing its immune functions.

Immediately following infection with HIV, billions of infectious particles are produced every day. For a time, the immune system keeps pace, also producing billions of new cells. Unlike the virus, however, the immune system cannot make new cells indefinitely; as long as the virus keeps replicating, it wins in the end. The destruction of the immune system is signaled by the loss of CD4 T cells. As CD4 cells decline, an infected person may begin to experience mild to moderately severe symptoms. A person is diagnosed with AIDS when he or she develops one of the conditions defined as a marker for AIDS or when the number of CD4 cells in the blood drops below a certain level (200/μl). People with AIDS are vulnerable to a number of serious—often fatal—**opportunistic (secondary) infections.**

The first weeks after being infected with HIV are called the *primary infection* phase. People have large amounts of HIV in the bloodstream and genital fluids, making it easier to transmit the virus. The next phase of HIV infection is the chronic, **asymptomatic** (symptom-free) stage, also called the *latency* phase. This period can last from 2 to 20 years, averaging 11 years in untreated adults. During this time, the virus progressively infects and destroys the cells of the immune system. People infected with HIV can transmit the disease to others, even if they are symptom-free.

Transmitting the Virus   HIV lives only within cells and body fluids, not outside the body. It is transmitted by blood and blood products, semen, vaginal and cervical secretions, and breast milk. It cannot live in air, in water, or on objects or surfaces such as toilet seats, eating utensils, or telephones.

The three main routes of HIV transmission are specific kinds of sexual contact, direct exposure to infected blood, and contact between an HIV-infected woman and her child during pregnancy, childbirth, or breastfeeding.

HIV is more likely to be transmitted by unprotected anal or vaginal intercourse than by other sexual activities. During vaginal intercourse, male-to-female transmission is more likely to occur than female-to-male transmission. HIV has been found in preejaculatory fluid, so transmission can occur before ejaculation. Being the receptive partner during unprotected anal intercourse is the riskiest of all sexual activities. Oral–genital contact carries some risk of transmission, although less than anal or vaginal intercourse.

The presence of lesions, blisters, or inflammation from other STDs in the genital, anal, or oral areas makes it two to nine times easier for the virus to be passed. Spermicides may also cause irritation and increase the risk of HIV transmission. Studies of the widely used spermicide nonoxynol-9 (N-9) have found that frequent use may cause vaginal and rectal irritation, increasing the risk of transmission of HIV and other STDs. The risk of HIV transmission during oral sex is generally considered to be low but may be increased if a person has oral sores or other damage to the gums or tissues in the mouth. Studies in developing nations with high rates of HIV infection have found that circumcised males have a lower risk of HIV infection than uncircumcised males.

Direct contact with the blood of an infected person is another major route of HIV transmission. Needles and syringes used to inject drugs (including heroin, cocaine, and anabolic steroids) are usually contaminated with the user's blood. In the past, before effective screening was available, some people were infected with HIV through blood transfusions and other medical procedures involving blood products. All blood in licensed U.S. blood banks and plasma centers is now thoroughly screened for HIV.

The final major route of HIV transmission is mother-to-child, also called *vertical* or *perinatal transmission*, which can occur during pregnancy, childbirth, or breastfeeding. Without intervention, the likelihood of HIV transmission from mother to child is 20–45%; however, testing and treatment can dramatically lower this incidence.

TERMS

HIV infection   A chronic, progressive viral infection that damages the immune system.

CD4 T cell   A type of white blood cell that helps coordinate the activity of the immune system; the primary target for HIV infection. The decrease in the number of these cells correlates with the severity of HIV-related illness.

opportunistic (secondary) infection   An infection caused when organisms take the opportunity presented by a primary (initial) infection to multiply and cause a new, different infection.

asymptomatic   Showing no signs or symptoms of a disease.

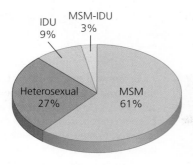

IDU 9%

MSM-IDU 3%

Heterosexual 27%

MSM 61%

* MSM = Men who have sex with men
  IDU = Injection drug users

FIGURE 13.3 **Routes of HIV transmission Among Americans**

SOURCE: Centers for Disease Control and Prevention. 2012. *AIDS in the United States: At a Glance* (http://www.cdc.gov/hiv/resources/factsheets/PDF/HIV_at_a_glance.pdf).

Populations of Special Concern for HIV Infection

Among Americans with AIDS, the most common means of HIV exposure is sexual activity between men (Figure 13.3). Each year the largest number of new cases of HIV infections is among men who have sex with men (MSM). In 2009 this group accounted for 61% of all HIV infections, even though they are estimated to represent just 2% of the population.

Young men in particular are at risk, in part because they tend to engage in unsafe sexual practices such as unprotected anal intercourse. Drug and alcohol use has also been associated with risky sexual behavior and is directly or indirectly associated with HIV acquisition in this population. Use of methamphetamine and club drugs, as well as the recreational use of erectile dysfunction drugs, has been associated with risky sexual behavior and HIV infection in MSM.

Disproportionately high rates of HIV infection also occur in certain racial and ethnic groups, as well as among the poor. In 2009 black men represented almost one-third of all new HIV infections. Black women accounted for 57% of new HIV infections among women; most were infected through heterosexual sex. Hispanics accounted for 20% of all new HIV infections. These patterns of HIV infection reflect complex social, economic, and behavioral factors. Reducing the rates of HIV transmission and AIDS death in minorities, women, and high-risk groups requires addressing problems of poverty, discrimination, and drug abuse.

Symptoms Within a few days or weeks of infection with HIV, most people will develop symptoms of primary (also called acute) HIV infection. These can include fever, fatigue, rashes, headache, swollen lymph nodes, body aches, night sweats, sore throat, nausea, and ulcers in the mouth. Diagnosis of HIV at this very early stage of infection is extremely beneficial. People with early-stage HIV can make lifestyle changes to improve their overall health during this period. They can also protect their partners during this phase, when viral levels are very high.

Other than the initial flulike symptoms, most people have few if any symptoms in the first months or years of HIV infection. As the immune system weakens, however, a variety of symptoms can develop—persistent swollen lymph nodes; lumps, rashes, sores, or other growths on or under the skin or on the mucous membranes; persistent yeast infections; unexplained weight loss; fever and drenching night sweats; dry cough and shortness of breath; persistent diarrhea; easy bruising and unexplained bleeding; profound fatigue; memory loss; difficulty with balance; tremors or seizures; changes in vision, hearing, taste, or smell; changes in mood and other psychological symptoms; and persistent or recurrent pain. Many of these symptoms can also occur with a variety of other illnesses.

People with HIV infection are highly susceptible to infections. The most common one in the United States is *Pneumocystis* pneumonia, a fungal infection. **Kaposi's sarcoma,** a previously rare form of cancer, is common in HIV-infected men. Women with HIV infection often have frequent and difficult-to-treat vaginal yeast infections. Cases of tuberculosis (TB) are increasingly being reported in people with HIV.

Diagnosis The most commonly used screening tests for HIV are **HIV antibody tests.** Standard testing involves an initial test called an **ELISA;** if it is positive, a second test—either a **Western blot** or immunofluorescence assay—is done to confirm the results (see the box "Getting an HIV Test"). Antibodies may not appear in the blood for weeks or months after infection, so people who are newly infected are likely to have a negative antibody test. In its early stages, the infection can be detected with an **HIV RNA assay,** which directly measures the presence of the virus in the blood.

TERMS

***Pneumocystis* pneumonia**   A fungal infection common in people infected with HIV.

Kaposi's sarcoma   A form of cancer characterized by purple or brownish lesions that are generally painless and occur anywhere on the skin; usually appears in men infected with HIV.

HIV antibody test   A blood test to determine whether a person has been infected by HIV; becomes positive within weeks or months of exposure.

ELISA (enzyme-linked immunosorbent assay)   A blood test that detects the presence of antibodies to HIV.

Western blot   A blood test that detects the presence of HIV antibodies; a more accurate and more expensive test used to confirm positive results from an ELISA test.

HIV RNA assay   A test used to determine the viral load (the amount of HIV in the blood).

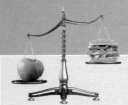

CRITICAL CONSUMER
Getting an HIV Test

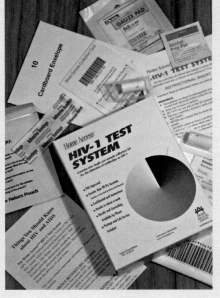

You should strongly consider being tested if any of the following apply to you or any past or current sexual partners:

- You have had unprotected sex (vaginal, anal, or oral) with more than one partner or with a partner who was not in a mutually monogamous relationship with you.

- You have used or shared needles, syringes, or other paraphernalia for injecting drugs (including steroids).

- You have exchanged sex for drugs or money.

- You received a transfusion of blood or blood products between 1978 and 1985.

- You have ever been diagnosed with hepatitis, tuberculosis, or an STD.

If you decide to be tested, you can have the test done by a health care provider or you can take a home test.

Physician or Clinic Testing

Your physician, student health clinic, Planned Parenthood, public health department, or local AIDS association can arrange your HIV test. Testing usually costs $50–$100, but public clinics often charge little or nothing. The standard test involves drawing a sample of blood that is sent to a lab, where it is checked for antibodies. If the first stage of testing is positive, a confirming test is done. This standard test takes one to two weeks, and you'll be asked to phone or come in personally to obtain your results, which should also include appropriate counseling.

Alternative tests are available at some clinics. The Orasure test uses oral fluid, which is collected by swabbing the inside of the mouth. Urine tests are also available. New rapid tests are now also available at some locations. These tests involve the use of blood or oral fluid and can provide results in as little as 20 minutes. If a rapid test is positive for HIV infection, a confirming test will be performed.

Before you get an HIV test, be sure you understand what will be done with the results. Results from confidential tests may still become part of your medical record and be reported to state and federal public health agencies. If you decide you want to be tested anonymously, ask your physician about an anonymous test, or use a home test.

Home Testing

Home test kits for HIV cost about $40–70. Avoid test kits sold on the Internet that are not FDA-approved. As of this printing, the only FDA-approved home test kit for HIV is manufactured by Home Access. To use the Home Access test, you prick a finger with a supplied lancet, blot a few drops of blood onto blotting paper, and mail it to the company's laboratory. In about a week (or within three business days for more expensive "express" tests), you call a toll-free number to find out your results. Anyone testing positive is routed to a trained counselor, who can provide emotional and medical support. Approval of another home test, the OraQuick HIV test, manufactured by Orasure, was recommended to the FDA by an FDA advisory panel in 2012. Like the Orasure test available to clinics, the OraQuick home test uses a sample taken from the mouth and returns results in 20 minutes. The results of home test kits are completely anonymous.

Understanding the Results

A negative test result means that no antibodies were found in your sample. However, as noted in the text, it usually takes at least a month after exposure to HIV (and possibly as long as six months in some people) for antibodies to appear. Therefore, an infected person may get a false negative result. If you test negative but your risk of infection is high, ask about obtaining an HIV RNA assay, which allows very early diagnosis.

A positive result means that you are infected. It is important to seek medical care and counseling immediately. Rapid progress is being made in treating HIV, and treatments are potentially much more successful when started early. For more information about testing, visit the CDC National HIV and STD Testing Resources website (www.hivtest.org).

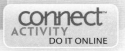
ACTIVITY DO IT ONLINE

If a person is diagnosed as **HIV-positive,** the next step is to determine the disease's severity to plan appropriate treatment. The status of the immune system can be gauged

by taking CD4 T cell measurements every few months. The infection itself can be monitored by tracking the viral load (the amount of virus in the body) through the HIV RNA assay. A new diagnostic test that may help guide treatment decisions is called HIV Replication Capacity. This test shows how fast HIV from a patient's blood sample can reproduce itself. The CDC currently recommends universal HIV testing as part of routine medical care for

HIV-positive A diagnosis resulting from the presence of HIV in the bloodstream; also referred to as *seropositive*.

TERMS

everyone aged 13–64. People at greater risk should be tested periodically.

A diagnosis of AIDS, the most severe form of HIV infection, is given if a person is HIV-positive and either has developed an infection defined as an AIDS indicator or has a severely damaged immune system (as measured by CD4 T-cell counts).

In the United States, every state has laws that require doctors, clinics, and laboratories to report all diagnosed cases of HIV and AIDS to public health authorities, who use this information to track the spread of the disease. Despite efforts to safeguard confidentiality and prohibit discrimination, mandatory reporting of HIV infection remains controversial. If people believe they are risking their jobs, friends, or social acceptability, they may be less likely to get tested. The CDC recommends that states continue to provide opportunities for people to be tested anonymously, including via home tests.

Treatment   Although there is no known cure for HIV infection, medications can significantly alter the course of the disease and extend life. The drop in the number of U.S. AIDS deaths that has occurred since 1996 is in large part due to the increasing use of combinations of new drugs.

The main types of antiviral drugs used against HIV/AIDS are reverse transcriptase inhibitors, protease inhibitors, integrase inhibitors, and entry inhibitors. These drugs either block HIV from replicating itself or prevent it from infecting other cells. More than 30 drugs are now available to treat HIV, including two once-a-day tablets (containing three combined HIV medications). In addition to antiviral drugs, most patients with low CD4 T cell counts take a variety of antibiotics to help prevent opportunistic infections such as pneumonia, tuberculosis, and other bacterial and fungal infections.

The cost of treatment for HIV continues to be an area of major concern. Pharmaceutical companies, the World Bank, and the international community are working to lower drug costs and provide aid for developing regions. HIV treatment is also challenging because taking the combination drugs is complicated, and the drugs have short-term side effects that may cause people to stop taking them. The drugs can also have long-term side effects, including serious health problems. The National Institutes of Health has issued guidelines for HIV treatment that help patients and their doctors with decisions about treatment.

Prevention   The best hope for stopping the spread of HIV worldwide is the development of a safe, effective, and inexpensive vaccine. However, no vaccine is likely to be ready for widespread use within the next decade. Researchers are making more rapid progress in producing a microbicide that could be used to prevent HIV and other STDs.

> In many people, combination therapies can **reduce HIV in the blood to undetectable levels.**

High Risk

Unprotected anal sex is the riskiest sexual behavior, especially for the receptive partner.

Unprotected vaginal intercourse is the next riskiest, especially for women, who are much more likely to be infected by an infected male partner than vice versa.

Oral sex is probably considerably less risky than anal and vaginal intercourse but can still result in HIV transmission.

Sharing of sex toys can be risky because they can carry blood, semen, or vaginal fluid.

Use of a condom reduces risk considerably but not completely for any type of intercourse. Anal sex with a condom is riskier than vaginal sex with a condom; oral sex with a condom is less risky, especially if the man does not ejaculate.

Hand-genital contact and deep kissing are less risky but could still theoretically transmit HIV; the presence of cuts or sores increases risk.

Sex with only one uninfected and totally faithful partner is without risk, but effective only if both partners are uninfected and completely monogamous.

Activities that don't involve the exchange of body fluids carry no risk: hugging, massage, closed-mouth kissing, masturbation, phone sex, and fantasy.

Abstinence is completely without risk. For many people, it can be an effective and reasonable method of avoiding HIV infection and other STDs during certain periods of life.

No Risk

FIGURE 13.4   What's risky and what's not: The approximate relative risk of HIV transmission of various sexual activities.

How Can You Protect Yourself?   Although AIDS cannot be cured, infection can be prevented. You can protect yourself by avoiding behaviors that may bring you into contact with HIV. In a sexual relationship, the current and past behaviors of you and your partner determine the amount of risk involved. For anyone not involved in a long-term, mutually monogamous relationship, abstinence from any sexual activity that involves the exchange of body fluids is the only sure way to prevent HIV infection (Figure 13.4).

People who inject drugs should avoid sharing needles, syringes, filters, or anything that might have blood on it. Needles

microbicide   Microbicide is a disinfectant that kills microorganisms and their spores.   **TERMS**

TAKE CHARGE
Preventing STD Infection

For those who aren't in a long-term monogamous relationship with an uninfected partner, abstinence is the only truly safe option for avoiding STDs. If you are sexually active, talk with potential partners about HIV, safer sex, and condom use before you begin a sexual relationship. The following guidelines can also help you avoid infection:

• Don't drink alcohol or use drugs in sexual situations. Mood-altering drugs can affect your judgment and make you more likely to take risks.

• Limit the number of partners. Avoid sexual contact with people who have HIV or an STD or who have engaged in risky behaviors in the past.

• Use condoms during every act of intercourse and oral sex. Condoms do not provide perfect protection, but they greatly reduce your risk of contracting an infection.

• Use condoms properly for maximum protection.

• Avoid sexual contact that could cause cuts or tears in the skin or tissue.

• Get periodic screening tests for STDs and HIV. Sexually active young women should be tested for STDs at least annually. Women should have a Pap test at age 21 and every three years thereafter.

• Get vaccinated. All sexually active men and women should be vaccinated against hepatitis B. All men who have sex with men should be vaccinated against hepatitis A. Young men and women aged 26 years and younger should consider getting vaccinated against HPV.

• Get prompt treatment for any STDs you contract. Make sure your partner gets treated, too. Don't have sex until both of you have completed your treatment.

If you inject drugs of any kind, don't share needles, syringes, or anything that might have blood on it. If your community has a syringe exchange program, use it. Seek treatment.

If you are at risk for HIV infection, don't donate blood, sperm, or body organs. Don't have unprotected sex or share needles or syringes. Get tested for HIV soon, and get treated. HIV-infected people who get early treatment generally feel better and live longer than those who delay.

---

can be decontaminated with a solution of bleach and water, but this is not a foolproof procedure, and HIV can survive in a syringe for a month or longer. HIV can also survive boiling. For more guidelines and tips, see the box "Preventing STD Infection."

Chlamydia

Chlamydia trachomatis causes **chlamydia,** the most prevalent bacterial STD in the United States. Both men and women are susceptible to chlamydia, but, as with most STDs, women bear the greater burden because of possible complications and consequences of the disease. For women, the highest rates of infection occur among 15- to 24-year-olds. For men, the highest rates occur among 20- to 24-year-olds.

If untreated, chlamydia can lead to pelvic inflammatory disease (PID). Chlamydia also greatly increases a woman's risk for infertility and ectopic pregnancy. The CDC currently recommends annual chlamydia testing for all sexually active women aged 25 or younger and for older women who are at increased risk (such as those who have multiple sex partners).

Chlamydia can also lead to infertility in men, although not as often as in women. In men under age 35, chlamydia is the most common cause of epididymitis, inflammation of the sperm-carrying ducts. In men, up to half of all cases of **urethritis,** inflammation of the urethra, are caused by chlamydia. Infants of infected mothers can acquire the infection through contact with the pathogen in the birth canal during delivery.

Symptoms Most people experience few or no symptoms from chlamydia infection, increasing the likelihood that they will inadvertently spread the infection to their partners. In men, chlamydia symptoms can include painful urination, a slight watery discharge from the penis, and sometimes pain around the testicles. Women may notice increased vaginal discharge, burning with urination, pain or bleeding with intercourse, and lower abdominal pain. Symptoms in both men and women can begin within five days of infection.

Diagnosis and Treatment Chlamydia is diagnosed through laboratory tests on a urine sample or a small amount of fluid from the urethra, cervix, rectum, or vagina. Once chlamydia has been diagnosed, the infected person and his or her partner(s) are given antibiotics. When it is unlikely that a partner will seek medical treatment, the CDC recommends that an extra prescription for antibiotics be provided to the patient to give to his or her partner. This strategy, called *expedited partner therapy,* is legal and encouraged under certain circumstances.

> **TERMS**
>
> **chlamydia** An STD transmitted by the bacterium *Chlamydia trachomatis.*
>
> **urethritis** Inflammation of the tube that carries urine from the bladder to the outside opening.

Gonorrhea

Gonorrhea is caused by the bacterium *Neisseria gonorrhoeae*. More than 300,000 new cases of gonorrhea were reported to the CDC in 2010, a slight increase from the previous year. The highest incidence is among 15- to 24-year-olds. Like chlamydia, untreated gonorrhea can cause PID in women and urethritis and epididymitis in men. An infant passing through the birth canal of an infected mother may contract *gonococcal conjunctivitis*, an infection in the eyes that can cause blindness if not treated.

Symptoms   In males the first symptoms are due to urethritis, which causes urinary discomfort and a thick, yellowish white or yellowish green discharge from the penis. Up to half of males have very minor symptoms or none at all. Most females with gonorrhea are asymptomatic. Those who have symptoms often experience pain with urination, increased vaginal discharge, and severe menstrual cramps. Gonorrhea can also infect the throat or rectum of people who engage in oral or anal sex.

Diagnosis and Treatment   Gonorrhea is detectable through several tests; depending on the test, samples of urine or cervical, urethral, throat, or rectal fluids may be collected. Antibiotics are used to treat gonorrhea, but increasing drug resistance is a major concern. Only one class of antibiotics, the cephalosporins, remains consistently effective against gonorrhea.

Although 80% of sexually active people become infected with HPV by age 50, **most have no symptoms at all.**

Pelvic Inflammatory Disease

Pelvic inflammatory disease (PID) is a major complication in 10–40% of women who have been infected with either gonorrhea or chlamydia and have not received treatment. PID occurs when the initial infection travels upward beyond the cervix into the uterus, oviducts, ovaries, and pelvic cavity. PID is often serious enough to require hospitalization and sometimes surgery. Even if the disease is treated successfully, about 25% of affected women will have long-term problems, such as a continuing susceptibility to infection, ectopic pregnancy, infertility, and chronic pelvic pain.

PID is the leading cause of infertility in young women, often going undetected until the inability to become pregnant leads to further evaluation. As with all STDs, the more sex partners a woman has had, the greater her risk of PID. Using IUDs for contraception increases the risk of PID, although this risk is greatly reduced for women with only one uninfected sexual partner.

Symptoms   Symptoms of PID vary greatly. Some women, especially those with chlamydia, may be asymptomatic; others may have abdominal pain, fever, chills, nausea, and vomiting. Early symptoms are essentially the same as those described for chlamydia and gonorrhea. Symptoms often begin or worsen during or soon after a woman's menstrual period. Many women have abnormal vaginal bleeding—either bleeding between periods or heavy and painful menstrual bleeding.

Diagnosis and Treatment   Diagnosis of PID is made on the basis of symptoms, physical examination, ultrasound, and laboratory tests. **Laparoscopy** may be used to confirm the diagnosis and obtain material for cultures. Antibiotics are usually started immediately; in severe cases, the woman may be hospitalized and antibiotics given intravenously. It is especially important that an infected woman's partners be treated. As many as 60% of the male contacts of women with PID are infected but asymptomatic.

Human Papillomavirus

As noted earlier in the chapter and in Chapter 12, **human papillomavirus (HPV)** infection causes several diseases, including common warts, **genital warts,** and genital cancers. HPV causes virtually all cervical cancers, as well as penile cancer and some forms of anal and oropharyngeal cancers (the oropharynx includes the back of the mouth and the throat). Genital HPV is quite contagious and is usually spread through sexual activity, including oral sex. HPV is the most common STD in the United States. In all, more than 80% of sexually active people will become infected with HPV by the age of 50. HPV is especially

Why Do College Students Have High Rates of STDs?

- Risky sexual behavior is common. One study of college students found that fewer than half used condoms consistently and one-third had had 10 or more sex partners. Another study found that 19% of male students and 33% of female students had consented to sexual intercourse simply because they felt awkward refusing.

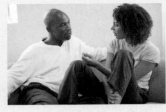

- College students underestimate their risk of STDs and HIV. Although students may have considerable knowledge about STDs, they often feel the risks do not apply to them—a dangerous assumption. One study of students with a history of STDs showed that more than half had unprotected sex while they were infected, and 25% of them continued to have sex without ever informing their partner(s).

- Many students are infected but don't know it. A 2006 study of asymptomatic college women revealed that nearly 10% were infected with chlamydia.

What Effect Does Alcohol or Drug Use Have on My Likelihood of Getting an STD?

- Between one-third and one-half of college students report participating in sexual activity as a direct result of being intoxicated. All too often, sexual activity while intoxicated leads to unprotected intercourse.

- Students who binge-drink are more likely to have multiple partners, use condoms inconsistently, and delay seeking treatment for STDs than are students who drink little or no alcohol. Sexual assaults occur more frequently when either the perpetrator or the victim has been drinking.

What Can Students Do to Protect Themselves against STDs?

- Limit the number of sex partners. Even people who are always in a monogamous relationship can end up with extensive potential exposure to STDs if, over the years, they have numerous relationships.

- Use condoms consistently, and don't assume it's safe to stop after you've been with a partner for several months. HIV infection, HPV infection, herpes, and chlamydia can be asymptomatic for months or years and can be transmitted at any time. If you haven't been using condoms with your current partner, start now.

- Enjoy sexuality on your own terms. Don't let the expectations of friends and partners cause you to ignore your own feelings. Let your own wellness be your first priority. If you choose to be sexually active, learn about safer sex practices.

- Get to know your partner, and talk to him or her before becoming intimate. Be honest about yourself, and encourage your partner to do the same. But practice safer sex no matter what.

---

common in young people, with some of the highest infection rates among college students (see the box "College Students and STDs").

There are more than 100 different strains of HPV, and different strains cause different types of infection. More than 30 types are likely to cause genital infection. Types 16 and 18 are most often implicated in anal and genital cancers; types 6 and 11 cause most visible genital warts. A person can be infected with several different strains of HPV.

Two HPV vaccines—Gardasil and Cervarix—have been approved by the FDA. Gardasil protects against four types of HPV virus that together account for 90% of genital warts, 70% of cervical cancers, and most anal cancers. Gardasil has also been shown to prevent cancers of the vagina, vulva, and anus. Cervarix protects against two types of HPV but not against the type that causes genital warts.

Gardasil was originally approved for girls and women, but in 2009 it was also approved for boys and men aged 9–26 to prevent anal cancer. Many experts believe that it makes sense to routinely vaccinate young males for HPV to protect them from HPV-related diseases and to protect their female partners. Cervarix is approved for girls and

women aged 10–25. The CDC recommends the vaccine for all children between the ages of 11 and 12. This age was chosen because the vaccine is most effective when given prior to exposure to genital HPV, and this virus is so common that many young people will be exposed to it shortly after becoming sexually active.

Symptoms   Most people infected with HPV have no visible warts or other symptoms and are not aware that they are infected and contagious to others. The good news is that the immune system usually clears the virus on its own, and infection disappears without any treatment. But in some cases, the infection persists and causes genital warts or cancers.

The types of HPV that cause cervical cancer do not produce any visible changes on the external genitals. The types that cause genital warts can produce anything from a small bump to a large, warty growth. In men, warts appear on the penis and often involve the urethra, appearing first at the opening and then spreading inside. In women, warts may appear on the labia or vulva and may spread to the *perineum*, the area between the vagina and the rectum. They may also appear on the cervix.

Diagnosis and Treatment Genital warts are usually diagnosed based on the appearance of the lesions. HPV infection of the cervix is often detected on routine Pap tests. Special tests are now available to detect the presence of HPV infection and to distinguish among the more common strains of HPV, including those that cause most cases of cervical cancer.

Treatment focuses on reducing the number and size of warts, through cryosurgery (freezing), electrocautery (burning), or laser surgery. Even after treatment and the disappearance of visible warts, the individual may continue to carry HPV in healthy-looking tissue and can probably still infect others. Cervical abnormalities that are cancerous or precancerous are treated surgically or with other techniques such as electrical excision, freezing, and laser.

Anyone who has ever had HPV infection should inform all partners and use condoms, even though they do not provide total protection. Whether or not they have had the vaccine, all women should have regular pelvic exams and PAP tests.

Genital Herpes

Up to one in five adults in the United States has **genital herpes.** Worldwide, genital herpes is extremely common, and it is a major factor in the transmission of HIV. Two types of herpes simplex viruses, HSV 1 and HSV 2, cause genital herpes and oral–labial herpes (cold sores). Infection with HSV is generally lifelong. After infection, the virus lies dormant in nerve cells and can reactivate at any time.

HSV 1 infection is so common that 50–80% of U.S. adults have antibodies to it (indicating previous exposure to the virus); most were exposed to HSV 1 during childhood. HSV 2 infection usually occurs during adolescence and early adulthood, often between ages 18 and 25.

HSV 2 is almost always sexually transmitted, including during oral sex. The infection spreads readily whether people have active sores or are completely asymptomatic. Because HSV is asymptomatic in 80–90% of people, the infection is often acquired from a person who does not know that he or she is infected. If you have ever had an outbreak of genital herpes, you should consider yourself always contagious and inform your partners. Avoid intimate contact when any sores are present, and use condoms during all sexual contact. One study showed that using condoms for every act of intercourse results in a 30% decrease in the transmission of herpes compared with no condom use. Condoms are more effective in preventing the transmission of other STDs than for herpes, but this study shows that they can make a significant difference in preventing the spread of genital herpes.

Newborns can occasionally be infected with HSV, usually during passage through the birth canal of an infected mother. Without treatment, 65% of newborns with HSV will die, and most who survive will have some degree of brain damage. Pregnant women who have been exposed to genital herpes should inform their physicians so that appropriate precautions can be taken to protect their babies from infection.

Symptoms Up to 90% of people who are infected with HSV have no symptoms. Those who develop symptoms often first notice them within 2–20 days of having sex with an infected partner. (However, it is not unusual for the first outbreak to occur months or even years after initial exposure.) The first episode of genital herpes frequently causes flulike symptoms in addition to genital lesions. The lesions tend to be painful or itchy and can occur anywhere on the genitals, inner thighs, or anal area. Depending on their location, they can cause considerable pain with urination. Lymph nodes in the groin may become swollen and tender. The sores usually heal within three weeks. On average, newly diagnosed people will experience five to eight outbreaks per year, with a decrease in the frequency of outbreaks over time. Recurrent episodes are usually less severe than the initial one, with fewer and less painful sores that heal more quickly. Outbreaks can be triggered by stress, illness, fatigue, sun exposure, sexual intercourse, and menstruation.

Diagnosis and Treatment Genital herpes can be diagnosed on the basis of symptoms, but laboratory testing is helpful if there is any question about the diagnosis. Several blood tests can detect the presence of HSV antibodies in the blood.

There is no cure for herpes. Once infected, a person carries the virus for life. Antiviral drugs such as acyclovir can be taken at the beginning of an outbreak to shorten the severity and duration of symptoms. Support groups are available to help people learn to cope with herpes. There is no vaccine to prevent herpes, but research is ongoing.

Hepatitis B

Hepatitis (inflammation of the liver) can cause serious and sometimes permanent damage to the liver, which can result in death in severe cases. One of the many types of hepatitis is caused by hepatitis B virus (HBV). Like HIV, HBV is found in most body fluids, including blood and blood products, semen, saliva, urine, and vaginal secretions. HBV is much more contagious than HIV. It is easily transmitted through any sexual activity that involves the exchange of body fluids. The

> **QUICK STATS**
> More than **80%** of people infected with genital herpes do not know they are infected.
> —CDC, 2009

> **TERMS**
> **genital herpes** A sexually transmitted infection caused by the herpes simplex virus.
>
> **hepatitis** Inflammation of the liver, which can be caused by infection, drugs, or toxins; some forms of infectious hepatitis can be transmitted sexually.

primary risk factors for HVB are sexual exposure and injection drug use; having multiple sex partners greatly increases risk. HBV can also be transmitted through nonsexual close contact, including the use of contaminated needles, razor blades, toothbrushes, and eating utensils. Because of crowded living conditions in many college settings, vaccination against HVB is recommended for incoming college students.

Other forms of viral hepatitis can also be sexually transmitted. Hepatitis A is of particular concern for people who engage in anal sex; a vaccine is available and is recommended for all people at risk. Less commonly, hepatitis C can be transmitted sexually. Experts believe that traumatic sexual activity that causes tissue damage is most likely to transmit hepatitis C.

Symptoms   Many people infected with HBV never develop symptoms; they have what are known as silent infections. Mild cases of hepatitis cause flulike symptoms such as fever, body aches, chills, and loss of appetite. As the illness progresses, there may be nausea, vomiting, dark-colored urine, abdominal pain, and jaundice.

Most adults who have acute hepatitis B recover completely within a few weeks or months. But about 5% of adults who are infected with HBV become chronic carriers of the virus, capable of infecting others for the rest of their life. Some chronic carriers remain asymptomatic, while others develop chronic liver disease. Chronic hepatitis can cause cirrhosis, liver failure, and a deadly form of liver cancer.

Diagnosis and Treatment   Hepatitis is diagnosed by blood tests used to analyze liver function, detect the infecting organism, and detect antibodies to the virus. There is no cure for HBV and no specific treatment for acute infections; antiviral drugs and immune system modulators may be used for chronic HBV infection. The vaccine for hepatitis B is safe and effective. Vaccination is recommended for everyone under age 19 and for all adults at increased risk for hepatitis B.

Syphilis

Syphilis, a disease that once caused death and disability for millions, can now be effectively treated with antibiotics. In 2010 overall rates of syphilis were lower than they had been in the previous 10 years. However, rates in young men who have sex with men were rising; rates of co-infection with HIV were also high in this group. Studies have found an association between syphilis infection and the use of the Internet as a means to meet sex partners among men who have sex with men. Another trend is an increase in the proportion of cases of syphilis transmitted through oral sex.

Syphilis is caused by a spirochete called *Treponema pallidum*, a thin, corkscrew-shaped bacterium. The disease is usually acquired through sexual contact, although infected pregnant women can transmit it to their fetuses. The pathogen passes through any break or opening in the skin or mucous membranes and can be transmitted by kissing, vaginal or anal intercourse, or oral–genital contact.

Symptoms   Syphilis progresses through several stages. *Primary syphilis* is characterized by an ulcer called a **chancre** that appears within 10–90 days after exposure. Chancres contain large numbers of bacteria and make the disease highly contagious when present; they are often painless and typically heal on their own within a few weeks. If the disease is not treated during the primary stage, about a third of infected individuals progress to chronic stages of infections.

Secondary syphilis is usually characterized by a skin rash that appears three to six weeks after the chancre. The rash may cover the entire body or only a few areas, but the palms of the hands and soles of the feet are usually involved. Areas of skin affected by the rash are highly contagious but usually heal within several weeks or months.

If the disease remains untreated, the symptoms of secondary syphilis may recur over a period of several years; affected individuals may then lapse into an asymptomatic latent stage in which they experience no further consequences of infection. However, in about one-third of cases of untreated secondary syphilis, the individual develops *late*, or *tertiary*, *syphilis*. Late syphilis can damage many organs of the body, possibly causing severe dementia, cardiovascular damage, blindness, and death.

In infected pregnant women, who aren't treated, the probable result is stillbirth, prematurity, or congenital deformity. In many cases the infant is also born infected (*congenital syphilis*) and requires treatment.

Diagnosis and Treatment   Syphilis is diagnosed by examination of infected tissues and with blood tests. All stages can be treated with antibiotics, but damage from late syphilis can be permanent.

Other STDs

Trichomoniasis (often called *trich*) is a common STD among young women. The single-celled organism that causes trich, *Trichomonas vaginalis*, thrives in warm, moist conditions,

---

Ask Yourself

QUESTIONS FOR CRITICAL THINKING AND REFLECTION

Have you ever had sex and regretted it later? If so, what were the circumstances, and what influenced you to act the way you did? Were there any negative consequences? What preventive strategies can you use in the future to make sure it doesn't happen again?

TERMS

syphilis   A sexually transmitted bacterial infection caused by the spirochete *Treponema pallidum*.

chancre   The sore produced by syphilis in its earliest stage.

trichomoniasis   A protozoal infection caused by *Trichomonas vaginalis*, transmitted sexually and externally.

making women particularly susceptible to these infections in the vagina. Women who become symptomatic with trich develop a greenish, foul-smelling vaginal discharge and severe itching and pain in the vagina. Men usually have no symptoms, but they may have mild irritation after urinating or a slight discharge. Prompt treatment with metronidazole (Flagyl) is important because studies suggest that trich may increase the risk of HIV transmission and, in pregnant women, premature delivery.

Bacterial vaginosis (BV) is the most common cause of abnormal vaginal discharge in women of reproductive age. BV occurs when healthful bacteria that normally inhabit the vagina become displaced by unhealthful species. BV is usually, but not always, associated with sexual activity and often occurs after a change in partners. Symptoms of BV include vaginal discharge with a fishy odor and sometimes vaginal irritation. BV is treated with topical and oral antibiotics.

Lymphogranuloma venereum (LGV) is an infection of the lymphatic system caused by three strains of the bacteria *Chlamydia trachomatis* (not the same strain that causes the genital STD chlamydia). LGV is more common in men than in women; the main risk factor is being HIV-positive. The first symptom is an ulcer at the site of sexual penetration that appears 3–30 days after exposure; there may also be swollen glands in the genital area. Among those who practice anal receptive intercourse, symptoms may include rectal ulcers, bleeding, and pain. If the infection is untreated, chronic symptoms may develop, so individuals with symptoms should see a physician.

Pubic lice (commonly known as *crabs*) and **scabies** are highly contagious parasitic infections. They are usually treated with topical medicines, but oral medications are sometimes needed as well.

WHAT YOU CAN DO ABOUT STDs

You can take responsibility for your health and contribute to a general reduction in the incidence of STDs in three major areas: education, diagnosis and treatment, and prevention.

Education

Educational campaigns about HIV/AIDS and other STDs have paid off in changing attitudes and sexual behaviors. Levels of awareness about HIV infection among the general population are quite high, although some segments of the population are harder to reach and continue to engage in very high-risk behaviors. Learning about STDs is still up to every person individually, as is applying that knowledge to personal situations.

Diagnosis and Treatment

Early diagnosis and treatment of STDs can help you avoid complications and help prevent the spread of infection.

• *Be alert for symptoms.* If you are sexually active, be alert for any sign or symptom of disease, such as a rash, a

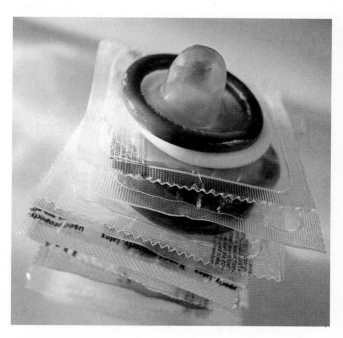

Condoms protect against STDs and should be used even if another form of contraception, such as birth control pills or an IUD, is being used.

discharge, sores, or pain. Although only a physician can make a proper diagnosis of an STD, you can perform a genital self-examination between check-ups to look for early warning signs of disease, such as bumps, sores, blisters, or warts.

• *Get vaccinated.* Every young, sexually active person should be vaccinated against hepatitis B. Men who have sex with men should be vaccinated against hepatitis A, and men and women aged 9–26 should be vaccinated against HPV.

• *Get tested.* The CDC recommends that everyone between the ages of 13 and 64 be tested for HIV at least once during routine medical care. If you are sexually active, be sure to get periodic STD checks, even if you have no symptoms. If you have a risky sexual encounter, see a physician as soon as possible.

• *Inform your partners.* Telling a partner that you have exposed him or her to an STD isn't easy. Despite the awkwardness and difficulty, it is crucial that your sex partner or

---

TERMS

bacterial vaginosis (BV) A condition linked to sexual activity; caused by an overgrowth of certain bacteria inhabiting the vagina.

lymphogranuloma venereum (LGV) An infection of the lymphatic system caused by three strains of the bacterium *Chlamydia trachomatis*, transmitted sexually.

pubic lice Parasites that infest the hair of the pubic region, commonly called crabs.

scabies A contagious skin disease caused by a type of burrowing parasitic mite.

partners be informed and urged to seek testing and/or treatment as quickly as possible.

• **Get treated.** With the exception of AIDS treatments, treatments for STDs are safe and generally inexpensive. If you are being treated, follow instructions carefully and complete all the medication as prescribed. Don't stop taking the medication just because you feel better or your symptoms have disappeared.

TIPS FOR TODAY AND THE FUTURE

Your immune system is a remarkable germ-fighting network, but it needs your help to work at its best.

RIGHT NOW YOU CAN:

- Move your bedtime up 15 minutes, starting tonight.
- Make an appointment with your health care provider if you are worried about possible STD infection.
- Resolve to discuss condom use with your partner if you are sexually active and are not already using condoms.

IN THE FUTURE YOU CAN:

- Learn how to communicate effectively with a partner who resists safer sex practices or is reluctant to discuss his or her sexual history. Support groups and educational classes can help.
- Make sure all your vaccinations are up-to-date; ask your doctor if you should be vaccinated against hepatitis A or B, HPV, or any other STDs.

connect™

Connect to Your Choices

Have you ever thought about where you get your behaviors and habits related to infectious diseases and STDs? Many factors can influence our behaviors and habits, some not as obvious as others. Was your family conscientious about making sure you got all the recommended vaccinations when you were growing up? Did you have comprehensive sex education in high school? Do the significant people in your peer group use condoms and practice safer sex? Does your campus health clinic promote HIV/AIDS awareness?

What are the external factors that influence your choices about sexually transmitted diseases? What are your inner motivations and core values, and how do they affect your choices? Based on what you learned in this chapter, will you make some different choices in the future? If so, what will they be?

Go online to Connect to complete this activity: www.mcgraw-hillconnect.com

Prevention

If you choose to be sexually active, think about prevention *before* you have a sexual encounter, and plan accordingly. By thinking and talking about responsible sexual behavior, you are expressing a sense of caring for yourself, your potential partner, and your future children.

SUMMARY

• The immune system includes both surface barriers and the cells, tissues, and organs that mount the immune response. Physical and chemical barriers to microorganisms include skin, mucous membranes, and the cilia lining the respiratory tract.

• The immune response is carried out by white blood cells that are continuously produced in the bone marrow. Cells of the innate immune system include neutrophils, eosinophils, macrophages, dendritic cells, and natural killer cells. Cells of the adaptive immune system are lymphocytes—in particular, T cells and B cells.

• The immune response has four stages: recognition of the invading pathogen; rapid replication of killer T cells and B cells; attack by killer T cells and macrophages; and suppression of the immune response.

• Immunization is based on the body's ability to remember previously encountered organisms and retain its strength against them.

• Allergic reactions occur when the immune system responds to harmless substances as if they were dangerous pathogens.

• The step-by-step process by which infections are transmitted from one person to another involves a pathogen, its reservoir, a portal of exit, a means of transmission, a portal of entry, and a new host. Infection can be prevented by breaking the chain at any point.

• Bacteria are single-celled organisms; some cause disease in humans. Significant bacterial infections include pneumonia, meningitis, strep throat, toxic shock syndrome, MRSA, tuberculosis, and Lyme disease.

• Viruses cannot grow or reproduce themselves; different viruses cause the common cold, influenza, chicken pox, cold sores, mononucleosis, hepatitis, and warts.

• Other infectious diseases are caused by certain types of fungi, protozoa, parasitic worms, and prions.

• Autoimmune diseases occur when the body identifies its own cells as foreign. A healthy immune system can target and destroy mutant cells that may become cancerous, but age and other conditions can cause the immune system to break down and allow cancer cells to grow unchecked.

• HIV affects the immune system, making an otherwise healthy person less able to resist a variety of infections. HIV is carried in blood and blood products, semen, vaginal and cervical secretions, and breast milk. The virus is transmitted through the exchange of these fluids.

- There is currently no cure or vaccine for HIV infection. Drugs have been developed to slow the course of the disease and to prevent or treat certain secondary infections.

- Chlamydia causes epididymitis and urethritis in men; in women, it can lead to PID and infertility if untreated.

- Untreated gonorrhea can cause PID in women and epididymitis in men, leading to infertility. In infants, untreated gonorrhea can cause blindness.

- Pelvic inflammatory disease (PID), usually a complication of untreated gonorrhea or chlamydia, is an infection of the uterus and oviducts that may extend to the ovaries and pelvic cavity. It can lead to infertility, ectopic pregnancy, and chronic pelvic pain.

- Human papillomavirus (HPV) causes genital warts and cervical cancer. The virus can be transmitted by asymptomatic people. Even after treatment, a person may continue to carry the virus in healthy-looking tissue. The immune system often clears HPV on its own.

- Genital herpes is a common viral infection that can cause painful blisters on the genitals. The virus remains in the body for life and causes recurrent outbreaks.

- Hepatitis B is an inflammation of the liver caused by one of the many types of hepatitis viruses. It is transmitted through both sexual and nonsexual contact.

- Syphilis is a highly contagious bacterial infection that can be treated with antibiotics. If left untreated, it can lead to deterioration of the central nervous system and death.

- Other diseases that can be transmitted sexually or are linked to sexual activity include trichomoniasis, bacterial vaginosis, lymphogranuloma venereum (LGV), pubic lice, and scabies. Any STD that causes sores or inflammation can increase the risk of HIV transmission.

- Individuals can contribute to a reduction in the incidence of STDs by educating themselves, being diagnosed and treated for any infections, and practicing preventive strategies.

FOR MORE INFORMATION

BOOKS

Barry, J. 2005. *The Great Influenza: The Epic Story of the Deadliest Plague in History*. New York: Penguin. *A compelling account of the medical, social, and political aspects of the influenza epidemic of 1918–1919.*

Grimes, J. 2008. *Seductive Delusions: How Everyday People Catch STDs*. Baltimore, MD: The Johns Hopkins University Press. *This very readable book debunks the widespread "it can't happen to me" attitude with real-life stories about young people who became infected with STDs.*

Nakazawa, D. J. 2009. *The Autoimmune Epidemic*. New York: Touchstone. *The author explores potential links between autoimmune disorders and environmental toxins.*

Pepin, J. 2011. The Origin of AIDS. Cambridge, UK: Cambridge University Press. *A highly readable investigation into the perplexing evolutionary origin and early epidemiology of the AIDS virus.*

Reid, E. 2012. *The Thriving Child: Parenting Successfully through Allergies, Asthma, and Other Common Challenges*. New York: Center Street. *A mother's description of raising two children with allergies and asthma in New York City and developing a healthy environment for her family.*

Shilts, R. 2007. *And the Band Played On: Politics, People, and the AIDS Epidemic*. 20th Anniversary Edition. New York: St. Martin's Griffin. *Originally published in 1987, this landmark book chronicles the early years of the AIDS epidemic, tracing the political, medical, and social forces that facilitated the spread of the epidemic.*

ORGANIZATIONS, HOTLINES, AND WEBSITES

American Academy of Allergy, Asthma, and Immunology. Provides information and publications; pollen counts are available from the website.

http://www.aaaai.org

American Autoimmune-Related Diseases Association. Provides background information, coping tips, and an online knowledge quiz about autoimmune diseases.

http://www.aarda.org

American Social Health Association (ASHA). Provides written information and referrals for STDs; sponsors support groups for people with herpes and HPV.

http://www.ashastd.org

Black AIDS Institute. Provides public health information about a variety of topics including testing, treatment, vaccines, and health care access; focuses on black people and the black community.

http://www.blackaids.org

CDC National Center for Emerging and Zoonotic Infectious Diseases. Provides extensive information on a wide variety of infectious diseases.

http://www.cdc.gov/ncezid/

CDC National Prevention Information Network. Provides extensive information and links for HIV/AIDS and other STDs.

http://www.cdcnpin.org

CDC National STD and AIDS Hotlines. Callers can obtain information, counseling, and referrals for testing and treatment. The hotlines offer information on more than 20 STDs and include Spanish and TTY service.

800-342-AIDS or 800-227-8922; 800-344-SIDA (Spanish)
800-243-7889 (TTY, deaf access)

CDC: Vaccines. Information and answers to frequently asked questions about immunizations.

http://www.cdc.gov/vaccines/

HIV InSite: Gateway to AIDS Knowledge. Provides information about prevention, education, treatment, statistics, clinical trials, and new developments; from the University of California, San Francisco.

http://hivinsite.ucsf.edu

Joint United Nations Programme on HIV/AIDS (UNAIDS). Provides statistics and information on the international HIV/AIDS situation.

http://www.unaids.org

MedlinePlus: Sexually Transmitted Diseases. Maintained by the CDC; a clearinghouse of links and information on STDs.

http://www.nlm.nih.gov/medlineplus/
sexuallytransmitteddiseases.html

The NAMES Project Foundation AIDS Memorial Quilt. Includes the story behind the quilt, images of quilt panels, and information and links relating to HIV infection.

http://www.aidsquilt.org

National Institute of Allergy and Infectious Diseases. Includes fact sheets about many topics relating to allergies and infectious diseases, including tuberculosis and STDs.

http://www.niaid.nih.gov

Planned Parenthood Federation of America. Provides information about STDs, family planning, and contraception.

http://www.plannedparenthood.org

World Health Organization: Infectious Diseases. Provides fact sheets about many emerging and tropical diseases as well as information about current outbreaks.

http://www.who.int/topics/infectious_diseases/en/

SELECTED BIBLIOGRAPHY

American College Health Association. 2011. *American College Health Association–National College Health Assessment II: Reference Group Executive Summary Spring 2011.* Linthicum, MD: American College Health Association.

Blaser, M. 2011. Antibiotic overuse: Stop the killing of beneficial bacteria. *Nature* 476: 393–394.

Buchbinder, Susan. 2010. HIV epidemiology, testing strategies and prevention interventions. *Topics in HIV Medicine.* 18(2): 38–44.

Butler, D., and H. Ledford. 2012. US biosecurity board revises stance on mutant-flu studies. *Nature,* March 30 (http://www.nature.com/news/us-biosecurity-board-revises-stance-on-mutant-flu-studies-1.10369).

Caskey, Rachel. 2009. Knowledge and early adoption of the HPV vaccine among girls and young women: Results of a national survey. *Journal of Adolescent Health* 45(5): 453–462.

Centers for Disease Control and Prevention. 2006. Revised recommendations for HIV testing of adults, adolescents, and pregnant women in health care settings. *Morbidity and Mortality Weekly Report* 55(RR-14): 1–17.

Centers for Disease Control and Prevention. 2010. *Expedited Partner Therapy* (http://www.cdc.gov/std/ept/).

Centers for Disease Control and Prevention. 2011. Asthma in the United States: Growing every year (http://www.cdc.gov/vitalsigns/Asthma).

Centers for Disease Control and Prevention. 2011. HIV risk, prevention, and testing behaviors among men who have sex with men—National HIV Behavioral Surveillance System, 21 U.S. Cities, United States, 2008. *Morbidity and Mortality Weekly Report* 60(14): 1–11.

Centers for Disease Control and Prevention. 2011. Methicillin-resistant *Staphylococcus aureus* (MRSA) infections (http://www.cdc.gov/mrsa).

Centers for Disease Control and Prevention. 2011. Recommendations on the use of quadrivalent human papillomavirus vaccine in males—Advisory Committee on Immunization Practices (ACIP), 2011. *Morbidity and Mortality Weekly Report* 60(50): 1705–1708.

Centers for Disease Control and Prevention. 2011. *Sexually Transmitted Disease Surveillance, 2010.* Atlanta: U.S. Department of Health and Human Services.

Centers for Disease Control and Prevention. 2012. Recommended adult immunization schedule—United States, 2012. *Morbidity and Mortality Weekly Report* 61(4): 1–7.

Centers for Disease Control and Prevention. 2012. Seasonal influenza: Questions & answers (http://www.cdc.gov/flu/about/qa/disease.htm).

Centers for Disease Control and Prevention. 2012. Trends in tuberculosis—United States, 2011. *Morbidity and Mortality Weekly Report* 61(11): 180–189.

Chhabra, N., et al. 2012. Pharmacotherapy for mulitdrug resistant tuberculosis. *Journal of Pharmacology and Pharmacotherapy* 3(2): 98–104.

Do Prado, M. F., et al. 2012. Antimicrobial efficacy of alcohol-based gels with a 30-s application. *Letters in Applied Microbiology* 54(6): 564–567.

Frieri, M, and A. Valluri. 2011. Vitamin D deficiency as a risk factor for allergic disorders and immune mechanisms. *Allergy Asthma Proceedings* 32(6): 438–444.

Garland, S. 2010. Prevention strategies against human papillomavirus in males. *Gynecologic Oncology* 117(2010): S20–25.

Goetz, M. B., et al. 2010. HIV replication capacity is an independent predictor of disease progression in persons with untreated chronic HIV infection. *Journal of Acquired Immune Deficiency Syndrome* 53(4): 472–479.

Gradison, M. 2012. Pelvic inflammatory disease. *American Family Physician* 85(8): 791–796.

Harmon, K. 2011. What will the next influenza pandemic look like? *Scientific American,* September 19.

Lam, C. B., and E. S. Lefkowitz. 2012. Risky sexual behaviors in emerging adults: Longitudinal changes and within-person variations. *Archives of Sexual Behaviors,* May 11 (epub ahead of print).

Mathers, C. D., and D. Loncar. 2006. Projections of global mortality and burden of disease from 2002 to 2030. *Public Library of Science, Medicine* 3(11): 2011–2030.

McRee, A. L., et al. 2012. Human papillomavirus vaccine discussions: An opportunity for mothers to talk with their daughters about sexual health. *Sexually Transmitted Diseases* 29(5): 394–401.

Pennell, LM., et al. 2012. Sex affects immunity. *Journal of Autoimmunity* 38(2): 1282–1291.

Rashid, H., et al. 2012. Vaccination and herd immunity: What more do we know? *Current Opinion in Infectious Diseases* 25(3): 243–249.

Tobian, A., et al. 2009. Male Circumcision for the prevention of HSV-2 and HPV infections and syphilis. *New England Journal of Medicine* 360: 1298–309.

Tohme, R., and S. D. Holmberg. 2012. Transmission of hepatitis C virus infection through tattooing and piercing: A critical review. *Clinical Infectious Diseases* 54(8): 1167–1178.

U.S. Preventive Services Task Force. 2012. *Screening for Cervical Cancer* (http://www.uspreventiveservicestaskforce.org/uspstf/uspscerv.htm).

World Health Organization. *Global HIV/AIDS response: Epidemic Update and Health Sector Progress towards Universal Access: Progress Report 2011.* Geneva: World Health Organization.

World Health Organization. 2011. *Malaria Deaths Are Down but Progress Remains Fragile* (http://www.who.int/mediacentre/news/releases/2011/malaria_report_20111213/en/index.html).

World Health Organization. 2012. *Pneumonia Is the Leading Cause of Death in Children* (http://www.who.int/maternal_child_adolescent/news_events/news/2011/pneumonia/en).

The time to talk about safer sex is before you begin a sexual relationship. But even if you've been having unprotected sex with your partner, you can still start practicing safer sex now.

There are many ways to bring up the subject of safer sex and condom use with your partner. Be honest about your concerns and stress that protection against STDs means that you care about yourself and your partner. You may find that your partner shares your concerns and also wants to use condoms. He or she may be happy and relieved that you have brought up the subject of safer sex.

However, if he or she resists the idea of using condoms, you may need to negotiate (see the dialogue suggestions). Stress that you both deserve to be protected and that sex will be more enjoyable when you aren't worrying about STDs. If you and your partner haven't used condoms before, buy some and familiarize yourselves with how to use them. Once you feel more comfortable handling condoms, you'll be able to use them correctly and incorporate them into your sexual activity. Consider trying the female condom as well.

If your partner still won't agree to use condoms, think carefully about whether you want to have a sexual relationship with this person. Maybe he or she is not the right partner for you.

IF YOUR PARTNER SAYS . . .	TRY SAYING . . .
"They're not romantic."	"Worrying about AIDS isn't romantic, and with condoms we won't have to worry." OR "If we put one on together, a condom could be fun."
"You don't trust me."	"I do trust you, but how can I trust your former partners or mine?" OR "It's important to me that we're both protected."
"I don't have any diseases. I've been tested."	"I'm glad you've been tested, but tests aren't foolproof for all diseases. To be safe, I always use condoms."
"I forgot to bring a condom. But it's OK to skip it just this once."	"I'd really like to make love with you, but I never have sex without a condom. Let's go get some."
"I don't like the way they feel."	"They might feel different, but let's try." OR "Sex won't feel good if we're worrying about diseases." OR "How about trying the female condom?"
"I don't use condoms."	"I use condoms every time." OR "I don't have sex without condoms."
"But I love you."	"Being in love can't protect us from diseases." OR "I love you, too. We still need to use condoms."
"But we've been having sex without condoms."	"I want to start using condoms now so we won't be at any more risk." OR "We can still prevent infection or reinfection."

SOURCE: Dialogue from San Francisco AIDS Foundation. 1998. *Condoms for Couples*. Reprinted with permission.

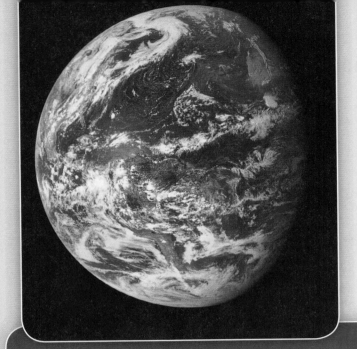

LOOKING AHEAD...

After reading this chapter, you should be able to

- Explain how population growth affects the earth's environment and contributes to pollution and climate change

- Discuss the causes and effects of air and water pollution, and describe strategies that people can take to protect these resources

- Discuss the issue of solid waste disposal and the impact it has on the environment and human health

- Identify some key sources of chemical and radiation pollution, and discuss methods for preventing such pollution

- Explain how energy use affects the environment, and describe steps everyone can take to use energy more efficiently

Environmental Health

14

We are constantly reminded of our intimate relationship with everything that surrounds us—our **environment.** Although the planet provides us with food, water, air, and everything else that sustains life, it also provides us with natural occurrences—earthquakes, tsunamis, hurricanes, drought, climate changes—that destroy life and disrupt society. In the past, humans frequently had to struggle against the environment to survive. Today, in addition to dealing with natural disasters, we also have to find ways to protect the environment from the by-products of our way of life.

This chapter introduces the concept of environmental health and explains how the environment affects us. The chapter also discusses the ways humans affect the planet and its resources, and describes steps you can take to improve your personal environmental health while reducing your impact on the earth.

ENVIRONMENTAL HEALTH DEFINED

The field of **environmental health** grew out of efforts to control communicable diseases. These efforts led to systematic garbage collection, sewage treatment, filtration and chlorination of drinking water, food inspection, and the establishment of public health enforcement agencies. Cleaning up the environment changed the health profile of the developed world, reducing or eliminating deaths from diseases like cholera and typhoid fever. Unfortunately, infectious diseases have not been eradicated worldwide.

In the United States a huge, complex public health system is constantly at work behind the scenes. Every time the system is disrupted, danger recurs. After any disaster that damages a community's public health system, prompt restoration of basic health services becomes crucial to human survival. Every time we venture beyond the boundaries of our everyday world, whether traveling to a less developed country or camping in a wilderness area, we are reminded of the importance of these basics: clean water, sanitary waste disposal, safe food, and insect and rodent control.

Over the last few decades, the focus of environmental health has expanded and become more complex. We now recognize that environmental pollutants contribute not only to infectious diseases but to many chronic diseases as well. Technological advances have increased our ability to affect and damage the environment. Rapid population growth, which has resulted partly from past environmental improvements, means that far more people are consuming and competing for resources than ever before, magnifying the effect of humans on the environment.

Environmental health encompasses all the interactions of humans with their environment and the health consequences

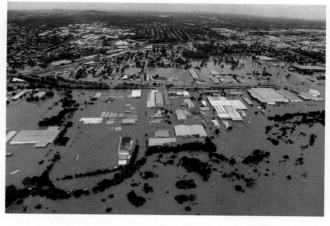

Natural events—such as the flooding that occurred in Queensland in 2012—can directly kill thousands of people while wiping out essential services, polluting water, and facilitating the spread of disease.

of these interactions. Fundamental to this definition is a recognition that we hold the world in trust for future generations and for other forms of life. Our responsibility is to pass on a world no worse, and preferably better, than the one we live in today. Although many environmental problems are complex and seem beyond the control of the individual, there are ways that people can make a difference to the future of the planet.

POPULATION GROWTH AND CONTROL

Throughout most of history, humans have been a minor pressure on the planet. About 300 million people were alive in the year AD 1; by the time Europeans were settling in the United States 1600 years later, the world population had increased

> **TERMS**
>
> **environment**   The natural and human-made surroundings in which we spend our lives.
>
> **environmental health**   The collective interactions of humans with the environment and the short-term and long-term health consequences of those interactions.

gradually to a little over 500 million. But then it began rising exponentially—zooming to 1 billion by about 1800, more than doubling by 1930, and then doubling again in just 40 years (Figure 14.1).

The United Nations projects that world population will reach 9.3 billion by 2050 and will continue to increase until it levels off above 10.1 billion in 2100. Virtually all of this increase is taking place in less developed regions. This rapid expansion of population, particularly in the past 50 years, is generally believed to be responsible for most of the stress humans put on the environment.

No one knows how many people the world can support, but most scientists agree that there is a limit. A 2011 report from the United Nation's Convention on Biological Diversity states that the population's demand for resources already exceeds the earth's capacity by 20%. The primary factors that may eventually put a cap on human population are likely to be the limits of the earth's resources—food, water, land, and energy.

FIGURE 14.1   World population growth. The United Nations estimates that the world's population will continue to increase dramatically until it stabilizes above 10 billion people in 2100.

SOURCES: United Nations Population Division. 2011. *World Population Prospects: The 2010 Revision.* (http://esa.un.org/unpd/wpp/) New York: United Nations; U.S. Bureau of the Census.

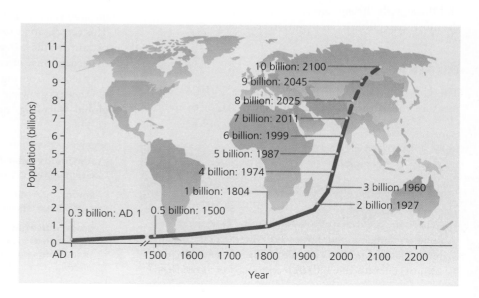

The mass media have exposed the entire world to the American lifestyle and raised people's expectations of living at a comparable level. But such a lifestyle is supported by levels of energy consumption that the earth cannot support indefinitely. The United States has about 5% of the world's population but uses 25% of the world's energy.

Although it is apparent that population growth must be controlled, population trends are difficult to influence and manage. A variety of interconnecting factors fuel the current population explosion, including high fertility rates, lack of family planning resources, and low death rates.

To be successful, population management policies must change the condition of people's lives, especially poverty, to remove the pressures to have large families. Research indicates that the combination of improved health, better education, and increased literacy and employment opportunities for women works together with family planning to decrease fertility rates. Unfortunately, in the fastest-growing countries, the needs of a rapidly increasing population use up financial resources that might otherwise be used to improve lives and ultimately slow population growth.

> The United States has about 5% of the world's population but **uses 25% of the world's energy.**

AIR QUALITY AND POLLUTION

Air pollution is not a human invention or even a new problem. The air is polluted naturally with every forest fire, pollen bloom, and dust storm, as well as with countless other natural pollutants. To these natural sources, humans have always contributed the by-products of their activities.

Air pollution is linked to a wide range of health problems. The very young, the elderly, and those with chronic diseases are among the most susceptible to air pollution's effects.

Air Quality and Smog

The U.S. Environmental Protection Agency (EPA) uses a measure called the **Air Quality Index (AQI)** to indicate

whether air pollution levels pose a health concern. The AQI is used for five major air pollutants: carbon monoxide (CO), sulfur dioxide (SO_2), nitrogen dioxide (NO_2), particulate matter (PM), and ground-level ozone. A major source of these pollutants is the burning of fossil fuels in vehicles and industrial processes. AQI values run from 0 to 500; the higher the AQI, the greater the level of pollution and associated health danger. Local AQI information is often available in newspapers, on television and radio, on the Internet, and from state and local telephone hotlines.

The term **smog** was first used in the early 1900s in London to describe the combination of smoke and fog. What we typically call *smog* today is a mixture of pollutants, with ground-level ozone being the key ingredient. Major smog occurrences are linked to the combination of several factors: heavy motor vehicle traffic, high temperatures, and sunny weather can increase the production of ozone. Pollutants are also more likely to build up in areas with little wind and/or where a topographic feature such as a mountain range or valley prevents the wind from pushing out stagnant air.

The Greenhouse Effect and Global Warming

The temperature of the earth's atmosphere depends on the balance between the amount of energy the planet absorbs from the sun (mainly as high-energy ultraviolet radiation) and the amount of energy radiated back into space as lower-energy infrared radiation. Key components of temperature regulation are carbon dioxide, water vapor, methane, and other **greenhouse gases**—so named because, like the glass panes in a greenhouse, they let through visible light from the sun but trap some of the resulting infrared radiation and reradiate it back to the earth's surface. This reradiation causes a buildup of heat that raises the temperature of the lower atmosphere, a natural process known as the **greenhouse effect.** (See page T1-5 of the color transparency insert "Touring Lifestyle Behaviors" in Chapter 10.)

There is growing consensus that human activity is causing **global warming,** or *climate change*. The concentration of

Air Quality Index (AQI)   A measure of local air quality and what it means for health.   TERMS

smog   Hazy atmospheric conditions resulting from increased concentrations of ground-level ozone and other pollutants.

greenhouse gas   A gas (such as carbon dioxide) or vapor that traps infrared radiation instead of allowing it to escape through the atmosphere, resulting in a warming of the earth (the *greenhouse effect*).

greenhouse gases is increasing because of human activity, especially the combustion of **fossil fuels.** Carbon dioxide levels in the atmosphere have increased rapidly in recent decades and currently stand at 396.18 parts per million. Many scientists and climate experts say that 350 parts per million is the target number for the safe upper limit of carbon concentration in our atmosphere. The use of fossil fuels pumps more than 20 billion tons of carbon dioxide into the atmosphere every year. Deforestation, often by burning, also sends carbon dioxide into the atmosphere and reduces the number of trees available to convert carbon dioxide into oxygen.

The 12-month period between May 2011 and April 2012 was the warmest period on record since record keeping began in 1895, and the 10 warmest periods have all occurred since June 1999. The average global temperature has risen more than 1 degree Fahrenheit since 1895. There is growing agreement among scientists that temperatures will continue to rise. Possible consequences include increased rainfall and flooding in some regions, and increased drought in others; increased mortality from heat stress, urban air pollution, and tropical diseases; a poleward shift of about 50–350 miles in the location of vegetation zones, affecting crop yields, irrigation demands, and forest productivity; and increasingly rapid and drastic melting of the earth's polar ice caps. Parties at the 2011 United Nations Climate Change Conference in Durban, South Africa, endorsed the scientific view that keeping the increase in global temperature below 2 degrees Celsius is necessary to stave off the worst effects of climate change.

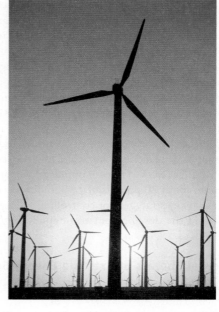

Wind power, generated from turbines, is a clean and renewable source of energy.

trialized nations agreed to eliminate CFC production in the year 2000. Ozone-depleting substances have very long lifetimes in the atmosphere, however, so despite these efforts, the ozone hole is not expected to disappear until 2070.

Thinning of the Ozone Layer

Another air pollution problem is the thinning of the **ozone layer** of the atmosphere, a fragile, invisible layer about 10–30 miles above the earth's surface that shields the planet from the sun's hazardous ultraviolet (UV) rays. Since the mid-1980s scientists have observed the seasonal appearance and growth of a hole in the ozone layer over Antarctica. More recently thinning over other areas has been noted.

The ozone layer is being destroyed primarily by **chlorofluorocarbons (CFCs)**, industrial chemicals that rise into the atmosphere and release chlorine atoms, which destroy ozone. In the Northern Hemisphere, ozone levels have declined by about 10% since 1980, and certain areas may be temporarily depleted in late winter and early spring by as much as 40%. Without the ozone layer to absorb the sun's UV radiation, life on earth would be impossible. The potential effects of increased long-term exposure to UV light for humans include skin cancer, wrinkling and aging of the skin, cataracts and blindness, and reduced immune response. UV light may interfere with photosynthesis and cause lower crop yields; it may also kill phytoplankton and krill—the basis of the ocean food chain.

Worldwide production and use of CFCs have declined rapidly since the danger to the ozone layer was recognized. Indus-

> Without the ozone layer to absorb the sun's UV radiation, **life on earth would be impossible.**

Energy Use and Air Pollution

Americans are the biggest energy consumers in the world. About 83% of the energy we use comes from fossil fuels—oil, coal, and natural gas. The remainder comes from nuclear power and renewable energy sources (such as hydroelectric, wind, and solar power).

TERMS

fossil fuels Buried deposits of decayed animals and plants that are converted into carbon-rich fuels by exposure to heat and pressure over millions of years; oil, coal, and natural gas are fossil fuels.

greenhouse effect A warming of the earth due to a buildup of greenhouse gases in the atmosphere.

global warming An increase in the earth's atmospheric temperature when averaged across seasons and geographical regions; also called *climate change.*

ozone layer A layer of ozone molecules (O_3) in the upper atmosphere that screens out UV rays from the sun.

chlorofluorocarbons (CFCs) Chemicals used as spray can propellants, refrigerants, and industrial solvents, which have been implicated in the destruction of the ozone layer.

Energy consumption is at the root of many environmental problems, especially those relating to air pollution. Automobile exhaust and the burning of oil and coal by industry and by electric power plants are primary causes of smog, acid precipitation, and the greenhouse effect. The mining of coal and the extraction and transportation of oil cause pollution on land and in the water. Nuclear power generation creates hazardous wastes and carries the risk of dangerous releases of radiation.

Despite increases in U.S. consumer gas prices, more than 70% of commuters drive alone to work, and low-fuel-economy sport utility vehicles (SUVs) remain popular. Every gallon of gas burned puts about 20 pounds of carbon dioxide into the atmosphere. Two key strategies for controlling energy use are conservation and the development of nonpolluting, renewable energy sources.

Environmental Threats of Extreme Energy Sources

As the worldwide demand for energy rises and supplies of easily accessible oil dwindle, some energy companies have turned to what are often called "extreme energy sources—fossil fuels that are relatively difficult to access and extract from the environment. Examples include deepwater oil rigs, tar sands oil extraction, and hydrofracking of natural gas.

The Deepwater Horizon oil rig that exploded in April 2011 in the Gulf of Mexico was a deepwater rig. As oil gushed into the waters of the Gulf at an estimated rate of 60,000 barrels a day, it became clear that BP, the company that owned the rig, did not know how to stop it. It took BP three months to plug the leak, after nearly 5 million barrels of oil were released into the Gulf. The disaster killed thousands of birds, hundreds of endangered sea turtles, and many dolphins and other marine mammals. The Gulf's ecosystems may need generations to recover fully, and some parts of it may never recover.

Tar sands (or oil sands) are sand deposits that are saturated with a dense form of petroleum called bitumen. The largest deposits are found in Canada, Kazakhstan, and Russia. Making liquid fuel from the oil in tar sands is a very energy-intensive process. When used as fuel, the resulting molasses-like product produces two to four times the amount of greenhouse gases per barrel compared to other conventional oils. In addition, Canada's tar sands oil will need to travel through thousands of miles of pipelines across pristine wildlife habitats in both Canada and the United States.

Hydraulic fracturing, or "fracking," uses pressurized mixes of fluids to create cracks in rock formations deep underground, releasing natural gas. Critics have raised concerns about the safety of the technique, and reports of groundwater contamination have been verified by independent third parties.

Renewable Energy

Renewable energy sources are those sources that are naturally replenished and essentially inex-

haustible, such as wind and sunlight. Together with technologies that improve energy efficiency, renewable energy sources contribute to sustainability—the capacity of natural or human systems to endure and maintain well-being over time. A common definition of *sustainable development* is development that meets society's present needs without compromising the ability of future generations to meet their needs.

Renewable energy sources include wind power, solar power, water and wave power, geothermal power, and biomass and biofuels from renewable sources, among others. Worldwide, renewable energy sources were providing one-quarter of power capacity from all sources and 19% of the global electricity supply in 2011, and 118 countries had enacted some type of policy target or promotion policy related to renewable energy. Many of these targets call for 15–25% of energy or electricity to be provided by renewable sources by 2020.

Alternative Fuels The U.S. Department of Energy (DOE) encourages researchers and automobile manufacturers to produce vehicles that can handle alternative fuels such as ethanol. Ethanol, a form of alcohol, is a renewable fuel produced from fermenting plant sugars such as corn, sugarcane, and other starchy agricultural products. Ethanol use reduces the amount of imported oil required to produce gasoline, reduces overall greenhouse gas emissions from automobiles, and supports the U.S. agricultural industry. Ethanol can be used alone or mixed with gasoline.

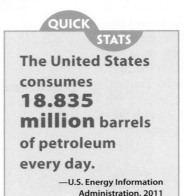

QUICK STATS

The United States consumes 18.835 million barrels of petroleum every day.
—U.S. Energy Information Administration, 2011

Ethanol, however, has its critics, who say the alternative fuel may do more harm than good. For one thing, some reports show that corn-based ethanol requires more energy to produce than it yields when burned as fuel. In addition, the production of ethanol diverts corn crops from the food supply and may be a factor in food shortages around the world. The food-related concerns prompted the United Nations to call for a moratorium on food-based ethanol production until nonfood sources of alternative fuels could be developed.

Another alternative fuel is biodiesel, a fuel made primarily from vegetable oils, fats, or greases. It is the fastest-growing alternative fuel in the United States, is biodegradable, and produces lower levels of most air pollutants than petroleum-based products. Biodiesel, like ethanol, can be problematic depending on its material source. If it is produced from waste animal fat and grease or as a by-product of other agricultural processes, it can be carbon-neutral. But in some parts of the world natural vegetation and forests have been cleared and burned to grow soybeans and palm oil trees to make biodiesel, and these negative environmental and social effects can outweigh any benefit.

Hybrid and Electric Vehicles Hybrid vehicles use two or more distinct power sources to propel the vehicle, such as a battery and an internal combustion engine. The hybrid vehicle typically realizes greater fuel economy than a conventional car does and produces fewer polluting emissions. Hybrids also

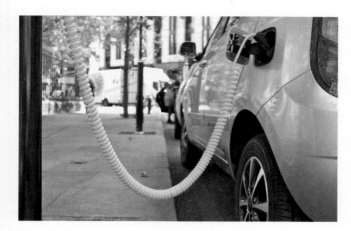

A new generation of electric vehicles is taking advantage of the development of infrastructure to support its use.

tend to run with less noise than conventional vehicles. All-electric vehicles are also gaining credibility and popularity. A new generation of all-electric vehicles has recently been introduced to consumer markets, taking advantage of better battery storage performance, "quick-charging station" infrastructure, and changing consumer perceptions of trip use and distance. Researchers hope that hybrid and battery technologies can be extended to all classes of vehicles.

Indoor Air Quality

Although most people associate air pollution with the outdoors, buildings may also harbor potentially dangerous pollutants. Some of these compounds trigger allergic responses, and others have been linked to cancer. Common indoor pollutants include environmental tobacco smoke (ETS); carbon monoxide and other combustion by-products from wood-stoves, fireplaces, kerosene heaters and lamps, and gas ranges; volatile organic compounds (VOCs), gases emitted from paints, lacquers, cleaning supplies, aerosols, building materials, furnishings, and office equipment; and biological pollutants like bacteria, dust mites, mold, and animal dander, which can cause health problems when inhaled, especially for people with asthma and other respiratory conditions.

Preventing Air Pollution

You can do a great deal to reduce air pollution. Here are a few ideas:

- Cut back on driving. Ride your bike, walk, use public transportation, or carpool in a fuel-efficient vehicle.

- Keep your car tuned up and well maintained. Keep your tires inflated at recommended pressures. To save energy when driving, avoid quick starts, stay within the speed limit, limit the use of air conditioning, and don't let your car idle unless absolutely necessary.

- Buy energy-efficient appliances and use them only when you have full loads. Do laundry in warm or cold water

instead of hot. Clean refrigerator coils and clothes dryer lint screens frequently.

- Replace incandescent bulbs with LED and compact fluorescent bulbs (CFLs). Although they cost more initially, they save you money in the long run. Burned-out CFLs should be recycled, not put in the trash, because they contain small amounts of mercury.

- Make sure your home is well-insulated with ozone-safe agents; use insulating shades and curtains to keep heat in during winter and out during summer.

- Plant and care for trees in your yard and neighborhood. They recycle carbon dioxide, so trees work against global warming. They also provide shade and cool the air so less air conditioning is needed.

- Before discarding a refrigerator, air conditioner, or humidifier, check with the waste hauler or your local government to ensure that ozone-depleting refrigerants will be removed prior to disposal.

- Keep paints, cleaning agents, and other chemical products tightly sealed in their original containers.

- Clean and inspect chimneys, furnaces, and other appliances regularly. Install carbon monoxide detectors.

WATER QUALITY AND POLLUTION

Few parts of the world have enough safe, clean drinking water, and yet few things are as important to human health.

Water Contamination and Treatment

Many cities rely at least in part on wells that tap local groundwater, but often it is necessary to tap lakes and rivers to supplement wells. Because such surface water is more likely to be contaminated with both organic matter and pathogenic microorganisms, it is purified in water treatment plants before being piped into the community. **Fluoridation,** a water treatment process that reduces tooth decay by 15–40%, has

---

Ask Yourself

QUESTIONS FOR CRITICAL THINKING AND REFLECTION

What are your views on the issue of climate change? Do you believe it is a real problem, or that it has been overly hyped by the media and some politicians and activist groups? How do you support your views?

---

fluoridation   The addition of fluoride to the water supply to reduce tooth decay.

been used successfully in the United States for more than 60 years. In most areas of the United States, water systems have adequate, dependable supplies, are able to control waterborne disease, and provide water without unacceptable color, odor, or taste. However, problems do occur. The CDC estimate that 1 million Americans become ill and 900–1000 die each year from microbial illnesses from drinking water.

Water Shortages

Water shortages are a growing concern in many regions of the world. Some parts of the United States, such as the desert West, are experiencing rapid population growth that outstrips the ability of local systems to provide adequate water to all. Groundwater pumping and the diversion of water from lakes and rivers for irrigation are further reducing the amount of water available to local communities.

Sewage

Most cities have sewage treatment systems that separate fecal matter from water in huge tanks and ponds and stabilize it so that it cannot transmit infectious diseases. After it is treated and biologically safe, the water is released back into the environment. The sludge that remains behind is often contaminated with **heavy metals** and is handled as hazardous waste. If not contaminated, sludge may be used as fertilizer, although this practice is being discouraged by scientists and some government agencies and is not permitted in organic agriculture.

Many cities have expanded sewage treatment measures to remove heavy metals and other hazardous chemicals. This action has resulted from many studies linking exposure to chemicals such as mercury, lead, and **polychlorinated biphenyls (PCBs)** with long-term health consequences, including cancer and damage to the central nervous system.

Protecting the Water Supply

By reducing your own water use, you help preserve your community's valuable supply. By taking steps to keep the water supply clean, you reduce pollution overall and help protect the land, wildlife, and other people from illness. Here are some simple steps you can take:

• Take showers, not baths, to minimize your water consumption. Don't let water run when you're not actively

QUICK STATS

The average American generates **4.5 pounds** of trash per day; about 1.5 pounds of this is recycled.

—Environmental Protection Agency, 2010

Ask Yourself

QUESTIONS FOR CRITICAL THINKING AND REFLECTION

How would you describe the quality of the water where you live? Are there lakes or streams where you can safely swim or fish? What local information sources can you find about water quality in your area?

using it while brushing your teeth, shaving, or hand-washing clothes.

• Install sink faucet aerators and water-efficient showerheads, which use two to five times less water with no noticeable decrease in performance. Purchase a water-saving toilet, or put a displacement device in your toilet tank to reduce the amount of water used with each flush.

• Fix any leaky faucets in your home. Leaks can waste thousands of gallons of water per year.

• Don't pour toxic materials such as cleaning solvents, bleach, or motor oil down the drain. Store them until you can take them to a hazardous waste collection center.

• Don't pour old medicines down the drain or flush them down the toilet. Some pharmacies will take back unused or expired medications for disposal, and many communities have drop-off days for these drugs.

SOLID WASTE POLLUTION

Humans generate huge amounts of waste, which must be handled appropriately to ensure environmental safety.

Solid Waste

The bulk of the organic food garbage produced in American kitchens is now dumped in the sewage system by way of the mechanical garbage disposal. The garbage that remains is not hazardous from the standpoint of infectious disease because there is very little food waste in it, but it does represent an enormous disposal and contamination problem.

What's in Our Garbage?   The biggest single component of household trash by weight is paper products, including junk mail, glossy mail-order catalogs, and computer printouts (Figure 14.2). About 1% of the solid waste is toxic; a new source of toxic waste is the disposal of computer components in both household and commercial waste. Burning, as opposed to burial, reduces the bulk of solid waste, but it can release hazardous material into the air, depending on what is being burned.

---

heavy metal   A metal with a high specific gravity, such as lead, copper, or tin.

polychlorinated biphenyl (PCB)   An industrial chemical used as an insulator in electrical transformers and linked to certain human cancers; banned worldwide since 1977 but persistent in the environment.

TERMS

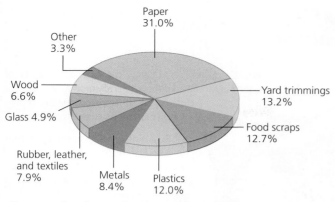

Paper
31.0%

Other
3.3%

Wood
6.6%

Glass 4.9%

Rubber, leather,
and textiles
7.9%

Metals
8.4%

Plastics
12.0%

Yard trimmings
13.2%

Food scraps
12.7%

Due to rounding, these numbers do not add up to 100%.

FIGURE 14.2   Components of municipal solid waste, by weight, before recycling.

SOURCE: Environmental Protection Agency, 2011. *Municipal Solid Waste Generation , Recycling and Disposal in the United States: Facts and Figures* for 2010. Washington, DC: Environmental Protection Agency. Pub. No. EPA-530-F-11-005.

Table 14.1	Biodegrading Times of Different Objects	
ITEM	**TIME REQUIRED TO BIODEGRADE**	
Banana peel	2–10 days	
Paper	2–5 months	
Rope	3–14 months	
Orange peel	6 months	
Wool sock	1–5 years	
Cigarette butt	1–12 years	
Plastic-coated milk carton	5 years	
Aluminum can	80–100 years	
Plastic six-pack holder ring	450 years	
Glass bottle	1 million years	
Plastic bottle	Forever	

Manufacturing, mining, and other industries all produce large amounts of potentially dangerous materials that cannot simply be dumped.

Disposing of Solid Waste   Since the 1960s, billions of tons of solid waste have been buried in **sanitary landfill** disposal sites. Sometimes protective liners are used around the site, and nearby monitoring wells are now required in most states. Layers of solid waste are regularly covered with thin layers of dirt until the site is filled. Some communities then plant grass and trees and convert the site into a park. Landfill is relatively stable; almost no decomposition occurs in the solidly packed waste. Much of this waste contains chemicals, ranging from leftover pesticides to paints and oils, that should not be released into the environment. Despite precautions, buried contaminants sometimes leak into the surrounding soil and groundwater. Burial is also expensive and requires huge amounts of space.

Biodegradation is the process by which organic substances are broken down naturally by living organisms. Items that are biodegradable can break down naturally, safely, and quickly into the raw materials of nature, then disappear back into the environment. Table 14.1 shows the amount of time required for different types of material to biodegrade.

Recycling   In **recycling,** many kinds of waste materials are collected and used as raw materials in the production of new

products. Recycling is a good idea because it puts unwanted objects back to good use and because it reduces the amount of solid waste sitting in landfills, some of which takes decades to decay naturally.

Discarded Technology: eWaste   Americans scrap about 400 million consumer electronic devices each year. This "e-waste" is the fastest-growing portion of our waste stream. Junked electronic devices are toxic because they contain varying amounts of lead, mercury, and other heavy metals. Many components of electronic devices are valuable, however, and can be recycled and reused. Local and state e-waste recycling programs are becoming more common, and private companies are also getting into the e-waste recycling business. If you recycle your electronic devices, look for a "green" program or one that is certified by e-stewards, an organization that advocates for responsible e-waste recycling (www.e-stewards.org).

Reducing Solid Waste

By reducing your consumption, recycling more, and throwing away less, you can conserve landfill space and put more reusable items back into service. Here are some ideas to help you reduce solid waste:

• Buy products with the least amount of packaging you can, or buy products in bulk (see the box "How to Be a Green Consumer") or packaged in recyclable containers.

Ask Yourself

QUESTIONS FOR CRITICAL THINKING AND REFLECTION

What are your own waste disposal habits like? Do you recycle everything you possibly can? Do you get rid of items that are still usable? Even if you are conscientious about the way you deal with waste, how could you improve your habits?

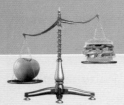

CRITICAL CONSUMER
How to Be a Green Consumer

You can quickly and easily develop habits that direct your consumer dollars toward environmentally friendly products and companies.

• Remember the four Rs of green consumerism:

    • Reduce the amount of trash and pollution you generate by consuming and throwing away less.

    • Reuse as many products as possible—either yourself or by selling them or donating them to charity.

    • Recycle all appropriate materials and buy recycled products whenever possible.

    • Respond by educating others about reducing waste and recycling, by finding creative ways to reduce waste and toxicity, and by making your preferences known.

• Choose products packaged in refillable, recycled, reusable containers, such as paper, cardboard, aluminum, or glass. Don't buy products that are excessively packaged or wrapped.

• Look for products made with the highest possible content of recycled paper, metal, glass, plastic, and other materials.

• Choose simple products containing the lowest amounts of bleaches, dyes, and fragrances. Look for organically grown foods and for clothing made from organically grown cotton or naturally colored cotton.

• Buy high-quality appliances that have an Energy Star seal from the EPA or some other type of certification indicating that they are energy- and water-efficient.

• Get a reusable cloth shopping bag. If you forget to bring your bag to the store, use paper bags to carry your purchases home—and reuse or recycle those bags.

• Look beyond the products to the companies that make them. Support those with good environmental records. If some of your favorite products are overpackaged or contain harmful ingredients, write to the manufacturer.

• Keep in mind that doing something is better than doing nothing. Even if you can't be a perfectly green consumer, doing your best on any purchase *will* make a difference.

SOURCES: U.S. Environmental Protection Agency. 2010. The *Consumer's Handbook for Reducing Solid Waste* (http://www.epa.gov/osw/wycd/catbook); Natural Resources Defense Council. 2012. *NRDC's Smarter Living* (http://www.nrdc.org/living/default.asp).

• Buy recycled or recyclable products. Avoid disposables; instead use long-lasting or reusable products such as refillable pens and rechargeable batteries.

• Avoid using foam or paper cups and plastic stirrers by bringing your own ceramic coffee mug and metal spoon to work or wherever you drink coffee or tea. Pack your lunch in reusable containers.

• To store food, use glass jars and reusable plastic containers rather than foil and plastic wrap.

• Recycle your newspapers, glass, cans, paper, and other recyclables. If you receive something packaged with foam pellets, take them to a commercial mailing center that accepts them for recycling.

• Do not throw electronic items, batteries, or fluorescent lights into the trash. Take these to state-approved recycling centers.

• Start a compost pile for your organic garbage (non-animal food and yard waste) if you have a yard. If you live in an apartment, you can take your organic wastes to a community composting center. Many communities now offer curbside collection of kitchen scraps for recycling into compost, which is sold to farms and wineries.

CHEMICAL POLLUTION AND HAZARDOUS WASTE

New chemical substances are constantly being introduced into the environment as pesticides, herbicides, solvents, and hundreds of other products. More people and wildlife are exposed to them than ever before.

Asbestos

A mineral-based compound, asbestos was widely used for fire protection and insulation in buildings until the late 1960s. Microscopic asbestos fibers can be released into the air when this material is applied or when it later deteriorates or is damaged. These fibers can lodge in the lungs, causing **asbestosis,** lung cancer, and other serious lung diseases. Similar conditions expose workers to risk in the coal mining industry, from coal and silica dust (black lung disease), and in the textile industry, from cotton fibers (brown lung disease).

Lead

Thanks to better preventive efforts, lead poisoning is not as serious a problem today as it was in the past. Still, the CDC estimates that about 435,000 children under age 6 may have unsafe lead levels in their blood; the actual number could be much higher. Many of these children live in poor, inner-city areas (see the box "Poverty, Gender, and Environmental Health"). When lead is ingested or inhaled, it can damage the central nervous system, cause mental impairment, hinder oxygen transport in the blood, create digestive problems, and cause coma or even death. Neurological damage can be permanent.

Lead-based paints are the chief culprit in lead poisoning of children. They were banned from residential use in 1978, but as many as 57 million American homes still contain lead paint. The EPA requires contractors to take special lead containment measures when doing renovations, repairs, or painting in certain buildings. The use of lead in plumbing is now also banned, but some old pipes and faucets contain lead.

Pesticides

Pesticides are used to prevent the spread of insect-borne diseases and to maximize food production by killing insects that eat crops. Both uses have risks as well as benefits. For example, DDT was extremely effective in controlling insect-borne diseases in tropical countries and in increasing crop yields throughout the world, but it was found to disrupt the life cycles of birds, fish, and reptiles and was banned in the United States in 1972. DDT also builds up in the food chain, increasing in concentration as larger animals eat smaller ones—a process known as **biomagnification.**

Mercury

A naturally occurring metal, mercury is a toxin that affects the nervous system and may damage the brain, kidneys, and gastrointestinal tract; increase blood pressure, heart rate, and heart attack risk; and cause cancer. Mercury slows fetal and child development and causes irreversible deficits in brain function. Coal-fired power plants are the largest producers of mercury; other sources include mining and smelting operations and the disposal of consumer products containing mercury. Mercury persists in the environment and, like pesticides, it is bioaccumulative. In particular, large, long-lived fish may carry high levels of mercury. Chapter 9 includes information about safe fish consumption.

Other Chemical Pollutants

Hazardous wastes are commonly found in the home and should be handled and disposed of properly. They include automotive supplies (motor oil, antifreeze, transmission fluid), paint supplies (turpentine, paint thinner, mineral spirits), art and hobby supplies (oil-based paint, solvents, acids and alkalis, aerosol sprays), insecticides, batteries, computer and electronic components, and household cleaners containing sodium hydroxide (lye) or ammonia. These chemicals are dangerous when inhaled or ingested, when they contact the skin or the eyes, or when they are burned or dumped. Many cities provide guidelines about approved disposal methods and have hazardous waste collection days.

Preventing Chemical Pollution

You can take steps to reduce the chemical pollution in your community.

• When buying products, read the labels, and try to buy the least toxic ones available. Choose nontoxic, nonpetrochemical cleansers, disinfectants, polishes, and other personal and household products.

• Dispose of your household hazardous wastes properly. If you are not sure whether something is hazardous or don't know how to dispose of it, contact your local environmental health office or health department.

• Buy organic produce and produce that has been grown locally.

TERMS

asbestosis   A lung condition caused by inhalation of microscopic asbestos fibers, which inflame the lung and can lead to lung cancer.

pesticides   Chemicals used to prevent the spread of diseases transmitted by insects and to maximize food production by killing insects that eat crops.

biomagnification   The accumulation of a substance in a food chain.

Ask Yourself

QUESTIONS FOR CRITICAL THINKING AND REFLECTION

Are there any hazardous chemicals in your home, such as cleaning products, solvents, paint, or batteries? Would you know what to do if one of these chemicals spilled? How would you clean it up?

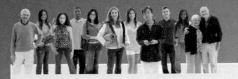

Residents of poor and minority communities are often exposed to more environmental toxins than are residents of wealthier communities, and they are more likely to suffer from health problems caused or aggravated by pollutants.

Poor neighborhoods are often located near highways and industrial areas that have high levels of air and noise pollution; they are also common sites for hazardous waste production and disposal. Residents of substandard housing are more likely to come into contact with lead, asbestos, carbon monoxide, pesticides, and other hazardous pollutants associated with peeling paint, old plumbing, and poorly maintained insulation and heating equipment.

In addition, poor people are more likely to have jobs that expose them to asbestos, silica dust, and pesticides, and they are more likely to catch and consume fish contaminated with PCBs, mercury, and other toxins.

The most thoroughly researched and documented link among poverty, the environment, and health is lead poisoning in children. Many studies have shown that children of low-income black families are much more likely to have elevated levels of lead in their blood than are white children. One survey found that two-thirds of urban African American children from families earning less than $6000 a year had elevated lead levels. The CDC and the American Academy of Pediatrics recommend annual testing of blood lead levels for all children under age 6, with more frequent testing for children at special risk.

Asthma is another health threat that appears to be linked with both environmental and socioeconomic factors. The number of Americans with asthma has grown dramatically in the past 20 years; most of the increase has occurred in children, with African Americans and the poor hardest hit. Researchers are not sure what accounts for this increase, but suspects include household pollutants, pesticides, air pollution, cigarette smoke, and allergens like cockroaches. These risk factors are likely to cluster in poor urban areas where inadequate health care may worsen asthma's effects.

Gender also influences exposure to environmental hazards. In many societies, women are more often involved in day-to-day activities associated with the environment, including food preparation, agricultural work, and tasks around the home. These activities can expose women to indoor air pollution, water pollution, foodborne pathogens, agricultural chemicals, and waste contamination. Indoor pollutants, especially soot from burning wood, charcoal, and other solid fuels used for home heating and cooking, are a particular risk. Exposure to this particulate pollution increases the risk of respiratory diseases, lung cancer, and reproductive problems. In 2010 U.S. Secretary of State Hillary Clinton launched the Global Alliance for Clean Cookstoves to help hundreds of millions of people, mostly women, avoid the toxic smoke produced by traditional stoves and open fires used in poorly ventilated indoor areas.

All humans are exposed to chemicals in air, food, and drinking water, and we all carry a body load of chemicals. Some of these chemicals bioaccumulate in our bones, blood, or fatty tissues. Women are smaller than men, on average, and have a higher percentage of body fat, so chemicals that accumulate in fatty tissue may pose a relatively greater risk for women. On the other hand, men may be more likely to work in industries that involve significant occupational exposures to disease-related toxins. For example, coal miners have an increased risk of lung cancer (black lung disease).

Although any chemical exposure can be a concern for health, women face the added risk of passing pollutants to a developing fetus during pregnancy or to an infant through breastfeeding. Even relatively low exposure to pollutants can result in a significant chemical body load in an infant or young child because of their small body size. And because infants and children are still developing, the effects of chemical exposure can be significant and devastating. It is not unusual for dangerous toxin exposures to be first recognized through noticeable effects on infants or children.

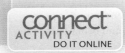

connect
ACTIVITY
DO IT ONLINE

• If you must use pesticides or toxic household products, store them in a locked place where children and pets can't get to them. Don't measure chemicals with food preparation utensils, and wear gloves whenever handling them.

• If you have your house fumigated for pest control, be sure to hire a licensed exterminator. Keep everyone, including pets, out of the house while the crew works and, if possible, for a few days after.

RADIATION POLLUTION

Radiation comes in different forms and from different sources, such as the sun, uranium, and nuclear weapons. Of most concern to health are gamma rays produced by radioactive sources such as nuclear weapons, nuclear energy plants, and radon gas. These high-energy waves are powerful enough to penetrate objects and break molecular bonds. Although gamma radiation cannot be seen or felt, its effects at high doses can include **radiation sickness** and death. At lower doses, chromosome damage, sterility, tissue damage, cataracts, and cancer can occur. Other types of radiation can also

> **TERMS**
>
> **radiation** Energy transmitted in the form of rays, waves, or particles.
>
> **radiation sickness** An illness caused by excess radiation exposure, marked by low white blood cell counts and nausea; possibly fatal.

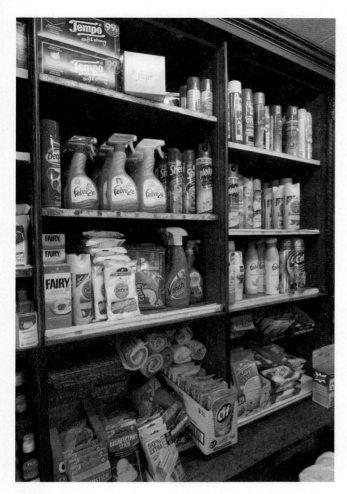

Hazardous chemicals accumulate in many homes, as well as in businesses and industrial sites

as an alternative to oil and coal, it was promoted as clean, efficient, inexpensive, and safe. In general, this has proven to be the case. Power systems in several parts of the world rely on nuclear power plants. However, despite all the built-in safeguards and regulating agencies, accidents in nuclear power plants do happen, whether as a result of human error or following a natural disaster. The 1986 fire and explosion at the Chernobyl nuclear power station in Ukraine caused hundreds of deaths and increased rates of genetic mutation and cancer in the surrounding population. The zone around Chernobyl has been sealed off to human habitation and could be unsafe for the next 24,000 years. In 2011, a 9.0 magnitude earthquake 15 miles below Japan's Honshu Island, followed by a powerful tsunami, severely damaged the Fukushima Daiichi nuclear power plant complex. Attempts to stabilize and completely shut down the reactors are ongoing.

An additional enormous problem is disposing of the radioactive wastes these plants generate. To date, no storage method has been devised that can provide infallible, infinitely durable shielding for nuclear waste. Despite these problems, nuclear power is gaining favor again as an alternative to fossil fuels.

Medical Uses of Radiation

Another area of concern is the use of radiation in medicine, primarily in X-rays. Studies have revealed that X-ray exposure is cumulative and that no level of exposure is absolutely safe. From a personal health point of view, no one should ever have a "routine" X-ray examination; each such exam should have a definite purpose, and its benefits and risks should be carefully weighed.

affect health. For example, exposure to UV radiation from the sun or from tanning salons can increase the risk of skin cancer. The effects of some sources of radiation, such as cell phones, remain controversial.

Nuclear Weapons and Nuclear Energy

Nuclear weapons pose a health risk of the most serious kind to all species. Reducing the stockpiles of nuclear weapons is a challenge and a goal for the 21st century. Power-generating plants that use nuclear fuel also pose health problems. When **nuclear power** was first developed

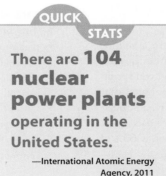

QUICK STATS

There are **104 nuclear power plants** operating in the United States.

—International Atomic Energy Agency, 2011

TERMS

nuclear power The use of controlled nuclear reactions to produce steam, which in turn drives turbines to produce electricity.

Radiation in the Home and Workplace

Recently there has been concern about electromagnetic radiation associated with common modern devices such as microwave ovens, computer monitors, and even high-voltage power lines. These forms of radiation do have effects on health, but research results are inconclusive.

Another controversial issue today is the effect of radiation from cell phones on health. Cell phones use electromagnetic waves (radio frequency radiation) to send and receive signals. This radiation is not directional, meaning that it travels in all directions equally, including toward the user. Factors such as the type of digital signal coding in the network, the antenna and handset design, and the position of the phone relative to the head all determine how much radiation is absorbed by a user. The CDC has undertaken a long-term study to determine whether cell phone use actually exposes users to harmful levels of radiation. Another area of concern is **radon,** a naturally occurring radioactive gas found in certain soils, rocks, and building materials.

Avoiding Radiation

• Get only X-rays that you need, and keep a record of the date and location of every X-ray exam. Don't have a full-body CT scan for routine screening; the radiation dose of one full-body CT scan is nearly 100 times that of a typical mammogram.

• Follow government recommendations for radon testing.

• Use sunscreen to protect yourself from the sun's UV radiation.

NOISE POLLUTION

Loud noise in the environment can cause both hearing loss and stress. Prolonged exposure to sounds above 80–85 **decibels** (a measure of the intensity of a sound wave) can cause permanent hearing loss. Hearing damage can occur after eight hours of exposure to sounds louder than 80 decibels. Regular exposure for longer than one minute to more than 100 decibels can cause permanent hearing loss. Children may suffer damage to their hearing at lower noise levels than those at which adults suffer damage.

Two common sources of excessive noise are the workplace and large gatherings of people at sporting events, rock concerts, and movie theaters. The Occupational Safety and Health Administration (OSHA) sets legal standards for noise in the workplace, but no laws exist regulating noise levels at concerts, which can be much louder than most workplaces. Here are some ways to avoid exposing yourself to excessive noise:

• Wear ear protectors when working around noisy machinery.

• When listening to music on a headset with a volume range of 1–10, keep the volume no louder than 6. Your headset is too loud if you are unable to hear people around you speaking in a normal tone of voice. Earmuff-style headphones may be easier on the ears than earbuds, which are inserted into the ear canal. Experts warn that earbuds should not be used more than 30 minutes a day unless the volume is set below 60% of maximum; headphones can be used up to one hour.

• Avoid loud music. Don't sit or stand near speakers or amplifiers at a concert, and don't play a car radio or stereo so high that you can't hear the traffic.

TERMS

radon A naturally occurring radioactive gas emitted from rocks and natural building materials that can become concentrated in insulated homes, causing lung cancer.

decibel A unit for expressing the relative intensity of sounds on a scale from 0 for the average least perceptible sound to about 120 for the average pain threshold.

Connect to Your Choices

Have you ever thought about where you get your behaviors and habits related to the environment? Many factors can influence our behaviors and habits, some not as obvious as others. When you were growing up, was your family aware of environmental issues and respectful of the environment? Do people in your peer group dispose of their trash when they're outdoors, or do they leave trash behind? Does your school promote environmental awareness and action, such as by participating in the green campus movement, providing for the proper recycling of old computers, cell phones, and other e-waste, and celebrating Earth Day in meaningful ways?

What are the external factors that influence your choices about the environment? What are your inner motivations and core values, and how do they affect your choices? Based on what you learned in this chapter, will you make some different choices in the future? If so, what will they be?

Go online to Connect to complete this activity: www.mcgraw-hillconnect.com

TIPS FOR TODAY AND THE FUTURE

Environmental health involves protecting ourselves from environmental dangers and protecting the environment from the dangers created by humans.

RIGHT NOW YOU CAN:
• Turn off the lights, televisions, and stereos in any unoccupied rooms.
• Turn off power strips when not in use.
• Turn down the heat a few degrees and put on a sweater, or turn off the air conditioner and change into cooler clothes.
• Check your trash for recyclable items and take them out for recycling. If your town does not provide curbside pickup for recyclable items, find out where the nearest community recycling center is.

IN THE FUTURE YOU CAN:
• As your existing lightbulbs burn out, replace them with LED or compact fluorescent lightbulbs.
• Have your car checked to make sure it runs as well as it can and puts out the lowest amount of polluting emissions possible.
• Go online and find one of the many calculators available that can help you estimate your environmental footprint. After calculating your footprint, figure out ways to reduce it.

- Environmental health encompasses all the interactions of humans with their environment and the health consequences of those interactions.

- The world's population is increasing rapidly, especially in the developing world. Factors that may eventually limit human population are food, availability of land and water, energy, and minimum acceptable standard of living.

- Increased amounts of air pollutants are especially dangerous for children, older adults, and people with chronic health problems.

- Factors contributing to the development of smog include heavy motor vehicle traffic, hot weather, and stagnant air.

- Carbon dioxide and other natural gases act as a greenhouse around the earth, increasing the temperature of the atmosphere. Levels of these gases are rising through human activity; as a result, the world's climate could change.

- Environmental damage from energy use can be limited through energy conservation and the development of nonpolluting, renewable sources of energy.

- Indoor pollutants can trigger allergies and illness in the short term and cancer in the long term.

- Concerns with water quality focus on pathogenic organisms and hazardous chemicals from industry and households, as well as on water shortages.

- Sewage treatment prevents pathogens from contaminating drinking water; it often must also deal with heavy metals and hazardous chemicals.

- The amount of garbage is growing all the time; paper is the biggest component. Recycling can help reduce solid waste disposal problems.

- Potentially hazardous chemical pollutants include asbestos, lead, pesticides, mercury, and many household products. Proper handling and disposal are critical.

- Radiation can cause radiation sickness, chromosome damage, and cancer, among other health problems.

- Loud or persistent noise can lead to hearing loss and/or stress.

FOR MORE INFORMATION

BOOKS

Ausenda, F. 2009. *Green Volunteers: The World Guide to Voluntary Work in Nature Conservation*, 7th ed. New York: Universe. *Describes a variety of opportunities to volunteer for environmental causes in many different parts of the world.*

Heinberg, R., and D. Lerch (eds.). 2010. *The Post Carbon Reader: Managing the 21st Century's Sustainability Crises*. Healdsburg, CA: Watershed Media. *A collection of diverse and provocative articles on pressing environmental problems and what can be done about them.*

Maslin, M. 2009. *Global Warming: A Very Short Introduction*, 2nd ed. New York: Oxford University Press. *A survey of the science and politics of global warming.*

Nadakavukaren, A. 2011. *Our Global Environment: A Health Perspective*, 7th ed. Prospect Heights, IL: Waveland Press. *A broad survey of major environmental issues and their effects on personal and community health.*

Wright, R. T. 2010. *Environmental Science: Toward a Sustainable Future*. New York: Pearson. *An easy-to-read introduction to the realm of environmental science and its importance to our future.*

ORGANIZATIONS, HOTLINES, AND WEB SITES

CDC National Center for Environmental Health. Provides brochures and fact sheets about a variety of environmental issues.

http://www.cdc.gov/nceh/default.htm

Earth Times. An international online newspaper devoted to global environmental issues.

http://www.earthtimes.org

Ecological Footprint. Calculates your personal ecological footprint based on your diet, transportation patterns, and living arrangements.

http://www.myfootprint.org

Indoor Air Quality Information Hotline. Answers questions, provides publications, and makes referrals.

800-438-4318

National Oceanic and Atmospheric Administration (NOAA): Climate. Provides information about a variety of issues related to climate, including global warming, drought, and El Niño and La Niña.

http://www.noaa.gov/climate.html

National Safety Council Environmental Health Center. Provides information about lead, radon, indoor air quality, hazardous chemicals, and other environmental issues.

http://www.nsc.org/international/env_hth_sty/Pages/EnvironmentalHealthSafety.aspx

Student Environmental Action Coalition (SEAC). A coalition of student and youth environmental groups; the website has contact information for local groups.

http://www.seac.org

United Nations. Several U.N. programs are devoted to environmental problems on a global scale; the websites provide information about current and projected trends and about international treaties developed to deal with environmental issues.

http://www.un.org/popin (Population Information Network)

http://www.unep.org (Environment Programme)

U.S. Department of Energy: Energy Efficiency and Renewable Energy (EERE). Provides information about alternative fuels and tips for saving energy at home and in your car.

http://www.eere.energy.gov/

U.S. Environmental Protection Agency (EPA). Provides information about EPA activities and many consumer-oriented materials. The website includes special sites devoted to global warming, ozone loss, pesticides, and other areas of concern.

http://www.epa.gov

Worldwatch Institute. A public policy research organization focusing on emerging global environmental problems and the links between the world economy and the environment.

http://www.worldwatch.org

There are many national and international organizations working on environmental health problems. A few of the largest and best known are listed below:

Greenpeace: 800-326-0959; http://www.greenpeace.org
National Audubon Society: 212-979-3000; http://www.audubon.org
National Wildlife Federation: 800-822-9919; http://www.nwf.org
National Resources Defense Council: (212) 727-2700; http://www.nrdc.org
Nature Conservancy: 800-628-6860; http://www.nature.org
Sierra Club: 415-977-5500; http://www.sierraclub.org
U.S. Green Building Council: 800-795-1747; http://www.usgbc.org/
World Wildlife Fund—U.S.: 800-960-0993; http://www.worldwildlife.org

SELECTED BIBLIOGRAPHY

Brown, M. J., et al. 2012. Lead in drinking water and human blood lead levels in the United States. *Morbidity and Mortality Weekly Report* 61: 1–9.

Centers for Disease Control and Prevention. 2011. Adult blood lead epidemiology and surveillance—United States, 2008–2009. *Morbidity and Mortality Weekly Report* 60(25)): 841–845.

Centers for Disease Control and Prevention. 2011. Surveillance for waterborne disease outbreaks and other health events associated with recreational water—United States, 2007–2008. *Morbidity and Mortality Weekly Report, Surveillance Summaries* 60(2212): 1–32.

Chew, G. L. 2012. Assessment of environmental cockroach allergen exposure. *Current Allergy and Asthma Reports* 12(5): 456–464.

De Coster, S., and N. van Larebeke, 2012. Endocrine-disrupting chemicals: Associated disorders and mechanisms of action. *Journal of Environmental and Public Health*, Sept. 6 (Epub ahead of print).

Delworth-Bart, J. E., and C. F. Moore. 2006. Mercy mercy me: Social injustice and the prevention of environmental pollutant exposures among ethnic minority and poor children. *Child Development* 77(2): 247–265.

Dissanayake, V. and T. B. Erickson. 2012. Ball and chain: The global burden of lead poisoning. *Clinical Toxicology* 50(6): 528–531.

Dominici, F., et al. 2006. Fine particulate air pollution and hospital admission for cardiovascular and respiratory diseases. *Journal of the American Medical Association* 295(10): 1127–1134.

Franchini, M. et al. 2012. Air pollution, vascular disease and thrombosis: Linking clinical data and pathogenic mechanisms. *Journal of Thrombosis and Haemostasis*, Sept. 25 (Epub ahead of prin).

Grasso, M.et al. 2012 The health effects of climate change: A survey of recent quantitative research. International *Journal of Environmental Research and Public Health* 9(5):1523–1547.

Griffith, G. P., et al. 2012. Predicting interactions among fishing, ocean warming, and ocean acidification in a marine system with whole-ecosystem models. *Conservation Biology*, Sept. 25 (Epub ahead of print).

Hegarty, M. J. 2012. Invasion of the hybrids. *Molecular Ecology* 21(19): 4669–4671.

Laden, F., et al. 2006. Reduction in fine particulate air pollution and mortality: extended follow-up of the Harvard Six Cities study. *American Journal of Respiratory and Critical Care Medicine* 173(6): 667–672.

Miller, M. R., C. A. Shaw, and J P. Langrish. 2012. From particles to patients: Oxidative stress and the cardiovascular effects of air pollution. *Future Cardiology* 8(4): 577–602.

National Oceanic and Atmospheric Administration. 2008. *Billion Dollar U.S. Weather Disasters, 1980–2007* (http://www.ncdc.noaa.gov/billions/).

Pennisi, E. 2012. Water reclamation going green. *Science* 337(6095): 674–676.

United Nations Population Division. 2011. *World Population Prospects: The 2010 Revision.* New York: United Nations.

U.S. Energy Information Administration. 2012. EIA's AEO2012 includes analysis of breakthroughs in vehicle battery technology (http://www.eia.gov/todayinenergy/detail.cfm?id=6930).

U.S. Energy Information Agency. 2012. *Gasoline and Diesel Fuel Update* (http://www.eia.gov/petroleum/gasdiesel/).

U.S. Environmental Protection Agency. 2012. Mercury: *Health Effects* (http://www.epa.gov/hg/effects.htm).

U.S. Environmental Protection Agency. 2011. *Municipal Solid Waste* (http://www.epa.gov/waste/nonhaz/municipal/index.htm).

Vehmas, T., P. Pallasaho, and P. Oksa. 2012. Lung and pleural fibrosis in asbestos-exposed workers: A risk factor for pneumonia mortality. *Epidemiology and Infection* 140(11): 1987–1992.

Virtanen, J. K., et al. 2005. Mercury, fish oils, and risk of acute coronary events and cardiovascular disease, coronary heart disease, and all-cause mortality in men in eastern Finland. *Arteriosclerosis, Thrombosis, and Vascular Biology* 25(1): 228–233.

Wasi, S., S. Tabrez, and M. Ahmad. 2012. Toxicological effects of major environmental pollutants: An overview. *Environmental Monitoring and Assessment*, July 6 (Epub ahead of print).

World Health Organization. 2010. Cholera, 2010. *Weekly Epidemiological Record* 85(13): 1177–1128.

Worldwatch Institute. 2012. *Vital Signs 2012.* New York: Norton. (http://vital-signs.worldwatch.org/).

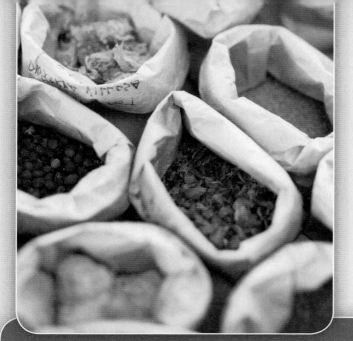

LOOKING AHEAD...

After reading this chapter, you should be able to

- Explain the self-care decision-making process and discuss options for self-treatment

- Describe the basic premises, practices, and providers of conventional medicine

- Describe the basic premises, practices, and providers of complementary and alternative medicine

- Explain how to communicate effectively with health care providers and use their input when evaluating different types of treatment

- Discuss different types of health insurance plans

15

Conventional and Complementary Medicine

Today people are becoming more empowered and confident in their ability to solve personal health problems on their own. People who manage their own health care gather information and learn skills from a variety of resources. They solicit opinions and advice, make decisions, and take action. They know how to practice safe, effective self-care, and they know how to make decisions about professional medical care—whether conventional Western medicine or complementary and alternative medicine.

This chapter will help you develop skills to identify and manage medical problems and to make the health care system work effectively for you.

SELF-CARE

Effectively managing medical problems involves developing several skills. First, you need to learn to be a good observer of your own body and assess your symptoms. You also must be able to decide when to seek professional advice and when you can safely deal with a problem on your own. You need to know how to safely and effectively self-treat common medical problems. Finally, you need to know how to develop a partnership with physicians and other health care providers and how to carry out treatment plans.

Self-Assessment

Symptoms are often an expression of the body's attempt to heal itself. A fever may be an attempt to inhibit the growth and reproduction of infectious agents. A cough can help clear the airways and protect the lungs. Carefully observing symptoms also helps you identify signals that suggest you need professional help. Begin by noting when the symptom began, how often and when it occurs, what makes it worse, what makes it better, and whether you have any associated symptoms or illnesses. You can also monitor your body's vital signs, such as temperature and heart rate. Medical self-tests for blood pressure, blood sugar, pregnancy detection, and urinary tract infections can also help you make a more informed decision about when to seek medical help and when to self-treat.

Knowing When to See a Physician

In general, you should see a physician for symptoms that you would describe as follows:

1. *Severe.* If the symptom is very severe or intense, medical assistance is advised. Examples include severe pains, major injuries, and other emergencies.

2. *Unusual.* If the symptom is peculiar and unfamiliar, it is wise to check it out with your physician. Examples

The act of writing down feelings and thoughts about stressful life events has been shown to help people improve their health. Investigators remain unsure why writing about one's feelings has beneficial effects. It is possible that expressing feelings about a traumatic event helps people work through the event and put it behind them. The resulting sense of release and control may reduce stress levels and have positive physical effects such as reduced heart rate and blood pressure, and improved immune function. Alternatively, expressive writing may change the way people think about previous stressful events in their lives and help them cope with new stressors. Whatever the mechanism, it's clear that expressive writing can be a safe, inexpensive, and effective supplement to standard treatment of certain illnesses.

What about the effects of expressive writing on otherwise healthy individuals? Other studies have, in fact, found a similar benefit: people who wrote about traumatic experiences reported fewer symptoms, fewer days off work, fewer physician visits, improved mood, and a more positive outlook.

If you'd like to try expressive writing to help you deal with a traumatic event, set aside a special time—15 minutes a day for four consecutive days, for example, or one day a week for four weeks. Write in a place where you won't be interrupted or distracted. Explore your deepest thoughts and feelings and why

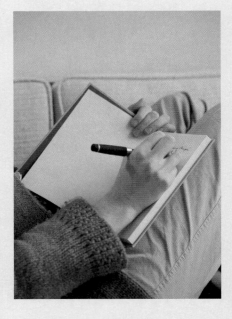

you feel the way you do. Write as rapidly as possible and don't worry about grammar or coherence or about what someone else might think about what you're writing; you are writing just for yourself. (Interestingly, writing by hand has been found to produce more beneficial health effects than writing using a keyboard.) You may find the writing exercise to be distressing in the short term—sadness and depression are common when dealing with feelings about a stressful event—but most people report relief and contentment after writing for several days.

---

include unexplained lumps, changes in a mole, problems with vision, difficulty swallowing, numbness, weakness, unexplained weight loss, and blood in the sputum, urine, or stool.

3. *Persistent.* If the symptom lasts longer than expected, seek medical advice. Examples in adults include fever for more than five days, a cough lasting longer than two weeks, a sore that doesn't heal within a month, and hoarseness lasting longer than three weeks.

4. *Recurrent.* If a symptom returns again and again, medical evaluation is advised. Examples include recurrent headaches, abdominal pain, and backache.

Sometimes a single symptom is not a cause for concern, but when the symptom is accompanied by other symptoms, the combination suggests a more serious problem. For example, a fever with a stiff neck suggests meningitis.

If you think you need professional help, you must decide how urgent the problem is. If it is a true emergency, you should go (or call someone to take you) to the nearest hospital emergency department. Emergencies include the following:

- Major trauma or injury to the head, a suspected broken bone, deep wound, severe burn, eye injury, or animal bite.

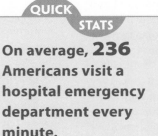

QUICK STATS

On average, **236** Americans visit a hospital emergency department every minute.

—National Hospital Ambulatory Medical Care Survey: 2008

- Uncontrollable bleeding or internal bleeding, as indicated by blood in the sputum, vomit, or stool.
- Intolerable and uncontrollable pain or severe chest pain.
- Severe shortness of breath.
- Persistent abdominal pain, especially if associated with nausea and vomiting.
- Poisoning or drug overdose.
- Loss of consciousness or seizure.
- Stupor, drowsiness, or disorientation that cannot be explained.
- Severe or worsening reaction to an insect bite or sting or to a medication, especially if breathing becomes difficult.

If your problem is not an emergency but still requires medical attention, call your physician's office. Often you can be given medical advice over the phone without needing a visit to the clinic.

Self-Treatment

In most cases, your body itself can relieve your symptoms and heal the disorder. Patience and careful self-observation are often the best choices in self-treatment.

Nondrug Options Nondrug options are often easy, inexpensive, safe, and highly effective. For example, massage, ice packs, and neck exercises may at times be more helpful than drugs in relieving headaches and other pains. Getting adequate rest, increasing exercise, drinking more water, eating more or less of certain foods, using humidifiers, changes in ergonomics when working at a desk, and similar remedies are just some of the hundreds of nondrug options for preventing or relieving many common health problems. For a variety of disorders caused or aggravated by stress, the treatment of choice may be relaxation or other stress management strategies (see the box "The Health Benefits of Expressive Writing").

Self-Medication Self-treatment with nonprescription medications is an important part of health care. Nonprescription or **over-the-counter (OTC) medications** are medicines that the Food and Drug Administration (FDA) has determined are safe for use without a physician's prescription. There are more than 100,000 OTC drugs on the market; about 60% of all medications are sold over the counter. Hundreds of products sold over the counter today use

> **Many ingredients in OTC drugs have not been proven effective,** a fact the FDA does not dispute.

ingredients or dosage strengths available only by prescription 20 years ago. With this increased consumer choice, however, comes increased consumer responsibility for using OTC drugs safely.

Although many OTC products are effective, others are unnecessary or divert attention from better ways of coping. Many ingredients in OTC drugs—perhaps 70%—have not been proven to be effective, a fact the FDA does not dispute. And any drug may have risks and side effects.

Follow these simple guidelines to self-medicate safely:

1. Always read labels and follow directions carefully. The information on most OTC drug labels now appears in a standard format developed by the FDA (Figure 15.1). If you have any questions, ask a pharmacist or a qualified health care provider before using a product.

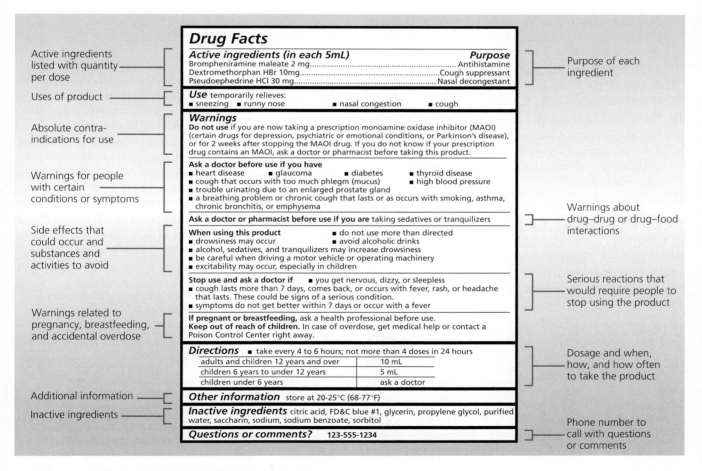

FIGURE 15.1 Reading and understanding OTC drug labels.

SOURCE: Food and Drug Administration. 1999. Over-the-counter human drugs: labeling requirements: final rule. *Federal Register* 64(51), 17 March, 13254–13303.

2. Do not exceed the recommended dosage or length of treatment unless you discuss this with your physician.

3. Use caution if you are taking other medications or supplements because OTC drugs and herbal supplements can interact with some prescription drugs. If you have questions about drug interactions, ask your doctor or pharmacist *before* you take medicines in combination.

4. Try to select medications with one active ingredient rather than combination products. A product with multiple ingredients is likely to include drugs for symptoms you don't have.

5. When choosing medications, try to buy **generic drugs,** which contain the same active ingredient as brand-name products but generally at a much lower cost.

6. Never take or give a drug from an unlabeled container or when you can't read the label.

7. If you are pregnant or nursing or have a chronic condition such as kidney or liver disease, consult your health care provider before self-medicating.

8. The expiration date marked on many medications is an estimate of how long the medication is likely to be safe and effective. However, an extensive study by the FDA found that 90% of all prescription and OTC medications are potent for several years after their stated expiration date. Exceptions include the antibiotic tetracycline, liquid antibiotics, nitroglycerine, and insulin. Expiration dates are very conservative. If you have any question about a medicine's expiration date, ask a pharmacist.

9. Store your medications in a cool, dry place that is out of the reach of children.

10. Use special caution with aspirin. Because of an association with a rare but serious problem known as Reye's syndrome, aspirin should not be used by children or adolescents who may have the flu, chicken pox, or any other viral illness.

PROFESSIONAL CARE

When self-treatment is not appropriate or sufficient, you need to seek professional medical care, whether by going to a hospital emergency department, by scheduling an appointment

---

Table 15.1 Use of Complementary and Alternative Therapies by Adults

	PERCENTAGE WHO USED THERAPY IN LAST 12 MONTHS
Natural products (nonvitamin, nonmineral)	17.7
Chiropractic care	8.6
Deep breathing exercises	12.7
Meditation	9.4
Massage	8.3
Yoga	6.1
Diet-based therapies	3.6
Progressive relaxation	2.9
Acupuncture	1.4
Homeopathic treatment	1.8
Guided imagery	2.2
T'ai chi	1.0
Hypnosis	0.2
Energy healing therapy/Reiki	0.5
Biofeedback	0.2
Any therapy	**38.3**

SOURCE: Barnes, P. M., et al. 2008. Complementary and alternative medicine use among adults and children: United States, 2007. *CDC National Health Statistics Report #12.* Hyattsville, MD: National Center for Health Statistics.

---

with your physician, or by accessing some other conventional health care. In recent years many Americans have also sought health care from practitioners of **complementary and alternative medicine (CAM)**—defined as those therapies and practices that do not form part of **conventional medicine**, which is defined as mainstream health care and medical practices taught in most U.S. medical schools and offered in most U.S. hospitals. The most frequently used CAM therapies are nonvitamin, nonmineral natural products; chiropractic care; deep breathing exercises; meditation; massage; and yoga (Table 15.1). Between 2002 and 2007 there was increased use of acupuncture, deep breathing exercises, massage therapy,

generic drug A drug that is not registered or protected by a commercial trademark; a drug that does not have an exclusive brand name.

complementary and alternative medicine (CAM) Health care practices and products that are not considered part of conventional, mainstream medical practice as taught in most U.S. medical schools and are not available at most U.S. health care facilities; examples of CAM practices include acupuncture and herbal remedies.

TERMS

conventional medicine A system of medicine based on the application of the scientific method; diseases are thought to be caused by identifiable physical factors and characterized by a representative set of signs and symptoms; also called *biomedicine* or *standard Western medicine.*

Ask Yourself

QUESTIONS FOR CRITICAL THINKING AND REFLECTION

Do you self-medicate for common medical problems, such as headaches or colds? If so, how careful are you about reading product labels and following directions? For example, would you know if you were taking two OTC medications that contained the same ingredient (such as ibuprofen) at the same time?

meditation, naturopathy, and yoga, among others, and an increased use of CAM overall. People often use CAM therapies in addition to their conventional medical treatments, but most do not tell their physicians about it.

CAM is the term widely used in the United States for safe and possibly effective complementary practices that are used together with (**complementary medicine**) or rather than (**alternative medicine**) conventional practices. The term **integrative medicine** to practicing conventional health care with the *addition* of unconventional modalities.

Consumers turn to CAM for a variety of purposes related to health and well-being, such as boosting their immune systems, lowering their cholesterol levels, losing weight, quitting smoking, or enhancing their memory. Despite their popularity, many CAM practices remain controversial, and consumers need to be aware of safety issues. The National Center for Complementary and Alternative Medicine (NCCAM), a branch of the National Institutes of Health (NIH), was established in the 1990s to apply rigorous scientific standards for proving or disproving the safety and effectiveness of CAM.

The following sections examine the principles and providers of both conventional medicine—the dominant medical system in the United States and Europe, also referred to as standard *Western medicine* or *biomedicine*—and complementary and alternative medicine, with particular attention to consumer issues.

CONVENTIONAL MEDICINE

Referring to conventional medicine as "standard Western medicine" draws attention to the fact that it differs from the various medical systems that have developed in China, Japan, India, and other parts of the world. Calling it "biomedicine" reflects conventional medicine's foundation in the biological and physical sciences.

TERMS

complementary medicine   Unconventional medical practices that are used together with conventional ones.

alternative medicine   Unconventional medical practices that are used instead of conventional methods.

integrative medicine   Conventional health care practice that is sometimes augmented by unconventional (CAM) modalities.

Premises and Assumptions of Conventional Medicine

One of the important characteristics of Western medicine is the belief that disease is caused by identifiable physical factors. Western medicine identifies the causes of disease as pathogens (such as bacteria and viruses), genetic factors, and unhealthful lifestyles that result in changes at the molecular and cellular levels. In most cases, the focus is primarily on the physical causes of illness rather than mental or spiritual imbalance.

Another feature that distinguishes Western biomedicine from other medical systems is the concept that almost every disease is defined by a certain set of signs (physical manifestations) and symptoms (the effects on an individual), and that they are similar in most patients suffering from the disease. Western medicine tends to treat diseases as biological disturbances occurring in humans, rather than being integral in some way to the individual with the illness.

A disease can be caused by either internal or external factors. Internal factors include anatomic or physiologic abnormalities, and defective genetic, hormonal, and immune

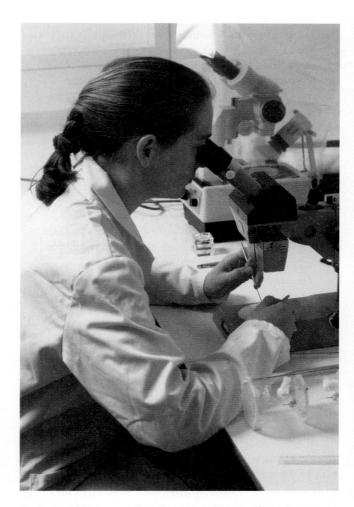

Conventional Western medicine is grounded in scientific explanations resulting from the application of the scientific method or through observable outcomes in randomized controlled studies.

mechanisms. External causes include infections by bacteria and viruses, and some cases of traumatic injury. The public health measures of the 19th and 20th centuries—chlorination of drinking water, sewage disposal, food safety regulations, vaccination programs, education about hygiene, and so on—were an outgrowth of this orientation.

The implementation of public health measures is one way to control disease; others include preventive lifestyle measures and the use of drugs and surgery. The discovery and development of sulfa drugs, antibiotics, and steroids in the 20th century, along with advances in chemistry that made it possible to identify the active ingredients in common plant-derived remedies, paved the way for the current close identification of Western medicine with **pharmaceuticals** (medical drugs, both prescription and over-the-counter). Western medicine also relies heavily on surgery and on advanced medical technology to discover a physical cause of an individual's disease and to correct, remove, or destroy it.

Further, Western medicine is based on the scientific method of obtaining knowledge and explaining health-related phenomena using scientific explanations that have these characteristics:

- *Empirical*—they are based on the evidence of the senses and on objective and systematic observation, often carried out under carefully controlled conditions; they must be capable of verification by other observers or through the use of technology (such as lab tests and physical measurement, such as blood pressure).
- *Rational*—they follow the rules of logic and are consistent with known facts.
- *Testable*—either they are verifiable through direct observation or they lead to predictions about what should occur under conditions not yet observed.
- *Parsimonious*—they explain phenomena with the fewest causes.
- *General*—they have broad explanatory power.
- *Rigorously evaluated*—they are constantly evaluated for consistency with the evidence and known principles, for parsimony, and for generality.
- *Tentative*—scientists are willing to entertain the possibility that their explanations are faulty, based on new, better, or connected evidence.

Western medicine translates the scientific method into practice through the research process, a highly refined and well-established approach to exploring the causes of disease and ensuring the safety and efficacy of treatments. Research ranges from case studies—descriptions of a single patient's illness and treatment—to randomized controlled trials (RTCs) conducted on large populations; RTCs are considered the highest level of scientific medical research. Drugs are developed and tested through an elaborate course that begins with preliminary research in the lab and continues through trials with human participants, review and approval by the FDA, and monitoring of the drug's effects even after it is on the market. The process may take 12 years or more, and only about 20% of drugs are eventually approved for marketing.

When results of research studies are published in medical journals, a community of scientists, physicians, researchers, and scholars has the opportunity to share the findings and enter a dialogue about the subject. Publication of research often prompts further research designed to replicate and confirm the findings, challenge the conclusions, or pursue related lines of thought or experimentation. (For guidelines on how to interpret research when it is reported in the popular press, see the box "Evaluating Health News.")

Pharmaceuticals and the Placebo Effect

A placebo is a chemically inactive substance that a patient believes is an effective therapy for his or her condition. (For procedures that don't involve drugs, a *sham* procedure is used.) By comparing the effects of the actual treatment with the effects of the placebo or sham, researchers can judge whether the treatment is effective.

The *placebo effect* occurs when a patient improves after receiving a placebo. In such cases, the effect of the placebo on the patient cannot be attributed to the specific actions or properties of the drug or procedure. Researchers have consistently found that 30–40% of all patients given a placebo show improvement. This result has been observed for a wide variety of conditions or symptoms, including coughing, seasickness, depression, migraines, and angina. Placebos are particularly effective when they are administered by a practitioner whom the patient likes and believes in.

Researchers hypothesize that positive expectations of a medication's effects may result in changes in nerve and muscle activity or in electrical or chemical activity in the brain. A positive aspect of the placebo effect is that a sense of confidence in a provider and hope about a treatment can add to the benefits of the treatment itself. Anatomy, physiology, emotions, hope, beliefs, and expectations all contribute to the way the body reacts to medical treatments and utilizes its own healing mechanisms.

The Providers of Conventional Medicine

Conventional medicine is practiced by a wide range of health care professionals in the United States. Several kinds of professionals are permitted to practice specific fields of medicine independently, including medical doctors, osteopaths, podiatrists, optometrists, and dentists.

- **Medical doctors** are practitioners who hold a doctor of medicine (MD) degree from an accredited medical school. In the United States, an education in medicine involves three

pharmaceuticals   Medical drugs, both prescription and over-the-counter.

TERMS

medical doctor   An independent practitioner who holds a doctor of medicine degree (MD) from an accredited medical school.

Health-related research published in scientific medical journals is often summarized for the public in the popular media, which may oversimplify, exaggerate, or sensationalize the results. The following questions can help you evaluate scientific health advice presented in popular media:

1. *Is the report based on scientific studies?* Information or advice based on carefully designed research studies has more validity than casual observations.

2. *What is the source of the information?* A study published in a respected peer-reviewed scientific journal has been examined by editors and researchers who are professionally prepared to evaluate the merits of a study and its results and its application to actual patients. Most journals include information on the funding source and the authors' affiliations that may introduce a bias or conflict of interest. Studies sponsored by drug companies or other commercial groups are suspect; information from universities, government agencies, and national research organizations is usually considered more reliable.

3. *How many subjects were included in the study?* A study involving many subjects is more likely to yield reliable results than a study involving only a few subjects. Most quality studies include a "statistical power analysis" section that specifies how many subjects were necessary. Too few subjects are suspect; too many subjects above the number specified in the power analysis may inflate the practical usefulness of the results even though "statistical significance" (usually a p-value less than or equal to 0.05 or 5%) was achieved.

4. *Who were the subjects?* Research findings are more likely to apply to you if you share important characteristics with the participants in the study.

5. *What kind of study was it?* Randomized controlled trials and meta-analyses are considered the most valid. Epidemiological studies (which involve noncontrolled observations) may *suggest* useful information, but they cannot always establish cause-and-effect relationships. Consider the following when deciding whether a study's results should be considered significant:

- *Were the treatment group results compared to the results in a control group?*

- *Were the subjects randomly assigned to the treatment and control groups?*

- *Was it a double-blind study?*

- *Was it a multicenter study or a meta-analysis?* A few randomized controlled trials are performed at more than one institution. A meta-analysis combines and recalculates data from several similar studies conducted in different locations by different researchers. A well-conducted meta-analysis is considered one of the most valid study designs.

6. *What do the statistics really say?* Are the results statistically significant (meaning there is a 5% or lower chance that the findings resulted from chance)? Does the study have the required number of subjects according to a statistical power analysis?

7. *Is new health advice being offered?* If the media report new guidelines for health behavior or medical treatment, examine the source. Be suspicious of absolutes and overstated words such as "certainty," "always," and "never." Scientifically accurate reports use words such as "results show," "for many people," and "the evidence suggests." Reliable information sources should present the limitations of a study's results and consider a great deal of evidence before offering health advice. Above all, use common sense, and check with your physician before making a major change in your health habits based on news reports.

connect
ACTIVITY
DO IT ONLINE

---

to eight years of study and residency beyond undergraduate premedical education.

- **Doctors of osteopathic medicine** (DO) receive their education and training at an osteopathic medical school, where there is an emphasis on structural and functional relationships and a whole-person approach to medicine. MDs and ODs are the two types of physicians in the United States who are trained and licensed to perform surgery and prescribe medication.

- **Podiatrists** are practitioners who specialize in the medical and surgical care of the feet. They hold a doctor of podiatric medicine (DPM) degree.

- **Optometrists** are practitioners trained to examine the eyes, detect eye diseases, and treat certain vision problems. They hold a doctor of optometry (OD) degree.

- **Dentists** focus on the care of the teeth and mouth. They are graduates of four-year dental schools and hold the doctor of dental surgery (DDS) or doctor of medical dentistry (DMD) degree.

TERMS

doctor of osteopathic medicine An independent medical practitioner (DO) who has graduated from an osteopathic medical school; osteopathy incorporates the theories and practices of scientific medicine and includes osteopathic manual therapy.

podiatrist A practitioner who holds a doctor of podiatric medicine degree (DPM) and specializes in the medical and surgical care of the feet.

optometrist A practitioner who holds a doctor of optometry degree (OD) and is trained to examine the eyes, detect eye diseases, and prescribe corrective lenses.

dentist A practitioner who holds a doctor of medical dentistry (DMD) or doctor of dental surgery degree (DDS) and who specializes in the prevention and treatment of diseases and injuries of the teeth, mouth, and jaws.

In addition to these practitioners, there are millions of other highly educated health care professionals. They include nursing professionals such as registered nurses (RNs), nurse practitioners (NPs), certified registered nurse anesthetists (CRNAs) and certified nurse midwives (CNM). **Allied health care providers** include physician assistants (PAs), physical therapists (PTs or DPTs), pharmacists (PPhs or PharmDs), medical social workers (MSWs), and registered dietitians (RDs).

Choosing a Primary Care Physician

Most experts believe it is best to have a primary care physician (PCP) who gets to know you, coordinates your medical care, and refers you to specialists when you need them. The primary care disciplines include family practice, internal medicine, pediatrics, and gynecology. These physicians are able to diagnose and treat the vast majority of common health problems and provide many preventive health services. The best time to look for a PCP is before you are sick.

To select a physician, begin by making a list of possible choices. If your insurance limits the health care providers you can see, check the plan's list first. If your health plan lets you choose a physician, ask for recommendations from family, friends, coworkers, local medical societies, and the physician referral service at a local clinic or hospital.

Once you have the names of a few physicians you might want to try, call their offices to find out information such as the following:

- Is the physician covered by your health plan and accepting new patients?

- What are the office hours, and when is the physician or office staff available? What do patients do if they need urgent care or have an emergency?

- Which hospitals does the physician use?

- How many other physicians are available to cover when he or she isn't available, and who are they?

- How long does it usually take to get a routine appointment?

- Does the office send reminders about preventive services and tests such as Pap tests?

- Does the physician (or a nurse or physician assistant) give advice online or over the phone for common problems and continued care of a diagnosed problem?

Schedule a visit with the physician you think you would most like to use. During that first visit, you'll get a sense of how well matched you are and how well he or she might meet your medical needs.

Getting the Most Out of Your Medical Care

The key to making the health care system work for you lies in good communication with your physician and other members of the health care team.

The Physician–Patient Partnership The image of the all-knowing physician and the passive patient is fading. What is emerging is a physician–patient *partnership* in which the physician acts more like a consultant and the patient participates more actively (see the box "Creating Your Own Health Record"). You should expect your physician to be attentive, caring, and able to listen and clearly explain health care matters to you. You also must do your part. You need to be assertive in a firm but nonaggressive manner. You need to express your feelings and concerns, ask questions and, if necessary, be persistent. If your physician is unable to communicate clearly with you despite your best efforts, you probably need to change physicians.

> The image of the all-knowing physician and the passive patient is fading. **What is emerging is a physician–patient partnership**.

Your Physician Appointment Prepare for your visit ahead of time by making a list of your questions and concerns, along with notes about your symptoms. Present your concerns at the beginning of the visit to set the agenda. Be specific and concise about your symptoms, and be open and honest about your concerns. Let your physician know if you are taking any drugs, are allergic to any medications, are breast-feeding, or may be pregnant. At the end of the visit, briefly repeat the physician's diagnosis, prognosis, and instructions to make sure you understand your next steps.

The Diagnostic Process The first step in the diagnostic process is the medical history, which includes your primary reason for the visit, your current symptoms, your past medical history, and your social history (job, family life, major stressors, living conditions, and health habits). Keeping

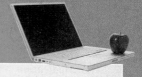

Many Americans believe that their medical records are compiled and maintained by their various health care providers over the years, but this is not necessarily the case. You may have records at several doctors' offices, at a student health clinic, at a hospital, and so on. The best way to keep track of your medical information is to keep your own records. Then you will have them when you move, when you're looking for a new provider, or in case of emergency. A personal health record should contain the following information:

- Your name, emergency contact, birth date, blood type, religious preference (if any), and the date this record was compiled or updated

- All known allergies (including medications)

- A list of all chronic conditions and the date of their diagnosis (diabetes, high blood pressure, asthma, emphysema, etc.)

- Any hereditary diseases

- The names and dosages of all medications you are taking and reasons for taking them

- The dates and reasons for all past hospitalizations and surgeries

- The date of physical exams and any major findings

- Vaccination schedules

- A record of laboratory test results, imaging studies, electrocardiograms, and any other tests, with dates

You have a right to view or receive a copy (or a summary) of your medical records. If you need help compiling your own

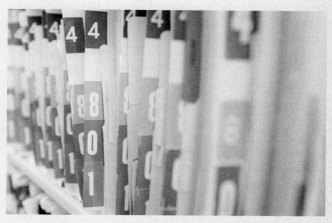

health record, you can request a copy of your medical record from your doctor. The only fee should be for the cost of copying and mailing. If you find any information in your medical record that you believe to be inaccurate, you can request an amendment. You have the right to have such an amendment permanently included in your record.

SOURCES: MedlinePlus. *Personal Health Records* (www.nlm.nih.gov/medlineplus/personalhealthrecords.html); AHIMA Foundation. *myPHR* (www.myphr.com).

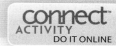
ACTIVITY
DO IT ONLINE

up-to-date records of your medical history can help you provide your physician with key facts about your health.

The next step is the physical exam, which usually begins with a review of vital signs: blood pressure, heart rate (pulse), breathing rate, and temperature. Depending on your primary complaint, your physician may give you a complete physical, or the exam may be directed to specific areas, such as your ears, nose, and throat.

Additionally, your physician may order medical tests to complete the diagnosis. Physicians can order imaging studies (such as X-rays, MRIs, or CAT scans), biopsies, blood and urine tests, and **endoscopies** to view, probe, or analyze almost any part of the body. If your physician orders a test for you, be sure you know why you need it, what the risks and benefits are for you, how you should prepare for it, and what the test will involve. Also ask what the test results mean because no test is 100% accurate—**false positives** and **false negatives** can occur—and interpretation of some tests is subjective.

> ### QUICK STATS
> **Americans spend more than $200 billion each year on prescription drugs.**
> —CDC, 2010

Medical and Surgical Treatments
Many conditions can be treated in a variety of ways; in some cases, lifestyle changes are sufficient. In other cases, the physician may prescribe a medication.

Thousands of lives are saved each year by antibiotics, insulin, and other drugs, but we pay a price for having such powerful tools. A report from the Institute of Medicine (IOM) estimates that 1.5 million prescription drug-related errors—called *adverse*

> ### TERMS
> **endoscopy**   A medical procedure in which a viewing instrument is inserted into a body cavity or opening.
>
> **false positive**   A test result that incorrectly detects a disorder or condition in a person who does not have the disorder or condition.
>
> **false negative**   A test result that fails to correctly detect a disease or condition.

drug events, or ADEs—occur each year in the United States. ADEs happen for several reasons:

• *Medication errors:* Physicians may overprescribe drugs, prescribe the wrong drug or prescribe a dangerous combination of drugs. Such problems are especially prevalent among older adults, who typically take multiple medications. At the pharmacy, patients may receive the wrong drug or may not be given complete information about drug risks, side effects, and interactions.

• *Off-label drug use:* Once a drug is approved by the FDA for one purpose, it can legally be prescribed (although not marketed) for purposes not listed on the label. Many off-label uses are safe and supported by some research, but both consumers and health care providers need to take special care with off-label use.

• *Online pharmacies:* Although convenient, some online pharmacies may sell products or engage in practices that are illegal in the offline world, putting consumers at risk for receiving adulterated, expired, ineffective, or counterfeit drugs. The FDA recommends that consumers avoid sites that prescribe drugs for the first time without a physical exam, sell prescription drugs without a prescription, or sell medications not approved by the FDA. You should also avoid sites that do not provide access to a registered pharmacist to answer questions or that do not provide a U.S. address and phone number to contact if there's a problem. The National Association of Boards of Pharmacy sponsors a voluntary certification program for Internet pharmacies. To be certified, a pharmacy must have a state license and allow regular inspections.

• *Costs:* Spending on prescription drugs is rising faster than the rate of inflation and is now the fastest-growing portion of U.S. health care spending. Consumers may be able to lower their drug costs by using generic versions of medications; by joining a drug discount program sponsored by a company, organization, or local pharmacy; and by investigating mail-order or Internet pharmacies.

There is ongoing controversy about the importation of lower-cost drugs from Canada. Canada imports U.S. drugs and regulates Canadian-produced drugs, so safety should theoretically not be a concern for drugs from Canada. However, companies in Canada may make drugs for export only, thus avoiding regulation, and online pharmacies may claim they are operating in Canada but may be located in another country where there is little or no regulation. In addition, shipping costs can be high, and U.S. generic drugs are often less expensive than Canadian drugs.

Patients share responsibility for their use of prescription drugs. Many people don't take their medications properly, skipping doses, taking incorrect doses, stopping too soon, or not taking the medication at all. An estimated 30–50% of the more than 3 billion prescriptions dispensed annually in the United States are not taken correctly and thus do not produce the desired results. Consumers can increase the safety and effectiveness of their treatment by carefully reading any prescription's label and fact sheets or brochures that come with the medication. Whenever a health care provider gives you a prescription, ask the following questions:

• Are there nondrug alternatives?
• What is the name of the medication, and what is it supposed to do, within what period of time?
• Can I take a generic drug rather than a brand-name one?
• Is there written information about the medication?

If written information is provided, check it for the following information:

• How and when do I take the medication, how much do I take, and for how long? What should I do if I miss a dose?
• What medications, foods, drinks, or activities should I avoid when taking this drug?
• What are the side effects, and what do I do if they occur?

Surgery is another staple of Western medical treatment. Each year more than 70 million operations and related procedures are performed. About 20% are in response to an emergency such as a severe injury, and 80% are **elective surgeries,** meaning the patient can generally choose when and where to have the operation, if at all. Many elective surgeries can be done on an **outpatient** basis, so the patient does not have to be admitted to a hospital for the procedure. If a health care provider suggests surgery for any reason, ask the following questions:

• Why do I need surgery at this time?
• Are any nonsurgical options available, such as medicine or physical therapy?
• What are the risks and complications of the surgery?
• Can the operation be done on an outpatient basis?
• What can I expect before, during, and after surgery?

Ask Yourself

QUESTIONS FOR CRITICAL THINKING AND REFLECTION

What sort of relationship do you have with your primary care physician? Do you think he or she understands your needs and is familiar enough with your history? Are you satisfied with this relationship?

TERMS

elective surgery   A nonemergency operation that the patient can choose to schedule.

outpatient   A person receiving medical attention without being admitted to the hospital.

COMPLEMENTARY AND ALTERNATIVE MEDICINE

Whereas conventional Western medicine tends to focus on the body, on the physical causes of disease, and on ways to eradicate pathogens in order to restore health, CAM tends to focus on an integration of mind, body, and spirit in seeking ways to restore the whole person to harmony so that he or she can regain health. This integration is referred to as **holistic health care**—considering the whole person as a mind–body–spirit entity when diagnosing, treating, or preventing any illness or disorder or promoting or maintaining health. The opposite of *holistic* is *dualistic*, which refers to treating the mind and body separately.

CAM therapies are slowly but steadily gaining momentum in the United States as new evidence emerges about the potential value of certain practices. More than 42 percent of hospitals offer one or more CAM therapies, and 40 major American universities have added integrative medical centers to their facilities. In addition, nearly all medical schools have curricular offerings on integrative therapies.

Although research studies on CAM modalities have been relatively small in size and conservative in their conclusions, some of their results are promising. For example, a 2010 study looked at the effects of tai chi on symptoms of fibromyalgia, a disorder that causes chronic pain and general fatigue. Patients in one group learned a variety of tai chi movements, and patients in another group practiced stretching exercises and received wellness counseling. Over the course of the study, the patients in the tai chi group reported significantly less pain than patients in the stretching group, and the benefits lasted well beyond the study's end.

Another 2010 study found that about 60% of adult Americans with back pain have tried at least one CAM therapy. The therapies most commonly used were chiropractic, massage, yoga, tai chi, gigong, and acupuncture. Nearly two-thirds of the respondents in this study said they experienced significantly reduced pain as a result of a CAM therapy.

NCCAM groups CAM practices into several broad categories: alternative medical systems, mind–body medicine, natural products, manipulative and body-based practices, and other CAM practices. What follows is a general introduction to the types of CAM available and a brief description of some of the more widely used ones.

Alternative Medical Systems

Many cultures formed complete systems of medical philosophy, theory, and practice long before the current Western biomedical approach was developed. The complete systems that are best known in the United States include traditional Chinese medicine (TCM), also known as traditional Oriental medicine, and homeopathy. Traditional medical systems have also been developed in many other regions of the world, including North, Central, and South America; the Middle East; India; Tibet; and Australia. In many countries, these medical approaches continue to be used today—frequently alongside Western medicine and quite often by physicians trained in Western medicine.

Alternative medical systems tend to have concepts in common. For example, the concept of life force or energy exists in many cultures. In traditional Chinese medicine, the life force contained in all living things is called *qi* (sometimes spelled chi). Most traditional medical systems think of disease as a disturbance or imbalance not just of physical processes but also of forces or energies within the body, the mind, and the spirit. Treatment aims at reestablishing equilibrium, balance, and harmony.

Because the whole patient, rather than an isolated body part or disease, is treated in most comprehensive alternative medical systems, it is rare that only a single treatment approach is used. Most commonly, multiple remedies and techniques are employed and are continually adjusted according to the changes in the patient's health status that occur naturally or are brought about by the treatment. Three of the best known alternative medical systems are traditional Chinese medicine, homeopathy, and naturopathy.

Traditional Chinese Medicine In **traditional Chinese medicine (TCM)**, the free and harmonious flow of qi defines health—a positive feeling of well-being and vitality in body, mind, and spirit. TCM works to restore and balance the flow of qi; the goal is not only to treat illnesses but also to increase energy, prevent disease, and support immunity.

Two of the primary treatment methods in TCM are **herbal remedies** and **acupuncture**. Chinese herbal remedies number about 5800. In addition to herbs, plant products, fungi (mushrooms), animal parts, and minerals may be used. The use of a single medicinal substance is rare in Chinese herbal medicine; rather, several different substances are combined in precise proportions, often to make a tea or soup.

Acupuncture is used to correct disturbances in the flow of qi through the insertion of thin needles at appropriate points

> The World Health Organization lists **more than 40 conditions that may benefit from acupuncture treatment**.

TERMS

holistic health care Practice that takes into account the whole person—body, mind, and spirit—when assessing, treating, and preventing illnesses and maintaining health.

traditional Chinese medicine (TCM) The traditional medical system of China, which views illness as the result of a problem in the quality, quantity, or flow of qi, the life force; therapies include acupuncture and herbal medicine.

herbal remedy A medicine prepared from plants.

acupuncture Insertion of thin needles through the skin at points along meridians—pathways through which qi is believed to flow.

through the skin. Qi is believed to flow through the body along several meridians, or pathways, and there are hundreds of acupuncture points located along these meridians. The points chosen for acupuncture are highly individualized for each patient, and they change during treatment as the patient's health status changes.

The World Health Organization has compiled a list of more than 40 conditions for which acupuncture may be beneficial. At a conference called by the National Institutes of Health, a panel of experts found that acupuncture was effective in relieving nausea and vomiting after chemotherapy, and pain after surgery, including dental surgery. Newer studies show that acupuncture may help relieve the painful symptoms of fibromyalgia and reduce the joint pain and stiffness of osteoarthritis. There is not yet enough evidence to show conclusively that acupuncture is effective for menstrual cramps, tennis elbow, carpal tunnel syndrome, asthma, or certain other conditions.

Almost no negative side effects have been reported with acupuncture. The FDA regulates acupuncture needles like other standard medical devices and requires that they be sterile. Most states require licensing for acupuncture practitioners, but requirements vary widely.

Homeopathy An alternative medical system of Western origin, **homeopathy** is based on the principles that "like cures like," and that remedies become more effective with greater dilution. "Like cures like" summarizes the concept that a substance that produces the symptoms of an illness in a healthy person can help cure the illness when given in very minute quantities. Remedies containing very small quantities of a particular substance are produced by repeatedly diluting the original solution. The extent of dilution varies, but the final extract can be so dilute that few, if any, of the original molecules remain.

More than 1000 different substances (plant and animal parts or products, minerals, and chemicals) are used to prepare homeopathic remedies, and each of these substances is thought to have different effects at different dilutions. That means a homeopathic practitioner must not only choose the correct remedy for a particular patient but also decide on the specific dilution of that remedy in order to achieve the desired effect.

To assess a patient's condition, homeopaths generally spend considerable time talking with a patient and assessing his or her physical, psychological, and emotional health before deciding on the correct remedy at the proper dilution. This long and intensive interaction between the practitioner and the patient might play an important role in the success of the therapy. Indeed, critics of homeopathy often attribute its reported effectiveness to this nonspecific placebo effect. However, when the results of 185 homeopathic trials were analyzed in a recent study, it was concluded that the clinical effects of homeopathy could not be completely explained by the placebo effect. Homeopathy remains one of the most controversial forms of CAM.

To date, the FDA has not reported any serious adverse effects associated with the use of homeopathy, with the possible exception of situations in which a patient might have been successfully treated with standard medical approaches but chose to rely solely on homeopathy. The FDA regulates some homeopathic remedies, but they are subject to many fewer restrictions than prescription or over-the-counter drugs. A few states require practitioners to have special licenses, but most providers practice homeopathy as a specialty under another license, such as a license to practice medicine or nursing.

Naturopathy The health care discipline of **naturopathy** is based in the premise that the body has the ability to restore and maintain optimal health. Naturopathic practitioners focus on removing barriers to good health and creating healing internal and external environments. They use nutritional counseling, acupuncture, herbology, homeopathic medicine, and other holistic approaches to treatment. The most frequently treated conditions include allergies, chronic pain, obesity, heart disease, fertility problems, and cancer. Naturopaths work in hospitals, clinics, and community health centers. They are licensed in several states.

Mind–Body Medicine

Mind–body interventions make use of the integral connection between mind and body and the effect each can have on the other. They include many of the stress management techniques discussed in Chapter 2, including meditation, yoga, visualization, taijiquan, and biofeedback. Psychotherapy, support groups, prayer, and music and art therapy can also be thought of as mind–body interventions. The placebo effect is one of the most widely known examples of mind–body interdependence.

Hypnotherapy is considered to be a CAM modality, although its use for certain conditions was accepted more than 40 years ago by the American Medical Association. Hypnotherapy involves the induction of a state of deep relaxation during which the patient is more likely to accept suggestions to influence health and overcome conditions such as chronic pain, pain during surgery or childbirth, unhealthy habits, and anxiety and phobias. The practitioner helps the patient change unwanted behavior or deal with pain and other

TERMS

homeopathy An alternative medical system that uses a holistic approach to diagnosis, and treatments that involve administering very small doses of remedies that would produce symptoms like those of the illness in larger doses.

naturopathy An alternative medical system based on supporting the body's ability to heal itself and maintain optimal health by removing barriers and creating a healing internal and external environment.

hypnotherapy The process by which a practitioner induces a state of relaxation in which the patient is more likely to achieve an agreed-upon health outcome; commonly used for managing pain, phobias, and addictions.

symptoms. An NIH-sponsored report found strong evidence for the effectiveness of relaxation techniques and hypnosis in reducing chronic pain stemming from a variety of medical conditions. Health professionals who are properly trained in hypnotherapy use this modality to augment their conventional treatments. Many states require hypnotherapists to be licensed, but the requirements for licensing vary substantially.

Natural Products

Natural products, also known as *biologically based therapies*, consist primarily of herbal therapies or remedies, botanicals, and extracts from animal tissues (such as shark cartilage). Herbal remedies are a major component of all indigenous forms of medicine. Prior to the development of pharmaceuticals at the end of the 19th century, people everywhere in the world relied on materials from nature for pain relief, wound healing, and treatment of a variety of ailments. Much of the **pharmacopoeia** of present-day scientific medicine originated in the folk medicine of native people, and many drugs used today are derived from plants.

Most natural products are sold as dietary supplements and are therefore largely unregulated by the FDA. Like foods, dietary supplements must carry ingredient labels, and manufacturers are responsible for ensuring that their dietary supplements are safe and properly labeled for marketing. The FDA is responsible for monitoring the labeling and accompanying literature of dietary supplements and for overseeing their safety once they are on the market.

Well-designed clinical studies have been conducted on a number of natural products. A few commonly used herbals, their uses, and the evidence supporting their efficacy are presented in Table 15.2. Participants in clinical trials with herbals such as St. John's wort, ginkgo biloba, and echinacea experienced only minor adverse events. New studies are also evaluating the effects of varying dosages and their interactions with conventional drugs.

Although most drug–herb interactions are relatively minor compared to conventional drug–drug interactions, some can be potentially serious. For example, herbs that have anticoagulant (anticlotting) properties, such as ginkgo biloba, when used concurrently with the commonly prescribed anticoagulant Coumadin, can result in delayed blood clotting or hemorrhage. St. John's wort interacts with drugs used to treat HIV infection and heart disease, and the herb may also reduce the effectiveness of oral contraceptives, antirejection drugs used in patients receiving organ transplants, and some medications used to treat infections, depression, asthma, and seizure disorders. Supplements containing kava kava have been linked to liver damage, and anyone who has liver problems, drinks large amounts of alcohol, or takes medications that can affect the liver is advised to consult a physician or pharmacist before using kava kava–containing supplements.

Another potential problem is the possibility of contaminants. Some herbal medicine products have been found to contain potentially harmful levels of lead, mercury, and arsenic. The content of herbal preparations is also variable.

Studies have shown that most people do not reveal their use of CAM therapies to their conventional health care providers, a problem that can have significant health consequences. Any herbs that are used in combination with conventional drugs should be evaluated for safety by a knowledgeable health care provider such as a pharmacist.

Manipulative and Body-Based Practices

Touch and body manipulation are longstanding forms of health care. Manual healing techniques are based on the concept that misalignment or dysfunction in one part of the body can cause pain or dysfunction in that or another part. Correcting these misalignments can help restore optimal health.

Many manipulative and body-based practices are integral components of physical therapy and osteopathic medicine, although certain techniques fit the definition of CAM because they are not a part of conventional health care practice, such as massage. The most commonly used CAM manual healing method is **chiropractic**, a method that focuses on the relationship between structure and function, primarily of the spine, joints, muscles, and the nervous system, to maintain or restore health. An important therapeutic procedure is the manipulation of joints, particularly those of the spinal column. However, chiropractors also use a variety of other techniques, including exercise, patient education and lifestyle modification, nutritional supplements, and orthotics (mechanical supports and braces) to treat patients.

Chiropractors, or doctors of chiropractic, are trained for a minimum of four years at accredited chiropractic colleges and can go on to postgraduate training in many countries. Although specifically listed by NCCAM as one of the manipulative and body-based practices of CAM, chiropractic is accepted by many health care and health insurance providers to a far greater extent than the other types of CAM therapies. Based on research showing the efficacy of chiropractic management in acute low-back pain, spinal manipulation has

TERMS

natural products   CAM therapies that include biologically based interventions and products; examples include herbal remedies, extracts from animal tissues, and dietary supplements.

pharmacopoeia   A collection of descriptions and formulas for drugs and medicinal preparations.

chiropractic   A system of manual healing most frequently used to treat musculoskeletal problems; the primary treatment is manipulation of the spine and other joints.

Table 15.2 · Commonly Used Herbals, Their Uses, Evidence for Their Effectiveness, and Contraindications

BOTANICAL	USE	EVIDENCE	EXAMPLES OF ADVERSE EFFECTS AND INTERACTIONS
Cranberry (*Vaccinium macrocarpon*)	Prevention or treatment of urinary tract disorders	May eliminate and prevent bacteria from infecting the urinary tract	None known
Dandelion (*Taraxacum officinale*)	As a "tonic" against liver or kidney ailments	None yet	May cause diarrhea in some users; people with gallbladder or bile duct problems should not take dandelion
Echinacea (*Echinacea purpurea, E. angustifolia, E. pallida*)	Stimulation of immune functions; to prevent colds and flulike diseases; to lessen symptoms of colds and flu	Some trials showed that it prevents colds and flu and helps patients recover faster from colds	Might cause liver damage if taken over long periods of time (more than 8 weeks); since it is an immune stimulant, it is not advisable to take it with immune suppressants (e.g., corticosteroids) or during chemotherapy
Evening primrose oil (*Oenothera biennis L.*)	Reduction of inflammation	Long-term supplementation effective in reducing symptoms of rheumatoid arthritis	None known
Feverfew (*Tanacetum parthenium*)	Prevention of headaches and migraines	Most trials indicate that it is more effective than placebo	Should not be used by people allergic to other members of the aster family; has the potential to increase the effects of warfarin and other anticoagulants
Garlic (*Allium sativum*)	Reduction of cholesterol	Short-term studies have found a modest effect	May interact with some medications, including anticoagulants, cyclosporine, and oral contraceptives
Ginkgo (*Ginkgo biloba*)	Improvement of circulation and memory	Improves cerebral insufficiency and slows progression of Alzheimer's disease and other types of senile dementia in some patients; improves blood flow in legs	Could increase bleeding time; should not be taken with nonsteroidal anti-inflammatory drugs or anticoagulants; gastrointestinal disturbance
Ginseng (*Panax ginseng*)	Improvement of physical performance, memory, immune function, and glycemic control in diabetes; treatment of herpes simplex 2	No conclusive evidence exists for any of these uses	Interacts with warfarin and alcohol in mice and rats, so should probably not be used with these drugs; may cause liver damage
St. John's wort (*Hypericum perforatum*)	Treatment of depression	There is strong evidence that it is significantly more effective than placebo, is as effective as some standard antidepressants for mild to moderate depression, and causes fewer adverse effects	Known to interact with a variety of pharmaceuticals and should not be taken together with digoxin, theophylline, cyclosporine, indinavir, and serotonin reuptake inhibitors
Saw palmetto (*Serenoa repens*)	Improvement of prostate health	Studies show that saw palmetto may reduce mild prostate enlargement	Has no known interactions with drugs, but should probably not be taken with hormonal therapies
Valerian (*Valeriana officinalis*)	Treatment of insomnia	Appears to help with sleep disorders	Interacts with thiopental and pentobarbital and should not be used with these drugs

been included in the federal guidelines for the treatment of this condition, and electrodiagnostic tests show that chiropractic is effective in controlling back pain. Promising results have also been reported with the use of chiropractic techniques in neck pain and headaches.

A word of caution is in order: Spinal manipulation must be performed only by a properly trained professional such as a chiropractor, osteopathic physician, or physical therapist who is specially trained and certified in orthopedic manual physical therapy.

Exercise for health maintenance, promotion, and disease prevention currently fits the definition of a CAM modality. However, the American College of Sports Medicine (ACSM) and the American Medical Association (AMA) are actively

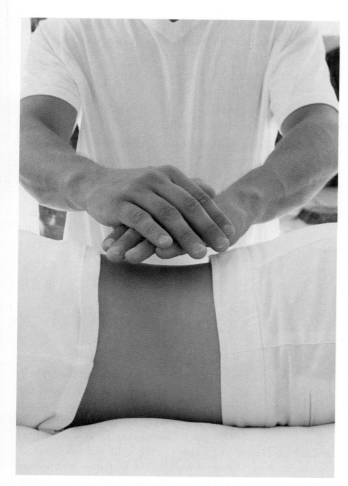

One of several energy medicine therapies, Reiki has bioenergetic and physical components.

are approaches that use movement to promote physical, mental, emotional, and spiritual well-being, such as the Feldenkrais method, the Alexander technique, and Pilates. Traditional healers use methods based on indigenous theories, beliefs, and experiences handed down from generation to generation. Examples are the Native American medicine man or woman and the shaman, the traditional healer in many cultures.

Energy therapies are forms of treatment that use energy originating from the patient's or therapist's body or from other sources such as therapeutic magnets. Energy therapies are based on the concept that energy surrounds and penetrates the body and can be influenced by movement, touch, pressure, or the placement of hands in or through the fields. **Qigong**, a component of traditional Chinese medicine, combines movement, meditation, and regulation of breathing to enhance the flow of qi to improve blood circulation and enhance immune function. **Therapeutic touch** is derived from ancient techniques involving using the hands to detect and transmit energy. It is based on the premise that healers can identify and correct energy imbalances by passing their hands over the patient's body. **Reiki** is another example of energy therapy; it is intended to correct disturbances in the flow of life energy (*ki* in the Japanese tradition) and enhance the body's healing powers through the use of specific hand positions on or near the patient's body to promote balance.

Bioelectromagnetics is the study of interactions between living organisms and electromagnetic fields, both those produced by the organism itself and those produced by outside sources. The recognition that the body produces electromagnetic fields has led to the development of many diagnostic procedures in Western medicine, including electroencephalography (EEG), electrocardiography (ECG), and nuclear magnetic resonance imaging (MRI).

Bioelectromagnetic-based therapies include the use of electromagnetic fields to manage pain, increase blood flow, and treat conditions such as arthritic pain.

trying to move exercise into the medical mainstream. A study has found that 65% of Americans would be more interested in exercising for staying healthy if advised to do so by their physicians.

A new program, Exercise Is Medicine™, encourages physicians to record a patient's exercise level as a routine vital sign during clinical visits, along with pulse, respiratory rate, temperature, and blood pressure. Those who are able will be advised to exercise for 30 minutes and to stretch and engag in light muscle training for an additional 10 minutes five days each week. The Exercise Is Medicine website (www.exerciseismedicine.com) advises physicians, other health care providers, medical educators, and the public about the benefits of exercise. Through efforts such as this, exercise is likely to become part of the curriculum in American medical schools and be recommended as a treatment in American health care institutions.

Other CAM Practices

CAM practices also include movement therapies, traditional healing practices, and energy therapies. Movement therapies

---

TERMS

energy therapies   Forms of CAM treatment that use energy fields originating either within the body or from outside sources to promote health and healing.

qigong   A component of traditional Chinese medicine that combines movement, meditation, and regulation of breathing to enhance the flow of qi, improve blood circulation, and enhance immune function.

therapeutic touch   A CAM practice based on the premise that healers can identify and correct energy imbalances by passing their hands over the patient's body.

Reiki   A CAM practice intended to correct disturbances in the flow of life energy and enhance the body's healing powers through the use of various hand positions on the patient.

bioelectromagnetic-based therapies   CAM therapies based on the notion that electromagnetic fields can be used to promote healing and manage pain.

Evaluating Complementary and Alternative Therapies

Because there is less information available about complementary and alternative therapies, as well as less regulation of associated products and providers, it is important for consumers to take an active role when they are thinking about using them.

Working with Your Physician When a health issue might be serious, the NCCAM advises consumers not to seek complementary therapies without first consulting a conventional health care provider. It's usually best to become informed and discuss conventional treatments that have been shown to be beneficial for your condition. If you are thinking of trying any complementary or alternative therapies, it is important to discuss this with your physician, pharmacist, or other conventional provider who is knowledgeable about your health status and is also informed about CAM. Areas to discuss include the safety of the treatment; evidence for its effectiveness, if any; issues of timing; and likely cost.

If appropriate, schedule a follow-up visit with your physician to assess your condition and your progress after a certain amount of time using a complementary therapy. Keep a symptom diary to track your symptoms and gauge your progress. (Symptoms such as pain and fatigue are difficult to recall with accuracy, so an ongoing symptom diary is an important tool.) If you plan to pursue a therapy against your physician's advice, you need to tell him or her.

Questioning the CAM Practitioner You can also get information from individual practitioners and from schools, professional organizations, and state licensing boards. Ask about education, training, licensing, and certification. If appropriate, check with local or state regulatory agencies or the consumer affairs department to determine if any complaints have been lodged against the practitioner. Some guidelines for talking with a CAM practitioner include the following:

- Ask the practitioner why he or she thinks the therapy will be beneficial for your condition. Ask for a full

> NCCAM advises consumers not to seek CAM treatment **without talking to their usual health care providers first**.

description of the therapy and any potential side effects. Ask if there is any research supporting the efficacy of the treatment for your condition.

- Describe in detail any conventional treatments you are receiving or plan to receive.
- Ask how long the therapy should continue before it can be determined if it is beneficial.
- Ask about the expected cost of the treatment. Does it seem reasonable? Will your health insurance pay some or all of the costs?

If anything an unconventional practitioner says or recommends directly conflicts with advice from your physician, discuss it with your physician before making any major changes in your current treatment regimen or lifestyle.

PAYING FOR HEALTH CARE

The American health care system is one of the most advanced and comprehensive in the world, but it is also the most expensive (Figure 15.2). In 2009 Americans spent $2.4 trillion on health care, or more than $8000 per person. Many factors contribute to the high cost of health care in the United States, including the cost of advanced equipment and new technology, expensive treatments for some illnesses, aging of the population, and the demand for profits by many commercial health care providers.

The Current System

Health care is financed by a combination of private and public insurance plans, patient out-of-pocket payments, and government assistance. Currently, private insurance and individual patients pay about 55% of the total; the government pays the rest, mainly through Medicare and Medicaid. Most nonelderly Americans receive health insurance through their employers.

By some estimates, as many as 50 million Americans—the vast majority of them employed—have no health insurance at all. Many more are underinsured, meaning they may be uninsured for periods of time, have health insurance that does not cover all needed services, and/or have high-out-of-pocket costs. New and extended government health insurance programs for children have reduced the number of Americans under age 18 who lack health insurance; still, 9.8 million American children were uninsured in 2010.

Health Insurance

Health insurance protects you against losses incurred for medical expenses. Health insurance enables people to receive

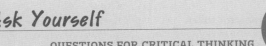

Ask Yourself

QUESTIONS FOR CRITICAL THINKING AND REFLECTION

Have you ever considered using a complementary or alternative treatment? If so, was it in addition to conventional treatment or instead of it? What kind of research did you do before having the treatment? What advice did your primary health care provider give you about it?

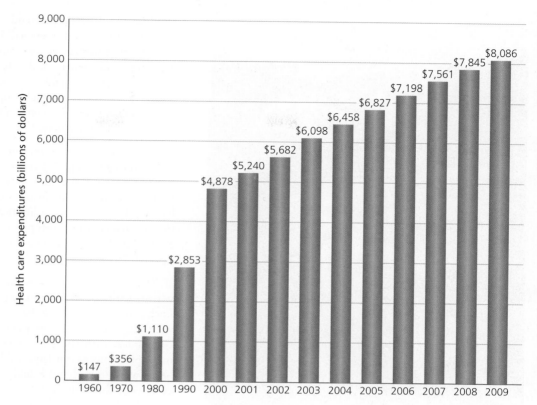

FIGURE 15.2 National health care expenditures (public and private), 1960–2007.

SOURCE: National Center for Health Statistics. 2010. *Health, United States: 2009*. Hyattsville, MD: National Center for Health Statistics.

health care they might not otherwise be able to afford. Health insurance is important for everyone, especially as health care costs continue to rise.

Traditional Fee-for-Service (Indemnity) Plans
In a fee-for-service, or indemnity, plan, you can use any physician or hospital you choose. You or the provider sends the bill to your insurance company, which pays part of it. Usually you have to pay a deductible amount each year, and then the plan will pay a percentage—often 80%—of what it considers the "usual and customary" charge for covered services.

Managed Care Plans
Managed care plans have agreements with a network of specified physicians, hospitals, and health care providers to offer a range of services to plan members at reduced cost. In general, you have lower out-of-pocket costs and less paperwork with a managed care plan than with an indemnity plan, but you also have less freedom in choosing your health care providers. Managed care plans may follow several different models:

• **Health maintenance organizations (HMOs)** offer members a range of services for a set monthly fee. You choose a primary care physician who manages your care and refers you to specialists if you need them.

• **Preferred provider organizations (PPOs)** have arrangements with physicians and other providers who have agreed to accept lower fees.

• **Point-of-service (POS) plans** are options offered by many HMOs in which you can see a physician outside the plan and still be partially covered.

Many managed care plans try to reduce costs over the long term by paying for routine preventive care, such as regular checkups and screening tests and prenatal care; they may also encourage prevention by offering health education and lifestyle modification programs for members.

Government Programs
Americans who are 65 or older and younger people with certain disabilities can be covered by **Medicare,** a federal health insurance program that helps

---

TERMS

managed care plan   A health care program that integrates the financing and delivery of services by using designated providers and incentives for following the plan's policies; HMOs, PPOs, and POS plans are managed care plans.

health maintenance organization (HMO)   A managed care plan that offers health care from designated providers.

preferred provider organization (PPO)   A managed care plan in which providers agree to deliver services for discounted fees; patients can go to any provider, but using nonparticipating providers results in higher costs to the patient.

point-of-service (POS) plan   A managed care plan that covers treatment by an HMO physician but permits patients to seek treatment elsewhere with a higher copayment.

Medicare   A federal health insurance program for people 65 or older and for younger people with certain disabilities.

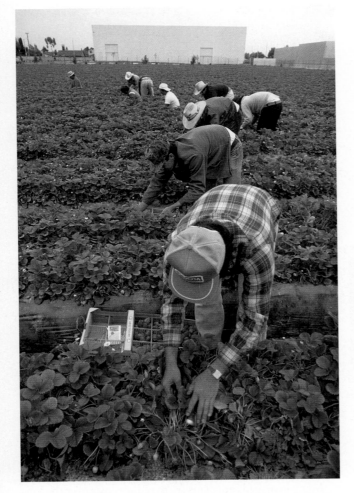

Some workers will still be uninsured under the new health care legislation.

families, the unemployed, and people with serious health conditions. The law also opens Medicaid to more Americans by loosening income requirements and other restrictions. The act provides federal and state funding to subsidize insurance coverage for qualified Americans who cannot access health care coverage through employer-sponsored or private plans. However, not everyone will qualify for free or low-cost coverage under the federal law.

• Placing tighter restrictions on the insurance industry. The Affordable Care Act restricts or bans certain insurance industry practices that have prevented millions of Americans from getting health care insurance. Some restrictions (such as banning lifetime coverage limits and prohibiting discrimination against children with preexisting health conditions) began in 2010; other regulations will gradually take effect through 2014.

The act also creates health care insurance "exchanges," where qualified Americans can purchase affordable coverage. Each state will ultimately have its own exchange. Exchanges will offer a variety of coverage options from private insurance companies, with the goal of creating competitive rates to make plans more affordable. In 2010 the federal government began working with individual states to create exchanges, and every state should have its own exchange in place by no later than 2014. In 2012, the U.S. Supreme Court upheld the constitutionality of the Affordable Care Act.

For more information about the health care reform act, visit the U.S. government's health care website at www. healthcare.gov.

pay for hospitalization, physician services, and prescription drugs. **Medicaid** is a joint federal–state health insurance program that covers some low-income people, especially children, pregnant women, and people with certain disabilities.

Health Care Reform

In 2010 Congress passed the Affordable Care Act, a sweeping reform of the health care industry that could ultimately extend health insurance coverage to some 32 million Americans who are currently uninsured. The law aims to make medical coverage more affordable and widely available through two broad types of action:

• Subsidizing insurance coverage for Americans who cannot afford it. Millions of Americans live without health care insurance simply because they cannot pay the premiums. This is particularly true for low-income Americans, large

Medicaid A federally subsidized state-run plan of health care for people with low income.

TERMS

TIPS FOR TODAY AND THE FUTURE

Most of the time you can take care of yourself without consulting a health care provider. When you need professional care, you can still take responsibility for yourself by making informed decisions.

RIGHT NOW YOU CAN:

- Make sure you have enough of your prescription medications on hand, and your prescriptions are up-to-date.
- If you take any supplements (dietary or herbal), ask your pharmacist if they can interact with any prescription drugs you are taking.

IN THE FUTURE YOU CAN:

- Thoroughly research complementary or alternative medical treatments you are using or considering to make sure they are considered safe and effective.
- Review your medical insurance policy and make sure you are familiar with your coverage and the policy's terms. If you don't have medical insurance, start investigating your options.

Connect to Your Choices

Have you ever thought about where you get your attitudes toward conventional medicine and complementary and alternative medicine? Many factors can influence our attitudes, some not as obvious as others. When you were growing up, was your family respectful of the medical establishment, or were they skeptical of it? Did your parents or grandparents use herbal remedies? Do any of your peers express strong opinions about physicians or CAM practices? Are there CAM practitioners in your community? Do you know people who see chiropractors or get acupuncture or massages?

What are the external factors that influence your choices about medicine? What are your inner motivations and core values, and how do they affect your choices? Based on what you learned in this chapter, will you make some different choices in the future? If so, what will they be?

Go online to Connect to complete this activity: www.mcgraw-hillconnect.com

SUMMARY

• Informed self-care requires knowing how to evaluate symptoms. It's necessary to see a physician if symptoms are severe, unusual, persistent, or recurrent.

• Self-treatment doesn't necessarily require medication, but OTC drugs can be a helpful part of self-care.

• Conventional medicine is characterized by a focus on the physical causes of disease; the identification of a set of signs and symptoms for different diseases; the development of public health measures to prevent disease and drugs and surgery to treat them; the use of scientific thinking to understand phenomena; and a well-established research methodology.

• Conventional practitioners include medical doctors, doctors of osteopathic medicine, podiatrists, optometrists, and dentists, as well as allied health care providers and nurses.

• The diagnostic process involves a medical history, a physical exam, and medical tests. Patients should ask questions about medical tests and treatments recommended by their physicians.

• Safe use of prescription drugs requires knowledge of what the medication is supposed to do, how and when to take it, and the possible side effects.

• Complementary and alternative medicine (CAM) is defined as those therapies and practices that do not form part of conventional health care and medical practice as taught in most U.S. medical schools and offered in most U.S. hospitals.

• CAM is characterized by a view of health as a balance and integration of body, mind, and spirit and a body of knowledge based on the accumulated observations and experience of practitioners.

• Alternative medical systems such as traditional Chinese medicine, homeopathy, and naturopathy are complete systems of medical philosophy, theory, and practice.

• Mind–body medicine includes meditation, biofeedback, group support, hypnosis, and prayer.

• Natural products include herbal remedies, botanicals, animal tissue products, and dietary supplements.

• Manipulative and body-based practices include massage and other healing techniques; the most frequently used is chiropractic.

• Other CAM practices include movement therapies, traditional healing practices, and energy therapies.

• Because there is presently less information available about CAM and less regulation of its providers and modalities, consumers must be proactive in researching and choosing treatments and using critical thinking skills.

• Health insurance plans can be fee-for-service or managed care plans. Indemnity plans allow consumers more choice in medical providers, but managed care plans are less expensive.

• Government programs include Medicaid for the poor, and Medicare for those aged 65 and over or chronically disabled.

• Recent government reforms of the health care industry aim to make affordable health care insurance coverage available to more Americans than ever before.

FOR MORE INFORMATION

BOOKS

American College of Physicians. 2009. *The ACP Evidence-Based Guide to Complementary and Alternative Medicine.* Washington, DC: American College of Physicians. *Highly regarded manual of CAM practices and evidence supporting them.*

Mayo Clinic. 2010. *The Mayo Clinic Book of Alternative Medicine*, 2nd edition. New York: Time-Life. *A concise review of currently popular CAM therapies and treatments.*

Micozzi, M. S. 2010. *Fundamentals of Complementary and Alternative Medicine*, 4th ed. New York: Saunders. *Detailed descriptions of the CAM modalities, with evidence supporting specific therapies for certain conditions.*

PDR. 2011. *PDR for Nonprescription Drugs, Dietary Supplements, and Herbs, 2011*, 32nd ed. Montvale, NJ: Thomson Healthcare. *A reference covering the safety and efficacy of over-the-counter medications and herbals.*

ORGANIZATIONS, HOTLINES, AND WEBSITES

American Board of Medical Specialties. Provides information about board certification, including information about specific physicians.
http://www.abms.org

American Chiropractic Association. Provides information about chiropractic care, consumer tips, and a searchable directory of certified chiropractors.
http://www.acatoday.org

American Medical Association (AMA). Provides information about physicians, including their training, licensure, and board certification.

http://www.ama-assn.org

American Osteopathic Association. Provides information about osteopathic physicians, including board certification.

http://www.osteopathic.org/Pages/default.aspx

ConsumerLab.com. Provides information about the results of tests of dietary supplements, including information about actual ingredients and concentrations.

http://www.consumerlab.com

Food and Drug Administration: Information for Consumers. Provides materials about dietary supplements, foods, prescription and OTC drugs, and other FDA-regulated products.

http://www.fda.gov/ForConsumers/default.htm

National Center for Complementary and Alternative Medicine (NCCAM). Provides general information packets, answers to frequently asked questions about CAM, consumer advice for safer use of CAM, research abstracts, and bibliographies.

http://nccam.nih.gov

National Council against Health Fraud. Provides news and information about health fraud and quackery and links to related sites.

http://www.ncahf.org

SELECTED BIBLIOGRAPHY

Abd Jalil, M. A., A. N. Shui, and N Muhammed. 2012. Role of medicinal plants and natural products on osteoporotic fracture healing. *Evidence-Based Complementary and Alternative Medicine*, September 2 (Epub ahead of print).

American Academy of Family Physicians. 2010. *Passage of Health Care Reform Only a Starting Point for Physicians* (http//www.aafp.org/online/en/home/publications/news/news-now/govenrment-medicine/2).

Ayers, S. L., and J. J. Kronenfeld. 2012. Delays in seeking conventional medical care and complementary and alternative medicine utilization. *Health Services Research* 47(5): 2081–096.

Baer, H. A. et al. 2012. A dialogue between naturopathy and critical medical anthropology: What constitutes holistic health? *Medical Anthropology Quarterly* 26(2): 241–256.

Bryan, S., G. Pitno Zipp, and R. Parasher. 2012. The effects of yoga on psychosocial variables and exercise adherence: A randomized, controlled pilot study. *Alternative Therapies in Health and Medicine* 18(5): 50–59.

Cramer, H., et al. 2012. Mindfulness-based stress reduction for low back pain: A systematic review. *BMC Complementary and Alternative Medicine* 12(1): 162.

Cyna, A. M., et al. 2006. Antenatal self-hypnosis for labour and childbirth: A pilot study. *Anaesthesia and Intensive Care* 34(4): 464–469.

Del Prete, A., et al. 2012 Herbal products: Benefits, limits and applications in chronic liver disease. *Evidence-Based Complementary and Alternative Medicine*, September 6 (Epub ahead of print).

D'Silva, S. et al. 2012. Mind-body medicine therapies for a range of depression severity: A systematic review. *Psychosomatics* 53(5): 407–423.

Fava, M. 2010. Using complementary and alternative medicines for depression. *Journal of Clinical Psychiatry* 71(9): e24.

Frazier, S. C. 2005. Health outcomes and polypharmacy in elderly individuals: An integrated literature review. *Journal of Gerontological Nursing* 31(9): 4–11.

Fronstin, P. 2012. Employment-based health benefits: Recent trends and future outlook. *Inquiry* 49(2): 101–115.

Gahche, J., et al. 2011. Dietary supplement use among U.S. adults has increased since NHANES III (1988–1994). *NCHS Data Brief*, no. 61. Hyattsville, MD: Naional Cener for Health Statistics.

Greene, J. A. 2010. What's in a name? Generics and the persistence of the pharmaceutical brand in American medicine. *Journal of the History of Medicine and Allied Sciences*. September 21, published online.

Grzywaca, J. G., et al. 2008. Age-related differences in the conventional health care–complementary and alternative medicine link. *American Journal of Health Behavior* 32(6): 650–663.

Hammer, D., et al. 2010. The intended—and unintended—consequences of healthcare reform. *Healthcare Financial Management* 64(10): 50–55.

Harris, P., et al. 2012. Prevalence of complementary and alternative medicine (CAM) use by the general population: A systematic review and update. *International Journal of Clinical Practice* 66(10): 924–939.

Jahnke, R., et al. 2010. A comprehensive review of health benefits of qigong and tai chi. *American Journal of Health Promotion* 24(6): e1–e25.

Kanodia, A.K., et al. 2010. Perceived benefit of complementary and alternative medicine (CAM) for back pain: a national survey. *Journal of the American Board of Family Medicine* 23(3): 354–362;

Litscher, G., et al. 2012. High-tech acupuncture and integrative laser medicine. *Evidence-Based Complementary and Alternative Medicine*, September 4 (Epub ahead of print).

Millet, J. D. 2010. Progress in complementary and alternative medicine research: Yale Research Symposium on Complementary and Integrative Medicine. *Yale Journal of Biology and Medicine* 83(3): 127–129.

National Center for Complementary and Alternative Medicine. *The Use of Complementary and Alternative Medicine in the United States* (http://nccam.nih.gov/news/camstats/2007/camsurvey_fs1.htm).

National Center for Health Statistics. 2010. *Health, United States, 2009.* Hyattsville, MD: National Center for Health Statistics.

O'Malley, P. A. 2012. Preventing and reporting adverse drug events: Pharmacovigilance for the clinical nurse specialist. *Clinical Nurse Specialist* 26(3): 136–137.

Radley, D. C., et al. 2006. Off-label prescribing among office-based physicians. *Archives of Internal Medicine* 166(9): 1021–1026.

Richmond, S. J., et al. 2009. Therapeutic effects of magnetic and copper bracelets in osteoarthritis: A randomized placebo-controlled crossover trial. *Complementary Therapies in Medicine* 17(5–6): 249–256.

Sarris, J., et al. 2012. Complementary medicine, exercise, meditation, diet, and lifestyle modification for anxiety disorders: A review of current evidence. *Evidence-Based Complementary and Alternative Medicine*, August 27 (Epub ahead of print).

Sasson, C. et al. 2012. The changing landscape of America's health care system and the value of emergency medicine. *Academy of Emergency Medicine*, September 20 (Epub ahead of print).

Shen, P. F., et al. 2012. Acupuncture intervention in ischemic stroke: A randomized controlled prospective study. *American Journal of Chinese Medicine* 40(4): 685–693.

Spears, W., et al. 2012. Parents' perspectives on their children's health insurance: Plight of the underinsured. *Journal of Pediatrics*, August 22 (Epub ahead of print).

Wahbeh, H., S. M. Elsas, and B. S. Oken. 2008. Mind–body interventions: applications in neurology. *Neurology* 70(24): 2321–2328.

Wang, C., et al. 2010. A randomized trial of tai chi for fibromyalgia. *New England Journal of Medicine* 363(8): 743–754.

Zhao, X. F., et al. 2012. Mortality and recurrence of vascular disease among stroke patients treated with combined TCM therapy. *Journal of Traditional Chinese Medicine* 32(2): 173–178.

Zhuang, L. X., et al. 2012 An effectiveness study comparing acupuncture, physiotherapy, and their combination in poststroke rehabilitation: A multicentered, randomized, controlled clinical trial. *Alternative Therapies in Health and Medicine* 18(3): 8–14.

Even though we sometimes have to entrust ourselves to the care of medical professionals, that doesn't mean we give up responsibility for our own behavior. Following medical instructions and advice often requires the same kind of behavioral self-management that's involved in quitting smoking, losing weight, or changing eating patterns. For example, if you have an illness or injury, you may be instructed to take medication at certain times of the day, do special exercises or movements, or change your diet.

The medical profession recognizes the importance of patient adherence and encourages different strategies to support it, such as the following:

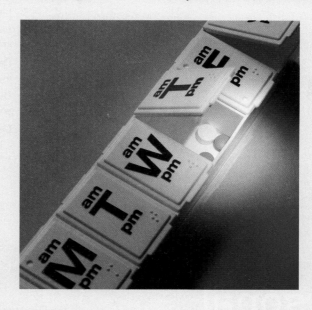

1 Use reminders placed at home, in the car, at work, on your computer screensaver, or elsewhere that improve follow-through in taking medication and keeping scheduled appointments. To help you remember to take medications,

   - Link taking the medication with some well-established routine, like brushing your teeth or eating breakfast.
   - Use a medication calendar, and check off each pill.
   - Use a medication organizer or pill dispenser.
   - Plan ahead; don't wait until the last pill to get a prescription refilled.

2. Use a journal or another form of self-monitoring to keep a detailed account of your health-related behaviors, such as taking pills on schedule, following dietary recommendations, following an exercise program, and so on.

3. Use a self-reward system so that desired behavior changes are encouraged, with a focus on short-term rewards.

4. Develop a clear image or explanation of how the medication or behavior change will improve your health, how you will look and feel, and your long-term well-being.

If these strategies don't help you stick with your treatment plan, you may need to consider other possible explanations for your lack of adherence. For example, are you confused about some aspect of the treatment? Do you find the schedule for taking your medications too complicated, or do the drugs have bothersome side effects that tempt you to avoid them? Do you feel that the recommended treatment is unnecessary or unlikely to help? Are you afraid of becoming dependent on a medication or that you'll be judged negatively if people know about your condition or treatment? A follow-up discussion with a health professional (your physician, a dietician, or a physical therapist) and an examination of your attitudes and beliefs about your condition and treatment plan can also help improve your adherence.

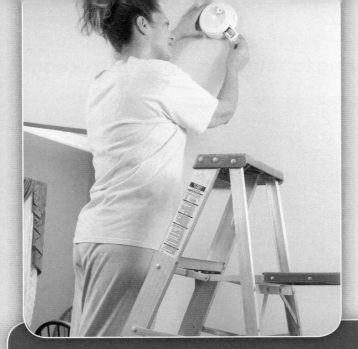

LOOKING AHEAD...

After reading this chapter, you should be able to

- Identify factors that contribute to unintentional injuries
- List the most common types of unintentional injuries and strategies for preventing them
- Describe factors that contribute to violence and intentional injuries
- Discuss different forms of violence and how to protect yourself from intentional injuries
- List strategies for helping others in an emergency situation

16

Personal Safety

Each year more than 185,000 Americans die from injuries, and many more are temporarily or permanently disabled. The economic cost of injuries is high, with nearly $700 billion spent each year for medical care and rehabilitation of injured people. Injuries also cause emotional suffering for injured people and their families, friends, and colleagues.

Engineering strategies such as safety belts can help lower injury rates, as can the passage and enforcement of safety-related laws, such as those requiring tamper-proof containers for OTC medications. Public education campaigns about risky behaviors such as texting while driving or driving under the influence of alcohol can also help prevent injuries. Ultimately, though, it is up to each person to take responsibility for his or her actions and make wise choices about safety behaviors.

DIFFERENTIATING INJURIES

An **intentional injury** is one that is purposely inflicted by oneself or by another person. If an injury occurs when no harm is intended, it is considered an **unintentional injury.** Motor vehicle crashes, falls, and fires often result in unintentional injuries. (Public health officials prefer not to use the word *accidents* to describe unintentional injuries because it

suggests events beyond human control. *Injuries* are predictable outcomes of factors that can be controlled or prevented.)

Although Americans tend to express more concern about intentional injuries, unintentional injuries are actually far more common. Unintentional injuries are the fifth leading cause of death among all Americans and the leading cause of death among people under age 45, as well as the leading cause of death among children and young adults. Because unintentional injuries are so common, they account for more **years of potential life lost** than any other cause of death.

UNINTENTIONAL INJURIES

Injury situations are generally categorized into four general classes, based on where they occur: motor vehicle injuries, home injuries, leisure injuries, and work injuries. The greatest number of deaths occur in motor vehicle crashes, but the greatest number of disabling injuries occur in the home (Table 16.1).

What Causes an Injury?

Most injuries are caused by a combination of human and environmental factors. Human factors are inner conditions or attitudes that lead to an unsafe state, whether physical, emotional, or psychological. Environmental factors are external

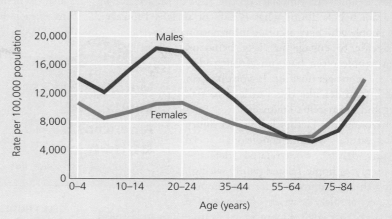

Overall, rates of injury are highest among young adults and seniors over age 85. Except among the oldest group of adults, the nonfatal injury rate is substantially higher in males than in females—and it peaks among young adult males (see figure). Males also significantly outnumber females in injury deaths, whether unintentional or intentional.

Why do men, especially young men, have such high rates of injury? Gender roles may be a key factor: traditional gender roles for males may associate masculinity with risk-taking behavior and a disregard for pain and injury, and risk-taking behavior may be particularly common among young men. Men are more likely to drive dangerously, drink and drive, binge-drink, and use aggressive behavior to control situations—all of which can lead to higher rates of fatal and nonfatal injury. Men may also have a lower perception of risk of dangerous behaviors compared with women.

Traditional gender roles may also make it more difficult for men to admit to injury or emotional vulnerability. Physical injuries may worsen or become chronic if care is not sought promptly. Untreated depression can lead to suicide.

In addition, men may have greater exposure to some injury situations. Compared with women, men may drive more miles, have greater access to firearms, and be more likely to ride motorcycles, operate machinery, and have jobs associated with

Nonfatal injury rate by age and sex.

high rates of workplace injuries. They may be more likely to engage in sports and other recreational activities that are associated with high rates of injuries. Greater access to and use of firearms plays a role in higher rates of deaths among men from assault and suicide. As described in Chapter 3, women are more likely than men to attempt suicide, but men are much more likely to succeed, primarily because they are more likely to use firearms.

Some researchers suggest that the male hormone testosterone may play a role in risky and aggressive behavior.

Differences in brain structure and activity may also influence how men and women respond to stressors and how quickly and to what degree they become verbally or physically aggressive in response to anger.

SOURCES: Centers for Disease Control and Prevention. 2004. Surveillance for fatal and nonfatal injuries—United States, 2001. *MMWR Surveillance Summaries* 53(SS07): 1–57; World Health Organization. 2002. *Gender and Road Traffic Injuries.* Geneva: World Health Organization; Courtenay, W. 1998. College men's health: an overview and a call to action. *Journal of American College Health* 46(6): 279–290.

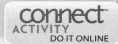

Table 16.1	Unintentional Injuries in the United States (2009)	
	DEATHS	DISABLING INJURIES
Motor vehicle	35,900	3,300,000
Home	65,200	21,100,000
Leisure	25,100	9,400,000
Work	3,582	5,100,000
All classes*	128,200	38,900,000

*Deaths and injuries for the four separate classes total more than the "All classes" figures because of rounding and because some deaths and injuries are included in more than one class.

SOURCE: National Safety Council. 2011. *Injury Facts, 2011 Edition.* Itasca, IL: National Safety Council.

conditions and circumstances, such as poor road conditions, a slippery surface, or the undertow of the ocean at the beach. A common human factor that leads to injuries is risk-taking behavior. People vary in the amount of risk they tend to take in life, but young men are especially prone to taking risks (see the box "Injuries among Young Men"). Alcohol and drug

TERMS

intentional injury   An injury that is purposely inflicted by either oneself or another person.

unintentional injury   An injury that occurs without harm being intended.

years of potential life lost   The difference between an individual's life expectancy and his or her age at death.

use is another common risk factor that leads to many injuries and deaths.

Psychological and emotional factors can also play a role in injuries. People sometimes act on the basis of inadequate or inaccurate beliefs about what is safe or unsafe. However, many people who have accurate information still decide to engage in risky behavior. Young people often have unsafe attitudes, such as "I won't get hurt" or "It won't happen to me." Attitudes like this can lead to risk taking and ultimately to injuries.

Environmental factors leading to injury may be natural (weather conditions), social (a drunk driver), work-related (defective equipment), or home-related (faulty wiring). Making the environment safer is an important aspect of safety. Laws are often passed to try to make our environment safer. Examples include speed limits on highways and workplace safety requirements.

Motor Vehicle Injuries

According to the National Safety Council (NSC), nearly 36,000 Americans were killed and nearly 3.3 million injured in motor vehicle crashes in 2009. Worldwide, motor vehicle crashes kill 1.2 million and injure up to 50 million people each year, making motor vehicle injuries the 11th leading cause of death overall. **Motor vehicle injuries** also result in the majority of cases of paralysis due to spinal injuries, and they are the leading cause of severe brain injury in the United States.

Factors Contributing to Motor Vehicle Injuries

Common causes of motor vehicle injuries are speeding, aggressive driving, fatigue, inexperience, cell phones and other distractions, the use of alcohol and other drugs, and the incorrect use of safety belts and other safety devices.

SPEEDING Nearly 63% of all motor vehicle crashes are caused by bad driving behaviors, especially speeding. As speed increases, momentum and the force of impact increase, and the time allowed for the driver to react (reaction time) decreases. Speed limits are posted to establish the safest maximum speed limit for a given area under ideal conditions; if visibility is limited or the road is wet, the safe maximum speed may be considerably lower.

AGGRESSIVE DRIVING Aggressive driving, includes frequent, erratic, and abrupt lane changes; tailgating; running red lights

> **QUICK STATS**
>
> **Motor vehicle injuries cost Americans $245 billion in 2009.**
>
> —NSC, 2011

or stop signs; passing on the shoulder; and blocking other cars trying to change lanes or pass. Aggressive drivers increase the risk of crashes for themselves and others. Injuries may also occur if aggressive drivers stop their vehicles and confront each other following an incident.

FATIGUE AND SLEEPINESS Driving requires mental alertness and attentiveness. Studies have shown that sleepiness causes slower reaction times, reduced coordination and vigilance, and delayed information processing. Research shows that even mild sleep deprivation causes a deterioration in driving ability comparable to that caused by a 0.05% blood alcohol concentration—a level considered hazardous when driving.

CELL PHONES AND OTHER DISTRACTIONS Anything that distracts a driver can increase the risk of a motor vehicle injury. Common distractions include talking to someone on a cell phone or in the vehicle, texting, eating, smoking, and reaching for controls in the car. Objects and activities outside the vehicle are a source of distraction, as well. More than a dozen U.S. cities have banned digital billboards because of their potential to distract drivers. Several common causes of crashes, such as disregarding stop signs, have been linked to driver distraction. Distraction is a contributing factor in 25–50% of all crashes. About 70% of distracted driver crashes involve noncollision (single-vehicle) or rear-end crashes.

Cell phones are a widely documented source of distraction for drivers. One highly regarded study showed that drivers who use cell phones are four times as likely to be involved in a crash as drivers who don't, primarily because the distraction increases reaction times. Estimates provided by the National Safety Council attribute 1.3 million traffic crashes (about 23% of all crashes) to the use of cell phones. So far, nine states (California, Connecticut, Delaware, Maryland, New Jersey, Nevada, New York, Oregon, and Washington); the District of Columbia, and the U.S. Virgin Islands have banned the use of handheld phones while driving. In 30 states and the District of Columbia, novice drivers are banned from using either handheld or hands-free cell phones while driving (see the box "Cell Phones, Texting, and Distracted Driving"). Thirty-five states, the District of Columbia, and Guam now ban all drivers from text messaging while driving; another eight states have no-texting laws that apply specifically to novice drivers. Given increasing concerns about distractions when driving, the National Transportation Safety Board (NTSB) recommended in December of 2011 that there be a full ban on use of portable electronic devices (including cell phones) while driving. Drivers could still use their GPS navigation systems and their cell phones in emergency situations.

ALCOHOL AND OTHER DRUGS Alcohol is involved in about one-third of all fatal crashes. Alcohol-impaired driving is illegal in all states and the District of Columbia. The legal limit for blood alcohol concentration (BAC) is 0.08%, but people

> **TERMS**
>
> **motor vehicle injuries** Unintentional injuries and deaths involving motor vehicles in motion, both on and off the highway or street; incidents causing motor vehicle injuries include collisions between vehicles and collisions with objects or pedestrians.

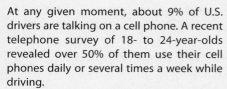

At any given moment, about 9% of U.S. drivers are talking on a cell phone. A recent telephone survey of 18- to 24-year-olds revealed over 50% of them use their cell phones daily or several times a week while driving.

Available evidence indicates that the distraction of using a cell phone while driving increases the risk of motor vehicle crashes. In a study using a driver training simulator, cell phone users were about 20% slower to respond to sudden hazards than were other drivers, and they were about twice as likely to rear-end a braking car in front of them. Among young adult drivers who used cell phones, reaction time was reduced to the level of a 70-year-old driver who was not using a phone.

More people are now being observed texting while driving, which is potentially more dangerous because most individuals need to look directly at the screen of their handheld devices to send and read messages. Results of a study of college-age students texting while operating a driving simulator revealed their risk of crashing was multiplied by a factor of 8 (compared to a group of college-aged cell phone users whose risk had increased by a factor of 4).

Several states have banned the use of cell phones while driving and even more prohibit the use of text messages or e-mail. Although using a cell phone while driving is still legal in some states, the safest strategy is not to do it. For people who live where cell phone use is legal while driving and who choose to

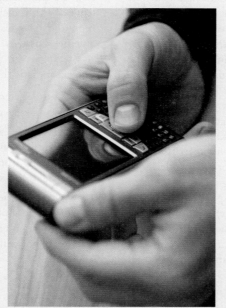

use a phone, the following strategies may help increase safety:

- Be familiar with your phone and its functions, especially speed dial and redial.

- Store frequently called numbers on speed dial so you can place calls without looking at the phone.

- If your phone has voice-activated dialing, use it.

- Use a hands-free device so you can keep both hands on the steering wheel.

- Let the person you are speaking to know you are driving and be prepared to end the call at any time.

- Don't place or answer calls in heavy traffic or hazardous weather conditions.

- Don't take notes or look up phone numbers while driving.

- Time calls so you can place them when you are at a stop.

SOURCES: AAA Foundation for Traffic Safety. 2009. *Safety Culture: Text Messaging and Cell Phone Use While Driving* (www.aaafoundation.org/pdf/TextingFS091012.pdf); TXTResponsibly. 2012. *Gauging Your Distraction* (www.txtresponsibly.org/resources/tools/); National Safety Council. 2012. *Distracted Driving* (www.nsc.org/safety_road/Distracted_Driving/Pages/distracted_driving.aspx).

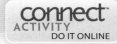

connect ACTIVITY DO IT ONLINE

---

can be impaired at much lower BACs. The combination of fatigue and alcohol use increases the risk even further. Because alcohol affects reason and judgment as well as the ability to make fast, accurate, and coordinated movements, a person who has been drinking will be less likely to recognize that he or she is impaired.

Use of many over-the-counter and all psychoactive drugs is potentially dangerous if you plan to drive.

SAFETY BELTS, AIR BAGS, AND CHILD SAFETY SEATS Although mandatory safety belt laws are in effect in 49 states (excluding New Hampshire) and the District of Columbia, only about 85% of motor vehicle occupants used safety belts in 2010, even though they are the single most effective way to reduce the risk of crash-related death. Combination lap and shoulder belts are even more effective in improving survival rates.

> Air bags are **not a replacement for safety belts;** everyone in a vehicle should buckle up.

Some people think that if they are involved in a crash they are better off being thrown free of their vehicle. In fact, the chances of being killed are 25 times greater if you are thrown from a vehicle, whether it is due to injuries caused by hitting a tree or the pavement or by being hit by another vehicle. Safety belts not only prevent you from being thrown from the car at the time of the crash but also provide protection from second collisions: If a car is traveling at 65 mph and hits another vehicle, the car stops first; then the occupants stop because they, too, are traveling at 65 mph. The second collisions occur when occupants hit something inside the car, such as the dashboard or windshield. The safety belts stop these second collisions from occurring and spreads the first collisions' force over the occupants' bodies.

Since 1998 all new cars and light trucks have been equipped with dual air bags—one for the driver and one for the front passenger. Many vehicles also offer side air bags, which further reduce the risk of injury. Although air bags provide supplementary protection in the event of a collision, most are useful only in head-on collisions. They also deflate immediately after inflating and therefore do not provide protection in collisions involving multiple impacts. Air bags are not a replacement for safety belts; everyone in a vehicle should buckle up.

Air bags deploy forcefully and can injure a child or short adult who is improperly restrained or sitting too close to the dashboard, although second-generation air bags are somewhat safer for children than older devices. To ensure that air bags work safely, always follow these basic guidelines: Place infants in rear-facing infant seats in the back seat, transport children aged 12 and under in the back seat, always use safety belts and appropriate safety seats, and keep 10 inches between the air bag cover and the breastbone of the driver or passenger. If necessary, adjust the steering wheel or use seat cushions to ensure that an inflating air bag will hit a person in the chest and not in the face. Children who have outgrown child safety seats but are still too small for adult safety belts alone (usually age 4–8) should be secured using booster seats that ensure that the safety belt is positioned low across the waist.

Preventing Motor Vehicle Injuries

About 75% of all motor vehicle collisions occur within 25 miles of home and at speeds lower than 40 mph. Strategies for preventing motor vehicle injuries include the following:

- Obey the speed limit.
- Always wear a safety belt.
- Never drive under the influence of alcohol or other drugs, and never ride with a driver who is.
- Keep your car in good working order.
- Always allow enough following distance. Use the three-second rule: When the vehicle ahead passes a reference point, count out three seconds. If you pass the reference point before you finish counting, drop back and allow more following distance. When traveling on highways or in poor weather conditions, allow four seconds.
- Choose interstate highways rather than rural roads. Highways are much safer because of better visibility, wider lanes, fewer surprises, and other factors.
- Always signal when turning or changing lanes.
- Stop completely at stop signs. Follow all traffic laws.
- Take special care at intersections. Look left, right, and then left again. Make sure you have time to complete your maneuver in the intersection.
- Don't pass on two-lane roads unless you're in a designated passing area and have a clear view ahead.

Motorcycles and Motorized Scooters   About one out of every seven traffic fatalities among people aged 15–34

involves someone riding a motorcycle. Injuries from motorcycle collisions are generally more severe than those involving automobiles because motorcycles provide little, if any, protection. People riding motorized scooters face additional challenges. Such vehicles usually have a maximum speed of 30–35 mph and have less power for maneuverability, especially in an emergency.

Strategies for preventing motorcycle and motor scooter injuries include the following:

- Wear light-colored clothing, drive with your headlights on, and correctly position yourself in traffic.
- Develop the necessary skills. Lack of skill is a major factor in motorcycle and motor scooter injuries. Skidding from improper braking is the most common cause of loss of control.
- Wear a helmet. Helmets should be marked with the DOT symbol, certifying that they conform to federal safety standards established by the Department of Transportation. Helmet use is required by law in most states.
- Protect your eyes with goggles, a face shield, or a windshield.
- Drive defensively, particularly when changing lanes and at intersections, and never assume that other drivers can see you.

Bicycles   Bicycle injuries result primarily from riders not knowing or understanding the rules of the road, failing to follow traffic laws, not having sufficient skill or experience to handle traffic conditions, or being intoxicated. Bicycles are considered vehicles; bicyclists must obey all traffic laws that apply to automobile drivers, including stopping at traffic lights and stop signs.

Head injuries are involved in about two-thirds of all bicycle-related deaths. Wearing a helmet reduces the risk of head injury by 85% (see the box "Choosing a Bicycle Helmet"). Safe cycling strategies include the following:

- Wear safety equipment, including a helmet, eye protection, gloves, and proper footwear. Secure the bottom of your pant legs with clips, and secure your shoelaces so they don't get tangled in the chain.
- Wear light-colored, reflective clothing. Equip your bike with reflectors, and use lights, especially at night or when riding in wooded or other dark areas.
- Ride with the flow of traffic, not against it, and follow all traffic laws. Use bike paths when they are available.
- Ride defensively; never assume that drivers have seen you. Be especially careful when turning or crossing at corners and intersections. Watch for cars turning right.
- Stop at all traffic lights and stop signs. Know and use hand signals.

> ### QUICK STATS
> About **54%** of all injuries that require medical attention occur in the home.
> —NSC, 2011

CRITICAL CONSUMER
Choosing a Bicycle Helmet

Wearing a bicycle helmet can help you avoid serious head injury, brain damage, or even death in the event of a collision or fall. Helmets have a layer of stiff foam, which absorbs shock and cushions a blow to your head, covered by a thin plastic shell that will skid along the ground. For maximum protection, it's important to select a correctly fitting helmet. When you go shopping, remember the four S's: size, strap, straight, and sticker.

• *Size:* Try on several different sizes before making your selection; it may take several tries before you find the most comfortable fit. The helmet should be very snug but not overly tight on your head. Pads are usually provided to help adjust the fit. A good salesperson can also help you get the right fit. When the helmet is strapped onto your head, it should not move more than an inch in any direction, and you should not be able to pull or twist it off no matter how hard you try.

• *Strap:* Be sure that the chin strap fits snugly under your chin and that the V in the strap meets under your ear. Avoid thin straps, which can be uncomfortable. Be sure that the buckle is strong and won't pop open and that the straps are sturdy.

• *Straight:* The helmet should sit straight on your head, not tilted back or forward. A rule of thumb is that the rim should be about two finger widths above your eyebrows (depending on the height of your forehead).

• *Sticker:* Helmets sold in the United States must meet uniform safety standards established by the U.S. Consumer Product Safety Commission (CPSC). Look for a sticker or label that says the helmet meets the CPSC standard. If a helmet does not have one, it does not meet federal safety standards and should not be used.

You are more likely to wear your helmet if it is comfortable, so be sure that vents on the helmet provide airflow to promote cooling and sweat control. You will be safer with a brightly colored helmet that makes you more visible to drivers, especially in rainy, foggy, or dark conditions. Reflective tape will also increase your visibility. Finally, a helmet is a good place to put emergency information (your name, address, and phone number, plus any emergency medical conditions and an emergency contact).

If you are involved in a crash, replace your helmet. Even if the helmet doesn't have any visible signs of damage, its ability to protect your head may be compromised.

SOURCES: Bicycle Helmet Safety Institute. 2010. *A Buyer's Guide to Bicycle Helmets* (www.helmets.org/guide.htm); Bicycle Helmet Safety Institute. 2010. *How to Fit a Bicycle Helmet* (www.helmets.org/fit.htm).

Pedestrians   About one in eight motor vehicle deaths involves pedestrians, and more than 60,000 pedestrians are injured each year. About 75% of pedestrian deaths occur when people cross or enter the roadway between intersections. Alcohol intoxication plays a significant role in up to half of all adult pedestrian fatalities. Walkers and joggers should face traffic and cross only at marked crosswalks and intersections.

Home Injuries

The most common fatal **home injuries** are the result of falls, fires, poisoning, suffocation, and unintentional shootings.

> **TERMS**
>
> **home injuries**   Unintentional injuries and deaths that occur in the home and on home premises to occupants, guests, and trespassers; falls, burns, poisonings, suffocations, unintentional shootings, drownings, and electrical shocks are examples.

Falls   Most deaths occurring from falls involve falling on stairs or steps or from one level to another. Falls also occur on the same level, from tripping, slipping, or stumbling. Alcohol is a contributing factor in many falls. Strategies for preventing falls include the following:

• Install handrails and nonslip surfaces in the shower and bathtub.

• Keep floors, stairs, and outside areas clear of objects or conditions that could cause slipping or tripping, such as ice, snow, electrical cords, and toys.

• Put a light switch by the door of every room so no one has to walk across a room to turn on a light. Use night lights in bedrooms, halls, stairs, and bathrooms.

• When climbing a ladder, use both hands. Never stand higher than the third step from the top. When using a stepladder, make sure the spreader brace is in the locked position. With straight ladders, set the base out one foot for every four feet of height. Don't use chairs to reach things.

- If there are small children in the home, place gates at the top and bottom of stairs. Never leave a baby unattended on a bed or table. Install window guards to prevent children from falling out of windows.

Fires Most fires begin in the kitchen, living room, or bedroom. Cooking is the leading cause of home fire injuries; careless smoking is the leading cause of fire deaths, followed by problems with heating equipment and arson. To prevent fires, it's important to dispose of all cigarettes in ashtrays and to never smoke in bed. Other strategies include proper maintenance of fireplaces, furnaces, heaters, chimneys, and electrical outlets, cords, and appliances. If you use a portable heater, keep it at least three feet away from curtains, bedding, or anything else that might catch fire. Never leave heaters on unattended.

It's important to be adequately prepared to handle fire-related situations. Plan at least two escape routes out of each room, and designate a location outside the home as a meeting place. For practice, stage a home fire drill; do this at night because that's when most deadly fires occur.

Install smoke detectors on every level of your home. Your risk of dying in a fire is almost twice as high if you do not use them. Clean the detectors and check the batteries once a month, and replace the batteries at least once a year. These strategies can help prevent injuries in a fire:

- Get out as quickly as possible, and go to the designated meeting place. Don't stop for a keepsake or a pet. Never hide in a closet or under a bed. Once outside, count heads to see if everyone is out. If you think someone is still inside the burning building, tell the firefighters. Never go back inside a burning building.

- If you're trapped in a room, feel the door. If it is hot or if smoke is coming in through the cracks, don't open it; use the alternative escape route. If you can't get out, go to the window and shout for help.

- Smoke inhalation is the primary cause of death and injury in fires. To avoid inhaling smoke, crawl along the floor away from the heat and smoke. Cover your mouth and nose, ideally with a wet cloth, and take short, shallow breaths.

- If your clothes catch fire, don't run. Drop to the ground, cover your face, and roll back and forth to smother the flames. Remember: stop–drop–roll.

Poisoning More than 2.5 million poisonings and over 39,000 poison-related deaths occur every year in the United States. Poisonous substances include cleaning agents, petroleum-based products, insecticides and herbicides, cosmetics, nail polish and remover, and many houseplants. Drug overdoses, whether from prescription drugs, recreational drugs, or combinations of drugs and alcohol, are classified as poisonings. All potentially poisonous substances should be used only as directed and stored out of the reach of children.

The most common type of poisoning by gases is carbon monoxide poisoning. Carbon monoxide gas is emitted by motor vehicle exhaust and some types of heating equipment. The effects of exposure to this colorless, odorless gas include headache, blurred vision, and shortness of breath, followed by dizziness, vomiting, and unconsciousness. Carbon monoxide detectors (similar to smoke detectors) are available for home use. To prevent poisoning by gases, never operate a vehicle in an enclosed space, have your furnace inspected yearly, and use caution with any substance or device that produces potentially toxic fumes.

Keep the national poison control hotline number (800-222-1222) in a convenient location. A call to the national hotline will be routed to a local poison control center, which provides expert emergency advice 24 hours a day. If a poisoning occurs, it's important that you act quickly. Remove the poison from contact with the victim's eyes, skin, or mouth, or move the victim away from contact with poisonous gases. Call the poison control center immediately for instructions; do not follow the emergency instructions on product labels because they may be incorrect. Depending on the situation, you may be instructed to give the victim water to drink, or to flush affected parts of the skin or eyes with water. Do not induce vomiting. If you are advised to go to a hospital emergency department, take the poisonous substance or container with you.

Suffocation and Choking Suffocation and choking account for over 6,000 deaths annually. Children can suffocate if they put small items in their mouth, get tangled in their crib bedding, or get trapped in airtight appliances like old refrigerators. Keep small objects out of reach of children under age 3, and don't give them raw carrots, hot dogs, popcorn, gum, or hard candy. Examine toys carefully for small parts that could come loose. Don't give plastic bags or balloons to small children.

Adults can also become choking victims, especially if they fail to chew food properly, eat hurriedly, or try to talk and eat at the same time. Many choking victims can be saved with the **Heimlich maneuver.** The American Red Cross recommends abdominal thrusts as the easiest and safest thing to do when an adult is choking. Back blows in conjunction with abdominal thrusts are an acceptable procedure for dislodging an object from the throat of an infant.

Firearms Over 40% of all unintended firearm deaths and nonfatal injuries involve children and young adults under 25 years of age. People who use firearms should remember the following:

- Always treat a gun as though it were loaded, even if you know it isn't.

> **Heimlich maneuver** A maneuver developed by Henry J. Heimlich, MD, to help force an obstruction from the airway.
>
> **TERMS**

- Never point a gun—loaded or unloaded—at anything you do not intend to shoot.
- Always unload a gun before storing it. Store unloaded firearms under lock and key, in a place separate from the ammunition.
- Always inspect firearms carefully before handling.
- If you ever plan to handle a gun, take a firearms safety course first.
- If you own a gun, buy and use a gun lock designed specifically for that weapon.

Proper storage is critical. Do not assume that young children cannot fire a gun. Every year about 120 Americans are unintentionally shot to death by children under 6. If you plan to handle a gun, avoid alcohol and drugs, which affect judgment and coordination.

Leisure Injuries

Leisure activities encompass a large part of our free time, so it is not surprising that **leisure injuries** are a significant health-related problem in the United States. Specific safety strategies for activities associated with leisure injuries include the following:

- Don't swim alone, in unsupervised places, under the influence of alcohol, or for an unusual length of time. Use caution when swimming in unfamiliar surroundings or in water colder than 70°F. Check the depth of water before diving. Make sure that residential pools are fenced and that children are never allowed to swim unsupervised.
- Always use a **personal flotation device** (also known as a life jacket) when on a boat.
- For all sports and recreational activities, make sure facilities are safe, follow the rules, and practice good sportsmanship. Develop adequate skill in the activity, and use proper safety equipment, including, where appropriate, a helmet, eye protection, correct footwear, and knee, elbow, and wrist pads.
- If using equipment such as skateboards, snowboards, mountain bikes, or all-terrain vehicles, wear a helmet and other safety equipment, and avoid excessive speeds and unsafe stunts. Playground equipment should be used only for those activities for which it is designed.
- Do not use alcohol or other drugs during recreational activities—such activities require coordination and sound judgment.

Weather-Related Injuries   Even though conditions may seem harmless at times, they can become very dangerous.

- *Heat:* Extreme heat is the leading weather-related killer in the United States, according to the National Weather Service. Heat-related illness such as heat stroke and heat exhaustion can be fatal, especially for children, older adults, and people with certain health conditions. Danger signals of heat stress include excessive perspiration, dizziness, headache, muscle cramps, nausea, weakness, rapid pulse, and disorientation. The best way to deal with excessive heat is to stay indoors as much as possible, with a fan or air conditioner on. Wear lightweight, light-colored clothing, drink plenty of water to stay hydrated, and avoid heavy meals.

- *Cold:* Conditions such as hypothermia (low body temperature) and frostbite (frozen skin or flesh) can be deadly. If you must go outdoors in very cold weather, dress in layers and cover your face, fingers, and ears to protect them from frostbite. Make sure your home and car are prepared with plenty of fuel, drinking water, warm clothes and blankets, batteries, and other emergency supplies.

- *Wind:* In extremely windy conditions, take cover in a sturdy shelter, preferably a permanent structure with a foundation. In a severe storm such as a tornado, move to the lowest portion of the building or to a small interior room away from windows. If you're outdoors when a severe storm or tornado strikes, lie flat in a low spot or ditch. Don't stay inside a car or hide under an open-sided structure such as a bridge; such structures can act as a funnel and make wind more intense.

- *Lightning:* About 300 Americans are struck by lightning every year, and about 10% of them die. When conditions are right for lightning, go indoors. Stay out of water, even indoors, because water pipes can conduct electricity. Don't use corded telephones or appliances because their wiring can also conduct the power from a lightning strike.

- *Flooding:* If you're near rapidly rising water, move to higher ground and call for help. Don't attempt to drive or walk through flooded streets, and don't traverse a bridge if it is being pounded by high, fast-moving water.

Work Injuries

According to the Bureau of Labor Statistics, 5.1 million Americans suffered injuries on the job in 2010. Certain types of **work injuries,** including skin disorders and repetitive

> Laborers constitute less than half of the American workforce but **suffer 75% of all work-related injuries**.

TERMS

leisure injuries   Unintentional injuries and deaths that occur in public places or places used in a public way, not involving motor vehicles; include most sports and recreation deaths and injuries; drownings, burns, and heat and cold stress are examples.

personal flotation device   A device designed to save a person from drowning by buoying up the body while in the water.

work injuries   Unintentional injuries and deaths that arise out of and in the course of gainful work, such as falls, electrical shocks, exposure to radiation and toxic chemicals, burns, cuts, back sprains, and loss of fingers or other body parts in machines.

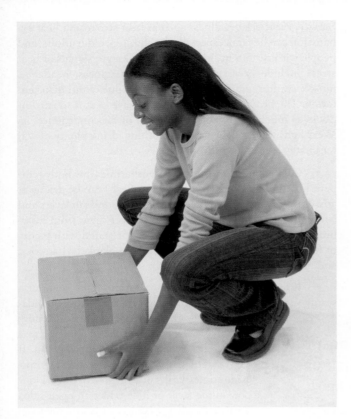

FIGURE 16.1 Correct lifting technique. Stay upright, bending at the knees and hips.

strain injuries, are increasing. Although laborers make up less than half of the workforce, they account for more than 75% of all work-related injuries and illnesses. Most fatal occupational injuries involve crushing injuries, severe lacerations, burns, and electrocutions; among women, the leading cause of workplace injury deaths is homicide.

Back problems accounted for over 450,000 work injuries in 2009; many of these could be prevented through proper lifting technique (Figure 16.1).

- Avoid bending at the waist. Remain in an upright position and crouch down if you need to lower yourself to grasp the object. Bend at the knees and hips.

- Place feet securely about shoulder-width apart; grip the object firmly.

- Lift gradually, with straight arms. Avoid quick, jerky motions. Lift by standing up or pushing with your leg muscles. Keep the object close to your body.

- If you have to turn, change the position of your feet. Twisting is a common and dangerous cause of injury. Plan ahead so that your pathway is clear and turning can be minimized.

- Put the object down gently, reversing the steps for lifting.

Musculoskeletal injuries and disorders in the workplace include **repetitive strain injuries (RSIs).** RSIs are caused by repeated strain on a particular part of the body. Twisting, vibrations, awkward postures, and other stressors may contribute to RSIs. **Carpal tunnel syndrome** is one type of RSI that has increased in recent years due to increased use of computers, both at work and in the home (see the box "Repetitive Strain Injury" for more information).

VIOLENCE AND INTENTIONAL INJURIES

Violence—the use of physical force with the intent to inflict harm, injury, or death upon oneself or another—is a major public health concern in the United States. According to the Federal Bureau of Investigation (FBI), over 1.3 million violent crimes occurred in the United States in 2009. Examples of violence are assault, homicide, sexual assault, domestic violence, suicide, and child abuse. In comparison to other industrialized countries, U.S. rates of violence are unusually high in only two areas—homicide and firearm-related deaths.

Factors Contributing to Violence

Most intentional injuries and deaths are associated with an argument or the committing of another crime. However, there are many forms of violence, and no single factor can explain all of them.

Social Factors Rates of violence vary by geographic region, neighborhood, socioeconomic level, and many other factors. According to the FBI, violence was highest in the South in 2009, followed by the West. Neighborhoods that are disadvantaged in status, power, and economic resources are typically the ones with the most violence. Rates of violence

repetitive strain injury (RSI) A musculoskeletal injury or disorder caused by repeated strain on the hand, arm, wrist, or other part of the body; also called *cumulative trauma disorder (CTD)*. **TERMS**

carpal tunnel syndrome Compression of the median nerve in the wrist, often caused by repetitive use of the hands, such as in computer use; characterized by numbness, tingling, and pain in the hands and fingers; can cause nerve damage.

Repetitive strain injuries (RSIs) impact the musculoskeletal and nervous systems of the body. Other terms to describe this condition include *repetitive motion disorder (RMD)*, *cumulative trauma disorder (CTD)*, and *occupational overuse syndrome (OOS)*.

An RSI can be caused by a combination of physical and psychosocial stressors, but the injury typically involves some kind of repetitive action or forceful exertion on the body over time. Pain in the extremities as well as the back and shoulders is commonly cited and tends to worsen with extended activity.

The task associated with an RSI may be something relatively simple and nonexertive like typing, writing, or clicking a computer mouse. One of the most common work-related injuries is *carpal tunnel syndrome (CTS)*, which is characterized by pressure on the median nerve in the wrist that also affects tendons and ligaments in the forearm. Symptoms of CTS include numbness, tingling, burning, and/or aching in the hand, particularly in the thumb and the first three fingers. The pain may worsen at night and may shoot up from the hand as far as the shoulder. If it does not clear up on its own, immobilization of the joint at night can be helpful; other options may involve anti-inflammatory drugs or even surgery in extreme cases.

There are complex and more physically destructive examples of an RSI. If a person is operating a jackhammer, the vibration of the equipment and the position in which it must be operated are contributory factors often recognized for that RSI. In terms of physical activity by an athlete, examples include conditions commonly referred to as "golfer's elbow" or "tennis elbow," where the joints are continually exposed to extreme stress in order to complete an action accurately with speed and force. Many people who use their thumbs to text are suffering from a condition referred to as "Blackberry thumb." Similarly, people who spend countless hours using handheld controls to play video games are experiencing "gamer's thumb."

In all cases, research indicates the primary risk factors are usually associated with poor posture, improper techniques for completing a activity, and overusing a certain part of the body. The good news is that a person can make adjustments to reduce the risk of an RSI, either in terms of what is being done or through modification of the environment. Warm up your wrists before you begin any repetitive motion activity, and take frequent breaks to stretch and flex your wrists and hands:

- Extend your arms out in front of you and stretch your wrists by pointing your fingers to the ceiling; hold for a count of five. Then straighten your wrists and relax your fingers for a count of five.

- With arms extended, make a tight fist with both hands and then bend your wrists so your knuckles are pointed toward the floor; hold for a count of five. Then straighten your wrists and relax your fingers for a count of five.

Repeat these stretches several times, and finish by letting your arms hang loosely at your sides and shaking them gently for several seconds. It's also important to maintain a physically active lifestyle, take plenty of breaks to avoid hours of sedentary activity, continue stretching during an activity, apply proper ergonomic principles, and try to minimize other stress factors.

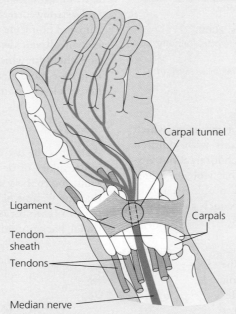

Carpal tunnel

Ligament

Tendon sheath

Tendons

Median nerve

Carpals

---

are highest among young people and minorities, groups that have relatively little power. In 2009 people under age 25 accounted for 44% of the arrests for violent crime in the United States and 56% of the arrests for property crime.

People who feel a part of society (have strong family and social ties), who are economically integrated (have a reasonable chance at getting a decent job), and who grow up in areas where there is a feeling of community (good schools, parks, and neighborhoods) are significantly less likely to engage in violence.

Studies have shown that the environment on college campuses can contribute to violence. The nature of college campuses—transitory communities rather than permanent places where people work and live together over the long term—means that there is less incentive for people to cooperate and coexist amicably.

Violence in the Media The mass media play a major role in exposing audiences of all ages to violence as an acceptable and effective means of solving problems. On the average, children in the United States watch about four hours of television daily and may view as many as 10,000 violent acts on television and in movies each year. Computer and video games also include many violent acts, leading to concern that children's exposure to violence will make them more accepting or tolerant of it. The consequences of violence are depicted much less frequently.

Researchers have found that exposure to media violence at least temporarily increases aggressive feelings in children, making them more likely to engage in violent or fearful behavior; the direct, short-term effects on teens and adults are less clear. Parents should monitor the TV shows, movies,

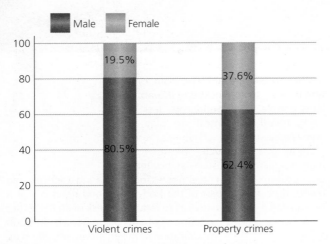

FIGURE 16.2   Arrests in the United States, 2009.
Males were arrested significantly more often than females for both violent and property crimes.

SOURCE: Federal Bureau of Investigation. 2011. *Crime in the United States 2010.* Washington, DC: U.S. Department of Justice.

video games, music, and other forms of media to which children are exposed. Watching programs with children gives parents the opportunity to talk to children about violence and its consequences, to explain that violence is not the best way to resolve conflicts or solve problems, and to point out examples of positive behaviors such as kindness and cooperation.

Gender   In most cases, violence is committed by men (Figure 16.2). Males are nine times more likely than females to commit murder, and four times more likely than females to be murdered. Male college students are twice as likely to be the victim of violence as female students. Women do commit acts of violence, including a small but substantial proportion of murders of spouses. This fact has been used to argue that women have the same capacity to commit violence as men, but most researchers note substantial differences. Men often kill their wives as the culmination of years of violence or after stalking them; they may kill their entire families and themselves at the same time. Women virtually never kill in such circumstances; rather, they kill their husbands after repeated victimization or while being beaten.

Interpersonal Factors   Although most people fear attack from strangers, the majority of victims are acquainted with their attacker. More than half of murders of women and three-fourths of sexual assaults are committed by someone the woman knows. Crime victims and violent criminals tend to share many characteristics—that is, they are likely to be young, male, in a minority, and poor.

Alcohol and Other Drugs   Substance abuse and dependence are consistently associated with interpersonal violence

and suicide. Intoxication affects judgment and may increase aggression in some people, causing a small argument to escalate into a serious physical confrontation. On college campuses, alcohol is involved in about 95% of all violent crimes.

Firearms   Many criminologists feel that the high rate of homicide in the United States is directly related to the fact that we are the only industrialized country in which handguns are widespread and easily available. The use of a handgun can change a suicide attempt to a completed suicide and a violent assault to a murder.

Over 100,000 deaths and injuries occur in the United States each year as a result of the use of firearms. Firearms are used in more than two-thirds of homicides, and studies reveal a strong correlation between the incidence of gun ownership and homicide rates for a given area of the country. Over half of all suicides involve a firearm, and people living in households in which guns are kept have a risk of suicide that is five or more times greater than that of people living in households without guns.

Assault

Assault is the use of physical force by a person or people to inflict injury or death on another; homicide, aggravated assault, and robbery are examples of assault. Research indicates that the victims of assaultive injuries and their perpetrators tend to resemble one another in terms of ethnicity, educational background, psychological profile, and reliance on weapons. In many cases, the victim actually magnifies the confrontation through the use of a weapon.

Homicide

The FBI estimates that more than 15,000 Americans were murdered in 2009. Men, teenagers, young adults, and members of minority groups, particularly African Americans and Latinos, are most likely to be murder victims. The murder rate for black males is several times higher than the rate for the U.S. population as a whole. Poverty and unemployment have been identified as key factors in homicide, and this may account for the high rates of homicide among minority groups.

Most homicides are committed with a firearm, occur during an argument, and occur among people who know one another. Intrafamilial homicide, where the perpetrator and victim are related, accounts for about one out of every eight homicides. About 40% of family homicides are committed by spouses, usually following a history of physical and emotional abuse directed at the woman.

Gang-Related Violence

Gangs are most frequently associated with large cities, but gang activity also extends to the suburbs and even to rural

> **QUICK STATS**
>
> In 2009, **21%** of aggravated assaults involved the use of a firearm.
> —FBI, 2010

areas. It is estimated that more than 1 million Americans belong to gangs; the average age for joining a gang is 14. Gang members are more likely than non–gang members to possess weapons, and violence may result from conflicts over territory or illegal activities. Gangs are more common in areas that are poor and suffer from high unemployment, population density, and crime. In these areas, a young person may feel that his or her hope of legitimate success in life is out of reach and knows that involvement in the drug market makes some gang members rich. Often gangs serve as a mechanism for companionship, self-esteem, support, and security. Indeed, in some areas gang membership may be viewed as the only possible means of survival.

Hate Crimes

When bias against another person's race or ethnicity, national origin, religion, sexual orientation, or disability motivates a criminal act, the offense is classified as a hate crime. Hate crimes may be committed against people or property. Those against people may include intimidation, assault, and even rape or murder. Crimes against property most frequently involve graffiti, the desecration of churches or synagogues, cross burnings, and other acts of vandalism or property damage.

Nearly 8,200 hate crimes were reported in 2009; many more go unreported. Crimes against people made up about 60% of all incidents; intimidation and assault are the most common offenses. Racial or ethnic bias was cited as a motivation in 54% of the hate crimes reported in 2009. National origin or ethnicity was cited in 11% of cases, religion in 18%, and sexual orientation in 16%.

Research indicates that a substantial number of hate crimes are committed by males under age 20. Hate crimes are frequently, but not always, associated with fringe groups that have extremist ideologies, such as the Ku Klux Klan and neo-Nazi groups. The rapid growth of hate sites on the Internet is another area of concern.

School Violence

According to the National School Safety Center, about 300 school-associated violent deaths of students, faculty, and administrators occurred in the last decade. Most of these deaths occurred in urban areas, at high schools, and involved use of a firearm. As with other types of violence, both victims and offenders were predominantly young men. Homicide and suicide are the most serious but least common types of violence in schools; an estimated 400,000 less serious incidents of violence and crime occur each year, including theft, vandalism, and fights not involving weapons.

Children are actually much safer at school than away from it. Fewer than 1% of all homicides among youths aged 5–19 occur at school, and 90% of schools report no incidents of serious violence. Children and adolescents are far more likely to be killed by an adult in their own homes or away from

school than they are to die as a result of school-associated violence. According to the National Institute of Justice (NIJ), the overall number of violent incidents has decreased steadily over the past two decades; however, the number of multiple-victim events may have increased.

Although schools are basically safe places overall, there are steps that can be taken to identify at-risk youths and improve safety for all students. Characteristics associated with youths who have caused school-associated violent deaths include uncontrollable angry outbursts, violent and abusive language and behavior, isolation from peers, depression and irritability, access to and preoccupation with weapons, and lack of support and supervision from adults. Being a victim of teasing, bullying, or social exclusion (rejection) may lead to aggressive behavior and violence.

Recommendations for reducing school violence include offering classroom training in anger management, social skills, and improved self-control; providing mental health and social services for students in need; developing after-school programs that help students build self-esteem and make friends; and keeping guns out of the hands of children and out of schools.

Workplace Violence

Each year U.S. workers experience an average of 1.5 million minor assaults, 400,000 serious assaults, 85,000 robberies, 50,000 sexual assaults, and 700 homicides. Most of the perpetrators of workplace violence are white males over age 21. Firearms are used in nearly 80% of workplace homicides, and the majority of these homicides occur during the commission of a robbery or other crime. Police and corrections officers have the most dangerous jobs, followed by taxi drivers, security guards, bartenders, mental health professionals, and workers at gas stations and convenience and liquor stores.

General crime prevention strategies, including use of surveillance cameras and silent alarms and limiting the amount of cash on hand, can help reduce workplace violence related to robberies. A highly stressed workplace is a risk factor in cases of violence between acquaintances or coworkers; clear guidelines about acceptable behavior and prompt action after any threats or incidents of violence can help control this type of workplace violence.

> Being a victim of teasing, bullying, or rejection may lead to **aggressive behavior or violence.**

Terrorism

In 2001 more Americans died as a result of terrorism than in any year before or since; the attacks on September 11 killed more than 3000 people, including citizens of 78 countries. The FBI defines *terrorism* as the unlawful use of force or violence against people or property to intimidate or coerce a government, the civilian population, or any segment thereof in furtherance of political or social objectives. Terrorism can be either domestic, carried out by groups based in the United

States, or international. It comes in many forms, including biological, chemical, nuclear, and cyber. Its intent is to promote helplessness by instilling fear of harm or destruction.

Terrorism prevention activities occur at all levels of government. U.S. government efforts include close work with the diplomatic, law enforcement, intelligence, economic, and military communities. The mission of the Department of Homeland Security is to help prevent, protect against, and respond to acts of terrorism on U.S. territory. It coordinates efforts to protect electric and water supply systems, transportation, gas and oil, emergency services, the computer infrastructure, and other systems.

Individuals have a role in preventing terrorism by making sure they are prepared in case of a terrorist attack or a disaster. They can also be proactive by reporting anything they see or hear that is suspicious or threatening. The best approach is taking personal responsibility and not letting the fear of terrorism immobilize or impede your ability to act.

Family and Intimate Violence

Family violence generally refers to any rough and illegitimate use of physical force, aggression, or verbal abuse by one family member toward another. Such abuse may be physical and/or psychological in nature. Based on reported cases, an estimated 6–8 million women and children are abused each year in the United States.

Battering   Studies reveal that over 85% of domestic violence victims are women. Violence against wives or intimate partners, or battering, occurs at every level of society but is more common at lower socioeconomic levels. It occurs more frequently in relationships with a high degree of conflict—an apparent inability to resolve arguments through negotiation and compromise. Over 25% of women report having been physically assaulted or raped by an intimate partner, and more than 50% report having experienced some type of abuse—physical or psychological—in a relationship. In more than 10% of cases, the domestic violence continues for 20 years or longer. The problem of intimate violence is even apparent among young people; each year, 1.7 million high school students are victims of physical violence while on a date, according to the CDC.

At the root of much of this abusive behavior is the need to control another person. Abusive partners are controlling partners. They not only want to have power over another person, but also believe they are entitled to it, no matter what the cost to the other person (see the box "Recognizing the Potential for Abusiveness in a Partner").

In abusive relationships, the abuser (in most cases a man) usually has a history of violent behavior, traditional beliefs about gender roles, and problems with alcohol abuse. He has low self-esteem and seeks to raise it by dominating and imposing his will on another person. Research has revealed a three-phase cycle of battering, consisting of a period of increasing tension, a violent explosion and loss of control, and a period of contriteness in which the man begs forgiveness and promises it will never happen again. The batterer is drawn back to this cycle over and over again, but he never succeeds in changing his feelings about himself.

Battered women often stay in violent relationships for years. They may be economically dependent on their partners, feel trapped or fear retaliation if they leave, believe their children need a father, or have low self-esteem themselves. They may love or pity their husband, or they may believe they'll eventually be able to stop the violence. They usually leave the relationship only when they become determined that the violence must end. Battered women's shelters offer physical protection, counseling, support, and other assistance.

Stalking and Cyberstalking   Battering is closely associated with **stalking,** characterized by harassing behaviors such as following or spying on a person and making verbal, written, or implied threats. In the United States it is estimated that 2.5 million women and 900,000 men are stalked each year; about two-thirds of stalkers are men. About one-third of female victims are stalked by current or former intimate partners; of these, 80% had been physically or sexually assaulted by that partner during the relationship. Stalking of female college students may be greater than that experienced by the general population. A stalker's goal may be to control or scare the victim or to keep her or him in a relationship. Most stalking episodes last a year or less.

The use of the Internet, e-mail, chat rooms, social media, and other electronic means to stalk another person is known as **cyberstalking.** As with offline stalking, the majority of cyberstalkers are men, and the majority of victims are women, although there have been same-sex cyberstalking incidents. Cyberstalkers may send harassing or threatening messages to the victim, or they may encourage others to harass the victim—for example, by impersonating the victim and posting inflammatory messages and personal information on bulletin boards or in chat rooms. Guidelines for staying safe online include the following:

- Avoid using your real name on the Internet. Select an age- and gender-neutral identity.

- Avoid filling out profiles for accounts with information that could be used to identify you.

- Do not share personal information in public spaces anywhere online or give it to strangers.

- Learn how to filter unwanted e-mail messages.

---

stalking   Repeatedly harassing or threatening a person through behaviors such as following a person, appearing at a person's residence or workplace, leaving written messages or objects, making harassing phone calls, or vandalizing property; frequently directed at a former intimate partner.   **TERMS**

cyberstalking   The use of e-mail, chat rooms, bulletin boards, or other electronic communication devices to stalk another person.

Recognizing the Potential for Abusiveness in a Partner

There are no sure ways to tell whether someone will become abusive or violent toward an intimate partner, but there are warning signs that you can look for. (Remember that, although most abusive relationships involve male violence directed at a woman, women can also be abusive, as can partners in a same-sex relationship. Because most abusers are male, the following material refers to the abuser as "he.") If you are concerned that a person you are involved with has the potential for violence, observe his or her behavior, and ask yourself these questions:

• What is this person's attitude toward women? How does he treat his mother and his sister? How does he work with female students, female colleagues, or a female boss? How does he treat your women friends?

• What is his attitude toward your autonomy? Does he respect the work you do and the way you do it? Or does he tell you how to do it better or encourage you to give it up?

• How self-centered is he? Does he want to spend all his leisure time on his interests?

• Is he possessive or jealous? Does he want to spend every minute with you? Does he cross-examine you about things you do when you're not with him?

• What happens when things don't go the way he wants them to? Does he always have to get his way?

• Is he moody, mocking, critical, or bossy? Do you feel as if you're walking on eggshells when you're with him?

• Do you feel you have to avoid arguing with him?

• Does he drink too much or use drugs?

• Does he refuse to use condoms or take other precautions for safer sex?

Listen to your own uneasiness, and stay away from any man who disrespects women, who wants or needs you intensely and exclusively, and who has a knack for getting his own way almost all the time.

If you are in a serious relationship with a controlling person, you may already have experienced abuse. Consider the following questions:

• Does your partner constantly criticize you, blame you for things that are not your fault, or verbally degrade you?

• Does he humiliate you in front of others?

• Is he suspicious or jealous? Does he accuse you of being unfaithful or monitor your mail or phone calls?

• Does he track all your time? Does he discourage you from seeing friends and family?

• Does he prevent you from getting or keeping a job or attending school? Does he control your shared resources or restrict your access to money?

• Has he ever pushed, pulled, slapped, hit, kicked, or restrained you? Thrown an object at you? Used a weapon on you?

• Has he ever destroyed or damaged your personal property or sentimental items, or threatened to do so?

• Has he ever forced you to have sex or to do something sexually you didn't want to do?

• Does he anger easily when drinking or taking drugs?

• Has he ever threatened to harm you or your children, friends, pets, or property?

• Has he ever threatened to blackmail you if you leave?

If you answered yes to one or more of these questions, you may be experiencing domestic abuse. If you believe you or your children are in imminent danger, look in your local telephone directory for a women's shelter, or call 911. If you want information, referrals to a program in your area, or assistance, contact one of the organizations listed in "For More Information" at the end of the chapter.

• Always use passwords that are unique and contain many characters—preferably an alphanumeric combination to make it more difficult for someone to hack into your account.

• If you use a social networking site, it is best to set your profile to "private" if that is an option.

• If you experience harassment online, do not respond to the harasser. Log off or go to a different site. If harassment continues, contact the harasser's Internet service provider (ISP) by identifying the domain of the stalker's account (after the "@" sign); most ISPs have an e-mail address for complaints. Often an ISP can try to stop the conduct by direct contact with the harasser or by

closing his or her account. Save all communications for evidence, and contact your ISP and your local police department. Many states have laws against cyberstalking.

Violence against Children   In 2009 there were 3.3 million reports of alleged child abuse and neglect in the United States, with the number of children involved being near 6 million. Nearly 1 million of the cases involved physical abuse, and over 4.5 million were a result of neglect. Parents who abuse children tend to have low self-esteem, to believe in physical punishment, to have a poor marital relationship, and to have been abused themselves (although many people who were abused as children do not grow up to abuse their own children). Poverty, unemployment, and social isolation are

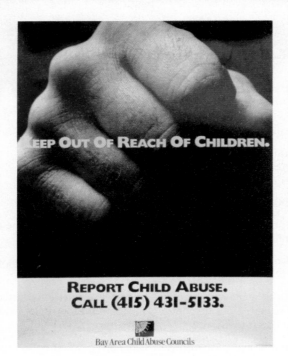

KEEP OUT OF REACH OF CHILDREN.

REPORT CHILD ABUSE.
CALL (415) 431-5133.

Bay Area Child Abuse Councils

Education, counseling, and support can help the victims of family violence.

characteristics of families in which children are abused. External stressors related to socioeconomic and environmental factors are most closely associated with neglect, whereas stressors related to interpersonal issues are more closely associated with physical abuse. Single parents, both men and women, are at especially high risk for abusing their children.

Elder Abuse   Each year over 2 million older adults are abused, exploited, or mistreated by someone who is supposed to be giving them care and protection; only one in six incidents is reported. Most abusers are family members who are serving as caregivers. Elder abuse can take different forms: physical, sexual, or emotional abuse; financial exploitation; neglect; or abandonment. Neglect accounts for about 59% of reported cases. Physical abuse accounts for about 16% of reported cases, and financial exploitation for about 12%. Abuse often occurs when caring for a dependent adult becomes too stressful for the caregiver. Many believe that the solution to elder abuse is support in the form of greater social and financial assistance, such as adult day care centers and education and public care programs.

Sexual Violence

The use of force and coercion in sexual relationships is one of the most serious problems in human interactions. The most extreme manifestation of sexual coercion—forcing a person to submit to another's sexual desires—is rape, but sexual coercion occurs in many subtler forms, including sexual harassment.

Sexual Assault: Rape   Sexual coercion that relies on the threat and use of physical force or takes advantage of circumstances that render a person incapable of giving consent (such as being drunk) constitutes **sexual assault** or **rape.** When the victim is younger than the legally defined age of consent, the act constitutes **statutory rape,** whether or not coercion is involved. Coerced sexual activity in which the victim knows or is dating the rapist is often referred to as **date rape,** or *acquaintance rape.* Most victims know their assailants, but fewer than 40% of all sexual crimes are reported.

Any woman—or man—can be a rape victim. Over 200,000 cases of rape are reported each year. It is estimated that at least 500,000 more women are raped each year. Research shows that 1 in 6 women and 1 in 33 men has experienced an attempted or completed rape at some point in their lives. A study of college students also found that between 1 in 4 and 1 in 5 college women experience a completed or attempted rape during their college years. Most male-on-male rapes do not occur in prison.

WHO COMMITS RAPE?   Men who commit rape may be any age and come from any socioeconomic group. Some rapists are exploiters in the sense that they rape on the spur of the moment and mainly want immediate gratification. Some attempt to compensate for feelings of sexual inadequacy and an inability to obtain satisfaction otherwise. Others are more hostile and sadistic and are primarily interested in hurting and humiliating a particular woman or women in general. Often the rapist is more interested in dominance, control, and power than in sexual satisfaction.

Most women are in much less danger of being raped by a stranger than of being sexually assaulted by a man they know or date. Surveys suggest that as many as 25% of women have had experiences in which the men they were dating persisted in trying to force sex despite pleading, crying, screaming, or resisting. Surveys have also found that more than 60% of all rape victims were raped by a current or former spouse, boyfriend, or date.

Most cases of date rape are never reported to the police. Usually no weapons are involved, and direct verbal threats may not have been made. Victims of date rape tend to shoulder much of the responsibility for the incident, questioning

> **QUICK STATS**
>
> Only **6%** of rapists ever spend a day in jail for their offenses.
>
> —Rape, Abuse, & Incest National Network, 2010

> **TERMS**
>
> **sexual assault** or **rape**   The use of force to have sex with someone against that person's will.
>
> **statutory rape**   Sexual interaction with someone under the legal age of consent.
>
> **date rape**   Sexual assault by someone the victim knows or is dating; also called *acquaintance rape.*

Guidelines for Women

• Believe in your right to control what you do. Set limits, and communicate these limits clearly, firmly, and early. Say no when you mean no.

• Be assertive with someone who is sexually pressuring you. Men often interpret passivity as permission.

• If you are unsure of a new acquaintance, go on a group date or double date. If possible, provide your own transportation.

• Remember that some men assume sexy dress and a flirtatious manner mean a desire for sex.

• Remember that alcohol and drugs interfere with clear communication about sex.

• Use the statement that has proven most effective in stopping date rape: "This is rape, and I'm calling the police."

Guidelines for Men

• Be aware of social pressure. It's OK to not score.

• Understand that no means no. Don't continue making advances when your date resists or tells you she wants to stop. Remember that she has the right to refuse sex.

• Don't assume sexy dress and a flirtatious manner are invitations to sex, that previous permission for sex applies to the current situation, or that your date's relationships with other men constitute sexual permission for you.

• Remember that alcohol and drugs interfere with clear communication about sex.

their own judgment and behavior rather than blaming the aggressor.

FACTORS CONTRIBUTING TO DATE RAPE Men and women tend to differ in their perception of romantic encounters and signals. In one study, researchers found that men interpreted women's actions on dates, such as smiling or talking in a low voice, as indicating an interest in having sex, whereas the women interpreted the same actions as just being friendly. Men's thinking about forceful sex also tends to be unclear. One psychologist reports that men find "forcing a woman to have sex against her will" more acceptable than "raping a woman," even though the former description is the definition of rape.

DATE-RAPE DRUGS The drugs used in date rapes include flunitrazepam (Rohypnol), gamma hydroxybutyrate (GHB), and ketamine ("Special K"). These drugs have a variety of effects, including sedation; if slipped surreptitiously into a drink, they can incapacitate a person within about 20 minutes and make her or him more vulnerable to assault. Rohypnol, GHB, and other drugs also often cause anterograde amnesia, meaning victims have little memory of what happened while they were under the influence of the drug. The Drug-Induced Rape Prevention and Punishment Act of 1996 adds up to 20 years to the prison sentence of any rapist who uses a drug to incapacitate a victim. Strategies such as the following can help ensure that your drink is not tampered with at a bar or party:

• Drink moderately and responsibly. Avoid group drinking and drinking games.

> Most rape victims are **assaulted by someone they know,** not by a stranger.

• Be wary of opened beverages—alcoholic or nonalcoholic— offered by strangers. When at an unfamiliar bar, watch the bartender pour your drink.

• If an opened beverage tastes, looks, or smells strange, do not drink it. If you leave your drink unattended, get a fresh drink when you return to your table.

• If you go to a party, club, or bar, go with friends and leave with them. Have a prearranged plan for checking on each other. If you feel giddy or light-headed, get assistance.

Both males and females can take actions that will reduce the incidence of acquaintance rape; see the box "Preventing Date Rape" for specific suggestions.

DEALING WITH A SEXUAL ASSAULT Each situation is unique, and a woman should respond in whatever way she thinks best. If a woman chooses not to resist, it does not mean that she has not been raped. If you are threatened by a rapist and decide to fight back, here is what Women Organized Against Rape (WOAR) recommends:

• Trust your gut feeling. If you feel you are in danger, don't hesitate to run and scream. It is better to feel foolish than to be raped.

• Yell—and keep yelling. It will clear your head and start your adrenaline going; it may scare your attacker and also bring help.

• If an attacker grabs you from behind, use your elbows for striking his neck, his sides, or his stomach.

• Try kicking. Your legs are the strongest part of your body, and your kick is longer than his reach. Kick with your rear foot and with the toe of your shoe. Aim low to avoid losing your balance.

- His most vulnerable spot is his knee; it's low, difficult to protect, and easily knocked out of place. Don't try to kick a rapist in the crotch; he has been protecting this area all his life and will have better protective reflexes there than at his knees.

- Once you start fighting, keep it up. Your objective is to get away as soon as you can.

- Remember that ordinary rules of behavior don't apply. It's OK to vomit, act crazy, or claim to have a sexually transmitted disease.

If you are raped, tell what happened to the first friendly person you meet. Call the police, tell them you were raped, and give your location. Try to remember as many facts as you can about your attacker; write down a description as soon as possible. Don't wash or change your clothes, or you may destroy important evidence. The police will take you to a hospital for a complete exam; show the physician any injuries. Tell the police simply, but exactly, what happened. If you decide that you don't want to report the rape to the police, see a physician as soon as possible to be checked for pregnancy and STDs.

THE EFFECTS OF RAPE Rape victims suffer both physical and psychological injury. For most, physical wounds heal within a few weeks. Psychological pain may endure and be substantial. Even the most physically and mentally strong are likely to experience shock, anxiety, depression, shame, and a host of psychosomatic symptoms after being victimized. Some victims experience rape trauma syndrome, a form of PTSD, characterized by fear, nightmares, fatigue, crying spells, and digestive upset. Self-blame is very likely; society has contributed to this tendency by perpetuating the myths that women can actually defend themselves and that no one can be raped if she doesn't want to be. Fortunately these false beliefs are dissolving in the face of evidence to the contrary.

Many organizations offer counseling and support to rape victims. Look online or in the telephone directory under Rape or Rape Crisis Center for a hotline number to call. Your campus may have counseling services or a support group.

Child Sexual Abuse Child sexual abuse is any sexual contact between an adult and a child who is below the legal age of consent. Adults and older adolescents are able to coerce children into sexual activity because of their authority and power over them. Threats, force, or the promise of friendship or material rewards may be used to manipulate a child. Sexual contacts are typically brief and consist of genital manipulation; genital intercourse is much less common.

Sexual abusers are usually male, heterosexual, and known to the victim. The abuser may be a relative, a friend, a neighbor, or another trusted adult acquaintance. Child abusers are often pedophiles, people who are sexually attracted to children. They may have poor interpersonal and sexual relationships with other adults and feel socially inadequate and inferior. One highly traumatic form of sexual abuse is **incest:** sexual activity between people too closely related to legally marry.

Child sexual abuse is often unreported. Surveys suggest that as many as 27% of women and 16% of men were sexually abused as children. An estimated 150,000–200,000 new cases of child sexual abuse occur each year. It can leave lasting scars; victims are more likely to suffer as adults from low self-esteem, depression, anxiety, eating disorders, self-destructive tendencies, sexual problems, and difficulties in intimate relationships.

If you were a victim of sexual abuse as a child and feel it may be interfering with your functioning today, you may want to address the problem. A variety of approaches can help, such as joining a support group of people who have had similar experiences, confiding in a partner or friend, or seeking professional help.

Sexual Harassment Unwelcome sexual advances, requests for sexual favors, and other verbal, visual, or physical conduct of a sexual nature constitute **sexual harassment** if such conduct explicitly or implicitly affects academic or employment decisions or evaluations; interferes with an individual's academic or work performance; or creates an intimidating, hostile, or offensive academic, work, or student living environment.

Extreme cases of sexual harassment occur when a manager, professor, or other person in authority uses his or her ability to control or influence jobs or grades to coerce people into having sex or to punish them if they refuse. A hostile environment can be created by conduct such as sexual gestures, displaying of sexually suggestive objects or pictures, derogatory comments and jokes, sexual remarks about clothing or appearance, obscene letters, and unnecessary touching.

If you have been the victim of sexual harassment, you can take action to stop it. Be assertive with anyone who uses language or actions you find inappropriate. If possible, confront your harasser and tell him or her that the situation is unacceptable to you and you want the harassment to stop. If assertive

> **QUICK STATS**
>
> About **12,000** sexual harassment charges are filed with the EEOC each year.
>
> —U.S. Equal Employment Opportunity Commission, 2010

> **TERMS**
>
> **incest**   Sexual activity between close relatives, such as siblings or parents and their children.
>
> **sexual harassment**   Unwelcome sexual advances, requests for sexual favors, and other conduct of a sexual nature that affects academic or employment decisions or evaluations; interferes with an individual's academic or work performance; or creates an intimidating, hostile, or offensive academic, work, or student living environment.

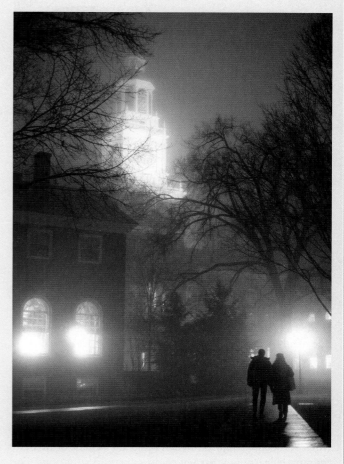

College campuses can be the site of criminal activity and violence just as any other environment or living situation can be—and so they require the same level of caution and awareness that you would use in other situations. Two key points to remember: 80% of campus crimes are committed by a student against a fellow student, and alcohol or drug use is involved in 90% of campus felonies. Drinking or drug use can affect judgment and lower inhibitions, so be aware if you or another person is under the influence. Here are some suggestions for keeping yourself safe on campus:

• Don't travel alone after dark. Many campuses have shuttle buses that run from spots on campus such as the library and the dining hall to residence halls and other locations. Escorts are often available to walk with you at night.

• Be familiar with well-lit and frequently traveled routes around campus if you do need to walk alone.

• If you have a car, follow the usual precautions about parking in well-lit areas, keeping the doors locked while you are driving, and never picking up hitchhikers.

• Always have your keys ready as you approach your residence hall, room, and car. Don't lend your keys to others.

• Let friends and family members know your schedule of classes and activities to create a sort of buddy system.

• Be sure the doors and windows of your dorm room have sturdy locks, and use them.

• Don't prop open doors or hold doors open for nonstudents or nonresidents trying to enter your dorm. Be aware of nonresidents around your dorm. If someone says that he or she is meeting a friend inside, that person should be able to call the friend from outside the building.

• Keep valuables and anything containing personal information—credit cards, wallets, jewelry, and so on—hidden. Secure expensive computer and stereo equipment with cables so that it can't be easily stolen. Use a quality U-shaped lock whenever you leave a bicycle unattended.

• Be alert when using an ATM, and don't display large amounts of cash.

• Stay alert and trust your instincts. Don't hesitate to call the police or campus security if something doesn't seem or feel right.

The Jeanne Clery Disclosure of Campus Security Policy and Campus Crime Statistics Act, named for a Lehigh University student who was murdered in her residence hall in 1986, requires colleges and universities to collect and report campus crime statistics. You can now review this information online at the Crime Statistics website of the U.S. Department of Education's Office of Postsecondary Education (ope.ed.gov/security/Search.asp).

communication doesn't work, assemble a file or log documenting the harassment, noting the details of each incident and information about any witnesses who may be able to support your claims. You may discover others who have been harassed by the same person, which will strengthen your case. Then file a grievance with the harasser's supervisor or employer.

If your attempts to deal with the harassment internally are not successful, you can file an official complaint with your city or state Human Rights Commission or Fair Employment Practices Agency, or with the federal Equal Employment Opportunity Commission. You may also wish to pursue legal action under the Civil Rights Act or under local laws prohibiting employment discrimination. Often the threat of a lawsuit or other legal action is enough to stop the harasser.

What You Can Do about Violence

Violence in our society is a serious threat to our collective health and well-being. This is especially true on college campuses (see the box "Staying Safe on Campus"). Schools are now providing training for conflict resolution and are educating people about the diverse nature of our society, thereby encouraging tolerance and understanding.

Reducing gun-related injuries may require changes in the availability, possession, and lethality of the 8–12 million firearms sold legally in the United States each year. As part of the Brady gun control law, computerized instant background checks are performed for most gun sales to prevent purchases by convicted felons, people with a history of mental instability, and certain other groups. In some states, waiting periods are required in addition to the background checks. Some groups advocate a complete and universal federal ban on the sale of all handguns.

PROVIDING EMERGENCY CARE

A course in **first aid** can help you respond appropriately when someone is injured. One important benefit of first aid training is learning what *not* to do in certain situations. For example, a person with a suspected neck or back injury should not be moved unless there are other life-threatening conditions. A trained person can assess emergency situations accurately before acting.

Emergency rescue techniques can save the lives of people who are choking, who have stopped breathing, or whose hearts have stopped beating. As described earlier, the Heimlich maneuver is used when a victim is choking. Pulmonary resuscitation (also known as rescue breathing, artificial respiration, or mouth-to-mouth resuscitation) is used when a person is not breathing. Cardiopulmonary resuscitation (CPR) is used when a pulse cannot be found. In 2010 the American Heart Association made significant changes in its CPR guidelines for lay persons. Previous guidelines were to clear the airway, check for breathing, and begin chest compressions (ABC). The new guidelines are to begin chest compressions, clear the airway, and check for breathing (CAB). Starting with compressions gets the blood circulating, which is critical to keeping the person alive until help arrives. Compressions should be delivered fast, about 100 times a minute. Courses in first aid and CPR are offered by the American Heart Association and the American Red Cross.

A new feature of some of these courses is training in the use of automated external defibrillators (AEDs), which monitor the heart's rhythm and, if appropriate, deliver an electrical shock to restart the heart. Because of the importance of early use of defibrillators in saving heart attack victims, these devices are being installed in public places, including casinos, airports, and many office buildings.

As a person providing assistance, you are the first link in the **emergency medical services (EMS) system.** The basic pattern for providing emergency care is check–call–care:

- *Check the situation:* Make sure the scene is safe for both you and the injured person. Don't put yourself in danger; if you get hurt too, you will be of little help to the injured person.

- *Check the victim:* Conduct a quick head-to-toe examination. Assess the victim's signs and symptoms, such as level of responsiveness, pulse, and breathing rate. Look for bleeding and any indications of broken bones or paralysis.

- *Call for help:* Call 911 or a local emergency number. Identify yourself and give as much information as you can about the condition of the victim and what happened.

- *Care for the victim:* If the situation requires immediate action (no pulse, shock, or the like), provide first aid if you are trained to do so.

Protecting yourself from injuries means taking sensible safety precautions every day and preparing yourself to deal with an emergency.

RIGHT NOW YOU CAN:

- Check your home for any object or situation that could cause an injury, such as a tripping hazard, top-heavy shelves, and so on.
- Test the batteries in your home's smoke detectors, and change them if necessary. Test the detectors to make sure they work properly.
- If you ride a bike, check your helmet to ensure that it fits properly and will protect you in a crash. If you have any doubts, throw it away and buy a new one.

IN THE FUTURE YOU CAN:

- Get trained in CPR, rescue breathing, and the use of an automated external defibrillator. If you have already had such training, take a refresher course.
- Be watchful for hazardous situations at your school and workplace. If you notice anything suspicious, report it to an appropriate person right away.
- Prepare for a poisoning emergency by putting the number of your local poison control hotline in a conspicuous place.

SUMMARY

- Injuries are caused by a dynamic interaction of human and environmental factors. Risk-taking behavior is associated with a high rate of injury.

- Key factors in motor vehicle injuries include aggressive driving, speeding, a failure to wear safety belts, alcohol and drug intoxication, fatigue, and distraction.

- Motorcycle, motor scooter, and bicycle injuries can be prevented by developing appropriate skills, driving or riding defensively, and wearing proper safety equipment, especially a helmet.

- Most fall-related injuries are a result of falls at floor level, but stairs, chairs, and ladders are also involved in a significant number of falls.

- Careless smoking and problems with cooking or heating equipment are common causes of home fires. Being prepared for fire emergencies means planning escape routes and installing smoke detectors.

- The home can contain many poisonous substances, including medications, cleaning agents, plants, and fumes from cars and appliances.

- Performing the Heimlich maneuver can prevent someone from dying from choking.

- The proper storage and handling of firearms can help prevent injuries; assume that any gun is loaded.

- Many injuries during leisure activities result from the misuse of equipment, lack of experience, use of alcohol, and a failure to wear proper safety equipment.

- Most work-related injuries involve manual labor; back problems and repetitive strain injuries are most common.

- Factors contributing to violence include poverty, the absence of strong social ties, the influence of the mass media, cultural attitudes about gender roles, problems in interpersonal relationships, alcohol and drug abuse, and the availability of firearms.

- Types of violence include assault, homicide, gang-related violence, hate crimes, school violence, workplace violence, and terrorism.

- Battering and child abuse occur at every socioeconomic level. The core issue is the abuser's need to control other people.

- Most rape victims are women, and most know their attackers. Factors in date rape include different standards of appropriate sexual behavior for men and women and different perceptions of actions.

- Child sexual abuse often results in serious trauma; usually the abuser is a trusted adult.

- Sexual harassment is unwelcome sexual advances or other conduct of a sexual nature that affects academic or employment performance or evaluations or that creates an intimidating, hostile, or offensive academic, work, or student living environment.

- Strategies for reducing violence include conflict resolution training, social skills development, and education programs that foster tolerance and understanding among diverse groups.

- Steps in giving emergency care include making sure the scene is safe for you and the injured person, conducting a quick examination of the victim, calling for help, and providing emergency first aid.

FOR MORE INFORMATION

BOOKS

American Medical Association. 2009. *American Medical Association Handbook of First Aid and Emergency Care*. New York: Random House Reference. *An everyday guide to first aid and emergency resuscitation techniques, with instructions for using automatic defibrillators.*

Carr, B., and E. Wondolowski. 2011. *The Prepper's Pocket Guide: 101 Easy Things You Can Do to Ready Your Home for a Disaster*. Berkeley, CA: Ulysses Press. *A practical guide to help prepare for potential disasters, both personal and environmental.*

Jones, S. A. 2011. *First Aid, Survival, and CPR: Home and Field Pocket Guide*. Philadelphia: F. A. Davis Company. A portable, waterproof guide for all kinds of first aid and survival emergencies; includes a section on pet first aid.

Lipman, I. A. 2010. *How to Be Safe: Survival Tactics to Protect Yourself, Your Home, Your Business and Your Family*. New York: Readers Digest Books. *A wide-ranging guide to safety, covering topics from home security to dealing with a terrorist attack.*

World Health Organization. 2010. *Preventing Intimate Partner and Sexual Violence against Women: Taking Action and Generating Evidence*. Geneva: World Health Organization. *The latest volume in a series of publications addressing the varying types of violence affecting our global society.*

ORGANIZATIONS, HOTLINES, AND WEBSITES

American Association of Poison Control Centers. Provides free, confidential, and expert advice related to poisoning (800-222-1222).

www.aapcc.org

American Automobile Association Foundation for Traffic Safety. Provides consumer information about all aspects of traffic safety; the website has online quizzes and extensive links.

www.aaafoundation.org/home

American Bar Association: Domestic Violence. Provides information about statistics, research, and laws relating to domestic violence.

http://www.americanbar.org/groups/domestic_violence/
resources/statistics.html

Consumer Product Safety Commission. Provides information and advice about safety issues relating to consumer products.

www.cpsc.gov

CyberAngels Internet Safety Program. Provides information about online safety and help and advice for victims of cyberstalking.

www.cyberangels.org

Insurance Institute for Highway Safety. Provides information about crashes on the nation's highways, as well as reports on topics such as speeding and crashworthiness of vehicles.

www.iihs.org

National Center for Injury Prevention and Control. Provides consumer-oriented information about unintentional injuries and violence.

www.cdc.gov/injury

National Center for Victims of Crime. An advocacy group for crime victims; provides statistics, news, safety strategies, tips on finding local assistance, and links to related sites.

www.ncvc.org

National Highway Traffic Safety Administration. Supplies materials about reducing deaths, injuries, and economic losses from motor vehicle crashes.

www.nhtsa.gov

National Safety Council. Provides information and statistics about preventing unintentional injuries.

www.nsc.org

National Violence Hotlines. Provide information, referral services, and crisis intervention.

800-799-SAFE (domestic violence)

800-422-4453 (child abuse)

800-656-HOPE (sexual assault)

Occupational Safety and Health Administration. Provides information about topics related to health and safety issues in the workplace.

www.osha.gov

Prevent Child Abuse America. Provides statistics, information, and publications relating to child abuse, including parenting tips.

www.preventchildabuse.org

Rape, Abuse, and Incest National Network (RAINN). Provides guidelines for preventing and dealing with sexual assault and abuse.

www.rainn.org

Tolerance.Org. Offers suggestions for fighting hate and promoting tolerance; sponsored by the Southern Poverty Law Center.

www.tolerance.org

World Health Organization: Violence and Injury Prevention and Disability. Provides statistics and information about the consequences of intentional and unintentional injuries worldwide.

www.who.int/violence_injury_prevention

The following sites provide statistics and background information about violence and crime in the United States:

Bureau of Justice Statistics: bjs.ojp.usdoj.gov
Federal Bureau of Investigation: www.fbi.gov
National Criminal Justice Reference Service: https://www.ncjrs.gov/

SELECTED BIBLIOGRAPHY

American College Health Association. 2008. *Shifting the Paradigm: Primary Prevention of Sexual Violence*. Linthicum, MD: American College Health Association.

Anderson, C. A., et al. 2010. Violent video game effects on aggression, empathy, and prosocial behavior in eastern and western countries: A meta-analytic review. *Psychological Bulletin* 136(2): 151–173.

Centers for Disease Control and Prevention. 2010. *Unintentional Drug Poisoning in the United States*. Atlanta, GA: Centers for Disease Control and Prevention.

Centers for Disease Control and Prevention. 2012. Youth risk behavior surveillance—United States, 2011. *Morbidity and Mortality Weekly Report Surveillance Summaries* 61(4): 1–162.

Cummings, P., et al. 2006. Changes in traffic crash mortality rates attributed to use of alcohol, or lack of a seat belt, air bag, motorcycle helmet, or bicycle helmet, United States, 1982–2001. *Injury Prevention* 12(3): 148–154.

Distracted driving: Fast lane to disaster. *Harvard Men's Health Watch* 16(10): 6–7.

Drysdale, D. et al. 2010. *Campus Attacks: Targeted Violence Affecting Institutions of Higher Education*. Washington, DC: U.S. Secret Service, U.S. Department of Education, and the Federal Bureau of Investigation.

Federal Bureau of Investigation. 2011. *Crime in the United States, 2010*. Washington, DC: U.S. Department of Justice.

Federal Bureau of Investigation. 2011. *Hate Crime Statistics, 2010*. Washington, DC: U.S. Department of Justice.

FIA Foundation for the Automobile and Society. 2010. *U.N. Decade of Action for Road Safety, 2011–2020* (www.fiafoundation.org/publications/Documents/decade_is_action_booklet.pdf).

Governors' Highway Safety Association. 2012. *Cell Phone and Texting Laws: February, 2012* (www.ghsa.org/html/stateinfo/laws/cellphone_laws.html).

Iqbal, S. et al. 2012. National carbon monoxide poisoning surveillance framework and recent estimates. *Public Health Reports* 127(5): 486–496.

Levinson, A. A., B. Lannert, and M. Yalch. 2012. The effects of intimate partner violence on women and children survivors: An attachment perspective. *Psychodynamic Psychiatry* 40(3): 397–433.

Liu, Y. C., and Y. K. Ou. 2011. Effects of age and the use of hands-free cellular phones on driving behavior and task performance. *Traffic Injury Prevention* 12(6): 550–558.

Narang, P., et al. 2010. Do guns provide safety? At what cost? *Southern Medical Journal* 103(2): 151–153.

National Center for Health Statistics. 2012. Deaths: Preliminary data for 2010. *National Vital Statistics Reports* 60(4):1–51.

National Highway Traffic Safety Administration. 2009. *Traffic Safety Facts Research Note: An Examination of Driver Distraction as Recorded in NHTSA Databases*. Washington, DC: National Highway Traffic Safety Administration.

What human and environmental factors are involved when you get injured? For the next 7–10 days, keep track of any mishaps you are involved in or injuries you sustain, recording them in a daily behavior record. Count each time you cut, burn, or injure yourself, fall down, run into someone, or have any other potentially injury-causing mishap, no matter how trivial. Also record any risk-taking behaviors, such as failing to wear your safety belt or bicycle helmet, drinking and driving, exceeding the speed limit, putting off home or bicycle repairs, and so on. For each entry (injury or incidence of unsafe behavior), record the date, the time, what you were doing, who else was there and how you were influenced by him or her, what your motivations were, and what you were thinking and feeling at the time.

At the end of the monitoring period, examine your data. For each incident, determine both the human factors and the environmental factors that contributed to the injury or unsafe behavior. Were you tired? Distracted? Did you not realize this situation was dangerous? Did you take a chance? Did you think this incident couldn't happen to you? Was visibility poor? Were you using defective equipment? Then consider each contributing factor carefully, determining why it existed and how it could have been avoided or changed. Finally, consider what preventive actions you could take to avoid such incidents or to change your behaviors in the future.

As an example, let's say that you usually don't use a safety belt when you run local errands in your car and that several factors contribute to this behavior: you don't really think you could be involved in a crash so close to home, you go on only short trips, you just never think to use it, and so on. One of the contributing factors to your unsafe behavior is inadequate knowledge. You can change this factor by obtaining accurate information about auto crashes (and their usual proximity to a victim's home) from this chapter and from library or Internet research. Just acquiring information about auto crashes and safety belt use may lead you to examine your beliefs and attitudes about safety belts and motivate you to change your behavior.

Once you're committed, you can use behavior change techniques described in Chapter 1, such as completing a contract and asking family and friends for support, to build a new habit. Put a note or picture reminding you to buckle up in your car where you can see it clearly. Recruit a friend to run errands with you and to remind you about using your safety belt. Once your habit is established, you may influence other people—especially people who ride in your car—to use safety belts all the time. By changing this behavior, you have reduced the chances that you or your passengers will suffer a serious injury or even die in a vehicle crash.

National Highway Traffic Safety Administration. 2012. High visibility enforcement demonstration programs in Connecticut and New York reduce hand-held phone use. *Annals of Emergency Medicine* 59(2): 141–142.

National Safety Council. 2012. *Injury Facts 2012.* Itasca, IL: National Safety Council.

National School Safety Center. 2010. *School Associated Violent Deaths.* Oak Park, CA: National School Safety Center.

National Weather Service. 2011. *Weather Safety* (www.weather.gov/safety.php).

Ross, T., et al. 2010. The bicycle helmet attitudes scale: Using the Health Belief Model to predict helmet use among undergraduates. *Journal of American College Health* 59(1): 29–36.

Roudsari, B., et al. 2009. Ethnicity, age, and trends in alcohol-related driver fatalities in the United States. *Traffic Injury Prevention* 10(5): 410–414.

Strayer, D. L., et al. 2006. A comparison of the cell phone driver and the drunk driver. *Human Factors* 48(2): 381–391.

Swogger, M. T., et al. 2012. Self-reported childhood physical abuse and perpetration of intimate partner violence: The moderating role of psychopathic traits. *Criminal Justice and Behavior* 39(7): 910–922.

U.S. Environmental Protection Agency. 2011. *Extreme Events* (www.epa.gov/climatechange/effects/extreme.html).

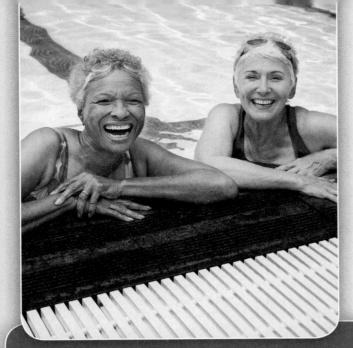

LOOKING AHEAD...

After reading this chapter, you should be able to

- List strategies for healthy aging

- Identify key physical, social, and mental changes that may accompany aging and explain how people can best confront these changes

- Describe practical considerations for older adults and caregivers, includ-ing housing, finances, health care, communication, and transportation

- Understand personal considerations in preparing for death, including making a will, assessing choices for end-of-life care, and making arrangements for a funeral or memorial service

- Describe the experience of living with a life-threatening illness and list ways to support a person who is dying

- Explain the grieving process and how support can be offered to adults and children who have experienced a loss

The Challenge of Aging

17

Aging does not begin at some specific point in life, and there is no precise age at which a person becomes "old." Rather, aging is a normal process of development that occurs throughout life. If you optimize wellness during young adulthood, you can exert great control over the physical and mental aspects of aging, and you can better handle your response to events that might be out of your control. This chapter discusses the aging process, and it also describes the process of dying and the issues that arise around death.

GENERATING VITALITY AS YOU AGE

Biological aging includes all the normal, progressive, irreversible changes to our bodies that begin at birth and continue until death. Psychological aging and social aging usually involve more abrupt changes in circumstance and emotion: relocating, changing homes, losing a spouse and friends, retiring, having a lower income, and changing roles and social status. These changes represent opportunities for growth throughout life.

Successful aging requires preparation. People need to establish good health habits in their teens and twenties. During their twenties and thirties, they usually develop important re-lationships and settle into a particular lifestyle. By their mid-forties, they generally know how much money they need to support the lifestyle they've chosen. At this point, they must assess their financial status and perhaps adjust their savings in order to continue enjoying that lifestyle after retirement. In their mid-fifties, they need to reevaluate their health insurance plans and may want to think about retirement housing. In their seventies and beyond, they need to consider ways of sharing their legacy with the next generation.

What Happens as You Age?

A significant number of older Americans describe themselves as being in poor health. Many of the characteristics associated with aging, however, are not due to aging at all. Rather, they result from the neglect and abuse of our bodies and minds. These assaults lay the foundation for later psychological problems and chronic conditions like arthritis, heart disease, diabetes, hearing loss, vision problems, and hypertension. But even with the healthiest behavior and environment, aging inevitably occurs as a result of biochemical processes we don't yet fully understand. Studies of healthy people indicate that functioning remains essentially constant until after age 70. Further research may help pinpoint the causes of aging and aid in the development of therapies to repair damage to aging organs.

Life-Enhancing Measures: Age-Proofing

You can prevent, delay, lessen, or even reverse some of the changes associated with aging through good habits. Simple things you can do daily will make a vast difference to your level of energy and vitality—your overall wellness.

Challenge Your Mind Numerous studies show that older adults who stay mentally active have lower levels of the brain protein linked to Alzheimer's and dementia. Reading, writing, doing puzzles, learning language, and studying music are good ways to stimulate the brain. The more complex the activity, the more protective it may be.

Develop Physical Fitness Exercise significantly enhances both psychological and physical health. A review of more than 70 scientific studies cited in the 2008 *Physical Activity Guidelines Advisory Committee Report* found that physically active people have about a 30% lower risk of dying prematurely compared with inactive people. Poor fitness and low physical activity levels were found to be better predictors of premature death than smoking, diabetes, or obesity. The committee found that about 150 minutes (2.5 hours) of physical activity per week is sufficient to decrease all-cause

> The aging process is genetically determined but **profoundly affected by our environment.**

mortality and that it is the overall volume of energy expended, regardless of what kinds of activities produce the energy expenditure, that makes a difference in risk of premature death.

The positive effects of exercise include lower blood pressure and healthier cholesterol levels; better protection against heart attacks and an increased chance of survival should one occur; sustained or increased lung capacity; weight control through less accumulation of fat; maintenance of strength, flexibility, and balance; improved sleep; longer life expectancy; protection against osteoporosis and type 2 diabetes; increased effectiveness of the immune system; and maintenance of mental agility and flexibility, response time, memory, and hand–eye coordination.

The stimulus that exercise provides also seems to protect against the loss of **fluid intelligence,** the ability to find solutions to new problems. Fluid intelligence depends on rapidity of responsiveness, memory, and alertness. Individuals who exercise regularly are also less susceptible to depression and dementia.

Regular physical activity is essential for healthy aging, as it is throughout life. The *2008 Physical Activity Guidelines for Americans* include recommendations for older adults that are the same as for all adults:

•   All older adults should avoid inactivity. Some physical activity is better than none.

•   For substantial health benefits, older adults should do at least 150 minutes a week of moderate-intensity activity, or 75 minutes a week of vigorous-intensity activity, or a combination of both. For additional and more extensive health benefits, older adults should increase their aerobic physical activity to 300 minutes a week of moderate-intensity, or 150 minutes a week of vigorous-intensity, aerobic physical activity.

•   Older adults should also do muscle-strengthening activities that are moderate or high intensity and involve all major muscle groups on two or more days a week because these activities provide additional health benefits.

There are also guidelines just for older adults:

•   When older adults cannot do 150 minutes of moderate-intensity aerobic activity a week because of chronic conditions, they should be as physically active as their abilities and conditions allow.

•   Older adults should do exercises that maintain or improve balance if they are at risk of falling.

•   Older adults with chronic conditions should understand whether and how their conditions affect their ability to do regular physical activity safely.

Regular exercise is a key to successful, healthy aging.

| **fluid intelligence**   The ability to develop a solution when confronted with a new problem. | TERMS |

- Older adults should maintain the flexibility necessary for regular physical activity and activities of daily life.

For more about the beneficial effects of exercise for older adults, see the box "Can Exercise Delay the Effects of Aging?"

Eat Wisely   Good health at any age is enhanced by eating a varied diet full of nutrient-rich foods. Special guidelines for older adults include the following:

- Get enough vitamin B-12 and extra vitamin D from fortified foods or supplements.
- Limit sodium intake to 1500 mg per day, and get enough potassium (4700 mg per day). Older adults tend to have higher blood pressure and to be salt-sensitive.
- Eat foods rich in dietary fiber and drink plenty of water to help prevent constipation.
- Pay special attention to food safety. Older adults are often more susceptible to foodborne illness.

Maintain a Healthy Weight   Weight management is especially difficult if you have been overweight most of your life. A sensible program of expending more calories through exercise, cutting calorie intake, or a combination of both will work for most people who want to lose weight, but there is no magic formula. Obesity is not physically healthy, and it leads to premature aging.

Control Drinking and Overdependence on Medications   Alcohol abuse ranks with depression as a common hidden mental health problem, affecting about 10% of older adults. (The ability to metabolize alcohol decreases with age.) The problem is often not identified because the effects of alcohol or drug dependence can mimic disease, such as Alzheimer's disease. Signs of potential alcohol or drug dependence include unexplained falls or frequent injuries, forgetfulness, depression, and malnutrition. Problems can be avoided by not using alcohol to relieve anxiety or emotional pain and not taking medication when safer forms of treatment are available.

Don't Smoke   The average pack-a-day smoker can expect to live about 13–14 fewer years than a nonsmoker. Furthermore, smokers suffer more illnesses that last longer, and they are subject to respiratory disabilities that limit their total vigor for many years before their death. Premature balding, skin wrinkling, and osteoporosis have been linked to cigarette smoking.

Ask Yourself

QUESTIONS FOR CRITICAL THINKING AND REFLECTION

How do you feel about the prospect of growing old? Would you say that you look forward to it, or are you anxious about it? What influences have shaped your feelings about aging?

Schedule Physical Examinations to Detect Treatable Diseases   When detected early, many diseases, including hypertension, diabetes, and many types of cancer, can be successfully controlled by medication and lifestyle changes. Regular testing for **glaucoma** after age 40 can prevent blindness from this eye disease. Recommended screenings and immunizations can protect against preventable chronic and infectious diseases.

Recognize and Reduce Stress   Stress-induced physiological changes increase wear and tear on your body. Cut down on the stresses in your life. Don't wear yourself out through lack of sleep, substance abuse or misuse, or overwork. Practice relaxation using the techniques described in Chapter 2.

DEALING WITH THE CHANGES OF AGING

Just as you can act now to prevent or limit the physical changes of aging, you can also begin preparing yourself psychologically, socially, and financially for changes that may occur later in life.

Planning for Social Changes

Retirement marks a major change in the second half of life in retirement. As Americans' longevity has increased, people spend a larger proportion of their lives in retirement.

Changing Roles and Relationships   Changes in social roles are a major feature of life as we age. Children become young adults and leave home, putting an end to daily parenting. Parents experiencing this empty-nest syndrome must adapt to changes in their customary responsibilities and personal identities. And although retirement may be a desirable milestone for most people, it may also be viewed as a threat to prestige, purpose, and self-respect—the loss of a valued or customary role—and often requires some adjustment.

Retirement and the end of child rearing also bring about changes in the relationship between marriage partners. The amount of time a couple spends together will increase, and activities will change. Couples may need a period of adjustment in which they get to know each other as individuals again. Discussing what types of activities each partner enjoys can help couples set up a mutually satisfying routine of shared and independent activities.

Increased Leisure Time   Although retirement confers the advantages of leisure time and freedom from deadlines, competition, and stress, many people do not know how to

glaucoma   A disease in which fluid inside the eye is under abnormally high pressure; can lead to the loss of peripheral vision and blindness.   **TERMS**

As people age, they often experience declines in functional health—the ability to perform the tasks of everyday life—and related declines in the quality of life. According to the CDC, more than 25% of Americans over age 65 report their health as only "fair" or "poor." Similarly, according to a Medicare survey, 31% of men and 42% of women aged 65–74 reported some sort of mobility limitation in 2003 (meaning they had difficulty walking one-quarter mile).

Can physical activity and exercise combat the degenerative effects of aging in middle-aged and older adults? The evidence indicates that they can. In reviewing the research, the U.S. government's Physical Activity Guidelines Advisory Committee concluded that physical activity can prevent or delay the onset of limitations and declines in functional health in older adults, can maintain or improve functional health in those who already have limitations, and can reduce the incidence of falls and fall-related injuries.

One mechanism by which physical activity prevents declines in functional health is through maintenance or improvement of the physiological capacities of the body, such as aerobic power, muscular strength, and balance—in other words, through im-

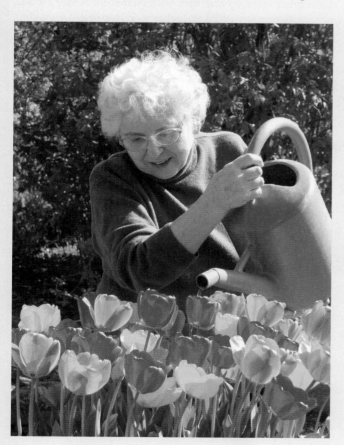

provements in physical fitness. Declines in these physiological capacities occur with biological aging and are often compounded by disease-related disability. But evidence shows that older adults who participate in regular aerobic exercise are 30% less likely than inactive individuals to develop functional limitations (such as a limited ability to walk or climb stairs) or role limitations (such as a limited ability to be the family grocery shopper). Although studies found that both physical activity and aerobic fitness were associated with reduced risk of functional limitations, aerobic fitness was associated with a greater reduction of risk. Evidence also suggests that regular physical activity is safe and beneficial for older adults who already have functional limitations.

Numerous studies have shown that regular exercise—particularly strength training, balance training, and flexibility exercises—can improve muscular strength, muscular endurance, and stability and provide some protection against falls. Aerobic activity, especially walking, also helps reduce risk of falls, and some evidence indicates that t'ai chi exercise programs are beneficial as well. Regular exercise not only reduces the incidence of falls but also greatly enhances mobility, allowing older people to live more independently and with greater confidence. Research also shows that regular physical activity can reduce anxiety and depression in older adults. Exercise stimulates blood flow to the brain and can even increase brain mass, helping the brain to function more efficiently and improving memory. There is some evidence that exercise may stave off mental decline and the occurrence of age-related dementia.

Current physical activity recommendations for older adults from the American Heart Association and the American College of Sports Medicine include moderate- to vigorous-intensity aerobic activity, strength training, and flexibility exercises, as well as balance exercises for older adults at risk for falls. Unfortunately more than 75% of Americans aged 65 and older do not get the recommended amounts of physical activity, and many get no exercise at all beyond the activities of daily living. Older adults are the least active group of Americans. Although it is important to exercise throughout life, the evidence indicates that older adults who become more active even late in life can experience improvements in physical fitness and functional health.

SOURCES: Centers for Disease Control and Prevention. 2007. Prevalence of regular physical activity among adults—United States, 2001 and 2005. *Morbidity and Mortality Weekly Report* 56 (46): 1209–1212; U.S. Department of Health and Human Services. 2008. 2008 Physical Activity Guidelines for Americans. Washington, DC: U.S. Department of Health and Human Services; Simonsick, E. M., et al. 2005. Just get out the door! Importance of walking outside the home for maintaining mobility: findings from the Women's Health and Aging Study. *Journal of the American Geriatrics Society* 53(2): 198–203.

enjoy their free time. If you have developed diverse interests, retirement can be a joyful and fulfilling period of your life. It can provide opportunities for expanding your horizons by giving you the chance to try new activities, take classes, and meet new people. Volunteering in your community can enhance self-esteem and allow you to be a contributing member of society.

The Economics of Retirement   Financial planning for retirement should begin early in life. People in their twenties and thirties should estimate how much money they need to support their standard of living, calculate their projected income, and begin a savings program. The earlier people begin such a program, the more money they will have at retirement.

Financial planning for retirement is especially critical for women. American women are much less likely than men to be covered by pension plans, reflecting the fact that many women have lower-paying jobs or work part-time during their childbearing years. They tend to have less money vested in other types of retirement plans as well. Although the gap is narrowing, women currently outlive men by about five to six years, and they are more likely to develop chronic conditions that impair their daily activities later in life. The net result of these factors is that older women are almost twice as likely as older men to live in poverty. Women should investigate their retirement plans and take charge of their finances to be sure they will be provided for as they get older.

Adapting to Physical Changes

Some changes in physical functioning are inevitable, and successful aging involves anticipating and accommodating these changes. Decreased energy and changes in health mean that older people have to develop priorities for how to use their energy. Rather than curtailing activities to conserve energy, they need to learn how to generate energy. This usually involves saying yes to enjoyable activities and paying close attention to the need for rest and sleep. Adapting, rather than giving up, favorite activities may be the best strategy for dealing with physical limitations. For example, if arthritis interferes with playing an instrument, a person can continue to enjoy music by taking up a different instrument or attending concerts.

Hearing Loss   The loss of hearing is a common physical change that can have a particularly strong effect on the lives of older adults. Hearing loss affects a person's ability to interact with others and can lead to a sense of isolation and depression. Hearing loss should be assessed and treated by a health care professional. In some cases hearing can be completely restored by dealing with the underlying cause of hearing loss. In other cases hearing aids may be prescribed.

Vision Changes   Vision usually declines with age. For some individuals this can be traced to conditions such as **glaucoma** or **age-related macular degeneration (AMD)** that can be treated medically. Glaucoma is caused by increased pressure within the eye due to built-up fluid. The optic nerve can be damaged by this increased pressure, resulting in a loss of side vision and, if untreated, blindness. Medication can relieve the pressure by decreasing the amount of fluid produced or by helping it drain more efficiently. Laser and conventional surgery are other options. People over 60, African Americans over 40, and anyone with a family history of glaucoma are at risk.

AMD is a slow disintegration of the *macula*—the tissue at the center of the retina where fine, straight-ahead detail is distinguished. AMD affects more than 1.5 million Americans over 40 and is the leading cause of blindness in people over age 75. Losing this vision makes it difficult to read, drive, or perform other close-up activities. Risk factors for AMD are age, gender (women may be at higher risk than men), smoking, elevated cholesterol levels, and family history. Some cases of AMD can be treated with laser surgery. Both glaucoma and AMD can be detected with regular screening.

By the time they reach their forties, many people have developed **presbyopia**—a gradual decline in the ability to focus on objects close to them. **Cataracts,** a clouding of the lens caused by lifelong oxidation damage (a by-product of normal body chemistry), may dim vision by the sixties.

Arthritis   More than 46 million American adults are estimated to have some form of **arthritis.** This degenerative disease causes joint inflammation leading to chronic pain,

> Financial planning for retirement should begin early in life—**as early as your twenties.**

QUICK STATS

120,000 Americans are blind due to glaucoma, accounting for 9–12% of all blindness.
—Glaucoma Research Foundation, 2010

TERMS

glaucoma   An increase in pressure in the eye due to fluid buildup that can result in loss of side vision and, if left untreated, blindness.

age-related macular degeneration (AMD)   A deterioration of the macula (the central area of the retina) leading to blurred vision and sensitivity to glare; some cases can lead to blindness.

presbyopia   The inability of the eyes to focus sharply on nearby objects, caused by a loss of elasticity of the lens that occurs with advancing age.

cataracts   Opacity of the lens of the eye that impairs vision and can cause blindness.

arthritis   Inflammation and swelling of a joint or joints, causing pain and swelling.

swelling, and loss of mobility. There are more than 100 different types of arthritis; osteoarthritis (OA) is by far the most common. In a person with OA, the cartilage that caps the bones in joints wears away, forming sharp spurs. It most often affects the hands and weight-bearing joints of the body—the knees, ankles, and hips.

Strategies for reducing the risk of arthritis and, for those who already have OA, for managing it include exercise, weight management, and avoidance of heavy or repetitive muscle use. Exercise lubricates joints and strengthens the muscles around them, protecting them from further damage. Swimming, walking, cross-country skiing, cycling, and t'ai chi are good low-impact exercises. Maintaining an appropriate weight is important to avoid placing stress on the hips, knees, and ankles.

Many people with OA take medication to relieve inflammation and reduce pain. Nonsteroidal anti-inflammatory drugs like ibuprofen can help but can irritate the digestive tract; prescription drugs that relieve pain without damaging the stomach have been found to have other dangerous side effects. Acetaminophen can also reduce pain without upsetting the stomach, but exceeding the recommended dosage can cause liver damage.

Menopause The natural process of menopause usually occurs during a woman's forties or fifties. The ovaries gradually stop functioning, estrogen levels drop, and eventually menstruation ceases. Several years before a woman stops menstruating, her periods usually become irregular, and she may experience hot flashes, vaginal dryness, sleep disturbances, and mood swings. This period, called *perimenopause*, can be troublesome for many women, some more than others.

Lifestyle strategies to reduce menopause-related problems include eating a healthy diet, exercising, losing weight, avoiding tobacco, and managing stress.

Sexual Functioning The ability to enjoy sex can continue well into old age, particularly if people make the effort to understand and respond to the various changes that age brings to the natural pattern of sexual response. All too often, older people give up sex because they mistakenly interpret these changes as signs of impending impotence. Lovemaking may become a more leisurely affair as a couple gets older, and the benefits of maintaining the sexual aspect of the relationship into old age can be great.

Osteoporosis As described in Chapter 9, **osteoporosis** is a condition in which bones become dangerously thin and fragile over time. Fractures are the most serious consequence of osteoporosis. Other problems associated with osteoporosis are loss of height and a stooped posture due to vertebral fractures, severe back and hip pain, and breathing problems.

Osteoporosis affects about 12 million Americans, 80% of whom are women. Women are at greater risk than men for

osteoporosis because they have 10–25% less bone in their skeletons and because bone loss accelerates during the first 5–10 years after the onset of menopause because of the drop in estrogen production. Black and Latino women have higher bone density and fewer fractures than white or Asian women but may be at increased risk of osteoporosis due to lack of vitamin D (a condition caused by high levels of melatonin). Other risk factors include a family history of osteoporosis, early menopause (before age 45), abnormal or irregular menstruation, a history of anorexia, and a thin, small frame. Thyroid medication, corticosteroid drugs for arthritis or asthma, and long-term use of certain contraceptives can also have a negative effect on bone mass.

Preventing osteoporosis requires building as much bone as possible during your young years and then maintaining it as you age. Girls aged 9–18 are in their critical bone-building years, and it is recommended that they eat more foods rich in calcium and vitamin D and get adequate exercise. Weight-bearing aerobic activities must be performed regularly throughout life to have lasting effects. Strength training improves bone density, muscle mass, strength, and balance, protecting against both bone loss and falls, a major cause of fractures. Even for people in their seventies, low-intensity strength training has been shown to improve bone density. Two other lifelong strategies for reducing the effects of osteoporosis are avoiding tobacco use and managing depression and stress. Bone mineral density testing can be used to gauge an individual's risk of fracture and help determine if any treatment is needed.

> A key to avoiding osteoporosis is to **build as much bone mass as you can while you're young.**

Handling Psychological and Mental Changes

Most older adults in good health remain mentally alert and retain their full capacity to learn and remember new information. Many people become smarter as they become older and more experienced in life.

Dementia **Dementia** is a loss of brain function that affects memory, thinking, language, judgment, and behavior. It affects about 1% of people aged 60–64 years and as many as 30–50% of people older than 85 years. Early symptoms of dementia include slight disturbances in a person's ability to

---

TERMS

osteoporosis The loss of bone density, causing bones to become weak, porous, and more prone to fractures.

dementia Deterioration of mental functioning (including memory, concentration, and judgment) resulting from a brain disorder; often accompanied by emotional disturbances and personality changes.

grasp the situation he or she is in. As dementia progresses, memory failure becomes apparent, and the person may forget conversations, the events of the day, or how to perform familiar tasks. It is important to have any symptoms evaluated by a health care professional because some of the over 50 known causes of dementia are treatable.

The most common forms of dementia among older people—**Alzheimer's disease** and multi-infarct dementia—are irreversible. The most common, **Alzheimer's disease** (AD), is a progressive brain disorder that damages and eventually destroys brain cells, leading to loss of memory, thinking, and other brain functions. About 5.3 million Americans have Alzheimer's disease, and that number is expected to quadruple in the next 50 years as more people live into their eighties and nineties.

Multi-infarct dementia results from a series of small strokes or changes in the brain's blood supply that deprive the brain of oxygen and destroy brain tissue. Symptoms may appear suddenly and worsen with additional strokes; they include disorientation in familiar locations; walking with rapid, shuffling steps; and difficulty following instructions. High blood pressure, cigarette smoking, and high cholesterol are some of the risk factors for stroke that may be controlled to prevent vascular dementia.

You can take lifestyle steps to help ward off dementia, such as controlling weight and blood pressure, eating a balanced diet (including adequate B vitamins and omega-3 fatty acids), exercising, not smoking, moderating your use of alcohol, practicing stress reduction techniques, maintaining social contacts, and cultivating a variety of mental pursuits, such as doing crossword puzzles.

Grief   Another psychological and emotional challenge of aging is dealing with grief and mourning. Aging is associated with loss—the loss of friends, family and spouse, peers, physical appearance, possessions, and health. Grief is the process of getting through the pain of loss, and it can be one of the loneliest and most emotionally intense times in a person's life. It can take years to completely come to terms with the loss of a loved one. Unresolved grief can have serious physical and psychological or emotional health consequences and may require professional help.

Depression and Suicide   Unresolved grief can lead to depression, a common problem in older adults. If you notice the signs of depression in yourself or someone you know, consult a mental health professional. A marked loss of interest in usually pleasurable activities, decreased appetite, insomnia, fatigue, and feelings of worthlessness are signs of depression. Listen carefully when an older friend or relative complains about being depressed; it may be a request for help.

Elderly Americans are more than twice as likely to commit suicide as any other demographic group. Among men over age 65, the rate of suicide among whites is more than double that of any other group. Depression is probably the single

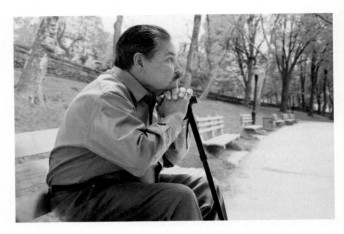

Suicide rates are relatively high among the elderly, and depression should be taken seriously.

most significant factor associated with suicidal behavior in older adults.

LIFE IN AN AGING AMERICA

Life expectancy is the average length of time we can expect to live. In 2009 life expectancy for the total population was 78.5 years, but those who reach age 65 can expect to live even longer—18.5 more years or longer—because they have already survived hazards to life in the younger years. Women have a longer life expectancy than men (see the box "Why Do Women Live Longer?"). Life expectancy also varies among ethnic groups; reasons for these differences include socioeconomic, genetic, and lifestyle factors.

As life expectancy increases, a larger proportion of Americans will be in their later years. This change will necessitate new government policies and changes in our general attitudes toward older adults.

America's Aging Minority

People over age 65 are a large minority in the American population—over 40.1 million people and about 13% of the total population in 2010. That number is expected to nearly double by the year 2030. The enormous increase in the over-65 population is markedly affecting our stereotypes of what it means to grow old. The misfortunes associated with aging—frailty, forgetfulness, poor health, isolation—occur in fewer

> **TERMS**
>
> **Alzheimer's disease**   A disease characterized by a progressive loss of mental functioning (dementia), caused by a degeneration of brain cells.
>
> **life expectancy**   The average length of time a person is expected to live.

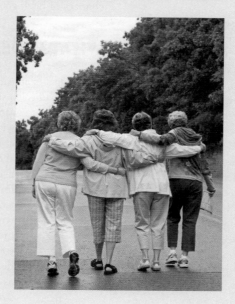

Women live longer than men in most countries around the world, even in places where maternal mortality rates are high. In the United States, women on average can expect to live about five years longer than men. Worldwide, among people over age 100, women outnumber men about nine to one.

The reason for the gender gap in life expectancy is not entirely understood but may be influenced by biological, social, and lifestyle factors. Estrogen production and other factors during a woman's younger years may protect her from early heart disease and from age-related declines in the heart's pumping power. Women may have lower rates of stress-related illnesses because they cope more positively with stress.

The news for women is not all good, however, because not all their extra years are likely to be healthy years. They are more likely than men to suffer from chronic conditions like arthritis and osteoporosis. Women's longer life spans, combined with the facts that men tend to marry younger women and that widowed men remarry more often than widowed women, mean there are many more single older women than men. Older men are more likely to live in family settings, whereas older women are more likely to live alone. Older women are also less likely to be covered by a pension or to have retirement savings, so they are more likely to be poor.

Increased male mortality can be traced in part to higher rates of behaviors such as smoking and alcohol and drug abuse. Testosterone production may be partly responsible in that it is linked to aggressive and risky behavior and to unhealthy cholesterol levels. Men have much higher rates of death than women from car crashes and other unintentional injuries, firearm-related deaths, homicide, suicide, AIDS, and early heart attack. Gender roles that promote risky behavior among young men are a factor in many of these causes of death. Indeed, among people who have made it to age 65, the gender longevity gap is smaller.

Social and behavioral factors may be more important than physiological causes in explaining the gender gap; for example, among the Amish, a religious sect that has strict rules against smoking and drinking, men usually live as long as women. This suggests that the longevity gap could be substantially narrowed through lifestyle changes.

SOURCES: U.S. Census Bureau. 2005. *We the People: Women and Men in the United States.* Washington, DC: U.S. Census Bureau; National Center for Health Statistics. 2009. *Health, United States, 2009.* Hyattsville, MD: National Center for Health Statistics; World Health Organization. 2003. *Gender, Health, and Aging.* Geneva: World Health Organization.

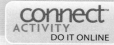

connect ACTIVITY DO IT ONLINE

---

people in their sixties and seventies and are shifting instead to burden the very old: those over age 85.

More than 80% of older Americans own their homes. Their living expenses are lower after retirement because they no longer support children and have fewer work-related expenses, and they consume and buy less food. They are more likely to continue practicing their expertise for years after retirement: thousands of retired consultants, teachers, technicians, and craftspeople work until their middle and late seventies. They receive greater amounts of assistance, such as Medicare, pay proportionately lower taxes, and have greater net worth from lifetime savings. As the aging population increases proportionally, however, the number of older people who are ill and dependent rises. Health care remains the largest expense for older adults. Most older Americans have at least one chronic condition; many have more than one.

Retirement finds many older people with their incomes reduced to subsistence levels. The majority of older Americans live with fixed sources of income, such as pensions, that are eroded by inflation. **Social Security** is the major source of income for most of the elderly. Social Security was intended to serve as a supplement to personal savings and private pensions, not as a sole source of income. It is vital to plan for an adequate retirement income.

Family and Community Resources for Older Adults

With help from friends, family members, and community services, people in their later years can remain active and independent. Over half of noninstitutionalized older Americans

Social Security A government program that provides financial assistance to people who are unemployed, disabled, or retired (and over a certain age); financed through taxes on business and workers. **TERMS**

live with a spouse; some live with a family member other than a spouse, and 30% live alone. Only 4% live in institutional settings, but among those over age 85, about 15% live in a nursing home.

In about three out of four cases, a spouse, a grown daughter, or a daughter-in-law assumes a caregiving role for elderly relatives.

Caregiving can be rewarding, but it is also hard work. If the experience is stressful and long-term, family members may become emotionally exhausted. Corporations are increasingly responsive to the needs of their employees who are family caregivers by providing services such as referrals, flexible schedules and leaves, and on-site adult care. Professional health care advice is another critical part of successful home care.

The best thing a family can do is talk honestly about the obligations, time, and commitment required by caregiving. Families should also explore the community resources and professional assistance that may be available to reduce the stress in this difficult job.

Government Aid and Policies

The federal government helps older Americans through several programs, such as food stamps, housing subsidies, Social Security, Medicare, and Medicaid.

Medicare is a major health insurance program for older adults and disabled persons. It provides basic health care coverage for acute episodes of illness that require skilled professional care, and it pays for some preventive services. Medicare pays less than 2% of nursing home costs, and private insurers pay less than 1%, creating a tremendous financial burden for nursing home residents and their families. When their financial resources are exhausted, people may apply for Medicaid, which provides medical insurance to low-income people of any age.

Health care policy planners hope that rising medical costs for older adults will shrink dramatically through education and prevention. Health care professionals, including **gerontologists** and **geriatricians,** are beginning to practice preventive medicine, just as pediatricians do. They advise older people about how to avoid and, if necessary, how to manage disabilities.

In sum, older adulthood can be a rewarding time of life, but its benefits don't come automatically. Planning and making wise lifestyle choices earlier in life can increase your chances of having a happy, healthy old age.

WHAT IS DEATH

Whether it is an earthquake and tsunami killing thousands in Japan, a man collapsing with a heart attack in a crowded restaurant, or a woman in her 90s dying peacefully with her family close by, images of death are easy to envision. Nevertheless, we rarely think about the inevitability of death in our own lives. Accepting and dealing with death are important tasks that present unique challenges to our sense of self, our relationships with others, and our understanding of the meaning of life itself. Although pain and distress may accompany the dying process, facing death also presents an opportunity for growth as well as affirmation of the preciousness of simple aspects of our daily lives.

Questions about the meaning of death and what happens when we die are central concerns of the great religions and philosophies. Some promise a better life after death. Others teach that everyone is evolving toward perfection or divinity, a goal reached after successive rounds of death and rebirth. There are also those who suggest that it is not possible to know what—if anything—happens after death and that any judgment about life's worth must be made on the basis of satisfactions or rewards that we create for ourselves in our lifetimes.

Even in modern secular societies, religion plays a major role in shaping our attitudes and behaviors toward death. The mourning ceremonies associated with various religious practices ease the pangs of grief for many people. Dying and death are more than biological events; they have social and spiritual dimensions.

Defining Death

Traditionally death has been defined as cessation of the flow of vital body fluids. This occurs when the heart stops beating and breathing ceases. These traditional signs are adequate for determining death in most cases. However, the use of ventilators, artificial heart pumps, and other **life support systems**

Ask Yourself

?

QUESTIONS FOR CRITICAL THINKING AND REFLECTION

What do you want your life to be like when you are old? Do you hope to retire, or keep working indefinitely? Where would you like to live? How much time do you spend thinking about these questions? Have you done any planning yet for old age?

TERMS

gerontologist   One who studies the biological, psychological, and social phenomena associated with aging and old age.

geriatrician   A physician specializing in the diseases, disabilities, and care of older adults.

life support systems   Medical technologies, such as a ventilator, that allow vital body functions to be artificially sustained.

allow many body functions to be artificially sustained. The concept of **brain death** was developed to determine whether a person is alive or dead when the traditional signs are inadequate because of supportive medical technology.

According to the standards published by a Harvard Medical School committee, brain death involves four characteristics: (1) lack of receptivity and response to external stimuli, (2) absence of spontaneous muscular movement and spontaneous breathing, (3) absence of observable reflexes, and (4) absence of brain activity, as signified by a flat **electroencephalogram (EEG).** The Harvard criteria require that a second set of tests be performed after 24 hours have elapsed, and they exclude cases of hypothermia (body temperature below 90°F) and situations involving central nervous system depressants, such as barbiturates.

In contrast to **clinical death,** which is determined by either the cessation of heartbeat and breathing or the criteria for establishing brain death, **cellular death** refers to a gradual process that occurs when heartbeat, respiration, and brain activity have stopped. It encompasses the breakdown of metabolic processes and results in complete nonfunctionality at the cellular level.

The way death is defined has potential legal and social consequences in a variety of areas, including criminal prosecution, inheritance, taxation, treatment of the corpse, and even mourning. It also affects the practice of organ transplantation because some organs—hearts, most obviously—must be harvested from a human being who is legally determined to be dead.

Learning about Death

Our understanding of death changes as we grow and mature, as do our attitudes toward it. Very young children view death as an interruption and an absence, but their lack of a mature time perspective means that they do not understand death as final and irreversible. A child's understanding of death evolves greatly from about age 6 to age 9. During this period, most children begin to understand that death is final, universal, and inevitable. A person who consciously recognizes these facts is said to possess a **mature understanding of death.**

It is important to add, however, that individuals who possess a mature understanding of death commonly hold nonempirical ideas about it as well. Such nonempirical ideas—that is, ideas not subject to scientific proof—deal mainly with the notion that human beings survive in some form beyond the death of the physical body. What happens to an individual's personality after he or she dies? Does the self or soul continue to exist after the death of the physical body? If so, what is the nature of this afterlife? Developing personally satisfying answers to such questions is also part of the process of acquiring a mature understanding of death.

Attitudes Toward Death

Our ability to find meaning and comfort in the face of mortality depends not only on our having an understanding of

Death awaits all of us at the end of our lives, and accepting and dealing with death are difficult but important tasks.

TERMS

brain death   A medical determination of death as the cessation of brain activity indicated by various diagnostic criteria, including a flat EEG reading.

electroencephalogram (EEG)   A record of the electrical activity of the brain (brain waves).

clinical death   A determination of death made according to accepted medical criteria.

cellular death   The breakdown of metabolic processes at the level of the body's cells.

mature understanding of death   The recognition that death is universal and irreversible, that it involves the cessation of all physiological functioning, and that there are biological reasons for its occurrence.

the facts of death, but also on our attitudes toward it. Many people seek to avoid any thought or mention of death. The sick and old are often isolated in hospitals and nursing homes. Relatively few Americans have been present at the death of a loved one. Where the reality of death is concerned, "out of sight, out of mind" often appears to be the rule of the day.

Although some commentators characterize the predominant attitude toward death in the United States as "death denying," others are reluctant to generalize so broadly. People often maintain conflicting or ambivalent attitudes toward death. Those who come to view death as a relief or release from insufferable pain may have at least a partial sense of welcoming death. Few people wholly avoid or wholly welcome death. In the last several decades, attitudes toward death in our culture have begun to slowly change, particularly as the hospice movement has grown.

PLANNING FOR DEATH

Acknowledging the inevitability of death allows us to plan for it. Adequate planning can help ensure that a sudden, unexpected death is not made even more difficult for survivors. Even when death is not sudden, many decisions can be anticipated, considered, and discussed with close relatives and friends.

Making a Will

Surveys indicate that about 7 out of 10 Americans die without leaving a will. A **will** is a legal instrument expressing a person's intentions and wishes for the disposition of his or her property after death. It is a declaration of how one's **estate**—that is, money, property, and other possessions—will be distributed after death. During the life of the **testator** (the person making the will), a will can be changed, replaced, or revoked. Upon the testator's death, it becomes a legal instrument governing the distribution of the testator's estate.

When a person dies **intestate**—that is, without having left a valid will—property is distributed according to rules set up by the state. If you haven't yet made a will, start thinking about how you'd like your property distributed in the case of your death. If you have a will, consider whether it needs to be updated in response to a key life event such as marriage, the birth of a child, or the purchase of a home.

You can also help your family members by completing a *testamentary letter*; this document includes information about your personal affairs, such as bank accounts, credit cards, the location of documents and keys, the names of your professional advisers, the names of people who should be notified of your death, and so on.

Considering Options for End-of-Life Care

An appropriate balance in end-of-life care may involve any combination of home care, hospital stays, nursing home care, and hospice care.

Home Care   The majority of people express a preference for at-home care during the end of life. An obvious advantage of home care is the fact that the person is in a familiar setting, ideally in the company of family and friends. Family members may or may not be capable of providing the level of care that is needed, and skilled professional caregivers may have to be hired. Currently about 25% of Americans die at home.

Hospice Programs   Terminally ill people who wish to die at home or in their assisted living residence are often aided by **hospice** programs, which are widely available throughout the United States. Hospice is a system of **palliative care** for patients who are likely to die within six months or less. The goal of palliative care is to reduce pain and other discomforting symptoms, allowing patients to function and enjoy the remainder of their lives as fully as possible. About two-thirds of hospice patients stay in their own homes, but hospice care is also offered in nursing homes, hospitals, and freestanding hospice facilities. Physicians, nurses, pharmacists, clergy, social workers, home health aides, and trained volunteers make up the core members of the hospice team.

More than 40% of people who died in the United States in 2010 were under the care of a hospice program. About 65% of hospice patients are over 75 years old, although hospice programs take care of patients of all ages, including children.

TERMS

will   A legal instrument expressing a person's intentions and wishes for the disposition of his or her property after death.

estate   The money, property, and other possessions belonging to a person.

testator   The person who makes a will.

intestate   Describes a person who dies without having made a legal will.

hospice   A program of care for dying patients and their families.

palliative care   A form of medical care aimed at reducing the intensity or severity of a disease by controlling pain and other discomforting symptoms.

Ask Yourself

QUESTIONS FOR CRITICAL THINKING AND REFLECTION

What situations or events make you think seriously about your own mortality? Is this something you consider now and then, or do you avoid thinking about death? What has influenced your willingness or reluctance to think about death?

In addition to helping patients achieve a good and peaceful death, an important gift of hospice care is the potential to help patients and families discover how much can be shared at the end of life through personal and spiritual connections.

Difficult Decisions at the End of Life

Modern medicine can sometimes keep the human organism alive despite the cessation of normal heart, brain, respiratory, or kidney function. But should a patient without any hope of recovery be kept alive by means of artificial life support? What if a patient has fallen into a **persistent vegetative state,** a state of profound unconsciousness, lacking any sign of normal reflexes and unresponsive to external stimuli, with no reasonable hope of improvement?

Ethical questions about a person's right to die have become prominent since the landmark case of Karen Ann Quinlan in 1975. At age 22 she was admitted in a comatose state to an intensive care unit, where her breathing was sustained by a mechanical ventilator. When she remained unresponsive, her parents asked that the respirator be disconnected, but the medical staff denied their request. The New Jersey Supreme Court eventually ruled that artificial respiration could be discontinued.

Since then courts have ruled on removing other types of life-sustaining treatment, including artificial feeding mechanisms that provide nutrition and hydration to permanently comatose patients who are able to breathe on their own. Notable was the case of Terri Schiavo in 2003. Terri had been diagnosed as being in a persistent vegetative state. Contending that she would not want to continue living on life support, Terri's husband requested that her feeding tube be removed. Terri's parents contested the request, and a series of legal actions ensued. Finally, in 2005, after intervention by the U.S. Supreme Court, physicians were allowed to remove the tube. Cases like this highlight the importance of expressing one's wishes about life-sustaining treatment, in writing, before the need arises.

Withholding or Withdrawing Treatment The right of a competent patient to refuse unwanted treatment is now generally established in both law and medical practice. The consensus is that there is no medical or ethical distinction between withholding (not starting) a treatment and withdrawing (stopping) a treatment once it has been started. The choice to forgo life-sustaining treatment involves refusing treatments that would be expected to extend life. The right to refuse treatment remains constitutionally protected even when a patient is unable to communicate. Although specific requirements vary, all states authorize some type of written advance directive to honor the decisions of individuals unable to speak for themselves but who have previously recorded their wishes in an appropriate legal document.

Physician-Assisted Suicide and Active Euthanasia

In contrast to withdrawing or withholding treatment, **physician-assisted suicide** and **active euthanasia** are practices that intentionally hasten the death of a person. **Physician-assisted suicide (PAS)** occurs when a physician provides lethal drugs—at the patient's request—with the understanding that the patient plans to use them to end his or her life. The patient administers the fatal dose.

Oregon was the first state to legalize physician-assisted suicide following a citizens' initiative called the Death with Dignity Act. Even though PAS has been legally available in Oregon since 1994, the practice remains rare; in 2011 only 71 deaths occurred in Oregan as a result of physician-assisted suicide. The states of Washington and Montana also now allow physician-assisted suicide.

Another ruling of importance by the Supreme Court involves the concept of **double effect** in the medical management of pain. The doctrine of double effect states that a harmful effect of treatment, even if it results in death, is permissible if the harm is not intended and occurs as a side effect of a beneficial action. Sometimes the dosages of medication needed to relieve a patient's pain must be increased to levels that can cause respiratory depression, which could hasten the patient's death. The doctrine of double effect allows physicians throughout the United States to do what is necessary to relieve pain, even if there is a chance that the medication may hasten death.

Unlike physician-assisted suicide, **active euthanasia** is the intentional act of killing someone who would otherwise suffer from an incurable and painful disease. *Voluntary euthanasia* (also known as voluntary active euthanasia, or VAE) is the intentional termination of life at the patient's request. In practice, this generally means that a competent patient requests

> ## QUICK STATS
>
> **114** prescriptions were written for lethal drugs under Oregon's Death with Dignity Act in 2011; **71** patients actually took the drugs.
>
> —Oregon Department of Human Services, 2012

> ## TERMS
>
> **persistent vegetative state** A condition of profound unconsciousness in which a person lacks normal reflexes and is unresponsive to external stimuli, lasting for an extended period with no reasonable hope of improvement.
>
> **physician-assisted suicide (PAS)** The practice of a physician intentionally providing, at the patient's request, lethal drugs or other means for a patient to hasten death with the understanding that the patient plans to use them to end his or her life. The patient administers the drug to himself or herself.
>
> **double effect** A situation in which a harmful effect occurs as an unintended side effect of a beneficial action, such as when medication intended to control a patient's pain has the unintended result of causing the patient's death.
>
> **active euthanasia** A deliberate act intended to end another person's life; voluntary active euthanasia involves the practice of a physician administering—at the request of a patient—medication or some other intervention that causes death.

direct assistance to die, and he or she receives assistance from a qualified medical practitioner. Voluntary active euthanasia is legal under very strict guidelines in Belgium, Luxembourg, and the Netherlands, but is currently unlawful in the United States. Taking active steps to end someone's life is a crime—even if the motive is mercy.

Completing an Advance Directive

To make your preferences known about medical treatment, you need to document them through a written **advance directive.** Two forms of advance directives are legally important. First is the **living will,** which enables individuals to provide instructions about the kind of medical care they wish to receive (or not receive) if they become incapacitated or otherwise unable to participate in treatment decisions. The second is the **health care proxy,** which is also known as a *durable power of attorney for health care.* This document makes it possible to appoint another person to make decisions about medical treatment if you become unable to do so. This decision maker may be a family member, close friend, or attorney with whom you have discussed your treatment preferences. The proxy is expected to act in accordance with your wishes as stated in an advance directive or as otherwise made known.

For advance directives to be of value, you must do more than merely complete the paperwork. Discuss your wishes ahead of time with caregivers and family members as well as with your physician.

Giving the Gift of Life

Each day about 77 people receive an organ transplant while another 18 people on the waiting lists die because not enough organs are available. As of February 2012, more than 113,000 Americans were waiting for organ transplants. If you decide to become an organ donor, the first step is to indicate your wish by completing a **Uniform Donor Card** (Figure 17.1); alternatively, you can indicate your wish on your driver's license in many states. Be sure to discuss your decision with your family.

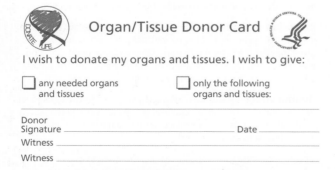

FIGURE 17.1   A sample organ/tissue donor card.
SOURCE: U.S. Department of Health and Human Services (http://www.organdonor.gov/donor/index.htm).

Planning a Funeral or Memorial Service

Funerals and memorial services are rites of passage that commemorate a person's life and acknowledge his or her passing from the community. Funerals and memorials allow survivors to support one another as they cope with their loss and express their grief. The presence of death rites in every human culture suggests that they serve innate human needs.

Disposition of the Body   People generally have a preference about the final disposition of their body. For most Americans, the choice is either burial or cremation. *Burial* involves a grave dug into the soil or entombment in a mausoleum. If the family wishes that the body be viewed during a wake or in an open casket funeral, **embalming** is generally done.

Cremation involves subjecting a body to intense heat. Cremated remains can be buried, placed in a columbarium niche, put into an urn kept by the family or interred in an urn garden, or scattered at sea or on land. Cremation is now the choice in about 40% of deaths in the United States, with the rate of cremation increasing rapidly in recent years.

Arranging a Service   A funeral or memorial service can be a healing experience that allows loved ones to honor the deceased, share memories, express their grief through ceremony, and support one another. The more the service fits the personality of the deceased person and meets the practical needs of the family, the better. People who have a terminal illness sometimes find comfort and satisfaction in helping to plan for their own memorial services. A memorial service can be the joint creation of the dying person and family members who wish to be part of the project. Making at least some plans

---

TERMS

advance directive   Any statement made by a competent person about his or her choices for medical treatment should he or she become unable to make such decisions or communicate them in the future.

living will   A type of advance directive that allows individuals to provide instructions about the kind of medical care they wish to receive, or not receive, if they become unable to participate in treatment decisions.

health care proxy   A type of advance directive that allows an individual to appoint another person as an agent in making health care decisions in the event he or she becomes unable to participate in treatment decisions; also known as a *durable power of attorney for health care.*

Uniform Donor Card   A consent form authorizing the use of the signer's body parts for transplantation or medical research upon his or her death.

embalming   The process of removing blood and other fluids and replacing them with chemicals to disinfect and temporarily retard deterioration of a corpse. Some of the chemicals used, such as formaldehyde, are toxic.

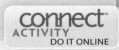

Some of the following tasks must be attended to soon after a death occurs, whereas others take weeks or months to complete. Many of these tasks, especially those that need to be dealt with in the first hours and days following the death, can be taken care of by friends and relatives of the immediate survivors. If the deceased person has been served by a hospice, the social worker has likely worked with the patient and family to make many of these plans ahead of time.

- Prepare a list of relatives, friends, and colleagues, and telephone them about the death as soon as possible. Friends can help with notifications.

- Find out if the deceased left instructions for disposition of the body or for a funeral or memorial service.

- If no prior plan exists, contact a funeral home, mortuary, or memorial society for help in making arrangements. Clergy, friends, and other family members can be asked to help decide what is most appropriate.

- If flowers are to be omitted from the funeral or memorial service, choose an appropriate charity or other memorial to which gifts can be made.

- Write the obituary. Consider including the deceased's age, birthplace, cause of death, occupation, academic degrees, memberships, military service, accomplishments, names and relationships of nearest survivors, and the time and place of the funeral or memorial service. If a small funeral is planned, and you are notifying people by phone or e-mail, you can wait to write the obituary later, or skip it entirely. You can also use an online obituary website, and even create an online memorial to a loved one.

- Ask friends to help coordinate the supplying of meals for the first few days following the death, as well as the management of other household tasks and child care, if necessary. You can also ask friends to coordinate a potluck or catered meal if you wish to have a gathering after the funeral.

- If you have relatives and friends who will be coming from out of town for the funeral, ask a friend or family member to help with arrangements for lodging and transportation to and from the airport.

- If a funeral ceremony is planned, choose the individuals who are to be pallbearers, and notify them that you would like their participation.

- Gather photos or other mementos for a memory book, memory board, or memorial website.

- Do you want to have a small booklet with information about the deceased and perhaps a photo or poem to give to mourners at the funeral or memorial service? If so, get help from family members and friends to create the pamphlet and have it printed.

connect ACTIVITY DO IT ONLINE

---

ahead of time can help ease the burden on survivors, who will undoubtedly face a great number of tasks and decisions when the death occurs (see the box "Tasks for Survivors").

COPING WITH DYING

There is no one right way to live with or die of a life-threatening illness. Every disease has its own set of problems and challenges, and each person copes with these problems and challenges in his or her own way. Much of the suffering experienced by people with a life-threatening illness comes from overwhelming feelings of loss on all levels.

Living with an illness that is life-threatening and incurable can be described as a living–dying experience. Hope and honesty are often delicately balanced—honesty to face reality as it is, and hope for a positive outcome. The early hope that the symptoms are not really serious gives way to hope that a cure is possible. When the illness is deemed incurable, there is hope for more time. As time begins to run out, one hopes for a pain-free death—a "good death" (see the box "In Search of a Good Death").

The Tasks of Coping

In her groundbreaking 1969 book *On Death and Dying*, Elisabeth Kübler-Ross, a Swiss American psychiatrist and one of the first medical experts to focus on the topic of end of life, suggested that the response to an awareness of imminent death involves five psychological stages: denial, anger, bargaining, depression, and acceptance. Individuals go back and forth among the stages during the course of an illness, and different stages can occur simultaneously. Today the notion of stages has been deemphasized in favor of highlighting the

Participants in a landmark study were asked to discuss the deaths of family members, friends, or patients and reflect on what made their deaths good or bad. From these discussions, six major themes emerged as components of a good death.

- *Pain and symptom management:* Many people fear dying in pain, and portrayals of bad deaths usually included inadequate pain management. When reassured that pain could be managed, patients were less anxious.

- *Clear decision making*: Both providers and families feared entering a medical crisis without knowing the patient's preferences. Patients and families who had good communication with health care providers and had discussed treatment decisions ahead of time felt empowered, and providers felt they were giving good care. Tolerance for uncertainty may increase if values and preferences are clarified.

- *Preparation for death:* Patients expressed satisfaction when they had time to prepare their wills and help plan their funeral arrangements. Patients and families also wanted to know what to expect during the course of the illness and what physical and psychosocial changes would take place as death approached. It was important for providers and families to have reached some personal comfort with death so they felt prepared when death occurred.

- *Completion:* the opportunity to review one's life, resolve conflicts, spend time with loved ones, and say good-bye. Participants confirmed the deep importance of spirituality or meaningfulness at the end of life. Many times, patients were able to view their experience of dying as part of a broader life trajectory and thus continue to grow emotionally and spiritually in their last days. Issues of faith were often mentioned as important to healing.

- *Contributing to others:* Patients wanted to know that they still had something to offer to others, whether it was making someone laugh or lightening the load of someone closer to death. Many patients found that as they reflected on their lives, what they valued most was their personal relationships with family and friends, and they were anxious to impart this wisdom to others.

- *Affirmation of the whole person:* Patients appreciated empathic health care providers, and family members were comforted by those who treated their loved ones as unique and whole people, rather than as a disease. The quality of dying is related to the acknowledgment that people die in character—that is, as an extension of who they have been in their lives.

The study affirmed that most people think of death as a natural part of life, not as a failure of technology. Although the biomedical aspects of end-of-life care are crucial, they merely provide a point of departure toward a good death. When pain is properly managed and the practical aspects of dying are taken care of, patients and their families have the opportunity to address the important emotional, psychological, and spiritual issues that all human beings face at the end of life.

---

tasks that require attention in order to cope well with a life-threatening illness. Psychologist and author Charles Corr, for example, distinguishes four primary dimensions in coping with dying:

1. *Physical:* satisfying bodily needs and minimizing physical distress.

2. *Psychological:* maximizing a sense of security, self-worth, autonomy, and richness in living.

3. *Social:* sustaining significant relationships and addressing the social implications of dying.

4. *Spiritual:* identifying, developing, or reaffirming sources of meaning and fostering hope.

People who apparently cope best with life-threatening illness often exhibit a fighting spirit that views the illness not only as a threat but also as a challenge. These people strive to inform themselves about their illness and take an active part in treatment decisions. They are optimistic and have a capacity to discover positive meaning in ordinary events. Holding to a positive outlook despite distressing circumstances involves creating a sense of meaning that is bigger than the threat. In the context of life-threatening illness, this encompasses a person's ability to comprehend the implications an illness has for the future, as well as for his or her ability to accomplish goals, maintain relationships, and sustain a sense of personal vitality, competence, and power.

Supporting a Person in the Last Phase of Life

People often feel uncomfortable in the presence of a person who is in the final stage of life. How should we act? What can

Ask Yourself

QUESTIONS FOR CRITICAL THINKING AND REFLECTION

What is your notion of a "good death"? In what setting does it take place, and who is there? In the last days of your life, what do you think you'll need to say, and to whom will you want to say it? If you were terminally ill, what would be the most supportive things others could do for you?

we say? Perhaps the most important and comforting thing we can do for a dying person is to simply be present. Sitting quietly and listening carefully, we can take our cues from the person who is dying. If the person is capable of speaking, and wishes to talk, attentive listening is an act of great kindness. If the person doesn't wish to talk, or is not able to, physical touch such as holding hands or putting a hand on the person's shoulder can be the most effective way to express your love and concern. As death is drawing near, simple steps—such as repositioning the patient, covering him or her with a light blanket, dimming the room's lighting, playing soft favorite music, or holding hands—can provide great relief and reassurance in the last moments.

COPING WITH LOSS

Even if we have not experienced the death of someone close, we are all survivors of losses that occur in our lives because of changes and endings. The loss of a job, the ending of a relationship, transitions from one school or neighborhood to another—these are examples of the kinds of losses that occur in all our lives. Such losses are sometimes called little deaths, and in varying degrees they all involve grief.

Experiencing Grief

Grief is the reaction to loss. It encompasses thoughts and feelings as well as physical and behavioral responses. Mental distress may involve disbelief, confusion, anxiety, disorganization, and depression. The emotions that can be present in normal grief include not only sorrow and sadness, but also relief, anger, guilt, and self-pity, among others. Common behaviors associated with grief include crying, searching for the deceased, and talking repetitively about the deceased and the circumstances of the death. Bereaved people may be restless, as if not knowing what to do with themselves. Outward signs of grief may involve frequent sighing, crying, inappropriate laughter, insomnia, loss of appetite, and marked fatigue. Grief may also evoke a reexamination of religious or spiritual beliefs as a person struggles to make meaning of the loss. Guilt is a common emotion after the death of a loved one. All such manifestations of grief can be present as part of our total response to **bereavement**—that is, the event of loss.

Mourning refers to the *reaction* to loss but to the *process* by which a bereaved person adjusts to loss and incorporates it

into his or her life. How this process is managed is determined, at least partly, by cultural and gender norms for the expression of grief.

The Course of Grief   Grieving, like dying, is highly individual. In the first hours or days following a death, a bereaved person is likely to experience shock and numbness, as well as a sense of disbelief. The cause or mode of death—natural, accidental, homicide, or suicide—influences how grief is experienced. Even when a death is anticipated, grief is not necessarily diminished when the loss becomes real.

The death of a loved one is frequently a severe physical as well as emotional stressor. Grieving people often have difficulty sleeping, may neglect to eat nourishing food, and may forget to take their usual medications. These factors add to the health risks associated with recent loss. People may also feel confused and have difficulty concentrating following a significant loss.

After the initial shock begins to fade, the course of grief is characterized by anxiety, apathy, and pining for the deceased. The pangs of grief are felt as the bereaved person deeply experiences the pain of separation. There is often a sense of despair as a person repeatedly goes over the events surrounding the loss, perhaps fantasizing that somehow everything could be undone and be as it was before.

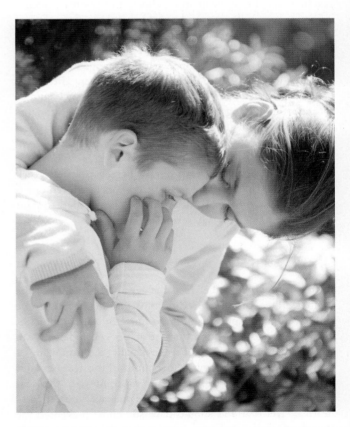

Children are better able to cope with loss when they are included in their family's experience of grief and mourning.

> **grief**   A person's reaction to loss as manifested physically, emotionally, mentally, and behaviorally.
>
> **bereavement**   The objective event of loss.
>
> **mourning**   The process whereby a person actively copes with grief in adjusting to a loss and integrating it into his or her life.

TERMS

As time goes on, the acute pain and emotional turmoil of grief begin to subside. Physical and mental balance are reestablished. The bereaved person becomes increasingly reintegrated into his or her social world. Sadness doesn't go away completely, but it recedes into the background much of the time. Although reminders of the loss stimulate waves of active grieving from time to time, the main focus is the present, not the past. Adjusting to loss may sometimes feel like a betrayal of the deceased loved one, but it is healthy to engage again in ongoing life and the future.

Social support for the bereaved is as critical during the later course of grief as it is during the first days after a loss. The first anniversary and major holidays following a significant loss can be times of renewed grieving when the support of others is important and appreciated. Knowing that others remember the loss and that they take time to connect is usually perceived as comforting.

Bereaved people may find it helpful to share their stories and concerns through organized support groups. Hospices provide bereavement support groups and counseling. Many online and in-person support groups are organized around specific types of bereavement, such as the loss of a child, the loss of a parent, or the loss of a loved one to suicide.

Supporting a Grieving Person

When a person finds out that a loved one has died, the initial reaction may be overwhelming shock and distress. Such a person may initially respond best to the physical comfort of hugging and holding. Later, simply listening may be the most effective way to help. Talking about a loss is an important way that many survivors cope with the changed reality, and they may need to tell their story over and over. The key to being a good listener is to avoid speaking too much, and to refrain from making judgments about whether the thoughts and feelings expressed by a survivor are right or wrong, good or bad.

If a grieving friend or relative talks about suicide, or seems in danger of causing harm to him or herself or others, seek professional help right away. The recent loss of a loved one is a major risk factor for suicide and self-harm. Be alert to signs that a grieving person is in serious danger.

When a Young Adult Loses a Friend

Among young people between the ages of 18 and 24 in the United States, the three leading causes of death tend to be sudden and unexpected: unintentional injuries, homicide, and suicide. Losing a close friend to an unexpected death can be particularly traumatic. There is usually an outpouring of sympathy and support toward the family of the deceased, but as a friend, you may feel left out and unsupported. Also, it is common to blame yourself in some way for your friend's death or feel that you should have somehow prevented the tragedy. If you lose a friend, be sure to look for support from friends, family, clergy, or health professionals, especially if the

intense sadness or guilt feelings last for more than a few days or weeks. Friends can often help each other by working together to create their own way of celebrating the life of their lost friend.

Helping Children Cope with Loss

Children tend to cope with loss in a healthier fashion when they are included as part of their family's experience of grief and mourning. Although adults may be uncomfortable about sharing potentially disturbing or painful news with children, a child's natural curiosity usually negates the option of withholding information. Mounting evidence shows that it is best to include children from the beginning—as soon as a terminal prognosis is made, for example—to help them understand what is happening. Children should spend time with the dying person, if possible, to learn, share, and offer and receive comfort.

In talking about death with children, the most important guideline is to be honest. Set the explanation you are offering at the child's level of understanding. Find out what the child wants to know. In general, it's advisable to keep the explanation simple, stick to basics, and verify what the child has understood from your explanation.

COMING TO TERMS WITH DEATH

We may wish we could keep death out of view and not make a place for it in our lives. But this wish cannot be fulfilled. With the death of a beloved friend or relative, we are confronted with emotions and thoughts that relate not only to the immediate loss but also to our own mortality. Our encounters with dying and death teach us that relationships are more important than things and that life offers no guarantees. In discovering the meaning of death in our own lives, we find that life is both precious and precarious.

Allowing ourselves to make room for death, we discover that it touches not only the dying or bereaved person and his or her family and friends but also the wider community of which we are all part. We recognize that dying and death offer opportunities for extraordinary growth in the midst of loss.

Ask Yourself

QUESTIONS FOR CRITICAL THINKING AND REFLECTION

Have you ever been in the position of being supportive to a bereaved person? What kind of support did he or she seem to appreciate most? How did the experience affect you?

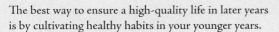

Connect to Your Choices

Have you ever thought about where you get your attitudes toward death? Many factors can influence our attitudes, some not as obvious as others. Were your grandparents part of your life growing up? Have they or your parents talked with you about advance directives or their end-of-life wishes? How susceptible are you to ageism, and how strongly are you influenced by the youth orientation of the media? Have you gotten the idea from the mainstream culture that it's best not to think or talk about death?

What are the external factors that influence your attitudes toward death? What are your inner motivations and core values, and how do they affect your attitudes? Based on what you learned in this chapter, will you make some different choices in the future? If so, what will they be?

Go online to Connect to complete this activity: www.mcgraw-hillconnect.com

TIPS FOR TODAY AND THE FUTURE

The best way to ensure a high-quality life in later years is by cultivating healthy habits in your younger years.

RIGHT NOW YOU CAN:
- Think about any unhealthy habits you have and resolve to change them. Review the information in this text to devise strategies for change.
- Think about how you want your body to be disposed of when you die.
- Consider organ donation as a lasting gift of life to others. If you want to be an organ donor, make the appropriate arrangements now, as described in this chapter.

IN THE FUTURE YOU CAN:
- Learn a new skill, such as a language or a game of strategy.
- Talk to your parents or grandparents about their wishes for the end of life. Let them know you care for them and want to be involved.

SUMMARY

- People who take charge of their health during their youth have greater control over the physical and mental aspects of aging.

- A lifetime of interests and hobbies helps maintain creativity and intelligence. Exercise and a healthful diet throughout life enhance physical and psychological health.

- Retirement can be a fulfilling and enjoyable time of life for those who adjust to their new roles, enjoy participating in a variety of activities, and have planned ahead for financial stability.

- Slight confusion and forgetfulness are not signs of a serious illness; however, severe symptoms may indicate Alzheimer's disease or another form of dementia.

- Resolving grief and mourning and dealing with depression are important tasks for older adults.

- People over age 65 form a large minority in the United States, and their status is improving.

- Family and community resources can help older adults stay active and independent.

- Government aid to the elderly includes food stamps, housing subsidies, Social Security, Medicare, and Medicaid.

- Although death makes rational sense in terms of species survival and evolution, there may be no completely satisfying answer to the question of why death exists from a personal point of view.

- Dying and death are more than biological events; they have social and spiritual dimensions.

- The traditional criteria for determining death focus on vital signs such as breathing and heartbeat. Brain death is characterized by a lack of physical responses other than breathing and heartbeat, with absence of brain activity as signified by a flat electroencephalogram (EEG).

- Between ages 6 and 9, most children begin to develop an understanding that death is final, universal, and inevitable.

- A mature understanding of death can include ideas about the survival of the human personality or soul after death. Problems arise when avoidance or denial of death fosters the notion that it happens only to others.

- A will is a legal instrument that governs the distribution of a person's estate after death.

- End-of-life care may involve a combination of home care, hospital stays, and hospice or palliative care.

- Palliative care is devoted to making dying patients comfortable by controlling pain and relieving suffering.

- Hospice programs apply a team-oriented approach to caring for dying patients and their families with the goal of helping people live as fully as possible until the end of their lives.

- Exercising choices about end-of-life care can involve making decisions about attempting to prolong life or choosing to allow natural death with comfort care.

- The practice of withholding or withdrawing potentially life-sustaining treatment is sometimes termed passive euthanasia.

- Physician-assisted suicide occurs when a physician provides lethal drugs or other interventions, at a patient's request, with the understanding that the patient plans to use them to end his or her life. Voluntary active euthanasia refers to the intentional ending of a patient's life, at his or her request, by someone other than the patient.

- Advance directives, such as living wills, are used to express people's wishes about the use of life-sustaining treatment and how they wish to be treated if they cannot speak for themselves.

- People can donate their bodies or specific organs for transplantation and other medical uses after death. People of all ages can make their wishes to donate their organs known on their driver's license or other state forms. They also need to let their families know that they wish to be organ donors.

- For Americans, the decision about what to do with the body after death usually involves either burial or cremation.

- Bereaved people usually benefit from participating in a funeral or other type of memorial service to commemorate a loved one's life and death.

- Coping with dying involves physical, psychological, social, and spiritual dimensions.

- It is useful for patients and caregivers to understand the trajectory, or course, of dying.

- In offering support to a dying person, the gift of listening can be especially important.

- Grief encompasses thoughts and feelings as well as physical and behavioral responses.

- Mourning, the process by which a person integrates a loss into his or her life, is determined partly by social and cultural norms for expressing grief.

- Children tend to cope with death in a healthier fashion when they are included in their family's experience of grief and mourning.

- Dying and death offer opportunities for growth in the midst of loss.

FOR MORE INFORMATION

BOOKS

Bonanno, G.A. 2009. *The Other Side of Sadness: What the New Science of Bereavement Tells Us about Life after Loss.* New York: Basic Books. *This book explains modern thinking about grief and resilience, with many vignettes.*

Byock, I. 2012. *The Best Care Possible: A Physician's Quest to Transform Care Through the End of Life.* New York: Avery. *A champion of palliative care argues that end-of-life care should meet the needs of the dying person, not those of the health care system, and that we need to move beyond our cultural aversion to talking about death.*

Callanan, M., and P. Kelley 2012. *Final Gifts: Understanding the Special Awareness, Needs, and Communications of the Dying.* New York: Simon & Schuster. *Real stories of the experience of dying people and their loved ones told by two hospice nurses.*

DeSpelder, L. A., and A. L. Strickland. 2011. *The Last Dance: Encountering Death and Dying*, 9th ed. New York: McGraw-Hill. *A comprehensive and readable text highlighting a broad range of topics related to dying and death.*

Hyams, J. 2011. *Time to Help Your Parents.* London: Piatkus. *A sympathetic overview of the many challenges facing adult children who must care for their aging parents.*

Johns Hopkins Medical Center. 2007. *The Johns Hopkins Medical Guide to Health after 50.* New York: Black Dog & Leventhal. *A practical guide to healthy aging for all wellness dimensions.*

Karnes, B. 1986, revised 2009. *Gone from My Sight: The Dying Experience.* Vancouver: BK Books. *This booklet, distributed to the families of dying patients by many hospices across the country, explains the process of dying in simple, straightforward terms.*

National Institute on Aging. 2010. *Exercise & Physical Activity: Your Everyday Guide from the National Institute on Aging*, book and DVD ed. New York: Hatherleigh Press. *A practical guide to physical activity and exercise, with specific guidelines for safe exercise for older adults.*

Pfeiffer, E. 2013. *Winning Strategies for Successful Aging.* New Haven, CT: Yale University Press. *A practical guide to maintaining one's health, happiness, spirituality, sexuality, and independence in the later years of life.*

Slocum, J and Carlson, L. 2011. *Final Rights: Reclaiming the American Way of Death.* Hinesburg VT: Upper Access Publishing. *Discusses how families can assert their rights by taking control of the funeral process. Topics include avoiding being taking advantage of by the funeral industry, green burial, home funerals, and a listing of funeral-related state laws.*

ORGANIZATIONS AND WEBSITES

AARP. Provides information about all aspects of aging, including health promotion, health care, and retirement planning.

http://www.aarp.org

Aging Well. A practical resource for seniors that includes information about diet, exercise, safety, and medical care.

http://www.aging.ny.gov

Aging with Dignity: Five Wishes. Source for an advanced directive that includes designation of a health care proxy (durable power of attorney), the kind of medical treatment you want or don't want, your wishes about pain control, how you want people to treat you, and what you want your loved ones to know when you are dying.

http://www.agingwithdignity.org/five-wishes.php

Alzheimer's Association. Offers tips for caregivers and patients and information on the causes and treatment of Alzheimer's disease.

http://www.alz.org

American Association of Suicidology. Information and help for people who have lost loved ones to suicide. Contains a variety of resources, including a directory of support groups.

http://www.suicidology.org/suicide-loss-survivors

Caring Connections (a program of the National Hospice and Palliative Care Organization). Provides resources for end-of-life decision making with the goal of planning before a crisis occurs. Information about state-specific advance directives. Hotline and multilingual line available.

http://www.caringinfo.org/i4a/pages/index.cfm?pageid=1

The Compassionate Friends. Provide grief support after the death of a child, including local chapters and online support groups.

http://www.compassionatefriends.org/home.aspx

The Dougy Center. Offers education about childhood bereavement and support groups for bereaved children, teens, young adults, and parents.

http://www.dougy.org

GriefNet. A site where you can communicate with others via e-mail support groups in the areas of death, grief, and major loss.

http://www.griefnet.org

Hospice Foundation of America. Promotes the hospice concept of care through education and leadership.

http://www.hospicefoundation.org

National Cancer Institute: Grief, Bereavement and Coping with Loss. Provides extensive information about types of grief reactions, complicated grief, treatment for complicated grief, children and loss, and cultural aspects of grief.

http://www.cancer.gov/cancertopics/pdq/supportivecare
/bereavement/Patient

National Funeral Directors Association (NFDA). Provides resources related to funerals and funeral costs, body disposition, and bereavement support.

http://www.nfda.org

National Hospice and Palliative Care Organization (NHPCO). Provides information about hospice care and advance directives, including an online national directory of hospices listed by state and city.

http://www.nhpco.org

National Institute on Aging. Provides fact sheets and brochures about aging-related topics.

http://www.nia.nih.gov

http://nihseniorhealth.gov

Nolo Press: Wills and Estate Planning. Provides answers to questions about planning for death, from writing a basic will to organ donation.

http://www.nolo.com

Organ Procurement and Transplantation Network. Provides information about organ donation and donor cards.

http://www.organdonor.gov/index.html

U.S. Administration on Aging. Provides fact sheets, statistical information, and Internet links to other resources on aging.

http://www.aoa.gov

SELECTED BIBLIOGRAPHY

Alzheimer's Association. 2012. *2012 Alzheimer's Disease Facts and Figures.* Chicago: Alzheimer's Association.

Beyond menopause: Life after estrogen. 2005. *Mayo Clinic Health Letter Supplement,* February.

Annas, G. J. 2005. "Culture of life" politics at the bedside—the case of Terri Schiavo. *New England Journal of Medicine,* 23 March [epub].

Casarett, D., et al. 2005. Making difficult decisions about hospice enrollment: What do patients and families want to know? *Journal of the American Geriatrics Society* 53(2): 249–254.

Chudyk, A. M., et al. 2012. Risk of hip fracture with hip or knee osteoarthritis: A systematic review. *Clinical Rheumatology* 31(5): 749–757.

Death with Dignity National Center. 2012. *Death with Dignity around the U.S.* (http://www.deathwithdignity.org/advocates/national/).

Doka, K. J., and A. S. Tucci (ed.). 2011. *Beyond Kubler-Ross: New Perspectives on Death, Dying and Grief.* Washington, DC: Hospice Foundation of America.

DuBois, J. M., and E. E. Anderson. 2006. Attitudes toward death criteria and organ donation among healthcare personnel and the general public. *Progress in Transplantation* 16(1): 65–73.

Field, N. P. 2006. Unresolved grief and continuing bonds: An attachment perspective. *Death Studies* 30(8): 739–756.

Fisher, J. E., P. J. Ballantye, and G. A. Hawker. 2012 Older adults living with osteoarthritis: Examining the relationship of age and gender to medicine use. *Canadian Journal on Aging* 31(3): 323–333.

Flaskerud, J. H. 2012. End-of-life preparation: Advance care planning. *Issues in Mental Health Nursing* 32(11): 720–722.

Goldstein, M., et al. 2012. Innovations in organ donation. *Mt. Sinai Journal of Medicine* 79(3): 351–364.

Gomez-Cabello, A., et al. 2012. Effects of training on bone mass in older adults: A systematic review. *Sports Medicine* 42(4): 301–325.

Harvard Medical School. 2005. Living wills and health care proxies. *Harvard Health Letter* 30(8): 1–3.

Harvard Medical School. 2006. Minding your mind: 12 ways to keep your brain young with proper care and feeding. *Harvard Men's Health Watch* 10(10): 1–4.

Izumi, S. S., et al. 2012. Defining end-of-life care from perspectives of nursing ethics. *Nursing Ethics* 19(5): 608-618.

Jager, R. D., et al. 2008. Age-related macular degeneration. *New England Journal of Medicine* 258(24): 2606–2617.

Kirkwood, T. 2010. Why women live longer: Stress alone does not explain the longevity gap. *Scientific American,* October.

Lannen, P. K., et al. 2008. Unresolved grief in a national sample of bereaved parents: Impaired mental and physical health 4 to 9 years later. *Journal of Clinical Oncology* 26(36): 5870–5876.

Manzari, Z. S. et al. 2012. Exploring families' experiences of an organ donation request after brain death. *Nursing Ethics* 19(5): 654–665.

Morrison, W. 2012. Organ donation prior to death—balancing benefits and harms. *American Journal of Bioethics* 12(6): 14–15.

Mostofsky, E., et al. 2012. Risk of acute myocardial infarction after the death of a significant person in one's life. *Circulation: Journal of the American Heart Association* 125: 491–496.

Mudge, A. M., et al. 2008. Exercising body and mind: An integrated approach to functional independence in hospitalized older people. *Journal of the American Geriatrics Society* 56(4): 630–635.

National Cancer Institute. 2012. *Grief, Bereavement, and Coping with Loss* (http://www.cancer.gov/cancertopics/pdq/supportivecare/bereavement/HealthProfessional).

National Hospice Foundation. 2012. *The History of Hospice* (http://www.nationalhospicefoundation.org/i4a/pages/index.cfm?pageid=218).

National Hospice and Palliative Care Organization. 2012. *Hospice Care in America* (http://www.nhpco.org/i4a/pages/index.cfm?pageid=5994).

National Kidney Foundation. 2012. *25 Facts about Organ Donation and Transplantation* (http://www.kidney.org/news/newsroom/fs_new/25factsorgdon&trans.cfm).

Nelson, H. D., et al. 2006. Nonhormonal therapies for menopausal hot flashes: Systematic review and meta-analysis. *Journal of the American Medical Association* 295(17): 2057–2071.

Norton, E. M., and P. J. Miller. 2012 What their terms of living and dying might be: Hospice social workers discuss Oregon's Death with Dignity Act. *Journal of Social Work in End-of-Life & Palliative Care* 8(3): 249–264.

Oregon Public Health Division. 2012. *Death with Dignity Act 2010* (http://public.health.oregon.gov/ProviderPartnerResources/EvaluationResearch/DeathwithDignityAct/Pages/index.aspx).

Owen, A. M., et al. 2006. Detecting awareness in the vegetative state. *Science* 313(5792): 1402.

Reid, M. C., R. Shengella, and S. Parker. 2012. Pharmacologic management of osteoarthritis-related pain in older adults. *American Journal of Nursing* 112: S38–43.

Scarre, G. 2012. Can there be a good death? *Journal of Evaluation in Clinical Practice* 18(5): 1082–1086.

Scarmeas, N., et al. 2006. Mediterranean diet, Alzheimer disease, and vascular mediation. *Archives of Neurology* 63: December.

Shear, M. K., et al. 2011. Complicated grief and related issues for DSM-5. *Depression and Anxiety* 28: 103–117.

Shubert, T. E. 2011. Evidence-based exercise prescription for balance and falls prevention: A current review of the literature. *Journal of Geriatric Physical Therapy* 34(3): 100–108.

Smith, T. J., and B. E. Hillner. 2011. Bending the cost curve in cancer care. *New England Journal of Medicine* 364: 2060–2065.

Sorrell, J. M. 2008. As good as it gets? Rethinking old age. *Journal of Psychosocial Nursing and Mental Health Services* 46(5): 21–24.

Souied, E. H., and N. Leveziel. 2012. Toward personalized medicine for age-related macular degeneration. *American Journal of Ophthalmology* 154(3): 427–428.

Steed, M. 2012. Palliative care: Are you asking the right questions? *Nursing* 42(10): 59–61.

Steinhauser, K. E., et al. 2000. In search of a good death: Patients, families and providers. *Annals of Internal Medicine* 132(10): 825–832.

Stern, C., and Z. Munn. 2010. Cognitive leisure activities and their role in preventing dementia: A systematic review. *International Journal of Evidence-Based Healthcare* 8(1): 2–17.

Sutter, C., and T. Reid. 2012. How do we talk to the children? Child life consultation to support the children of seriously ill adult inpatients. *Journal of Palliative Medicine*, Sept. 14 (Epub ahead of print).

Syed, F. A., and A. C. Ng. 2010. The pathophysiology of the aging skeleton. *Current Osteoporosis Reports* 8(4): 235–240.

Tallman, K., et al. 2012. Living with advanced illness: Longitudinal study of patient, family, and caregiver needs. *The Permanente Journal* 16(3): 28–35.

United Network for Organ Sharing. 2012. *Fact Sheets* (http://www.unos.org/donation/index.php?topic=fact_sheets).

Yuhas, D. 2012. Cracks in the plaques: Mysteries of Alzheimer's slowly yielding to new research. *Scientific American*, February.

Zager, B. S., and M. Yancy. 2011. A call to improve practice concerning cultural sensitivity in advance directives: A review of the literature. *Worldviews on Evidence-Based Nursing* 8(4): 202–211.

NUTRITIONAL CONTENT OF COMMON FOODS

If you are developing a behavior change plan to improve your diet, or if you simply want to choose more healthful foods, you may want to know more about the nutritional content of common food items. You can look up the nutrient content of the foods you eat in the USDA Agricultural Research Service National Nutrient Database for Standard Reference (http://www.ars.usda.gov/Services/docs. htm?docid=17477), which lists foods both by description and by nutrient content. For example, under "protein," you can find out how much protein there is in a chicken pot pie or what foods have the most protein per serving. Although cumbersome, the database is comprehensive.

You can also track your daily food intake, calculate your nutrient intake from foods, and compare your intake with MyPlate recommendations for your age, sex, height, and weight at the MyPlate SuperTracker website (https://www.choosemyplate. gov/SuperTracker/default.aspx). This site provides tools for tracking your activity level, weight goals, and other aspects of your health status.

NUTRITIONAL CONTENT OF POPULAR ITEMS FROM FAST-FOOD RESTAURANTS

Although most foods served at fast-food restaurants are high in calories, fat, saturated fat, cholesterol, sodium, and sugar, some items are more healthful than others. If you eat at fast-food restaurants, knowing the nutritional content of various items can help you make better choices. Fast-food restaurants provide nutritional information both online and in print brochures available at most restaurant locations. To learn more about the items you order, visit the restaurants' websites. Here are some popular fast-food restaurants and their web addresses:

Arby's	http://www.arbys.com
Burger King	http://www.bk.com/en/us/index.html
Chipotle	http://www.chipotle.com
Domino's Pizza	http://www.dominos.com
Hardees	http://www.hardees.com
Jack in the Box	http://www.jackinthebox.com
KFC	http://www.kfc.com
McDonald's	http://www.mcdonalds.com
Starbucks	http://www.starbucks.com
Subway	http://www.subway.com
Taco Bell	http://www.tacobell.com
Wendy's	http://www.wendys.com
White Castle	http://www.whitecastle.com

Click here to view a larger image of the Healthy Eating Plate

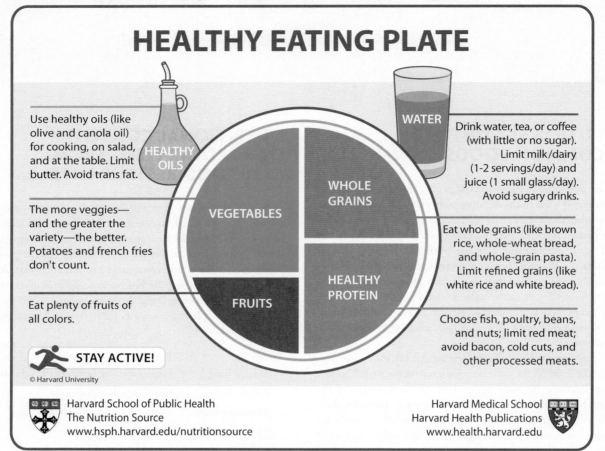

HEALTHY EATING PLATE

WATER

HEALTHY OILS

VEGETABLES

WHOLE GRAINS

FRUITS

HEALTHY PROTEIN

Use healthy oils (like olive and canola oil) for cooking, on salad, and at the table. Limit butter. Avoid trans fat.

The more veggies— and the greater the variety—the better. Potatoes and french fries don't count.

Eat plenty of fruits of all colors.

STAY ACTIVE!

© Harvard University

Drink water, tea, or coffee (with little or no sugar). Limit milk/dairy (1-2 servings/day) and juice (1 small glass/day). Avoid sugary drinks.

Eat whole grains (like brown rice, whole-wheat bread, and whole-grain pasta). Limit refined grains (like white rice and white bread).

Choose fish, poultry, beans, and nuts; limit red meat; avoid bacon, cold cuts, and other processed meats.

Harvard School of Public Health
The Nutrition Source
www.hsph.harvard.edu/nutritionsource

Harvard Medical School
Harvard Health Publications
www.health.harvard.edu

Chapter One

Opener: Purestock/Getty Images RF; p. 9: CATHERINE URSILLO/Getty Images; p. 12: © JGI/Blend Images LLC RF; p. 18: © Cindy Charles/PhotoEdit.

Chapter Two

Opener: Brand X Pictures/Punchstock RF; p. 29: RubberBall/SuperStock RF; p. 31: © Tim Boyle/Getty Images; p. 32: © Scott Olsen/Getty Images; p. 33: Camille Tokerud Photography Inc./Getty Images; p. 34: © Nick Daly/PhotoDisc/Getty Images RF; p. 40: BananaStock/JupiterImages RF; p. 44: Erik Dreyer/Getty Images.

Chapter Three

Opener: Cohen/Ostrow/Getty Images RF; p. 49: © Purestock/PunchStock RF; p. 52: © PhotoAlto/Laurence Mouton/Getty Images RF; p. 58: Design Pics/Patrick Kociniak RF; p. 64: Lisa Peardon/Getty Images.

Chapter Four

Opener: Emma Innocenti/Getty Images; p. 71: © Chris Robbins/Digital Vision/Getty Images RF; p. 72: © JLP/Jose L. Pelaez/Corbis; p. 73: © Mirko Iannace/Corbis; p. 76: Design Pics/Kristy-Anne Glubish RF; p. 77: Image Source/Getty Images RF; p. 78: © Brook Slezak/Stone/Getty Images; p. 81: © AP Photo/Eric Risberg; p. 82: © Big Cheese Photo/PunchStock RF; p. 85: © Royalty-Free/Corbis.

Chapter Five

Opener: © Stockbyte/PunchStock RF; p. 97: © Royalty-Free/Corbis; p. 100: Ingram publishing/SuperStock RF; p. 110: © RubberBall/Getty Images RF; p. 111: Tim Platt/Getty Images; p. 118: Image Source/Getty Images RF

Chapter Six

Opener: The McGraw-Hill Companies, Inc./Christopher Kerrigan, photographer; p. 125: © Joel Gordon; p. 127: SIU BIOMED COMM Custom Medical Stock Photo/Newscom; p. 132: The McGraw-Hill Companies, Inc./Christopher Kerrigan, photographer; p. 140: Getty Images;

Chapter Seven

Opener: Ingram publishing/SuperStock RF; p. 150: © Fancy Collection/SuperStock RF;

p. 155: Tracy Montana/PhotoLink/PhotoDisc/Getty Images RF; p. 160: Doug Menuez/Getty Images RF; p. 164: SW Productions/Getty Images RF; p. 169: © Veer RF.

Chapter Eight

Opener: © John Rensten/Riser/Getty Images; p. 177: © Rachel Weill/UpperCut Images/Getty Images; p. 184: Ingram Publishing RF; p. 185: Warner Bros./Getty Images; p. 188: © Morgan David de Lossy/Corbis; p. 189: © Jeff Greenberg/The Image Works.

Chapter Nine

Opener: © Rolf Bruderer/Blend Images LLC RF; p. 209: Nash Photos/Getty Images RF; p. 221: Joe Madeira/Getty Images RF.

Chapter Ten

Opener: © Liane Cary/age fotostock RF; p. 231: © artparadigm/Digital Vision/Getty Images RF; p. 235: © Brendan Smialowski/Getty Images; p. 240: © Glow Wellness RM 26/Alamy; p. 243: © Siede Preis/Photo-Disc/Getty Images RF.

Chapter Eleven

Opener: © Fancy Collection/SuperStock RF; p. 253: © 3660 Group, Inc./Getty Images; p. 263: Digital Vision/Getty Images RF.

Chapter Twelve

Opener: Ingram Publishing RF/age fotostock RF; p. 270: © 2007 Getty Images, Inc. RF; p. 273: Stephan Gladieu/Getty Images; p. 275: © Topham/The Image Works; p. 278: © Paul Seheult/Eye Ubiquitous/Corbis; p. 293: © AP Photo/John Amis; p. 294: © Stockbyte/Getty Images RF.

Chapter Thirteen

Opener: © moodboard/Getty Images; p. 312: Doug Menuez/Getty Images RF; p. 318: © Joel Gordon; p. 322: © Image Source/Corbis RF; p. 325: © Royalty-Free/Corbis.

Chapter Fourteen

Opener: Courtesy NASA; p. 331: AFP/Getty Images; p. 333: Digital Vision/PunchStock RF; p. 335: Martin Pickard/Getty Images RF; p. 338: Photodisc/Getty Images RF; p. 341: © Tony Hobbs/Alamy.

Chapter Fifteen

Opener: Ryan McVay/Getty Images RF; p. 346: © Meredith Heuer/Riser/Getty Images; p. 349: Andrew Wakeford/Getty Images RF; p. 353: Image Source/Jupiterimages RF; p. 359: Image Source/Getty Images RF; p. 362: © Mark Richards/PhotoEdit; p. 365: © John Wilkes Studio/Corbis RF.

Chapter Sixteen

Opener: The McGraw-Hill Companies, Inc./Ken Karp, photographer; p. 369: Glowimages/Getty Images RF; p. 371: © Michael Blann/PhotoDisc/Getty Images; p. 374: The McGraw-Hill Companies, Inc./Ken Karp, photographer; p. 380: © Rachel Epstein/PhotoEdit; p. 383: © George Robinson/Alamy.

Chapter Seventeen

Opener: Brand X Pictures/Jupiterimages RF; p. 389: © Markku Heikkilä/Flickr/Getty Images RF; p. 391: Pixtal/age fotostock RF; p. 394: Jose Luis Pelaez Inc/Getty Images RF; p. 395: © Mary Kate Denny/Photographer's Choice/Getty Images; p. 397: © Tom Mareschal/Photographer's Choice/Getty Images; p. 403: © PhotoAlto/Alamy.

Transparency Insert One

Students talking: Photodisc Red/Getty Images; Drinking on couch: George Doyle/Getty Images; Beer: ©iStockphoto.com/Bjorn Heller; Tequila: © iStockphoto.com/Chris Hutchison; Wine: © iStockphoto.com/plainview; Girl smoking: Image Source; Girl running: Rubberball/Getty Images; View of Earth from Space: © Planetary Vision Limited; Globe in space: © Planetary Vision Limited; Carrying bike: Creatas/ PictureQuest; CFL bulb: Mike Kemp/Getty Images; Electric car: © iStockphoto.com/Christian Waadt; Produce stand: Blend Images/Getty Images; Girl on computer: Comstock/ Corbis; Bike rack: Masterfile/Royalty Free

Transparency Inset Two

Mountain Biking: Joaquin Palting/Getty Images; Girl eating: © iStockphoto.com/webphotographeer; Jumping jacks: Mike Powell/Getty Images

INDEX